Biopsy: Interpretation of the Liver

Biopsy: Interpretation of the Liver

Editor: Kate Holland

FOSTER ACADEMICS
www.fosteracademics.com

www.fosteracademics.com

FOSTER ACADEMICS

Cataloging-in-Publication Data

Biopsy : interpretation of the liver / edited by Kate Holland.
p. cm.
Includes bibliographical references and index.
ISBN 978-1-63242-678-9
1. Liver--Biopsy. 2. Liver--Diseases--Diagnosis. 3. Biopsy. I. Holland, Kate.
RC847.5.B56 B56 2019
616.36--dc23

Foster Academics,
118-35 Queens Blvd., Suite 400,
Forest Hills, NY 11375, USA

ISBN 978-1-63242-678-9 (Hardback)

Printed and bound in China.

Contents

Preface

A biopsy is a medical procedure, performed by an interventional radiologist or cardiologist, or a surgeon, involving the extraction of tissue or cell samples for determining the presence or extent of a disease. The tissue is then examined by a pathologist and analyzed chemically. A biopsy is performed on a liver in patients with hepatitis, for determining response to therapy. In this, it is assessed if the inflammation of the liver has been reduced and the progression of the disease based on the degree of fibrosis is determined. A liver biopsy may also be performed in the case of Wilson's disease to determine the quantitative copper level in the body. This book is compiled in such a manner, that it will provide a clinical perspective of biopsy. It covers in detail some existing techniques and innovative practices concerning liver biopsy. As this field is emerging at a rapid pace, the elaborate content of this book will help the readers understand the modern concepts of this subject.

Various studies have approached the subject by analyzing it with a single perspective, but the present book provides diverse methodologies and techniques to address this field. This book contains theories and applications needed for understanding the subject from different perspectives. The aim is to keep the readers informed about the progresses in the field; therefore, the contributions were carefully examined to compile novel researches by specialists from across the globe.

Indeed, the job of the editor is the most crucial and challenging in compiling all chapters into a single book. In the end, I would extend my sincere thanks to the chapter authors for their profound work. I am also thankful for the support provided by my family and colleagues during the compilation of this book.

Editor

Factors Affecting the Accuracy of Controlled Attenuation Parameter (CAP) in Assessing Hepatic Steatosis in Patients with Chronic Liver Disease

Kyu Sik Jung[1], Beom Kyung Kim[1,2,4*], Seung Up Kim[1,2,4*], Young Eun Chon[1], Kyung Hyun Cheon[1], Sung Bae Kim[1], Sang Hoon Lee[1], Sung Soo Ahn[1], Jun Yong Park[1,2,4], Do Young Kim[1,2,4], Sang Hoon Ahn[1,2,4,5], Young Nyun Park[3], Kwang-Hyub Han[1,2,4,5]

1 Department of Internal Medicine, Yonsei University College of Medicine, Seoul, Korea, **2** Institute of Gastroenterology, Yonsei University College of Medicine, Seoul, Korea, **3** Department of Pathology, Yonsei University College of Medicine, Seoul, Korea, **4** Liver Cirrhosis Clinical Research Center, Seoul, Korea, **5** Brain Korea 21 Project of Medical Science, Seoul, Korea

Abstract

Background & Aims: Controlled attenuation parameter (CAP) can measure hepatic steatosis. However, factors affecting its accuracy have not been described yet. This study investigated predictors of discordance between liver biopsy (LB) and CAP.

Methods: A total of 161 consecutive patients with chronic liver disease who underwent LB and CAP were enrolled prospectively. Histological steatosis was graded as S0 (<5%), S1 (5–33%), S2 (34–66%), and S3 (>66% of hepatocytes). Cutoff CAP values were calculated from our cohort (250, 301, and 325 dB/m for ≥S1, ≥S2, and S3). Discordance was defined as a discrepancy of at least two steatosis stages between LB and CAP.

Results: The median age (102 males and 59 females) was 49 years. Repartition of histological steatosis was as follows; S0 26.1% (n = 42), S1 49.7% (n = 80), S2 20.5% (n = 33), and S3 3.7% (n = 6). In multivariate linear regression analysis, CAP value was independently associated with steatosis grade along with body mass index (BMI) and interquartile range/median of CAP value (IQR/M_{CAP}) (all $P<0.05$). Discordance was identified in 13 (8.1%) patients. In multivariate analysis, histological S3 (odd ratio [OR], 9.573; 95% confidence interval [CI], 1.207–75.931; $P = 0.033$) and CAP value (OR, 1.020; 95% CI, 1.006–1.034; $P = 0.006$) were significantly associated with discordance, when adjusting for BMI, IQR/M_{CAP}, and necroinflammation, reflected by histological activity or ALT level.

Conclusions: Patients with high grade steatosis or high CAP values have a higher risk of discordance between LB and CAP. Further studies are needed to improve the accuracy of CAP interpretation, especially in patients with higher CAP values.

Editor: James Fung, The University of Hong Kong, Hong Kong

Funding: This study was supported by the Liver Cirrhosis Clinical Research Center, in part by a grant from the Korea Healthcare technology R & D project, Ministry of Health and Welfare, Republic of Korea (no. A102065), and by the Yonsei Liver Blood Bank (YLBB), in part by a grant from sanofi-aventis Korea. BioPredictive kindly provided the complimentary service for calculation of FT score. The funders had no role in study design, data collection and analysis, decision to publish, or preparation of the manuscript.

Competing Interests: This study was supported by the Liver Cirrhosis Clinical Research Center, in part by a grant from the Korea Healthcare technology R & D project, Ministry of Health and Welfare, Republic of Korea (no. A102065), and by the Yonsei Liver Blood Bank (YLBB), in part by a grant from sanofi-aventis Korea. BioPredictive kindly provided the complimentary service for calculation of FT score.

* E-mail: beomkkim@yuhs.ac (BKK); ksukorea@yuhs.ac (SUK)

Introduction

Currently, the clinical implications of hepatic steatosis are gaining more attention not only in Western countries, but also in Asian countries with a westernized lifestyle such as Japan, China, and Korea. [1,2] Indeed, the incidence of non-alcoholic fatty liver disease (NAFLD), the most common condition of steatosis, is increasing worldwide and it is now the most common cause of abnormal liver function tests and chronic liver disease (CLD) in both developed and developing countries. [3].

Severe forms of NAFLD can cause serious liver-related complications such as liver failure and hepatocellular carcinoma. [4,5] Furthermore, fatty burden can negatively influence the prognosis of patients with CLD, as reported by recent studies revealing that coexistent steatosis in chronic hepatitis C is associated with fibrosis progression and decreased treatment response, and that steatosis may lead to a poor postoperative outcome such as a graft failure after liver transplantation or high mortality after hepatectomy. [6–9] Moreover, these studies also suggested that even low burden of hepatic steatosis could affect treatment outcome or prognosis. Thus, an accurate diagnosis and objective estimation of hepatic steatosis is important for clinical decision-making and estimating the prognosis.

To date, the gold standard for diagnosing and assessing the severity of hepatic steatosis has been liver biopsy (LB). [10] However, LB is an invasive and costly procedure with potential limitations such as sampling error and unsatisfactory reproducibility. [11,12] Moreover, LB is difficult to repeat and it allows only semiquantitative grading of steatosis. Although several non-invasive methods such as ultrasonography, computed tomography (CT), and magnetic resonance imaging (MRI) have been investigated for this purpose, their clinical use is limited by high cost, restrictive availability, operator dependence, and poor sensitivity. [13,14].

Recently, interest has shifted towards controlled attenuation parameter (CAP), which is based on the properties of ultrasonic signals acquired by transient elastography (TE). [15] Previous studies have demonstrated that CAP can be performed rapidly, and painlessly with high patient acceptance and that it can accurately grade the severity of steatosis in patients with CLDs. [15–18] However, in contrast to a situation that several confounding factors which determines the accuracy of liver stiffness (LS) values such as interquartile range/median value (IQR/M) or necroinflammatory activity have been identified, factors that affect the accuracy of CAP in assessing hepatic steatosis have not yet been identified. [19–22] Here, this study investigated factors which can influence the diagnostic accuracy of CAP for estimating the severity of hepatic steatosis.

Patients and Methods

Patients

Between November 2011 and August 2013, patients with CLD of any etiology who were scheduled to undergo LB and CAP were recruited for this prospective study at Severance Hospital, Yonsei University College of Medicine, Seoul, Korea. The indications of LB were (i) assessing the degree of inflammatory activity and the extent of liver fibrosis in patients with viral hepatitis B and C, and (ii) establish the cause of the liver disease in patients without viral hepatitis. Exclusion criteria were as follows; (1) TE measurement failure (no valid shot); (2) unreliable LS measurement; (3) non-interpretable biopsies including insufficient specimen size < 10 mm in length. Written informed consent was obtained from all patients before enrollment. The study protocol was consistent with the ethical guidelines of the 1975 Declaration of Helsinki. Written informed consent was obtained from each participant. This study was approved by the Ethics Committee/independent institutional review board of Severance Hospital, Yonsei University College of Medicine, Seoul, Korea. The cohort of this study included subjects recruited in our previous study [23] and we enrolled additional subjects in the currnet study.

Measurement of Liver Stiffness and Controlled Attenuation Parameter

All patients underwent TE using the Fibroscan M probe on the same day as LB after fasting for at least 8 hour. [24] TE was performed on the right lobe of the liver through the intercostal spaces with the patient lying in the dorsal decubitus position with the right arm in maximal abduction. Only one experienced technician blind to the patients' clinical data, was allowed to perform TE. The principles of CAP measurement have been described previously. [15] Briefly, the CAP measures ultrasonic attenuations at 3.5 MHz using signals acquired by TE.

TE results were expressed as kilopascals (kPa) for LS and dB/m for CAP. The interquartile range (IQR) was defined as an index of the intrinsic variability of LS and CAP values corresponding to the interval of LS and CAP results containing 50% of the valid measurements between the 25th and 75th percentiles. The median value of the successful measurements was selected as representative of LS and CAP values for a given patient. As an indicator of variability, the ratio of the IQR of LS and CAP values to the median (IQR/M and IQR/M_{CAP}, respectively) was calculated.

At the same time, hepatic steatosis was assessed using CAP value, only when LS measurement was valid for the same signals, ensuring that the liver ultrasonic attenuation was obtained simultaneously from the same volume of liver parenchyma as LS measurement. In this study, only TE measurement with at least 10 valid shots, and a success rate of at least 60% were considered reliable and used for statistical analysis.

Clinical Data

Before TE examination, demographics, liver disease etiology and anthropometric measurements were obtained. Biochemical parameters including aspartate aminotransferase (AST), alanine aminotransferase (ALT), platelet count, serum fasting glucose, total cholesterol, and triglycerides were measured on the same day as the LB.

Liver Biopsy

All patients underwent ultrasound-guided percutaneous LB. The LB specimens were fixed in formalin and embedded in paraffin. Then, 4-μm-thick sections were subjected to hematoxylin-eosin and Masson's trichrome staining. All liver tissue samples were evaluated by an experienced hepatopathologist (YN Park) who had no access to the clinical data on the study population. Liver fibrosis stage and necroinflammation were evaluated using the Metavir or Brunt scoring system, according to the liver disease etiology. [25,26] Steatosis was assessed as the percentage of hepatocytes containing lipid droplets and categorized according to the NAFLD Activity Score (S0, <5%, S1, 5–33%; S2, 34–66%; and S3, >66%). [27].

Statistical Analyses

Data are expressed as means ± SD, median (range), or n (%), as appropriate. '***Discordance***' was defined as a difference of at least two steatosis stages between LB and CAP. Correlations between variable were described using Spearman correlation coefficients (ρ). Comparisons between patients with discordance and those without were made using the Student *t*-tests or Mann-Whitney test for continuous variables and chi-squared or Fisher's exact test for categorical variables. Cutoff CAP values to determine discordance were calculated from our cohort, which maximized the sum of the sensitivity (Se) and specificity (Sp) (Youden index). Positive and negative predictive values (PPV and NPV) were also computed. Areas under the receiver operating characteristic curves (AUROC) were computed with 95% confidence intervals (CI). Univariate and subsequent multivariate binary logistic regression analyses were performed to identify independent factors of discordance between LB and CAP. Odd ratios (ORs) and corresponding 95% CI were also indicated. A *P* value <0.05 on a two-tailed test was considered significant. Data analyses were performed using the SAS program (ver. 9.1; SAS Inc., Cary, NC, USA).

Results

Baseline Characteristics

During the study period, 170 patients with CLD (135 patients who were recruited in our previous study [23] and additional 35 patients) were enrolled. However, after excluding 9 patients based on our exclusion criteria, 161 patients were selected for statistical analysis (**Fig. 1**). The baseline characteristics of the study are summarized in **Table 1**. The majority were male (n = 102, 63.4%) and the median age was 49 years. The median body mass index (BMI) was 24.4 kg/m2 and 28 (17.4%) patients had diabetes mellitus. The main etiologies of CLD were NAFLD (n = 72, 44.7%), followed by chronic viral hepatitis including chronic hepatitis B (n = 49, 30.4%) and C (n = 28, 17.4%), autoimmune hepatitis (n = 8, 5.0%) and primary biliary cirrhosis (n = 4, 2.5%). The median LS and CAP values were 8.1 (range, 2.9–75.0) kPa and 255 (range, 149–400) dB/m, respectively. The median IQR/M and IQR/MCAP were 0.12 (range, 0.01–0.35) and 0.12 (range, 0.02–0.33), respectively and IQR/M was higher than 0.3 in only one patient.

Liver Histology and Corresponding CAP Value

The median length of the LB specimens was 18.5 (range, 16.1–24.2) mm. The histological steatosis grade was S0 in 42 (26.1%) patients, S1 in 80 (49.7%), S2 in 33 (20.5%), and S3 in 6 (3.7%), respectively. The median CAP values for patients with S0, S1, S2, and S3 steatosis on LB were 217 (range, 149–288), 258 (range, 150–345), 331 (range, 234–400), and 326 (range, 230–347) dB/m, respectively. The median and range of CAP values according to fibrosis stage and activity grade are listed in **Table S1 in File S1**. CAP values were not significantly different between each fibrosis stage and activity grade (all $P>0.05$).

The cutoff CAP values determining ≥S1, ≥S2, and S3 were calculated as 250 dB/m (AUROC, 0.863 [95% CI, 0.807–0.920]; Se, 68.9%; Sp, 92.9%; PPV, 96.5%; NPV, 51.3%), 301 dB/m (AUROC, 0.898 [95% CI, 0.841–0.954]; Se, 82.1%; Sp, 87.7%; PPV, 68.1%; NPV, 93.9%), and 325 dB/m (AUROC, 0.738 [95% CI, 0.562–0.914]; Se, 50.3%; Sp, 81.3%; PPV, 9.4%; NPV, 97.7%), respectively.

Correlation between CAP and Clinicopathological Variables

In univariate linear regression, CAP value was significantly associated with BMI ($P<0.001$), ALT ($P=0.003$), total cholesterol ($P=0.002$), IQR/M_{CAP} ($P<0.001$), fibrosis stage ($P=0.001$), activity grade ($P<0.001$), and steatosis grade ($P<0.001$). In subsequent multiple linear regression analysis, CAP value was independently associated with BMI ($\rho=0.214$, $P=0.001$) and IQR/M_{CAP} ($\rho=-0.216$, $P=0.001$) along with histological steatosis grade ($\rho=0.455$, $P<0.001$). (**Table S2 in File S1**).

Discordance between LB and CAP

Discordance between LB and CAP was observed in 13 (8.1%) patients, whereas steatosis was underestimated on CAP in 5 (38.5%) patients and overestimated in 8 (61.5%) (**Table 2**). When patients with and without discordance between LB and CAP were compared, only the proportions of steatosis grade 3 and CAP values were significantly higher in patients with discordance (all $P<0.05$) (**Table 3**). Other clinical variables including distribution of etiologies for CLD did not significantly differ between two groups (**Table 3**).

Predictors of Discordance

In the first place, to identify independent risk factors for discordance, we performed multivariate analysis using histological parameters; the steatosis grade was entered into a multivariate analysis along with other two variables (BMI and IQR/M_{CAP}) which showed an independent correlation with CAP value on linear regression analysis. The histological activity grade was entered simultaneously as a covariate into multivariate analysis to adjust for the well-known overestimating influence of TE, given that CAP is measured on the basis of TE. [22] Finally, on multivariate analysis, only steatosis grade 3 was significantly related to discordance ($P=0.033$; OR, 9.573; 95% CI, 1.207–75.931) (**Table 4**). The percentages of discordance were significantly higher in patients with steatosis grade 3 than in those with steatosis grade 0–2 (2 of 6 [33.3%] *vs.* 11 of 155 [7.1%], $P=0.021$) (**Fig. 2**).

Similarly, we performed multivariate analysis using clinical parameters; CAP value was entered into multivariate analysis along with two other variables (BMI and IQR/M_{CAP}) which were independently correlated with CAP value in linear regression analysis. The ALT level, instead of the histological activity grade, was entered simultaneously as a covariate into multivariate analysis to adjust for the well-known overestimating influence of TE, since CAP is measured on the basis of TE. [28,29] Finally, on multivariate analysis, only CAP value was the only independent predictor of discordance ($P=0.006$; OR, 1.020; 95% CI, 1.006–1.034). The most discriminative CAP cutoff value to predict discordance by maximizing the Youden index was 323 dB/m. Patients with CAP>323 dB/m had a higher percentage of discordance than those with CAP≤323 dB/m. (8 of 33 [24.2%] vs. 5 of 128 [3.9%], $P=0.001$) (**Fig. 2**).

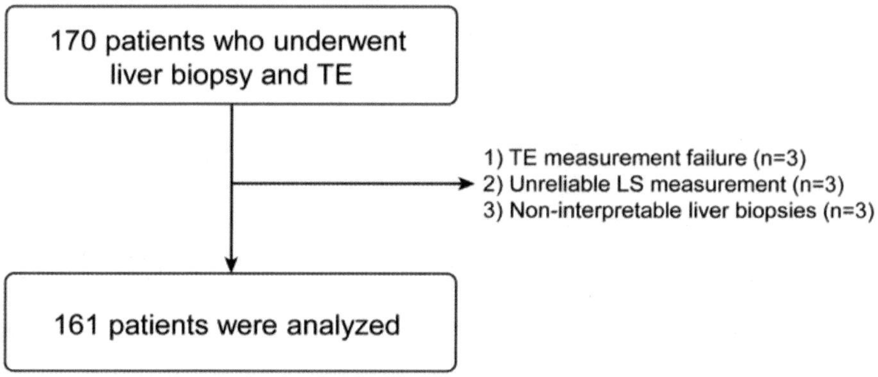

Figure 1. Recruitment algorithm. A total of 170 patients with CLD were consecutively enrolled. However 9 patients were excluded due to TE measurement failure (n = 3), unreliable LS measurement (n = 3), non-interpretable liver biopsies (n = 3), leaving 161 patients to be included in the statistical analysis. CLD, chronic liver disease; TE, transient elastography; LS, liver stiffness.

Table 1. Baseline characteristics (n = 161).

Variables	Values
Demographic variables	
Age (years)	49 (18–81)
Male gender	102 (63.4)
Body mass index (kg/m^2)	24.4 (14.3–34.3)
Diabetes mellitus	28 (17.4)
Etiology, NAFLD/HBV/HCV/Others	72 (44.7)/49 (30.4)/28 (17.4)/12 (7.5)
Biochemical parameters	
Aspartate aminotransferase (IU/L)	45.2±36.2
Alanine aminotransferase (IU/L)	49.8±43.8
Serum albumin (g/dL)	4.1±0.5
Fasting glucose (mg/mL)	109.6±35.2
Total cholesterol (mg/mL)	172.2±40.5
Triglycerides (mg/mL)	128.5±60.3
Liver biopsy	
Fibrosis stage	
F0–1/F2/F3/F4	65 (40.4)/44 (27.3)/22 (13.7)/30 (18.6)
Activity grade	
A0/A1/A2/A3	23 (14.3)/27 (16.8)/74 (46.0)/37 (23.0)
Steatosis	
S0/S1/S2/S3	42 (26.1)/80 (49.7)/33 (20.5)/6 (3.7)
Biopsy length (cm)	18.5 (16.1–24.2)
Liver stiffness measurement	
Liver stiffness value (kPa)	8.1 (2.9–75.0)
Interquartile range (kPa)	1.0 (0.1–14.0)
IQR/M	0.12 (0.01~0.35)
Controlled attenuation parameter	
Controlled attenuation parameter value (dB/m)	255 (149–400)
Interquartile range (dB/m)	29.0 (6–76)
IQR/M_{CAP}	0.12 (0.02–0.33)

Variables are expressed as median (range) or n (%). NAFLD, non-alcoholic fatty liver disease; HBV, hepatitis B; HCV, hepatitis C; kPa, kilopascal; IQR/M, interquartile range/median liver stiffness value; CAP, controlled attenuation parameter; IQR/M_{CAP}, interquartile range/median of CAP value.

Discussion

Although CAP showed promising results for non-invasive diagnosis of the significant steatosis, it is not obvious whether quantification of steatosis assessed by CAP could stratify severity of steatosis accurately in patients with severe steatosis. [15–18] Myer *et al.* reported that the diagnostic performance of CAP to identify severe steatosis was sub-optimal [16], and the ability to differentiate between steatosis grade 2 and 3 was not satisfactory in the studies by Sasso *et al.* and Ledinghen *et al.* [15,17] Consistent with these results, a high steatotic burden (steatosis grade 3 or high CAP

Table 2. Distribution of steatosis according to liver biopsy and CAP.

Steatosis according to liver biopsy	Steatosis according to calculated cutoff CAP value			
	S0 (<250 dB/m, n = 75)	**S1 (≥250 dB/m, n = 37)**	**S2 (≥301 dB/m, n = 19)**	**S3 (≥325 dB/m, n = 30)**
S0 (n = 42)	39	3	**0**	**0**
S1 (n = 80)	32	31	9	**8**
S2 (n = 33)	**3**	2	9	19
S3 (n = 6)	**1**	**1**	1	3

CAP, controlled attenuation parameter.
Bold cells indicate the number of patients with discordance between LB and CAP values.

Table 3. Comparison of patients with and without discordance.

Variables	Patients without discordance (n = 148, 91.9%)	Patients with discordance (n = 13, 8.1%)	*P* value
Demographic variables			
Age (years)	49 (18–81)	52 (35–70)	NS
Male gender	95 (64.2)	7 (53.8)	NS
Body mass index (kg/m^2)	24.4 (14.3–34.3)	24.5 (21.6–29.8)	NS
Diabetes mellitus	23 (15.5)	5 (38.5)	NS
Etiology, NAFLD/HBV/HCV/Others	64 (43.9)/45 (30.4)/26 (17.6)/12 (8.1)	7 (53.8)/4 (30.8)/2 (15.4)/0 (0.0)	NS
Biochemical parameters			
Aspartate aminotransferase (IU/L)	46.1±37.1	34.5±21.2	NS
Alanine aminotransferase (IU/L)	50.9±45.0	36.6±25.8	NS
Serum albumin (g/dL)	4.1±0.5	4.2±0.4	NS
Fasting glucose (mg/mL)	108.2±34.6	124.0±39.5	NS
Total cholesterol (mg/mL)	171.5±40.9	180.1±36.0	NS
Triglycerides (mg/mL)	126.2±60.4	153.7±54.9	NS
Liver biopsy			
Fibrosis stage			
F0–2/F3–4	99 (66.9)/49 (33.1)	10 (76.9)/3 (23.1)	NS
Activity grade			
A0–2/A3	114 (77.0)/34 (23.0)	9 (69.2)/4 (30.8)	NS
Steatosis			
S0–2/S3	144 (97.3)/4 (2.7)	11 (84.6)/2 (15.4)	0.021
Biopsy length (cm)	18.2 (16.4–24.2)	18.6 (16.1–23.5)	NS
Liver stiffness measurement			
Liver stiffness value (kPa)	8.2 (2.9–75.0)	7.4 (3.0–17.5)	NS
Interquartile range (kPa)	1.0 (0.1–14.0)	1.5 (0.4–2.6)	NS
IQR/M	0.12 (0.01–0.35)	0.15 (0.06–0.26)	NS
Controlled attenuation parameter			
Controlled attenuation parameter value (dB/m)	250 (149–400)	327 (230–345)	0.010
Interquartile range (dB/m)	29.0 (6–72)	30.0 (15–76)	NS
IQR/M_{CAP}	0.12 (0.02–0.28)	0.10 (0.05–0.33)	NS

Variables are expressed as median (range) or n (%).
NS, not significant; NAFLD, non-alcoholic fatty liver disease; HBV, hepatitis B; HCV, hepatitis C; kPa, kilopascal; IQR/M, interquartile range/median liver stiffness value; CAP, controlled attenuation parameter; IQR/M_{CAP}, interquartile range/median of CAP value.

values) was selected as the independent risk factor of discordant results between LB and CAP in our study.

To our knowledge, this is the first study to identify the factors that influence the accuracy of CAP by using the end point of discordance between LB and CAP values. Generally, it has been known that LS values become more reliable when advanced fibrosis or cirrhosis exists and that TE can diagnose liver cirrhosis with higher accuracy. [21,30] In contrast, CAP was more accurate in assessing less severe hepatic steatosis (≤S2) in our study as well as in those by Sasso *et al.* and Ledinghen *et al.*, although LS and CAP values were simultaneously measured from the same device. [15,17] The reason for this opposite phenomenon of LS and CAP is unclear. However, it can be hypothesized that the correlation between ultrasonic attenuation and the amount of hepatic steatosis may be diminished, especially when the steatosis is severe. Indeed, steatosis grade 3 was selected as the only influencing factor in discordance between LB and CAP. In addition, when only clinical factors including CAP values were adjusted, only CAP values independently influenced the discordance and its most discriminative cutoff was similar to the cutoff value for diagnosing steatosis grade 3 (323 vs. 325 dB/m). These results suggest that high CAP values can be used as the single most significant factor in determining the accuracy of CAP and thus, careful diagnosis considering clinical correlations may be required when a patient shows unexpectedly high CAP values. However, since a small sample size of S3 with potential spectrum bias and interpretational variability in grading histological hepatic steatosis may have lowered the diagnostic performance of CAP in patients with high steatotic burden, [31] further studies with a well-balanced distribution of hepatic steatosis stages using objective assessment tools such as computerized morphometry are required to clarify the accuracy of CAP. [14,31].

A high ALT levels has been identified as one of the most important confounders of LS values. [21] However, in the present study, there was no significant correlation between ALT level and CAP values, and ALT level was similar in patients with and without discordance (mean 50.9 vs. 36.6 IU/L; $P>0.05$). Similarly, histological necroinflammatory activity did not significantly

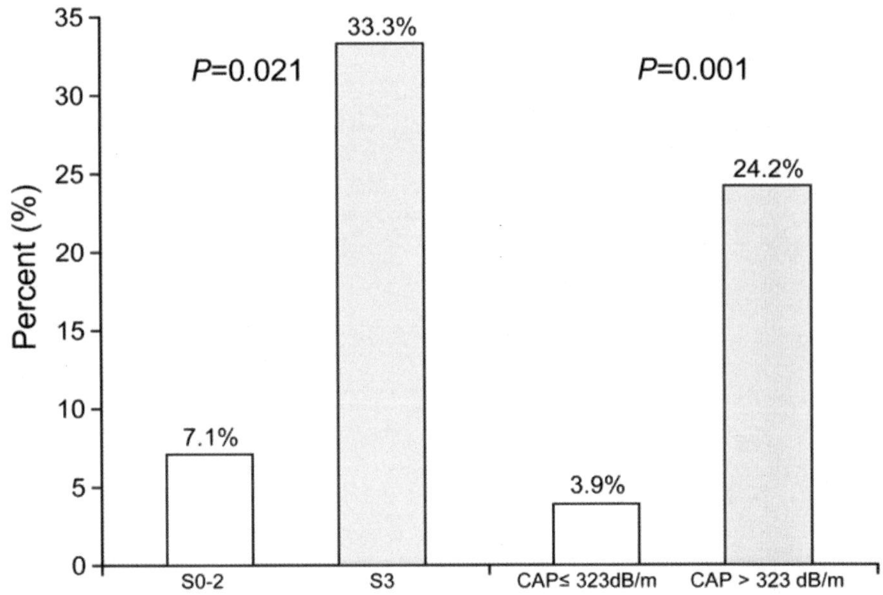

Figure 2. Percentage of patients with discordance according to histological steatosis grade and CAP value. The percentages of discordance between liver biopsy and CAP were significantly higher in patients with steatosis grade 3 than in those with steatosis grade 0–2 (2 of 6 [33.3%] vs. 11 of 155 [7.1%], $P=0.021$). Additionally, patients with CAP>323 dB/m had a higher percentage of discordance than those with CAP≤ 323 dB/m. (8 of 33 [23.1%] vs.5 of 128 [4.9%], $P=0.001$). CAP, controlled attenuation parameter.

influence discordance in our study, although previous studies reported overestimation due to necroinflammation. [22] Although there is still a chance that the influence of the high ALT level may have been masked due to the relatively low mean ALT level (49.8 IU/L) in our study population, our data suggest that the influence of a high ALT level or necroinflammation on CAP values seems negligible.

In our study, the effects of other clinical parameters on discordance were also investigated. First, the influence of IQR/M_{CAP} on the accuracy of CAP was explored and assessed for use as a surrogate marker for so called "reliable" criteria for CAP value as IQR/M is currently used to determine the reliability of LS value. [19] However, IQR/M_{CAP} was not selected as an independent predictor of discordance. In addition, we also tested the influence of IQR/M on discordance, but it is not associated with the diagnostic accuracy of CAP. Thus, it should be further investigated whether IQR/M_{CAP} or IQR/M can be incorporated into "reliable" criteria for CAP, although IQR/M can influence the accuracy of LS value. [19] Second, the influence of histological necroinflammatory activity and ALT level were also tested, but neither was associated with discordance, although previous studies revealed that a higher activity grade or high ALT level can cause significant overestimation of LS value. [22,32,33] These findings suggest that CAP has different characteristics from LS measurement and despite simultaneous measurement, should be interpreted independently in terms of the accuracy of CAP and the influence of necroinflammatory activity and ALT level. Lastly, although we hypothesized that the BMI can be a surrogate marker

Table 4. Independent predictors of discordance between liver biopsy and CAP.

Variables	*P* value	Odd ratio (95% CI)
Model using histological parameters		
Steatosis grade 3	0.033	9.573 (1.207–75.931)
Activity grade 3	NS	–
*Body mass index (kg/m^2)	NS	–
*IQR/M_{CAP}	NS	–
Model using clinical parameters		
CAP value (dB/m)	0.006	1.020 (1.006–1.034)
Alanine aminotransferase (IU/L)	NS	–
*Body mass index (kg/m^2)	NS	–
*IQR/M_{CAP}	NS	–

CAP, controlled attenuation parameters; CI, confidence interval; NS, not significant; IQR/M_{CAP}, interquartile range/median of CAP value.
*Body mass index and IQR/M_{CAP} were incorporated into multivariate analysis due to their significant correlations with CAP value in multivariate linear regression analysis.

to predict the accuracy of CAP values considering a significant association between BMI and CAP in our cohort, the BMI was not correlated with the discordance. However, because the overall BMI of our study population was not relatively high, the potential influence of high BMI might have been masked. Thus, our results did not clarify whether adjusting for BMI would increase the accuracy of CAP interpretation; this should be investigated in future.

Our study had several limitations. First, our cohort included patients with CLDs due to various etiologies. As the diagnostic performance could vary according to the etiology, the results may have been influenced. However, other clinical variables including steatosis grade and fibrosis stage did not significantly differ according to etiologies. Additionally, recent studies demonstrated that the accuracy of CAP was similar among different etiologies including viral hepatitis and NAFLD, suggesting that heterogeneous etiologies may not have a major influence on our results. [34] Second, the small sample size of severe steatosis and relatively low mean BMI might also have led to a bias, which could be related to the low diagnostic accuracy of CAP values for diagnosis of S3 steatosis. Furthermore, the AUROC can vary according to the prevalence of each steatosis grade. Thus, our results should be confirmed in future studies with a good balance of sample size in each steatosis grade and even BMI distribution. Third, the relationship between metabolic syndrome and CAP could not be fully evaluated in this study, as the assessment of metabolic syndrome was feasible only in 60 of 161 (37.2%) patients. Although, sub-group analysis revealed that metabolic syndrome did not influence the risk of discordance between LB and CAP (data not shown, $P>0.05$), further large scale study is required to investigate the potential influence of metabolic syndrome on CAP. Lastly, we defined our end point as "discordance of two steatosis stages between LB and CAP". Although these analytical methods have been used in several previous cross-sectional studies, [19,22] this definition still seems to be obscure.

In conclusion, histological steatosis grade 3 and high CAP values were identified as significant factors to decrease the diagnostic performance of CAP. Thus, our results suggest that high CAP values should be interpreted carefully and that additional complementary diagnostic modality such as ultrasonography or serological steatosis prediction indices, should be used to avoid errors in this area.

Acknowledgments

The authors are grateful to Dong-Su Jang, (Medical Illustrator, Medical Research Support Section, Yonsei University College of Medicine, Seoul, Korea) for his help with the figures.

Author Contributions

Conceived and designed the experiments: BKK SUK. Analyzed the data: KSJ BKK SUK. Contributed reagents/materials/analysis tools: YEC KHC JYP DYK SHA YNP KHH SBK SHL SSA. Wrote the paper: KSJ BKK SUK.

References

1. Angulo P (2002) Nonalcoholic fatty liver disease. N Engl J Med. 346: 1221–1231.
2. Oh MK, Winn J, Poordad F (2008) Review article: diagnosis and treatment of non-alcoholic fatty liver disease. Aliment Pharmacol Ther. 28: 503–522. doi: 510.1111/j.1365-2036.2008.03752.x. Epub 02008 Jun 03753.
3. Yilmaz Y (2012) Review article: is non-alcoholic fatty liver disease a spectrum, or are steatosis and non-alcoholic steatohepatitis distinct conditions? Aliment Pharmacol Ther. 36: 815–823. doi: 810.1111/apt.12046.
4. Ratziu V, Bonyhay L, Di Martino V, Charlotte F, Cavallaro L, et al. (2002) Survival, liver failure, and hepatocellular carcinoma in obesity-related cryptogenic cirrhosis. Hepatology. 35: 1485–1493.
5. Ong JP, Pitts A, Younossi ZM (2008) Increased overall mortality and liver-related mortality in non-alcoholic fatty liver disease. J Hepatol. 49: 608–612. Epub 2008 Jul 2009.
6. Leandro G, Mangia A, Hui J, Fabris P, Rubbia-Brandt L, et al. (2006) Relationship between steatosis, inflammation, and fibrosis in chronic hepatitis C: a meta-analysis of individual patient data. Gastroenterology. 130: 1636–1642.
7. Poynard T, Ratziu V, McHutchison J, Manns M, Goodman Z, et al. (2003) Effect of treatment with peginterferon or interferon alfa-2b and ribavirin on steatosis in patients infected with hepatitis C. Hepatology. 38: 75–85.
8. Spitzer AL, Lao OB, Dick AA, Bakthavatsalam R, Halldorson JB, et al. (2010) The biopsied donor liver: incorporating macrosteatosis into high-risk donor assessment. Liver Transpl. 16: 874–884. doi: 810.1002/lt.22085.
9. de Meijer VE, Kalish BT, Puder M, Ijzermans JN (2010) Systematic review and meta-analysis of steatosis as a risk factor in major hepatic resection. Br J Surg. 97: 1331–1339. doi: 1310.1002/bjs.7194.
10. Dowman JK, Tomlinson JW, Newsome PN (2011) Systematic review: the diagnosis and staging of non-alcoholic fatty liver disease and non-alcoholic steatohepatitis. Aliment Pharmacol Ther. 33: 525–540. doi: 510.1111/j.1365-2036.2010.04556.x. Epub 02010 Dec 04529.
11. Ratziu V, Charlotte F, Heurtier A, Gombert S, Giral P, et al. (2005) Sampling variability of liver biopsy in nonalcoholic fatty liver disease. Gastroenterology. 128: 1898–1906.
12. Regev A, Berho M, Jeffers LJ, Milikowski C, Molina EG, et al. (2002) Sampling error and intraobserver variation in liver biopsy in patients with chronic HCV infection. Am J Gastroenterol. 97: 2614–2618.
13. Schwenzer NF, Springer F, Schraml C, Stefan N, Machann J, et al. (2009) Non-invasive assessment and quantification of liver steatosis by ultrasound, computed tomography and magnetic resonance. J Hepatol. 51: 433–445. Epub 2009 Jun 2011.
14. Boursier J, Cales P (2012) Controlled attenuation parameter (CAP): a new device for fast evaluation of liver fat? Liver Int. 32: 875–877. doi: 810.1111/j.1478-3231.2012.02824.x.
15. Sasso M, Beaugrand M, de Ledinghen V, Douvin C, Marcellin P, et al. (2010) Controlled attenuation parameter (CAP): a novel VCTE guided ultrasonic attenuation measurement for the evaluation of hepatic steatosis: preliminary study and validation in a cohort of patients with chronic liver disease from various causes. Ultrasound Med Biol. 36: 1825–1835. Epub 2010 Sep 1827.
16. Myers RP, Pollett A, Kirsch R, Pomier-Layrargues G, Beaton M, et al. (2012) Controlled Attenuation Parameter (CAP): a noninvasive method for the detection of hepatic steatosis based on transient elastography. Liver Int. 32: 902–910. doi: 910.1111/j.1478-3231.2012.02781.x. Epub 02012 Mar 02721.
17. de Ledinghen V, Vergniol J, Foucher J, Merrouche W, le Bail B (2012) Non-invasive diagnosis of liver steatosis using controlled attenuation parameter (CAP) and transient elastography. Liver Int. 32: 911–918. doi: 910.1111/j.1478-3231.2012.02820.x.
18. Sasso M, Tengher-Barna I, Ziol M, Miette V, Fournier C, et al. (2012) Novel controlled attenuation parameter for noninvasive assessment of steatosis using Fibroscan((R)): validation in chronic hepatitis C. J Viral Hepat. 19: 244–253. doi: 210.1111/j.1365-2893.2011.01534.x. Epub 02011 Oct 01513.
19. Lucidarme D, Foucher J, Le Bail B, Vergniol J, Castera L, et al. (2009) Factors of accuracy of transient elastography (fibroscan) for the diagnosis of liver fibrosis in chronic hepatitis C. Hepatology. 49: 1083–1089. doi: 1010.1002/hep.22748.
20. Myers RP, Crotty P, Pomier-Layrargues G, Ma M, Urbanski SJ, et al. (2010) Prevalence, risk factors and causes of discordance in fibrosis staging by transient elastography and liver biopsy. Liver Int. 30: 1471–1480. doi: 1410.1111/j.1478-3231.2010.02331.x. Epub 02010 Aug 02330.
21. Kim SU, Seo YS, Cheong JY, Kim MY, Kim JK, et al. (2010) Factors that affect the diagnostic accuracy of liver fibrosis measurement by Fibroscan in patients with chronic hepatitis B. Aliment Pharmacol Ther. 32: 498–505. doi: 410.1111/j.1365-2036.2010.04353.x. Epub 02010 May 04311.
22. Kim SU, Kim JK, Park YN, Han KH (2012) Discordance between liver biopsy and Fibroscan(R) in assessing liver fibrosis in chronic hepatitis b: risk factors and influence of necroinflammation. PLoS One. 7: e32233. doi: 32210.31371/journal.pone.0032233. Epub 0032012 Feb 0032223.
23. Chon YE, Jung KS, Kim SU, Park JY, Park YN, et al. (2014) Controlled attenuation parameter (CAP) for detection of hepatic steatosis in patients with chronic liver diseases: a prospective study of a native Korean population. Liver Int 34: 102–109.

24. Mederacke I, Wursthorn K, Kirschner J, Rifai K, Manns MP, et al. (2009) Food intake increases liver stiffness in patients with chronic or resolved hepatitis C virus infection. Liver Int. 29: 1500–1506. doi: 1510.1111/j.1478-3231.2009.02100.x. Epub 02009 Sep 02103.
25. (1994) Intraobserver and interobserver variations in liver biopsy interpretation in patients with chronic hepatitis C. The French METAVIR Cooperative Study Group. Hepatology. 20: 15–20.
26. Brunt EM, Janney CG, Di Bisceglie AM, Neuschwander-Tetri BA, Bacon BR (1999) Nonalcoholic steatohepatitis: a proposal for grading and staging the histological lesions. Am J Gastroenterol. 94: 2467–2474.
27. Kleiner DE, Brunt EM, Van Natta M, Behling C, Contos MJ, et al. (2005) Design and validation of a histological scoring system for nonalcoholic fatty liver disease. Hepatology. 41: 1313–1321.
28. Kim SU, Kim do Y, Park JY, Lee JH, Ahn SH, et al. (2010) How can we enhance the performance of liver stiffness measurement using FibroScan in diagnosing liver cirrhosis in patients with chronic hepatitis B? J Clin Gastroenterol. 44: 66–71. doi: 10.1097/MCG.1090b1013e3181a1095c1097f.
29. Arena U, Vizzutti F, Corti G, Ambu S, Stasi C, et al. (2008) Acute viral hepatitis increases liver stiffness values measured by transient elastography. Hepatology. 47: 380–384.
30. Chon YE, Choi EH, Song KJ, Park JY, Kim do Y, et al. (2012) Performance of transient elastography for the staging of liver fibrosis in patients with chronic hepatitis B: a meta-analysis. PLoS One. 7: e44930. doi: 44910.41371/journal.pone.0044930. Epub 0042012 Sep 0044925.
31. El-Badry AM, Breitenstein S, Jochum W, Washington K, Paradis V, et al. (2009) Assessment of hepatic steatosis by expert pathologists: the end of a gold standard. Ann Surg. 250: 691–697. doi: 610.1097/SLA.1090b1013e3181bcd1096dd.
32. Wong GL, Wong VW, Choi PC, Chan AW, Chim AM, et al. (2009) Clinical factors associated with liver stiffness in hepatitis B e antigen-positive chronic hepatitis B patients. Clin Gastroenterol Hepatol. 7: 227–233. doi: 210.1016/j.cgh.2008.1010.1023. Epub 2008 Oct 1030.
33. Kim SU, Han KH, Park JY, Ahn SH, Chung MJ, et al. (2009) Liver stiffness measurement using FibroScan is influenced by serum total bilirubin in acute hepatitis. Liver Int. 29: 810–815. doi: 810.1111/j.1478-3231.2008.01894.x. Epub 02008 Oct 01824.
34. Kumar M, Rastogi A, Singh T, Behari C, Gupta E, et al. (2013) Controlled Attenuation Parameter for Non-invasive Assessment of Hepatic Steatosis: Does aetiology affect performance. J Gastroenterol Hepatol 21: 12134.

2

The Treatment Cascade for Chronic Hepatitis C Virus Infection in the United States: A Systematic Review and Meta-Analysis

Baligh R. Yehia[1,2,3*], Asher J. Schranz[4], Craig A. Umscheid[1,2,3,5], Vincent Lo Re III[1,3]

1 Department of Medicine, University of Pennsylvania Perelman School of Medicine, Philadelphia, Pennsylvania, United States of America, **2** Leonard Davis Institute of Health Economics, University of Pennsylvania, Philadelphia, Pennsylvania, United States of America, **3** Center for Clinical Epidemiology and Biostatistics, Department of Biostatistics and Epidemiology, University of Pennsylvania Perelman School of Medicine, Philadelphia, Pennsylvania, United States of America, **4** Department of Medicine, New York University School of Medicine, New York, New York, United States of America, **5** Center for Evidenced-Based Practice, University of Pennsylvania Health System, Philadelphia, Pennsylvania, United States of America

Abstract

Background: Identifying gaps in care for people with chronic hepatitis C virus (HCV) infection is important to clinicians, public health officials, and federal agencies. The objective of this study was to systematically review the literature to provide estimates of the proportion of chronic HCV-infected persons in the United States (U.S.) completing each step along a proposed HCV treatment cascade: (1) infected with chronic HCV; (2) diagnosed and aware of their infection; (3) with access to outpatient care; (4) HCV RNA confirmed; (5) liver fibrosis staged by biopsy; (6) prescribed HCV treatment; and (7) achieved sustained virologic response (SVR).

Methods: We searched MEDLINE, EMBASE, and the Cochrane Database of Systematic Reviews for articles published between January 2003 and July 2013. Two reviewers independently identified articles addressing each step in the cascade. Studies were excluded if they focused on specific populations, did not present original data, involved only a single site, were conducted outside of the U.S., or only included data collected prior to 2000.

Results: 9,581 articles were identified, 117 were retrieved for full text review, and 10 were included. Overall, 3.5 million people were estimated to have chronic HCV in the U.S. Fifty percent (95% CI 43–57%) were diagnosed and aware of their infection, 43% (CI 40–47%) had access to outpatient care, 27% (CI 27–28%) had HCV RNA confirmed, 17% (CI 16–17%) underwent liver fibrosis staging, 16% (CI 15–16%) were prescribed treatment, and 9% (CI 9–10%) achieved SVR.

Conclusions: Continued efforts are needed to improve HCV care in the U.S. The proposed HCV treatment cascade provides a framework for evaluating the delivery of HCV care over time and within subgroups, and will be useful in monitoring the impact of new screening efforts and advances in antiviral therapy.

Editor: Stacey A. Rizza, Mayo Clinic, United States of America

Funding: This work was supported by the National Institutes of Health [K23 MH097647 to BRY and K01 AI070001 to VLR]. The funders had no role in study design, data collection and analysis, decision to publish, or preparation of the manuscript.

Competing Interests: BRY receives investigator-initiated research support (to the University of Pennsylvania) from Gilead Sciences; AJS has no such interests; CAU has no such interests; VLR receives investigator-initiated research support (to the University of Pennsylvania) from AstraZeneca, Bristol Myers-Squibb, Merck, and Gilead Sciences.

* Email: byehia@upenn.edu

Introduction

The HIV treatment cascade (diagnosis, linkage to care, retention in care, prescription of antiretroviral therapy, and viral suppression) is an effective tool for improving the health of people living with HIV (PLWH) and for achieving the public health benefits of antiretroviral therapy [1,2]. It has been used by federal, state, and local agencies to identify gaps in the delivery of care, prioritize and target resources, and monitor the United States (U.S.) *National HIV/AIDS Strategy* [2–6]. As different patient behaviors and health system mechanisms are required to successfully complete each step of the cascade, it also demonstrates the need for coordinated action to meet treatment goals [7].

Similar to PLWH, people with chronic hepatitis C virus (HCV) infection need to fulfill several steps along a care continuum to achieve optimal health outcomes [8,9]. First, individuals must be diagnosed and aware of their HCV infection and seek care [10]. Once in care, patients should have HCV RNA confirmation testing and undergo liver fibrosis staging to help inform prognosis and make decisions regarding HCV therapy [11]. Lastly, individuals must receive and adhere to HCV treatment to achieve a sustained virologic response (SVR) [12]. Throughout this continuum, patients should receive recommended screenings, vaccinations, and care as outlined by national guidelines [11,13].

This HCV treatment cascade aligns with the goals of the U.S. *Action Plan for the Prevention, Care, and Treatment of Viral Hepatitis,* which established early identification, linkage to care and treatment, and improved quality of care as top priorities for combating the silent epidemic of chronic HCV infection [14]. As antiviral therapy for chronic HCV advances to become more convenient, effective, and better-tolerated, monitoring the HCV treatment cascade will become increasingly important to clinicians, public health officials, and federal agencies [15]. This systematic review and meta-analysis builds on prior studies evaluating rates of HCV detection, referral to care, and treatment [16,17], and integrates published data to provide estimates of the number of chronic HCV-infected persons living in the U.S. completing each step along the HCV treatment cascade. These data will help identify key deficits in chronic HCV care that will be important for the development of programs to improve diagnosis, linkage to care, and management of this disease.

Methods

Data Sources and Searches

We examined data addressing 7 key steps along the HCV treatment cascade to identify the number of people with: (1) chronic HCV infection; and the proportion of chronic HCV-infected individuals: (2) diagnosed and aware of their infection; (3) with access to outpatient care; (4) HCV RNA confirmed; (5) disease staged by liver biopsy; (6) prescribed HCV treatment; and (7) achieving SVR [16,17]. We searched MEDLINE, EMBASE, and the Cochrane Database of Systematic Reviews for English language articles published between January 2003 and July 2013 using keywords and structured language representing each step along the HCV treatment cascade [18]. Details appear in **Table S1**.

Study Selection

Titles and abstracts were screened by a single reviewer (BRY or AS). Articles were selected for full-text review if they were relevant to HCV treatment cascade steps. Two independent reviewers (BRY and VLR) evaluated articles selected for full-text review using a standardized form. Disagreements were resolved by consensus.

Studies were included if they addressed one or more steps along the HCV treatment cascade, were conducted inside the U.S., presented original data, and used data collected after January 1, 2000. We intentionally focus on studies conducted inside the U.S., and not in other developed counties, as multiple steps in the treatment cascade are directly influenced by the healthcare delivery system and these systems vary widely across countries [19]. The use of data collected after January 1, 2000 corresponds with the introduction of dual therapy with a pegylated interferon and ribavirin for the treatment of chronic HCV infection that occurred in the early 2000 s, and was also selected to ensure the use of the most current data available. To improve generalizability, single site studies and those exclusively focusing on specific populations (e.g., only immigrants, injection drug users, those with HIV/HCV co-infection) were excluded. If multiple publications resulted from the same patient sample or longitudinal cohort, we selected the most inclusive and current study. Bibliographies of included studies were reviewed for additional studies, and three experts in chronic HCV infection were contacted to ensure no relevant studies were missed.

Data Extraction

Data from each included study were extracted by one author (BRY) into tables stratified by HCV treatment cascade step and verified by another author (VLR) for accuracy. Discrepancies were resolved through consensus. We extracted information on study design, period, population, sample size, definition of outcome measure(s), and raw data to permit calculation of estimates of chronic HCV-infected persons completing each cascade step.

Data Synthesis and Analysis

The number of chronic HCV-infected persons completing each step along the HCV treatment cascade was determined. After ascertaining the initial estimate of chronic HCV-infected persons in the U.S. (cascade step 1), we estimated the number of chronic HCV-infected persons diagnosed and aware of their infection (cascade step 2). Among those diagnosed and aware of their chronic HCV infection, we estimated the number with access to outpatient care (cascade step 3). Next, among chronic HCV-infected persons diagnosed and aware of their infection and with access to outpatient care, we estimated the number who had: HCV RNA confirmed (cascade step 4), underwent a liver biopsy (cascade step 5), and antiviral therapy prescribed (cascade step 6). Since cascade steps 4–6 had the same denominator, the proportion of persons prescribed HCV treatment was not conditioned on the number with HCV RNA confirmation and liver biopsy. Finally, among persons prescribed HCV treatment, we estimated the number that achieved a sustained virologic response (cascade step 7). Using the above estimates, we calculated the proportion of chronic HCV-infected persons completing each step along the HCV treatment cascade by dividing the number of people who completed each step (numerator) by the number of chronic HCV-infected persons in the U.S. (denominator, obtained from cascade step 1).

Since multiple studies were identified for HCV treatment cascade steps 5–7, we performed random-effects meta-analyses for these steps to determine pooled prevalence estimates with 95% confidence intervals (CIs). We assessed the heterogeneity between study results using the I^2 statistic. Significant heterogeneity was defined as an I^2 statistic $\geq$50% [20]. Analyses were performed in OpenMeta[Analyst] [21].

The U.S. Veterans Health Administration (VA) is the largest single provider of HCV care in the U.S., currently caring for approximately 165,000 veterans with chronic HCV infection [13]. Because of differences in the prevalence of comorbid diseases, as well as the management and treatment of chronic HCV infection between U.S. Veterans and non-Veterans [13], we distinguished VA and non-VA studies. The primary analysis focused on non-VA studies. In a secondary analysis, we preferentially selected VA studies when available.

Results

Our literature search yielded 9,581 citations (excluding duplicates), of which 117 met eligibility for full text review (**Figure 1**). Of those, 107 were excluded because they did not address any of the study questions, were conducted outside of the U.S., did not present original data, only analyzed data collected prior to 2000, involved a single site, focused on special populations, or examined study subjects used in a more recent study. Among the remaining 10 articles [22–31], three focused exclusively on U.S. Veterans. Details on the study populations, periods, and sample sizes of included studies by cascade step are shown in **Table 1**.

Based on National Health and Nutrition Examination Survey (NHANES) data from 1999 through 2002, approximately 3.2 million people in the U.S. have chronic HCV infection [22]. Since NHANES did not sample high-risk groups, particularly incarcerated, homeless, or institutionalized individuals, the actual preva-

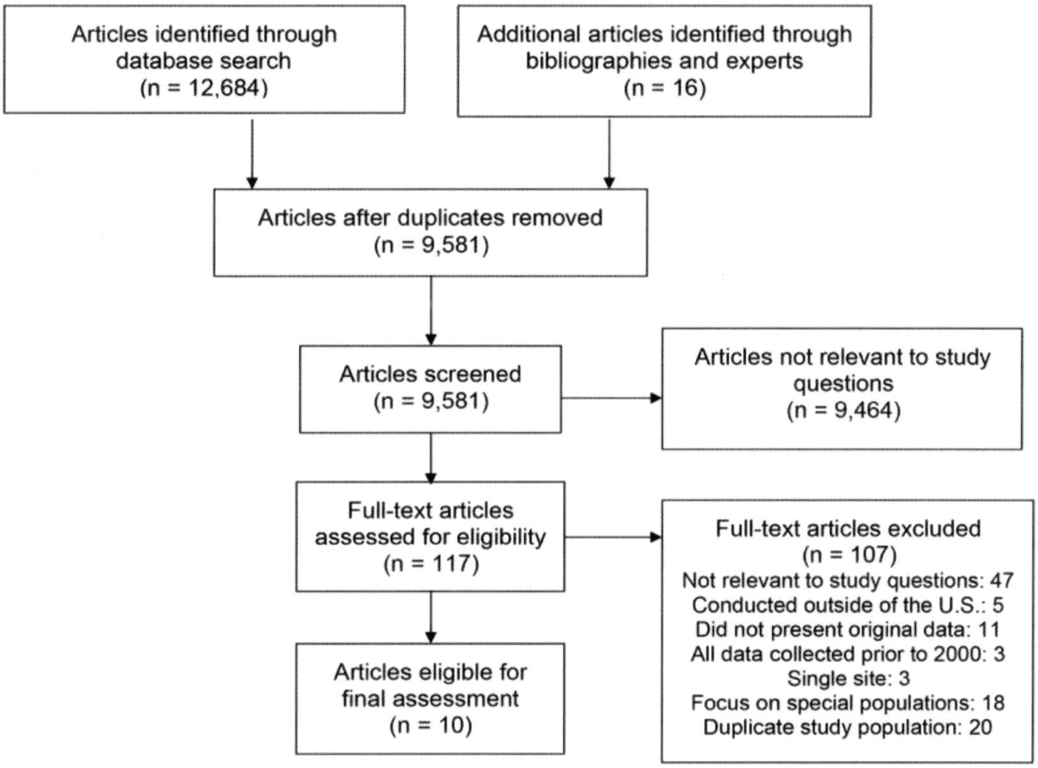

Figure 1. Summary of Article Search, Screening, and Selection Process.

Table 1. Evaluation of chronic hepatitis C virus treatment cascade studies eligible for final assessment.

Author, Year	Data Source	Time Period	Sample Size	Estimate (95% CI)	Pooled Prevalence Estimate (95% CI)*
Study Question 1: Number of people with chronic HCV infection					
Armstrong et al, 2006	NHAS	1999–2002	15,079	3,500,000 people	–
Study Question 2: Proportion aware of their infection					
Younossi et al, 2013	NHAS	2001–2010	203	49.8% (42.9–56.7)	–
Study Question 3: Proportion with access to healthcare, among those aware of their infection					
Younossi et al, 2013	NHAS	2001–2010	101	86.9% (80.3–93.5)	–
Study Question 4: Proportion HCV RNA confirmed, among those in care					
Moorman et al, 2013	4 HCOs	2001–2010	8,810	62.9% (61.9–63.9)	–
Study Question 5: Proportion disease staged by liver biopsy, among those in care					
Moorman et al, 2013	4 HCOs	2001–2010	8,810	38.4% (37.4–39.4)	–
Groessl et a, 2012	*VA*	*1996–2006*	*171,893*	*16.7% (16.5–16.9)*	
Study Question 6: Proportion prescribed HCV treatment, among those in care					
Moorman et al, 2013	4 HCOs	2001–2010	8,810	36.4% (35.4–37.4)	36.7% (35.8–37.6)
Kanwal et al, 2010	Insurance claims	2003–2006	2,893	37.5% (35.7–39.3)	
Kanwal et al, 2012	*VA*	*2003–2006*	*34,749*	*17.9% (17.5–18.3)*	–
Study Question 7: Proportion achieving SVR, among those in care and prescribed HCV treatment					
Mitra et al, 2010	Insurance claims	2002–2006	575	58.4% (54.4–62.4)	58.8% (56.1–61.5)
Arora et al, 2011	22 clinics	2004–2009	407	58.0% (53.2–62.8)	
Russell et al, 2012	Health system	2002–2008	259	60.1% (54.1–66.1)	
Backus et al, 2011	*VA*	*2001–2009*	*16,864*	*44.1% (43.4–44.9)*	–

Abbreviations: HCOs = healthcare organization; NHANES = National Health and Nutrition Examination Survey; VA = Veterans Administration.
*Obtained from meta-analyses. These estimates do not include Veterans Administration-based studies (*in italics*).

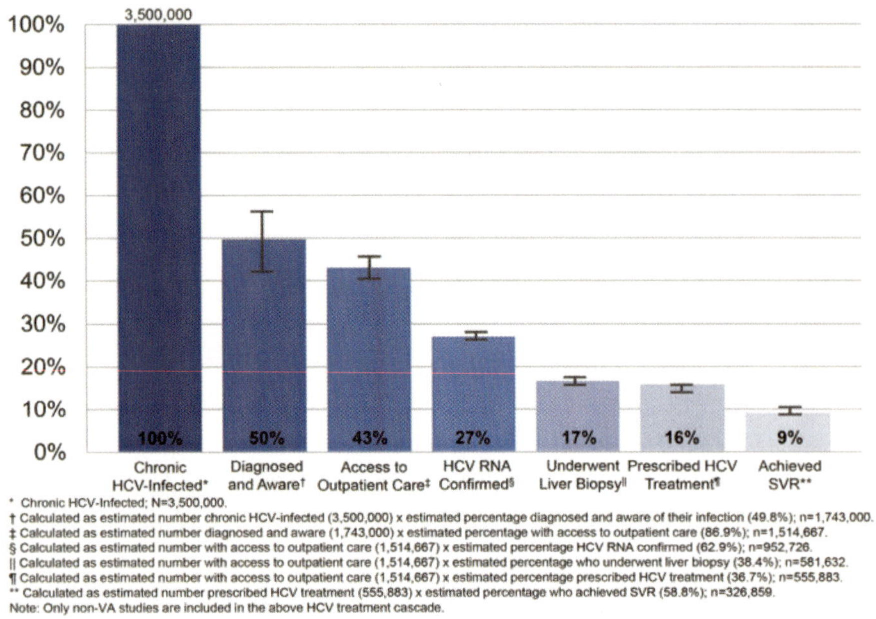

Figure 2. Treatment Cascade for People with Chronic Hepatitis C Virus (HCV) Infection, Prevalence Estimates with 95% Confidence Intervals. * Chronic HCV-Infected; N = 3,500,000. † Calculated as estimated number chronic HCV-infected (3,500,000) x estimated percentage diagnosed and aware of their infection (49.8%); n = 1,743,000. ‡ Calculated as estimated number diagnosed and aware (1,743,000) x estimated percentage with access to outpatient care (86.9%); n = 1,514,667. § Calculated as estimated number with access to outpatient care (1,514,667) x estimated percentage HCV RNA confirmed (62.9%); n = 952,726. || Calculated as estimated number with access to outpatient care (1,514,667) x estimated percentage who underwent liver biopsy (38.4%); n = 581,632. ¶ Calculated as estimated number with access to outpatient care (1,514,667) x estimated percentage prescribed HCV treatment (36.7%); n = 555,883. ** Calculated as estimated number prescribed HCV treatment (555,883) x estimated percentage who achieved SVR (58.8%); n = 326,859. Note: Only non-VA studies are included in the above HCV treatment cascade.

lence of chronic HCV infection was estimated to be 3.5 million [22]. This estimate was used for cascade step 1 (**Figure 2**).

Among those living with chronic HCV, approximately 50% are unaware of their diagnosis based on data from the NHANES Hepatitis C Follow-Up Survey [31,32]. A total of 500 participants who tested positive for HCV RNA between 2001 and 2010 were asked if they were aware of their HCV status before being notified by NHANES. Half of the 203 respondents were unaware of their HCV status [31,32]. Thus, 1,743,000 chronic HCV-infected persons (49.8% [95% CI, 42.9–56.7%] of 3.5 million) are estimated to be diagnosed and aware of their infection (cascade step 2).

In this same study, participants who were aware of their chronic HCV status were also asked about their health insurance status [31,32]. Among those aware of their chronic HCV infection, 86.9% had health insurance compared to 60.4% of those unaware of their HCV infection. Thus, 1,514,667 persons (43.3% [95% CI, 39.9–46.6%] of 3.5 million) are estimated to be aware of their chronic HCV diagnosis and have access to outpatient healthcare (cascade step 3).

Once in care, measurement of HCV RNA is needed to confirm diagnosis of chronic HCV infection, and staging of liver disease is important for guiding HCV treatment decisions. Data from the Chronic Hepatitis B and C Cohort Study, which included 8,810 patients with chronic HCV receiving care at four health systems in the U.S. (Detroit, Michigan; Danville, Pennsylvania; Honolulu, Hawaii; and Portland, Oregon), reported that 5,540 (62.9%) of these patients had confirmatory HCV RNA testing, and 3,380 (38.4%) had hepatic fibrosis staging with a liver biopsy during 2001–2010 [29]. Based on these data, 952,726 persons (27.2% [95% CI, 26.8–27.7%] of 3.5 million) are estimated to be aware of their chronic HCV diagnosis, have access to healthcare, and received confirmatory HCV RNA testing (cascade step 4) and 581,632 (16.6% [95% CI, 16.2–17.1%] of 3.5 million) are estimated to be aware of their chronic HCV diagnosis, have access to healthcare, and have underwent a liver biopsy for hepatic fibrosis staging (cascade step 5). In contrast, an evaluation of the national VA Hepatitis C Clinical Case Registry from 1997 to 2006 indicated that only 16.7% (28,677 of 171,893) of VA patients with chronic HCV received a liver biopsy [25]. Using these VA-based data, 252,949 persons (7.2% [95% CI, 7.1–7.3%] of 3.5 million) are estimated to be aware of their chronic HCV diagnosis, have access to healthcare, and received a liver biopsy (cascade step 5).

Two non-VA studies evaluated prescription of pegylated interferon plus ribavirin treatment among patients with chronic HCV infection [27,29]. Given the recent introduction of direct-acting antiviral agents, we did not identify any population-based studies evaluating these agents that met our selection criteria. Kanwal and colleagues examined prescription rates among 2,893 patients enrolled in one of the largest commercial health insurance carriers in the U.S. [27], while Moorman et al. focused on 8,810 patients receiving care within four U.S. health systems [29]. The proportion of chronic HCV-infected patients prescribed pegylated interferon plus ribavirin ranged from 36–38%, with a pooled proportion of 36.7% (95% CI, 35.8–37.6%; $I^2 = 4\%$). Thus, 555,883 persons (15.9% [95% CI, 15.5–16.3%] of 3.5 million) are estimated to be aware of their chronic HCV diagnosis, have access to healthcare, and have received HCV therapy (cascade step 6). This estimate differed from data reported by the VA system, where 17.9% (6,224 of 34,749) of chronic HCV-infected patients have been prescribed pegylated interferon plus ribavirin treatment [26]. Using these VA-based data, 271,125 people (7.7% [95% CI, 7.6–7.9%] of 3.5 million) are estimated to be aware of their chronic

HCV diagnosis, have access to healthcare, and received HCV treatment (cascade step 6).

Three non-VA studies examined SVR rates among chronic HCV-infected patients who received antiviral therapy [23,28,30]. These included an analysis of 575 patients (71% HCV genotype 1, 29% HCV genotype 2/3) within 40 managed care plans [28]; a study of 407 patients (57% HCV genotype 1, 42% HCV genotype 2/3) in care within a network composed of 21 community clinics and one academic health center [23]; and an evaluation of 258 patients in an integrated health care system (55% HCV genotype 1/4/6, 45% HCV genotype 2/3) [30]. The proportion of treated chronic HCV-infected patients who achieved SVR varied by genotype, with a pooled proportion of 47.0% (95% CI, 42.0–52.1%; $I^2 = 0\%$) for genotype 1, 75.1% (95% CI, 65.3–84.9%; $I^2 = 74\%$) for genotype 2/3, and 58.8% (95% CI, 56.1–61.5%; $I^2 = 0\%$) for all genotypes. Using the overall pooled proportion, 326,859 people (9.3% [95% CI, 8.9–9.8%] of 3.5 million) are estimated to be aware of their chronic HCV diagnosis, have access to healthcare, have been prescribed antiviral therapy, and achieved SVR (cascade step 7). In comparison, a national study of 16,864 chronic HCV-infected Veterans who received antiviral therapy (72% HCV genotype 1, 28% HCV genotype 2/3) reports an overall SVR rate of 44.1% [24]. Using these VA-based data, 245,144 people (7.0% [95% CI, 6.9–7.1%] of 3.5 million) are estimated to be aware of their chronic HCV diagnosis, have access to healthcare, received HCV treatment (based on the VA estimate reported above), and achieved SVR (cascade step 7).

Discussion

This review identifies large gaps between current practice and treatment goals for people with chronic HCV infection. It also highlights multiple opportunities for improving engagement along the HCV treatment cascade, particularly in the diagnosis and awareness of infection, prescription of antiviral therapy, and achievement of SVR. Our study confirms findings reported in a commentary by Holmberg *et al.* that only 5–6% of all people with chronic HCV infection in the U.S. successfully progressed from detection of HCV infection to achievement of SVR [16] and extends this work by rigorously reviewing and meta-analyzing the literature, highlighting differences between U.S. Veteran and non-Veteran populations. In addition, the proposed HCV treatment cascade provides a framework for evaluating the delivery of HCV care over time and within subgroups, which will be necessary to monitor the impact of new screening efforts [33,34] and advances in antiviral therapy [34,35] which will likely increase the number of people completing each step along the cascade.

In 2012, the Centers for Disease Control and Prevention recommended one-time HCV testing without prior ascertainment of risk for persons born between 1945 and 1965 - a group estimated to account for three-fourths of all HCV infections in the U.S. [34]. Implementation of this recommendation, which also calls for referral of newly identified HCV-infected persons for management, may improve the proportion of individuals diagnosed and aware of their infection and referred to care.

Hepatic fibrosis assessment via liver biopsy is not required for HCV therapy, as per current professional guidelines [11]. However, staging of liver fibrosis remains important for determining the urgency and timing of HCV therapy and for identification of cirrhosis, which should prompt screening for hepatocellular carcinoma and monitoring for the development of hepatic decompensation [36,37]. We therefore included hepatic fibrosis assessment as a step in the HCV treatment cascade. While liver biopsy has traditionally been the "gold standard" for assessing liver disease, noninvasive tests, including serum biochemical markers (e.g., aspartate aminotransferase-to-platelet ratio index, FIB-4, HCV FibroSure [LabCorp, Burlington, NC], Hepascore [San Juan Capistrano, CA], Fibrotest [Biopredictive, Paris, France]) and imaging modalities (e.g., transient elastometry [FibroScan, Echosens, Paris, France]), are increasingly playing a role in staging liver fibrosis screening [11,33,38]. As these noninvasive and more convenient tests evolve, it is likely that the number of patients undergoing hepatic fibrosis staging will increase.

The advent of new direct-acting antiviral agents will shorten treatment duration, likely increase the number of people offered treatment, and improve HCV cure rates (final two steps of the HCV treatment cascade) [15,35]. However, educating providers and the general public about HCV prevention, care, and treatment; ensuring access to providers skilled in the treatment of HCV infection; and addressing the high cost of these agents will be critical to maximizing the benefits of these new therapies [14,39]. In a recent cost-effectiveness simulation evaluating birth-cohort HCV screening and subsequent treatment of HCV-infected adults, Rein and colleagues note that birth-cohort screening followed by HCV treatment including direct-acting antiviral agents will increase quality-adjusted life-years (QALYs) by $532,200 and medical costs by $19.0 billion, for an incremental cost-effectiveness ratio of $35,700 per QALY saved (95% credible interval, $28,200 to $47,200) [40]. While these simulations accounted for common HCV-associated complications, funders, public health administrators, and providers should be aware of the financial burden of untreated HCV infection. Using data from the 2010 U.S. National Health and Wellness Survey, El Khoury et al. note that persons with untreated HCV infection had significantly ($p<0.001$) higher annual productivity losses ($10,316 vs. $5,459 per employed person) and annual all-cause healthcare costs ($22,818 vs. $15,362 per person) compared to HCV-uninfected individuals. [41] Evaluating the trade-off between the benefits and costs of these new agents will be critical to scaling up HCV treatment [35].

Individuals' progression along the HCV treatment cascade varied widely, with large drop-offs occurring at diagnosis and awareness of infection, prescription of antiviral therapy, and achievement of SVR. Studies are needed to evaluate and compare the population-level benefits and costs of interventions, such as screening and treatment efforts, at each step. These data can further assist public health officials in allocating resources to increase the proportion of chronic HCV-infected patients completing the cascade steps. In addition, monitoring the HCV treatment cascade over time will be critically important to defining overall progress and identifying persistent barriers at individual steps.

Since the VA system is the largest single provider of HCV care in the U.S. and because of potential differences in the management of chronic HCV infection among U.S. Veterans [42], we conducted a separate analysis to estimate the numbers of chronic HCV-infected people completing steps 5–7 in the HCV treatment cascade using VA-specific data. Among chronic HCV-infected Veterans in care, the proportion of those who received hepatic fibrosis staging by liver biopsy and who were prescribed HCV treatment was 22% and 19% lower, respectively, compared to the general population. Similarly, among Veterans with chronic HCV infection who were prescribed pegylated interferon plus ribavirin, a smaller proportion achieved SVR compared to the general population (44% vs. 58%). These variations may be due to differences in patient populations or in VA provider practices. Prior studies indicate that Veterans with chronic HCV have higher rates of absolute and relative contraindications to HCV treatment than persons seen at non-VA clinics [43–45]. In addition, differences in medication adherence [12], provider management, and health system factors may contribute to the lower proportion of Veterans completing the final steps of the HCV treatment cascade. Future studies should evaluate how the HCV treatment cascade changes for Veterans and non-Veterans with the advancement of new direct-acting antiviral therapies.

This study has several potential limitations. First, our treatment cascade included seven steps, as identified by prior research [8,9], evaluated at one time point. Future studies should explore the addition (e.g. linkage to and retention in HCV care) and deletion (e.g., liver biopsy) of cascade steps to best assist public health officials in monitoring HCV care in the U.S. Further, since patients receive care over time, the studies included in this analysis may not have allowed sufficient time for certain steps in the HCV treatment cascade to take place. Monitoring the steps of the cascade over time may help to define overall progress toward population-based goals and barriers at individual steps. Second, our systematic review was limited by the relatively small number of studies identified, particularly for cascade steps 1–3. Many studies excluded prisoners and homeless individuals, populations heavily affect by chronic HCV infection. These exclusions may underestimate cascade steps, particularly access to outpatient care. Third, we broadly focused on estimating the number of chronic HCV-infected people in the general population. Estimates for each step in the HCV treatment cascade could not be determined by sex, race/ethnicity, socioeconomic status, injection drug use, and HIV status because these data were not available in the included studies. Future studies should determine the cascade within these subgroups. Fourth, HCV RNA confirmation in evaluated studies was restricted to patients' healthcare network. This may underestimate HCV RNA testing, particularly for patients who transfer care between providers. Similarly, liver biopsy was used as the marker for HCV disease staging; however, this may underestimate the number of people who were staged through the use of noninvasive tests. Fifth, not all patients immediately require or are eligible to receive antiviral therapy for chronic HCV, which may underestimate the proportion of patients treated. Further, failure to achieve SVR may be a consequence of biological factors, including HCV genotype, treatment efficacy and tolerability, or adherence to therapy. Differentiating between these causes may be important because each requires a different intervention strategy. In addition, data on prescription and SVR rates of newer direct-acting anti-HCV medications were not available. Monitoring how these steps change as providers increasingly use these new therapies will be critical. Lastly, we present the treatment cascade for people with chronic HCV infection living in the U.S., but evaluating the treatment cascade in other countries will be important and may help identify models for improving HCV monitoring and public health in those areas.

In summary, our results suggest that continued efforts are needed to improve HCV care in the U.S. In a field that is changing rapidly, with increased attention on HCV screening and approval of new, effective direct-acting antiviral agents, this proposed HCV treatment cascade provides a framework for identifying gaps in care. This framework will be useful in monitoring the impact of new public health initiatives, care models, and treatments. Only by increasing the number of persons completing each step in the cascade can the goals of the U.S. *Action Plan for the Prevention, Care, and Treatment of Viral Hepatitis* be achieved.

Acknowledgments

We are grateful to Drs. K. Rajender Reddy, Jay R. Kostman, and Stacey Trooskin for their advice and support, and to Dr. Matthew D. Mitchell for his assistance with data analysis.

Author Contributions

Conceived and designed the experiments: BRY AJS CAU VLR. Performed the experiments: BRY AJS CAU VLR. Analyzed the data: BRY AJS CAU VLR. Wrote the paper: BRY AJS CAU VLR.

References

1. Gardner EM, McLees MP, Steiner JF, Del Rio C, Burman WJ (2011) The spectrum of engagement in HIV care and its relevance to test-and-treat strategies for prevention of HIV infection. Clin Infect Dis 52: 793–800.
2. Vital Signs (2011) HIV prevention through care and treatment–United States. MMWR Morb Mortal Wkly Rep 60: 1618–1623.
3. Hull MW, Wu Z, Montaner JS (2012) Optimizing the engagement of care cascade: a critical step to maximize the impact of HIV treatment as prevention. Curr Opin HIV AIDS 7: 579–586.
4. Mahle Gray K, Tang T, Shouse L, Li J, Mermin J, et al. (2013) Using the HIV surveillance system to monitor the National HIV/AIDS Strategy. Am J Public Health 103: 141–147.
5. Yehia B, Frank I (2011) Battling AIDS in America: an evaluation of the National HIV/AIDS Strategy. Am J Public Health 101: e4–8.
6. Fleishman JA, Yehia BR, Moore RD, Korthuis PT, Gebo KA, et al. (2012) Establishment, retention, and loss to follow-up in outpatient HIV care. J Acquir Immune Defic Syndr 60: 249–259.
7. Mugavero MJ, Amico KR, Horn T, Thompson MA (2013) The State of Engagement in HIV Care in the United States: From Cascade to Continuum to Control. Clin Infect Dis 57(8):1164–71.
8. Insitute of Medicine (2010) Hepatitis and Liver Cancer: A National Strategy for Prevention and Control of Hepatitis B and C. Washington, DC.
9. Edlin BR (2011) Perspective: test and treat this silent killer. Nature 474: S18–19.
10. Brau N (2013) Evaluation of the hepatitis C virus-infected patient: the initial encounter. Clin Infect Dis 56: 853–860.
11. Ghany MG, Strader DB, Thomas DL, Seeff LB, American Association for the Study of Liver Disease (2009) Diagnosis, management, and treatment of hepatitis C: an update. Hepatology 49: 1335–1374.
12. Lo Re V III, Teal V, Localio AR, Amorosa VK, Kaplan DE, et al. (2011) Relationship between adherence to hepatitis C virus therapy and virologic outcomes: a cohort study. Ann Intern Med 155: 353–360.
13. Yee HS, Chang MF, Pocha C, Lim J, Ross D, et al. (2012) Update on the management and treatment of hepatitis C virus infection: recommendations from the Department of Veterans Affairs Hepatitis C Resource Center Program and the National Hepatitis C Program Office. Am J Gastroenterol 107: 669–689; quiz 690.
14. US Department of Health and Human Services (2011) Combating the Silent Epidemic of Viral Hepatitis: Action Plan for the Prevention, Care & Treatment of Viral Hepatitis. Washington, DC. pp. 1–76.
15. Aghemo A, De Francesco R (2013) New horizons in Hepatitis C antiviral therapy with direct-acting antivirals. Hepatology 58(1):428–38.
16. Holmberg SD, Spradling PR, Moorman AC, Denniston MM (2013) Hepatitis C in the United States. N Engl J Med 368(20):1859–1861.
17. Kramer JR, Kanwal F, Richardson P, Mei M, El-Serag HB (2012) Gaps in the achievement of effectiveness of HCV treatment in national VA practice. J Hepatol 56: 320–325.
18. Umscheid CA (2013) A Primer on Performing Systematic Reviews and Meta-analyses. Clin Infect Dis 57: 725–734.
19. Cornberg M, Razavi HA, Alberti A, Bernasconi E, Buti M, et al. (2011) A systematic review of hepatitis C virus epidemiology in Europe, Canada and Israel. Liver Int 31 Suppl 2: 30–60.
20. Higgins JP, Thompson SG (2002) Quantifying heterogeneity in a meta-analysis. Stat Med 21: 1539–1558.
21. OpenMeta[Analyst] (2012). Accessed at http://www.cebm.brown.edu/open_meta. on Dec 15, 2013.

22. Armstrong GL, Wasley A, Simard EP, McQuillan GM, Kuhnert WL, et al. (2006) The prevalence of hepatitis C virus infection in the United States, 1999 through 2002. Ann Intern Med 144: 705–714.
23. Arora S, Thornton K, Murata G, Deming P, Kalishman S, et al. (2011) Outcomes of treatment for hepatitis C virus infection by primary care providers. N Engl J Med 364: 2199–2207.
24. Backus LI, Boothroyd DB, Phillips BR, Belperio P, Halloran J, et al. (2011) A Sustained Virologic Response Reduces Risk of All-Cause Mortality in Patients With Hepatitis C. Clin Gastroenterol Hepatol 9: 509–516.e501.
25. Groessl EJ, Liu L, Ho SB, Kanwal F, Gifford AL, et al. (2012) National patterns and predictors of liver biopsy use for management of hepatitis C. J Hepatol 57: 252–259.
26. Kanwal F, Hoang T, Chrusciel T, Kramer JR, El-Serag HB, et al. (2012) Process of care for hepatitis C infection is linked to treatment outcome and virologic response. Clin Gastroenterol Hepatol 10: 1270–1277.
27. Kanwal F, Schnitzler MS, Bacon BR, Hoang T, Buchanan PM, et al. (2010) Quality of care in patients with chronic hepatitis C virus infection: a cohort study. Ann Intern Med 153: 231–239.
28. Mitra D, Davis KL, Beam C, Medjedovic J, Rustgi V (2010) Treatment patterns and adherence among patients with chronic hepatitis C virus in a US managed care population. Value Health 13: 479–486.
29. Moorman AC, Gordon SC, Rupp LB, Spradling PR, Teshale EH, et al. (2013) Baseline characteristics and mortality among people in care for chronic viral hepatitis: the chronic hepatitis cohort study. Clin Infect Dis 56: 40–50.
30. Russell M, Pauly MP, Moore CD, Chia C, Dorrell J, et al. (2012) The impact of lifetime alcohol use on hepatitis C treatment outcomes in privately insured members of an integrated health care plan. Hepatology 56: 1223–1230.
31. Younossi ZM, Stepanova M, Afendy M, Lam BP, Mishra A (2013) Knowledge about infection is the only predictor of treatment in patients with chronic hepatitis C. J Viral Hepat 20: 550–555.
32. Denniston MM, Klevens RM, McQuillan GM, Jiles RB (2012) Awareness of infection, knowledge of hepatitis C, and medical follow-up among individuals testing positive for hepatitis C: National Health and Nutrition Examination Survey 2001–2008. Hepatology 55: 1652–1661.
33. Moyer VA, on behalf of the USPSTF (2013) Screening for Hepatitis C Virus Infection in Adults: U.S. Preventive Services Task Force Recommendation Statement. Ann Intern Med 159(5): 349–57.
34. Smith BD, Morgan RL, Beckett GA, Falck-Ytter Y, Holtzman D, et al. (2012) Recommendations for the identification of chronic hepatitis C virus infection among persons born during 1945–1965. MMWR Recomm Rep 61: 1–32.
35. Thomas DL (2012) Advances in the treatment of hepatitis C virus infection. Top Antivir Med 20: 5–10.
36. Garcia-Tsao G (2001) Current management of the complications of cirrhosis and portal hypertension: variceal hemorrhage, ascites, and spontaneous bacterial peritonitis. Gastroenterology 120: 726–748.
37. Bruix J, Sherman M, American Association for the Study of Liver D (2011) Management of hepatocellular carcinoma: an update. Hepatology 53: 1020–1022.
38. Chou R, Wasson N (2013) Blood tests to diagnose fibrosis or cirrhosis in patients with chronic hepatitis C virus infection: a systematic review. Ann Intern Med 158: 807–820.
39. Chan K, Lai MN, Groessl EJ, Hanchate AD, Wong JB, et al. (2013) Cost effectiveness of direct-acting antiviral therapy for treatment-naive patients with chronic HCV genotype 1 infection in the veterans health administration. Clin Gastroenterol Hepatol 11: 1503–1510.
40. Rein DB, Smith BD, Wittenborn JS, Lesesne SB, Wagner LD, et al. (2012) The cost-effectiveness of birth-cohort screening for hepatitis C antibody in U.S. primary care settings. Ann Intern Med 156: 263–270.
41. El Khoury AC, Vietri J, Prajapati G (2012) The burden of untreated hepatitis C virus infection: a US patients' perspective. Dig Dis Sci 57: 2995–3003.
42. Veterans Health Administration. (2009) The State of Care for Veterans with HIV/AIDS. Available: http://www.hiv.va.gov/provider/policy/state-of-care/. Accessed 2013 Dec 15.
43. Butt AA, Khan UA, Shaikh OS, McMahon D, Dorey-Stein Z, et al. (2009) Rates of HCV treatment eligibility among HCV-monoinfected and HCV/HIV-coinfected patients in tertiary care referral centers. HIV Clin Trials 10: 25–32.
44. Butt AA, Justice AC, Skanderson M, Good C, Kwoh CK (2006) Rates and predictors of hepatitis C virus treatment in HCV-HIV-coinfected subjects. Aliment Pharmacol Ther 24: 585–591.
45. Kanwal F, Hoang T, Spiegel BM, Eisen S, Dominitz JA, et al. (2007) Predictors of treatment in patients with chronic hepatitis C infection - role of patient versus nonpatient factors. Hepatology 46: 1741–1749.

Nonresponse to Interferon-α Based Treatment for Chronic Hepatitis C Infection Is Associated with Increased Hazard of Cirrhosis

Myrna L. Cozen[1*], James C. Ryan[1], Hui Shen[1], Robert Lerrigo[1], Russell M. Yee[2], Edward Sheen[3], Richard Wu[1], Alexander Monto[1]

1 Department of Medicine, Veterans Affairs Medical Center and University of California San Francisco, San Francisco, California, United States of America, 2 Department of Epidemiology, Mailman School of Public Health, Columbia University, New York, New York, United States of America, 3 Department of Medicine, Stanford University School of Medicine, Stanford, California, United States of America

Abstract

Background: The long-term consequences of unsuccessful interferon-α based hepatitis C treatment on liver disease progression and survival have not been fully explored.

Methods and Findings: We performed retrospective analyses to assess long-term clinical outcomes among treated and untreated patients with hepatitis C virus in two independent cohorts from a United States Veterans Affairs Medical Center and a University Teaching Hospital. Eligible patients underwent liver biopsy during consideration for interferon-α based treatment between 1992 and 2007. They were assessed for the probability of developing cirrhosis and of dying during follow-up using Cox proportional hazards models, stratified by pretreatment liver fibrosis stage and adjusted for known risk factors for cirrhosis and characteristics affecting treatment selection. The major predictor was a time-dependent covariate for treatment outcome among four patient groups: 1) patients with sustained virological response to treatment; 2) treatment relapsers; 3) treatment nonresponders; and 4) never treated patients. Treatment nonresponders in both cohorts had a statistically significantly increased hazard of cirrhosis compared to never treated patients, as stratified by pretreatment liver fibrosis stage and adjusted for clinical and psychosocial risk factors that disproportionately affect patients who were ineligible for treatment (Veterans Affairs HR = 2.35, CI 1.18–4.69, mean follow-up 10 years, and University Hospital HR = 5.90, CI 1.50–23.24, mean follow-up 7.7 years). Despite their increased risk for liver disease progression, the overall survival of nonresponders in both cohorts was not significantly different from that of never treated patients.

Conclusion: These unexpected findings suggest that patients who receive interferon-α based therapies but fail to clear the hepatitis C virus may have an increased hazard of cirrhosis compared to untreated patients.

Editor: Hans Tillmann, Duke University, United States of America

Funding: Funding provided by National Institutes of Health (NIH) RO1 AI 083113-01; NIH U19 AI 088790; NIH P30 DK026743 (University of California San Francisco Liver Center); Veterans Affairs Merit Award Program and the Veterans Affairs Hepatitis C Resource Center. The funders had no role in study design, data collection and analysis, decision to publish, or preparation of the manuscript.

* E-mail: Myrna.Cozen@va.gov

These authors contributed equally to this work.

Introduction

More than 3.2 million people in the United States (1% of the population) are chronically infected with hepatitis C virus (HCV) [1,2]. Until 2011, standard antiviral treatment consisted of subcutaneous pegylated interferon-α (IFNα and oral ribavirin (RBV), which failed to achieve a sustained virological response (SVR, or cure) in approximately half of patients. The proportion of treatment failures is greater among patients with HCV genotype 1, the most prevalent HCV subspecies in the U.S. [3,4,5,6]. The recent addition of an oral protease inhibitor, either boceprevir or telaprevir, to pegylated IFNα/RBV treatment for genotype 1 patients, has increased SVR rates to nearly 75% in treatment naïve patients [7,8,9]. SVR has been repeatedly associated with reduced rates of cirrhosis, hepatic decompensation and hepatocellular carcinoma, but the long-term impact of treatment failure on liver disease progression has not been fully explored [10,11,12].

Among treatment failures, it has been postulated that transient reductions in viral load during treatment or anti-fibrotic effects of IFNα may attenuate liver disease progression [13]. Alternatively, immunostimulatory influences of IFNα could accelerate liver injury in some patients by triggering hepatic inflammation and scarring [14]. Early observational studies suggested altered short-term progression of liver fibrosis in some treated patients who fail to clear HCV [12,15,16,17,18]. Pockros, et al, pooled data from eight IFNα-based clinical trials that analyzed paired liver biopsy specimens taken immediately prior to treatment and up to 24 weeks post-treatment, but long-term outcomes were not examined

[15]. Short term histologic improvement was seen in some, but not all, treatment failures, and fibrosis progressed in some patients [5,12,15,16,17,18]. The evidence from these treatment and from recent retreatment trials, such as HALT-C and EPIC[3], suggests that failed IFNα-based therapy might have either beneficial, null, or detrimental effects on liver related outcomes in HCV treatment failures [19,20]. There have been no prospective studies, however, comparing long-term clinical outcomes among chronic HCV patients with IFNα-based treatment failure to that of never treated patients. In the present study, we compared long-term clinical outcomes in two independent cohorts of treated and untreated patients with HCV. Our primary aims were to assess the long-term hazards of cirrhosis and death among the following treatment groups: those who achieved SVR, relapsers, nonresponders, and those who were never treated.

Methods

Ethics Statement

This study was conducted in accordance with the ethical principles stated in the Declaration of Helsinki and is consistent with good clinical practice and applicable regulatory requirements [21]. Specific approval was granted by the University of California, San Francisco (UCSF) Institutional Review Board and the SFVA Research and Development Committee for this retrospective records review.

Study Design and Patient Recruitment

We conducted a medical records review of patients with chronic HCV who were first seen at the San Francisco Veterans Affairs (SFVA) Medical Center Liver Clinic between January, 1992 and July 2007. Most patients had been prospectively consented at the time of liver biopsy for inclusion in a longitudinal database. Eligible patients were ≥18 years of age, had documented chronic HCV, underwent a pre-treatment liver biopsy, received follow-up care at the SFVA Liver Clinic for at least one year after the initial visit, and had at least one follow-up liver imaging study, biopsy or clinic visit. Patients were excluded if they were co-infected with either HIV-1 or hepatitis B virus or if they had decompensated cirrhosis, hepatocellular carcinoma, or liver transplantation prior to their first clinic visit. The study was replicated using an independent cohort of HCV patients from the UCSF Liver Clinic to which the same selection criteria were applied. Each cohort is comprised of all patients meeting study eligibility criteria who were evaluated and followed in these two clinics during this time period.

Assessment of Clinical Parameters

The SFVA and UCSF electronic medical records were the major sources of data for the study. Deaths were confirmed by cross reference with the national Social Security Death Index (SSDI). Data abstraction was performed by two teams, each including one clinician and one research staff member, using a standardized search algorithm. Two additional raters performed data validation on a random sample of patient charts to confirm the reliability of values for select variables.

Clinical parameters including body mass index (BMI), alanine aminotransferase (ALT), and HCV viral load were collected from the electronic medical record on the date closest to the initial liver clinic visit. Follow-up ALT was obtained from the laboratory test taken closest to 52 weeks following the end of treatment for treated patients. To obtain a comparable ALT value for the never treated patients, we used the ALT closest to 170.7 weeks following initial liver clinic visit. This interval corresponds to the average time between the first liver clinic visit and the completion of one year of post therapy follow-up among treated patients.

Psychosocial, demographic, and behavioral risk factors were assessed and recorded by clinic staff at the time of first liver clinic visit. This assessment and subsequent progress notes were used to determine the presence of risk factors affecting treatment eligibility such as current injection drug use, other substance abuse, history of depression and post-traumatic stress disorder (PTSD). Heavy alcohol use was defined as five or more years of daily alcohol use exceeding the equivalent of four to five drinks per day by patient self-report [22,23]. Indicators of social instability included recent or current homelessness, housing instability, familial dissolution, social isolation or incarceration.

The Batts-Ludwig system was used to assess fibrosis stage and inflammatory grade from liver biopsies [24,25]. These measures were obtained from the biopsy taken closest to the first liver clinic visit, although biopsies taken more than five years before or one year following this visit were not considered. Cirrhosis was defined as either (i) stage 4 fibrosis on biopsy or (ii) a nodular liver contour plus at least one of three previously validated criteria: ascites, evidence of venous collateral vessels, or splenomegaly as visualized on CT scan, MRI, and/or ultrasound [26].

Patients were categorized into four HCV treatment-related groups using previously described standard definitions: SVR, relapsers, nonresponders, and never treated [6,27,28]. Relapsers achieved undetectable viral load during treatment with detectable virus found during a six month follow-up period. Nonresponders were null and partial responders who were detectably viremic throughout therapy. Those treated for <12 weeks were designated "early treatment discontinuation" (ETD) patients. Patients who were treated more than once were assigned the treatment category corresponding to their last course of therapy.

Major Predictor and Outcome Measures

The primary outcome variables were time-to-cirrhosis and time-to-all-cause-death during the follow-up period. Never treated patients comprised the reference category. Time zero for all time-to-event analyses was the date of first liver clinic visit. To overcome the temporal bias associated with variations in treatment start time, we constructed a time-dependent covariate, using standard methods as previously described [29,30]. This covariate modifies the major predictor (treatment outcome) by adjusting for differences in waiting times between time zero and the beginning of treatment. Time-to-cirrhosis was calculated from time zero to the date cirrhosis was first diagnosed or to the date of last liver clinic visit. Patients diagnosed with cirrhosis prior to time zero were excluded from the time-to-cirrhosis analysis, but were included in time-to-death analysis. For time-to-death analysis, the study length extended from time zero to the date of either death or liver transplantation. In surviving patients, the right censoring time was the date of last medical service encounter or six months before the date that the SSDI was searched, whichever was later. As the SSDI only includes date but not cause of death, all-cause death was used as the outcome variable. March 31, 2012 was the cut-off date for all observations.

Statistical Methods

All analyses were performed using SAS version 9.2 (SAS Institute Inc., Cary, NC). Chi square tests were performed for categorical data analysis, and the Student's t test or Wilcoxon rank sum test was used to evaluate the association of continuous predictors on categorical dependent variables (such as patient treatment group). Cox proportional hazards models were used to analyze both univariate and multivariate effects on the outcomes of interest. Since differences in baseline fibrosis stage likely have nonlinear influences on long-term fibrosis progression, and because the distribution of fibrosis stage violated the proportional hazards assumption, all Cox proportional hazards models were stratified by fibrosis stage groupings (0–1 and 2–3 in time-to-cirrhosis analyses and 0–1, 2–3 and 4 in time-to-death analysis). Time-to-cirrhosis analysis was repeated using an alternate fibrosis stratification strategy to allow a closer examination of advanced stage 3 compared to stages 0–2.

We used two strategies to adjust for the non-random distribution of characteristics differentiating treated from untreated patients, including age at initial liver biopsy, race/ethnicity, HCV genotype, history of heavy alcohol use, other substance use, psychiatric comorbidities, and social stability. First, these factors were assessed individually in univariate hazards models and incorporated into the full multivariate model through backward stepwise regression, as described in Statistical Methods S1. Second, propensity scores were derived from non-collinear risk factors and substituted into the final time-to-event models using previously described methods to estimate a composite effect from the factors related to treatment selection [31,32]. Adjusted hazard ratios resulting from the two approaches were compared. After stratification by fibrosis stage, age-adjusted proportional hazards curves were generated to graph the hazard function for cirrhosis and death or liver transplantation among the four treatment outcome groups. These models assume proportional hazards for age, but not for treatment group.

Results

Demographic and Clinical Characteristics

Among SFVA patients screened, 358 (99% male) met the study inclusion criteria, and 159 patients (44.4%) received antiviral treatment for HCV. Approximately 80% were between the ages of 45 and 65 at initial liver clinic visit, with a mean age of 51 (Table 1). This age distribution corresponds to the birth cohort of Vietnam era veterans, a risk group known to have higher rates of prior IDU and HCV seroprevalence than other groups of veterans, which reflects likely exposure to HCV during and shortly after their service years in the 1960s and 1970s [33] [34]. Approximately 55% of the cohort had little or no liver disease at baseline, as measured by Batts-Ludwig fibrosis score, while 7.3% were cirrhotic. Mean follow-up time was 10 years, and 22% (n = 78) died during follow-up. One patient underwent liver transplantation. Deaths occurred among 8.7% of patients achieving SVR, 18.2% of relapsers, 28.6% of nonresponders, and 23.8% of the never treated patients ($p<0.01$).

Treated SFVA patients had higher liver fibrosis stage and inflammation score at baseline, however when stratified by fibrosis stage the influence of inflammation lost significance, suggesting effect modification by fibrosis. Treated patients were followed for a longer period than never treated patients (10.8 versus 9.4 years, $p<0.0001$) and treatment nonresponders and relapsers had more follow-up liver imaging (or liver biopsies) than never treated patients ($\bar{x} = 1.77$, 2.77, 3.88 and 1.74 for SVR, relapsers, nonresponders and never treated patients, respectively, $p<0.0001$) (Table 1). Never treated patients were older (52 versus 50 years, $p = 0.04$), more likely to be African American and more likely to be infected with "difficult to clear" genotypes HCV genotypes 1 or 4 than 2 or 3 (Table 1). Treated patients had a higher mean BMI at baseline than never treated patients (Table 1). The most common reasons cited for the decision not to treat during follow-up were minimal liver disease (21.6%), ongoing alcohol and substance use (19.1%), active mental health problems (11.1%), African American race (5.0%), advanced liver disease (3.0%), and advanced age with or without other comorbidities (8.5%). Compared with treated patients, never treated patients were more likely to be active substance users and to have at least one indicator of social instability (Table 2).

No statistically significant difference was found in mean baseline ALT between treated and never treated groups ($p = 0.15$, data not shown), although the SVR group had a marginally higher baseline value as compared to the other treatment outcome groups (Table 1). We compared the mean change in ALT before and after treatment for nonresponders and relapsers (grouped together) to that of never treated patients for a comparable time interval. We found that nonresponders and relapsers had a mean decrease in ALT of 15.0 U/L, while never treated patients had a mean increase of ALT of 17.6 U/L ($p = 0.05$) (data not shown). In further analysis we found that 69.2% of nonresponders and relapsers had a decrease in ALT ≥25% following treatment as compared to 45.2% of never treated patients, while 19.2% of nonresponders and relapsers and 41.9% of never treated patients had an increase in ALT of ≥25% ($p = 0.03$) (data not shown).

Predictors of treatment success. Among treated SFVA patients, African Americans were less likely to achieve SVR than other races/ethnic groups ($p = 0.03$) as were patients with HCV genotypes 1 or 4 ($p = 0.007$) and those with higher pretreatment fibrosis stage ($p = 0.004$). No significant difference was noted in treatment success between the small number of SFVA patients who received IFNα monotherapy and those treated with IFNα or pegylated IFNα/RBV combination therapy (Table 1).

Cumulative incidence of cirrhosis. We examined the cumulative incidence of cirrhosis among SFVA patients with baseline fibrosis stages 2 and 3 using age adjusted proportional hazards curves stratified by treatment group (Figure 1). A greater proportion of treatment relapsers and nonresponders developed cirrhosis than never treated patients. The overall incidence of cirrhosis in the SFVA cohort was 25.8 cases per 1,000 person years. While SVR and never treated patients had incidence rates of 16.2 and 20.5 cases per 1,000 person years, respectively, these rates rose to 28.9 and 58.9 cases per 1,000 person years among relapsers and nonresponders. These differences, however, were not statistically significant.

Time-to-cirrhosis analysis. In univariate proportional hazards models stratified by baseline fibrosis stage (0–1 and 2–3) and employing the time dependent covariate for SFVA treatment group, nonresponders were twice as likely to develop cirrhosis when compared to never treated patients (HR = 2.02, CI 1.11–3.67, Table 3). Patients achieving SVR did not realize appreciable protection from cirrhosis in these models, although their hazard ratios trended in that direction. Histological inflammation score was not predictive of cirrhosis once the cohort was stratified by baseline fibrosis stage. As expected, age incrementally increased the cirrhosis risk; for every additional year there was a 5% increase in the hazard of developing cirrhosis (HR, 1.05 CI 1.01–1.09). History of blood transfusion prior to 1992 was also associated with an increased the hazard of cirrhosis (HR 2.04, CI 1.16–3.59). African American patients were at considerably lower risk of developing cirrhosis than were Caucasians (HR = 0.47, CI 0.20–1.10), but this difference did not achieve statistical significance, probably due to the low number of cirrhosis events among African Americans. In contrast, Latinos were at greater risk of cirrhosis compared to Caucasians, but again this increased hazard did not attain statistical significance (HR = 1.82, CI 0.88–3.77). Neither BMI, diabetes mellitus, history of heavy alcohol use or lack of social stability were significantly associated with the hazard of cirrhosis in univariate models. ALT was not entered into the

Table 1. Demographic and Clinical Characteristics of the SFVA HCV Cohort.

Variable	Total	SVR	NR	Relapser	ETD/ Unknown	No Treatment	p-value
	(N = 358)	(N = 69)	(N = 49)	(N = 22)	(N = 19)	(N = 199)	
Age at 1st Liver Clinic Visit (Yr), Mean (SD)	50.98 (6.68)	49.13 (6.87)	50.38 (5.18)	51.06 (4.82)	50.47 (7.68)	51.81 (6.92)	0.20**
Male Gender	354 (98.9%)	66 (95.7%)	49 (100.0%)	22 (100.0%)	19 (100.0%)	198 (99.5%)	0.16*
Race/Ethnicity							
Caucasian	236 (66.1%)	59 (85.5%)	31 (64.6%)	18 (81.8%)	10 (52.6%)	118 (59.3%)	0.01
African-American	72 (20.2%)	4 (5.8%)	11 (22.9%)	3 (13.6%)	3 (15.8%)	51 (25.6%)	
Latino	31 (8.7%)	3 (4.3%)	4 (8.3%)	1 (4.5%)	4 (21.1%)	19 (9.5%)	
Asian/API/Native American	18 (5.0%)	3 (4.3%)	2 (4.2%)	0 (0.0%)	2 (10.5%)	11 (5.5%)	
HCV Genotype†							
Genotype 1	246 (68.7%)	33 (47.8%)	40 (81.6%)	13 (59.1%)	10 (52.6%)	150 (75.4%)	<0.0001
Genotype 2	52 (14.5%)	16 (23.2%)	3 (6.1%)	5 (22.7%)	3 (15.8%)	25 (12.6%)	
Genotype 3	30 (8.4%)	10 (14.5%)	5 (10.2%)	3 (13.6%)	1 (5.3%)	11 (5.5%)	
Genotype 4	6 (1.7%)	0 (0.0%)	0 (0.0%)	0 (0.0%)	1 (5.3%)	5 (2.5%)	
Mixed genotype	2 (0.6%)	0 (0.0%)	1 (2.0%)	1 (4.5%)	0 (0.0%)	0 (0.0%)	
Baseline Fibrosis Stage							
0	111 (31.0%)	13 (18.8%)	5 (10.2%)	7 (31.8%)	2 (10.5%)	84 (42.2%)	<0.0001
1	87 (24.3%)	20 (29.0%)	10 (20.4%)	2 (9.1%)	5 (26.3%)	50 (25.1%)	
2	92 (25.7%)	26 (37.7%)	13 (26.5%)	5 (22.7%)	3 (15.8%)	45 (22.6%)	
3	42 (11.7%)	7 (10.1%)	13 (26.5%)	4 (18.2%)	6 (31.6%)	12 (6.0%)	
4	26 (7.3%)	3 (4.3%)	8 (16.3%)	4 (18.2%)	3 (15.8%)	8 (4.0%)	
Baseline Inflammation Grade‡							
0	17(4.9%)	1(1.5%)	0(0.0%)	0(0.0%)	2(11.1%)	14(7.3%)	0.003
1	107(31.0%)	17(25.0%)	9(20.0%)	6(28.6%)	2(11.1%)	73(37.8%)	
2	195(56.5%)	42(61.8%)	33(73.3%)	11(52.4%)	14(77.8%)	95(49.2%)	
3	26(7.5%)	8(11.8%)	3(6.7%)	4(19.0%)	0(0.0%)	11(5.7%)	
Baseline ALT, Mean (SD)	94.01 (71.91)	109.84 (74.59)	92.89 (71.06)	99.69 (75.38)	76.47 (65.28)	89.17 (71.56)	0.09**
Baseline BMI, Mean (SD)	28.42 (5.25)	29.86 (5.10)	29.04 (5.23)	28.20 (4.71)	28.74 (7.62)	27.75 (5.02)	0.02**
Diabetes Mellitus	56 (15.6%)	9 (13.0%)	10 (20.4%)	5 (22.7%)	4 (21.1%)	28 (14.1%)	0.50*
Blood Transfusion before 1992	71 (21.1%)	14 (22.2%)	8(17.8%)	6 (30.0%)	3 (15.8%)	40 (21.2%)	0.82*
Number of Follow-up Images/Liver Biopsy, Mean (SD)	2.10 (1.96)	1.77 (2.09)	3.88 (2.25)	2.77 (1.63)	1.68 (1.83)	1.74 (1.62)	<0.0001**
Cirrhosis during Follow-up	60 (18.1%)	7 (10.6%)	20 (48.8%)	4 (22.2%)	2 (12.5%)	27 (14.1%)	<0.0001*
HCC during Follow-up	20 (5.6%)	2 (2.9%)	6 (12.2%)	1 (4.5%)	2 (10.5%)	9 (4.5%)	0.14*
Liver Transplant during Follow-up	1 (0.3%)	0 (0.0%)	0 (0.0%)	0 (0.0%)	1 (5.3%)	0 (0.0%)	0.05*
Died during Follow-up	78 (21.8%)	6 (8.7%)	14 (28.6%)	4 (18.2%)	7 (36.8%)	47 (23.6%)	0.01*
Years of Follow-Up, Mean (SD)	10.00 (3.05)	10.76 (2.88)	11.72 (2.89)	10.46 (3.12)	8.97 (4.27)	9.36 (2.78)	<0.0001**
Treated Patients Only	**N = 159**						
Courses of IFNα Treatment							
1	133 (83.6%)	62 (89.9%)	36 (73.5%)	19 (86.4%)	16 (84.2%)	NA	0.13*
≥2	26 (16.4%)	7 (10.1%)	13 (26.5%)	3 (13.6%)	3 (15.8%)	NA	
Length of IFNα treatment (wk), Mean (SD)	40.45 (22.32)	43.38 (17.11)	40.00 (22.27)	51.18 (27.68)	18.53 (19.25)	NA	<0.0001**
Therapeutic Regimen							
IFNα monotherapy	20 (12.6%)	6 (8.7%)	9 (18.4%)	2 (9.1%)	3 (15.8%)	NA	0.41*
IFNα/RBV therapy	139 (87.4%)	63 (91.3%)	40 (81.6%)	20 (90.9%)	16 (84.2%)	NA	

P-values were calculated from Chi-square test for category variables and ANOVA for continuous variables unless otherwise marked.
*P-values were calculated from Fisher's Exact test.
**Variable was rank transformed.
†22 cases missing HCV genotype data.
‡13 cases missing baseline inflammation grade.

Table 2. Risk Factors Characterizing Treated and Untreated Patient Groups (SFVA Cohort).

Variable	Total (N = 358)	SVR (N = 69)	NR (N = 49)	Relapse (N = 22)	ETD/ Unknown (N = 19)	No Treatment (N = 199)	p-value
History of Heavy Drinking	224 (62.6%)	35 (50.7%)	33 (67.3%)	13 (59.1%)	12 (63.2%)	131 (65.8%)	0.23
Active IDU	19 (5.3%)	1 (1.5%)	1 (2.0%)	0 (0.0%)	1 (5.3%)	16 (8.1%)	0.16*
Active Substance Use (non-IDU)	60 (17.2%)	6 (9.2%)	5 (10.9%)	4 (18.2%)	1 (5.3%)	44 (22.4%)	0.05*
Current Methadone	44 (12.4%)	5 (7.4%)	9 (18.4%)	1 (4.5%)	3 (15.8%)	26 (13.2%)	0.31*
History of Depression	133 (38.0%)	27 (39.7%)	24 (50.0%)	9 (42.9%)	8 (42.1%)	65 (33.5%)	0.45
PTSD	59 (16.9%)	14 (20.6%)	12 (24.5%)	4 (19.0%)	2 (10.5%)	27 (14.0%)	0.43
Social Stability	307 (86.5%)	67 (97.1%)	47 (97.9%)	20 (90.9%)	19 (100.0%)	154 (78.2%)	<0.0001

*P-values were calculated from Fisher's Exact test.

model as it was not a significant predictor of the hazard of cirrhosis.

Results of multivariate proportional hazards analysis stratified by pretreatment fibrosis stage in the SFVA cohort are presented in Table 3. The increased hazard of progression to cirrhosis among treatment nonresponders relative to never treated patients remained significant in this model, after adjustment for demographic and clinical characteristics and the factors that differentiated treated from never treated groups (HR = 2.35, CI 1.18–4.69). Latino ethnicity now became significantly associated with cirrhosis (HR = 2.50, CI 1.12–5.56), while African American race was protective (HR = 0.30, CI 0.13–0.72). Age continued to have an incremental effect as did BMI. Patients with HCV genotypes 1 or 4 were at increased risk of cirrhosis, even after correcting for the interaction between genotype and treatment initiation. Restratifying to compare more advanced baseline fibrosis stage 3 against stages 0–2 and repeating these analyses, we found that treatment nonresponders continued to exhibit an increased hazard of cirrhosis compared to never treated patients (HR = 2.95, CI 1.34–6.52, in the multivariate model, data not shown).

Since fibrosis progression is thought to proceed more slowly in African Americans compared to Caucasian patients with chronic HCV, we attempted to reanalyze these data separately for African American and non-African American patient groups [35,36,37]. There were too few cirrhosis events to develop a proportional hazards model for cirrhosis development using the multivariate modeling strategy described above, however when using a prefitted model, we found that treatment non-response (HR = 2.05, CI 0.99–4.26), age (HR = 1.07, CI 1.02–1.12) and BMI (HR = 1.08, CI 1.02–1.15) were each significant predictors of an increased hazard of cirrhosis among African Americans (data not shown).

Finally, as an alternative strategy to account for the inherent differences between treated and never treated groups, we

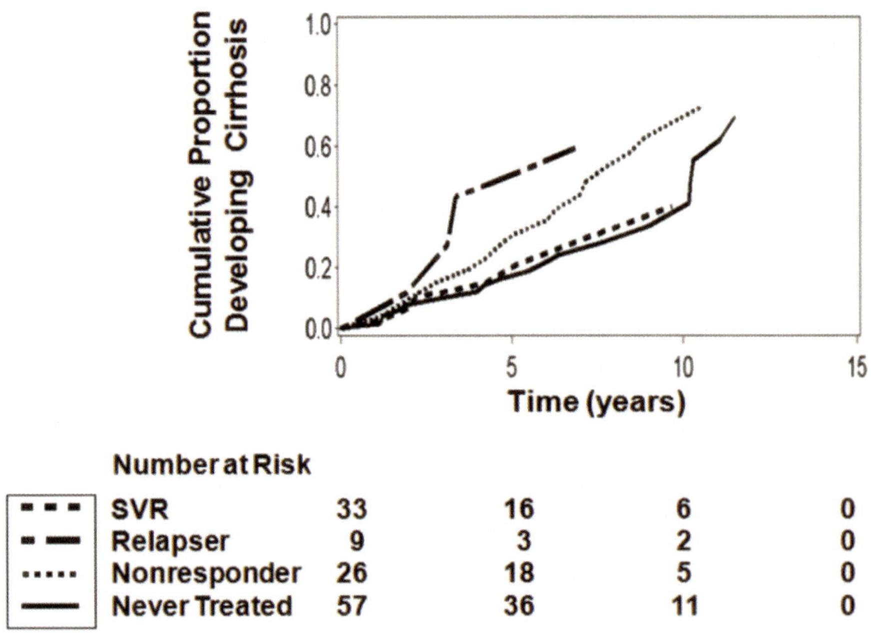

Figure 1. Cumulative incidence of cirrhosis among SFVA patients with baseline fibrosis stages 2 and 3. Age adjusted proportional hazards curves indicate that treatment relapsers and nonresponders had a higher incidence of cirrhosis over the study period compared to never treated patients, but these differences were not statistically significant unadjusted for other risk factors.

Table 3. Predictors of Development of Cirrhosis Stratified by Fibrosis Stage (SFVA Cohort, N = 332)*.

Characteristics‡	Univariate Model	Multivariate Model
	HR† (95% CI)	HR† (95% CI)
Treatment outcome		
SVR	0.67 (0.23–1.56)	0.68 (0.26–1.80)
Nonresponder	2.02 (1.11–3.67)	2.35 (1.18–4.69)
Relapser	1.24 (0.43–3.55)	1.00 (0.28–3.56)
ETD or Lost to Follow-up	1.07 (0.25–4.52)	1.28 (0.29–5.69)
Never Treated	ref	
Age at first liver clinic visit-per year increase§	1.05 (1.01–1.09)	1.09 (1.04–1.14)
Race§		
African American	0.61 (0.27–1.36)	0.30 (0.13–0.72)
Latino	1.82 (0.88–3.77)	2.50 (1.12–5.56)
Asian/API/Native American	0.41 (0.06–3.09)	0.42 (0.06–3.17)
Caucasian	ref	Ref
HCV genotype 1 or 4§	1.40 (0.77–2.56)	2.33 (1.10–4.93)
BMI-per unit increase§	1.03 (0.98–1.08)	1.07 (1.02–1.13)
Active Substance Use (non-IDU)§	1.10 (0.56–2.18)	NA
Social Stability§	0.72 (0.35–1.46)	0.48 (0.21–1.09)
Transfusion before 1992	2.04 (1.16–3.59)	NA

*Cox Proportional Hazards Models using time dependent covariate correcting for differences in waiting times from baseline to treatment initiation.
†Hazard Ratio (HR) calculated using Cox Proportional Hazards Modeling.
‡Interaction terms not shown.
§Risk factors that significantly differentiate the treated from never treated groups.

substituted a propensity score for statistically significant psychosocial risk factors in our multivariate proportional hazards models as described in Statistical Methods S1. These results differed little from the findings above, and again treatment nonresponders had a significantly increased hazard of cirrhosis compared to never treated patients (HR 2.68, CI 1.27–5.63, data not shown).

Replication Cohort

In order to confirm these unexpected findings, we used identical data collection and analytic methods to replicate the study in an independent cohort of patients with chronic HCV from the UCSF Liver Clinic (N = 265, Replication Cohort S1, Table S1). These patients were subject to the same eligibility criteria as the SFVA patients. All UCSF patients had a baseline liver biopsy and follow-up liver imaging or biopsy. UCSF cohort patients were significantly younger than the SFVA group (baseline age 48 versus 51 years for the SFVA) and included 46% female patients, whereas the SFVA group was 99% male (Table 4). There was a significantly higher proportion of Caucasian and Asian patients and a lower proportion of African American and Latino patients in the UCSF cohort ($p<0.0001$). The mean follow-up time was 7.7 years as compared to 10 years for the SFVA ($p<0.0001$) (Table 4). Descriptive characteristics of the UCSF cohort are provided in Tables S1 and S2.

Cumulative incidence of cirrhosis among UCSF patients with baseline fibrosis stages 2 and 3 was examined using age adjusted proportional hazards curves (Figure S1), which indicate that there were no differences in the incidence of cirrhosis among treatment groups, when unadjusted for other risk factors. In univariate proportional hazards models stratified by baseline liver fibrosis stage (0–1 and 2–3), UCSF treatment nonresponders showed an increased hazard for developing cirrhosis when compared to the never treated group, but this result fell just short of statistical significance (HR = 2.28, CI 0.93–5.59, Table S3). SVR was not significantly protective against cirrhosis. In multivariate proportional hazards models stratified by fibrosis stages (0–1 and 2–3) and adjusted for other risk factors, treatment nonresponse independently increased the long-term hazard of cirrhosis (HR = 5.90, CI 1.50–23.24, Table S3). Consistent with the SFVA cohort, incremental increases in age and BMI also contributed to the hazard of cirrhosis. In this model, social stability was significantly protective against cirrhosis (HR = 0.23, CI 0.07–0.79, Table S3). Restratifying to compare patients with advanced baseline fibrosis stage 3 to those with stages 0–2 still resulted in a significantly increased hazard of progression to cirrhosis among treatment non-responders in the final multivariate model (HR = 4.30, CI 1.16–15.93, data not shown).

Survival

Figure 2 depicts the survival experience for SFVA patients in age adjusted proportional hazards curves for two groups defined by baseline liver fibrosis stage. No differences in survival were observed among treatment groups for patients with baseline fibrosis stage 0–1 (Figure 2, panel A), whereas SVR led to a significant survival benefit compared to never treated patients among those with baseline fibrosis stage 2–4 ($p = 0.006$) (Figure 2, panel B).

Cox proportional hazards models were developed to examine the contribution of multiple risk factors on time-to-death (Table 5). Time-to-death models were stratified by baseline fibrosis stage 0–1, 2–3, and 4, and incorporated the time dependent covariate described above. In univariate analysis of the SFVA cohort, both SVR and nonresponder patients had a lower hazard of dying compared with never treated patients (HR = 0.24, CI 0.10–0.58

Table 4. Selected Characteristics of SFVA and UCSF HCV Cohorts.

Variable	SFVA	UCSF	p-value
	(N = 358)	(N = 265)	
Age at 1st Liver Clinic Visit (Yr), Mean (SD)	50.98 (6.68)	48.42 (8.39)	<0.0001*
Gender			
Female	4 (1.1%)	123 (46.4%)	<0.0001
Male	354 (98.9%)	142 (53.6%)	
Ethnicity			
Caucasian	236 (66.1%)	186 (72.4%)	<0.0001
African-American	72 (20.2%)	21 (8.2%)	
Latino	31 (8.7%)	11 (4.3%)	
Asian/API/Native American	18 (5.0%)	39 (15.2%)	
Cirrhosis during Follow-up	60 (18.1%)	28 (11.7%)	0.04
Death	78 (21.8%)	27 (10.2%)	0.0001
Liver Transplant	1 (0.3%)	12 (4.5%)	0.0002
Years of Follow-up, Mean (SD)	10.00 (3.05)	7.55 (4.09)	<0.0001*
Treatment Groups			
Never treated	199 (55.6%)	134 (50.6%)	0.21
Treated	159 (44.4%)	131 (49.4%)	
Treated Patients Only†			
Length of all IFNα treatment (wk), Mean (SD)	40.45 (22.32)	44.82 (36.13)	0.77*
Treatment Outcome			
Nonresponder	49 (30.8%)	42 (32.1%)	0.17
Relapser	22 (13.8%)	21 (16.0%)	
ETD or Lost to Follow-up	19 (11.9%)	25 (19.1%)	
SVR	69 (43.4%)	43 (32.8%)	

P-values were calculated from Chi-square test for category variables and ANOVA for continuous variables unless otherwise marked.
*Variable was rank transformed.
†Including 159 treated patients at VA and 131 treated patients at Moffitt.

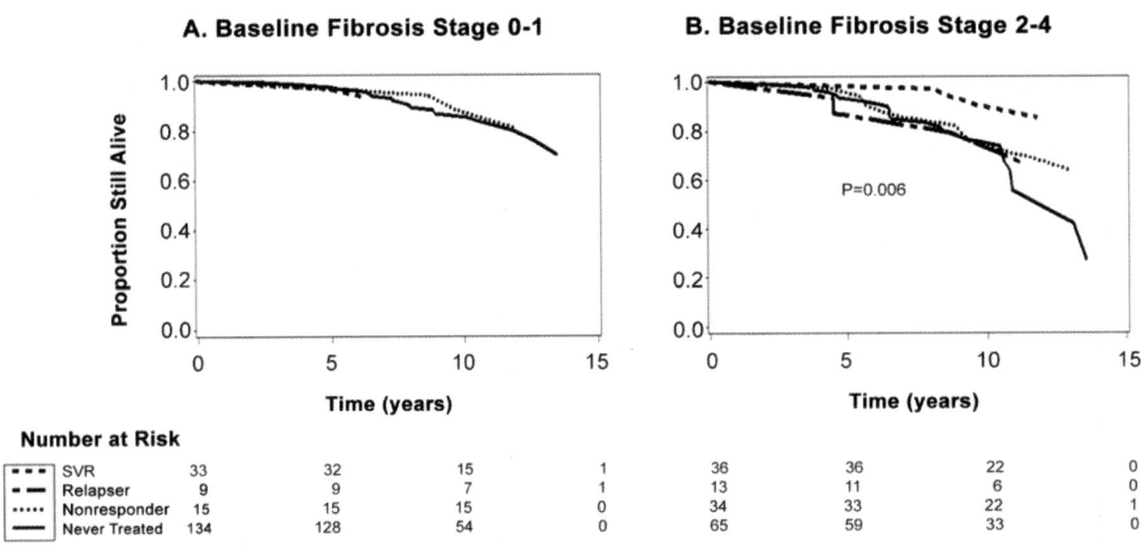

Figure 2. Proportion remaining alive among SFVA patients with baseline liver fibrosis stage 0–1 (panel A) and stage 2–4 (panel B). Age adjusted proportional hazards curves indicate that there were no significant differences in survival among the four treatment groups in patients with fibrosis stage 0–1 (panel A). Among patients with fibrosis stage 2–4, SVR significantly improved survival compared to never treated patients (p = 0.006), unadjusted for other risk factors (panel B).

and HR = 0.51, CI 0.26–0.98, respectively, Table 5). The hazard ratio for treatment relapsers also tended toward protection, but did not achieve significance. Older age at baseline liver biopsy, Latino ethnicity, heavy alcohol use, and prior blood transfusion each significantly increased the hazard of death during follow-up in univariate models (Table 5). After adjusting for psychosocial and clinical risk factors in multivariate proportional hazards analysis, SVR patients and relapsers each had a significant survival advantage (HR = 0.23, CI 0.07–0.75 and HR = 0.11, CI 0.01–0.95, respectively) compared to never treated patients. While the hazard ratio for nonresponders tended toward protection, it did not achieve statistical significance. Substituting propensity scores for individual psychosocial risk factors did not affect the directionality or significance of the hazard ratios for the major predictors in time-to-death analysis (data not shown).

Time-to-death or liver transplantation analyses were repeated for the UCSF cohort. Proportionally fewer UCSF patients died and more underwent liver transplantation than SFVA patients (Table 4). We examined the proportion remaining alive among UCSF patients with baseline liver fibrosis stage 0–1 and stage 2–4 in age adjusted proportional hazards curves (Figure S2, panels A and B, respectively). There were no deaths among treated patients with baseline fibrosis stage 0–1 (panel A). Among patients with baseline fibrosis stage 2–4, a greater proportion of relapsers and never treated patients died during follow-up compared with either SVR or nonresponder patients, but these differences were not statistically significant (panel B). In univariate proportional hazards models, stratified by baseline fibrosis stage, patients achieving SVR had a marginally significant reduction in death compared to never treated patients (HR = 0.24, CI 0.05–1.06, Table S4). This advantage did not extend to either nonresponders or relapsers. Incremental increases in baseline age were also contributory (HR = 1.07, CI 1.02–1.12, Table S4). In multivariate survival analysis, however, no risk factors achieved statistical significance.

Discussion

The present study measured long-term outcomes in patients with chronic HCV in two independent cohorts followed over the course of 7.7 to 10 years. Cohort patients were heterogeneous with regard to demographic and psychosocial characteristics, representing typical clinical practice, and data collection methods were optimized to maximize validity and measure known confounders. Unlike previously published studies, SVR was not associated with significant protection against cirrhosis in either cohort, even after stratifying for baseline levels of liver fibrosis and adjusting for liver inflammation [16,17,38,39,40]. Surprisingly, we found that the hazard of cirrhosis among treatment nonresponders was more than twice that of never treated patients in both cohorts. These results persisted after adjustment for clinical and psychosocial risk factors using two alternative adjustment strategies. Also, unlike previous studies, neither baseline ALT level nor change in ALT before and after completion of treatment was associated with progression to cirrhosis.

Although our study is not intended to identify an explanatory mechanism for this finding, it raises the question of whether hepatic inflammation and fibrosis could be increased by immunostimulatory IFNα-based antiviral therapies in cases where HCV is not eradicated. IFNα/RBV can trigger broad and robust antiviral T cell responses, which are beneficial when they result in SVR, but might contribute to worsened inflammation and scarring (cirrhosis) in the continued presence of viral antigens [41,42,43,44]. Lower rates of both cirrhosis and SVR among African Americans illustrate the point that lower inflammatory responses may be favorable in certain circumstances [35,37]. Further research is needed to explore this possibility.

The long-term effects of IFNα-based anti-HCV treatment on liver disease progression in noncirrhotic patients have been difficult to quantify from previous studies. In a meta-analysis of HCV cohort studies with greater than one year of follow-up,

Table 5. Predictors of Death or Liver Transplant Stratified by Fibrosis Stage (SFVA Cohort, N = 358)*.

Characteristics‡	Univariate Model	Multivariate Model
	HR† (95% CI)	HR† (95% CI)
Treatment Outcome		
SVR	0.24 (0.10–0.58)	0.23 (0.07–0.75)
Nonresponder	0.51 (0.26–0.98)	0.56 (0.24–1.32)
Relapser	0.48 (0.17–1.35)	0.11 (0.01–0.95)
ETD or Lost to Follow-up	1.32 (0.59–2.94)	1.44 (0.52–4.03)
Never Treated	ref	Ref
Age at 1st liver clinic visit-per year increase	1.08 (1.05–1.12)	1.1 (1.06–1.15)
Race		
African American	1.07 (0.59–1.97)	0.43 (0.20–0.93)
Latino	1.89 (1.00–3.57)	1.73 (0.74–4.02)
Asian/API/Native American	0.25 (0.03–1.82)	0.5 (0.07–3.77)
Caucasian	ref	Ref
BMI–per unit increase	1.02 (0.97–1.06)	1.07 (1.02–1.12)
History of Active Alcohol Abuse	1.67 (1.01–2.75)	1.82 (0.99–3.35)
Transfusion before 1992	1.66 (0.97–2.82)	3.36 (1.20–9.44)

*Cox Proportional Hazards Models.
†Hazard Ratio (HR) calculated using Cox Proportional Hazards Modeling.
‡Interaction terms not shown.

nearly 70% tracked subjects for less than seven years, whereas the mean duration of follow-up among patients in our SFVA cohort was 10 years [40]. Few previous studies have specifically compared the experience of treated patients to those who were never treated, and none specifically explored the hypothesis that failed IFNα-based treatment could increase the long-term risk of cirrhosis [38,45].

In recent years, there has been an emphasis on studies of IFNa-based retreatment in previous nonresponders and relapsers and their outcomes compared to those achieving SVR [46,47]. The most notable of these were the HALT-C and EPIC[3] trials which enrolled previously treated patients with advanced fibrosis. These two prospective studies examined histologic effects of low dose maintenance pegylated IFNα in prior HCV treatment failures with METAVIR F2 and F3 fibrosis at study initiation [48]. Patients were randomized to low dose maintenance pegylated IFNα therapy or observation and assessed for fibrosis response using repeat liver biopsies after a mean interval of 3.7 years. Results from the EPIC[3] study showed no statistically significant differences between METAVIR fibrosis scores of the treated and observation groups at the end of the study period [48]. HALT-C investigators extended the study for up to an 8 year period of observation and found that the annual rate of initial liver-related complications was higher among the pegylated IFNα group than among the controls [49]. Moreover, histologic features on sequential liver biopsies led the HALT-C investigators to speculate that pegylated IFNα might be associated with a long-term worsening of liver related morbidity in treatment nonresponders and in excess mortality among those with advanced liver disease [50].

In one of the few large-scale studies to compare outcomes between IFNα treated and untreated patients, the Japanese IHIT Study Group followed patients who had been previously treated with IFNα monotherapy over a median period of 3.7 years, using paired biopsies to compare liver fibrosis progression among SVR patients, patients without SVR and untreated patients, stratified by fibrosis stage at initial biopsy [51,52]. Among patients with initial METAVIR F2 or F3 fibrosis, a *post hoc* analysis of primary data presented in this report found no significant difference in cirrhosis development among patients without SVR and untreated patients [51]. None of the patients with initial F2 or F3 fibrosis who achieved SVR developed cirrhosis. These data suggest that failed therapy may not increase the risk of cirrhosis during intermediate (3–5 year) follow-up.

Unlike the patients in the Japanese cohort, the majority of our patients were treated with IFNα/RBV combination therapy, rather than with IFNα monotherapy, and our follow-up period was more than twice as long. Our study included few Asian patients, who have a higher probability of achieving SVR, but also are more likely to progress to cirrhosis [28]. Our finding that treatment failures have an increased long-term hazard of cirrhosis is thus neither directly supported nor contradicted by this or any other published report.

Previously published studies also found that never treated HCV patients had a greater mortality risk than patients who achieve SVR, and in some cases, those who fail treatment [38,52]. In another IHIT study, Yoshida et al. found that the overall risk of death was reduced among IFNα treated patients, including treatment nonresponders, as compared to patients not receiving treatment [52]. Their multivariate Cox proportional hazards models were adjusted by gender, age and IFNα therapy outcome. When survival analysis was further stratified by cirrhotic and noncirrhotic patients, IFNα therapy was associated with improved survival among the noncirrhotic patients only [52]. A recent Cochrane Review of seven trials, including the HALT-C and EPIC[3] studies, found a significant increase in all-cause mortality in IFNα maintenance patients and concluded that patients with severe fibrosis who failed previous IFNα treatment did not derive a survival benefit from further therapy with pegylated IFNα [46].

These studies did not assess the effects of clinical and behavioral risk factors on liver disease outcomes as comprehensively as ours did. Our multivariate time-to-death analyses reveal that, even though nonresponders had more than twice the hazard of cirrhosis, their survival was not significantly different from that of never treated patients. The effects of cirrhosis on survival in our cohort may be offset by the relatively younger age and more beneficial clinical and psychosocial risk factor profile of nonresponders compared with never treated patients. Our findings suggest that some previously reported benefits of therapy among treatment failures might be attributable to the lower concomitant risks associated with treatment candidacy, rather than to disease modifying benefits of pharmacologic therapy [38,52].

As is the case in most nonrandomized studies, the presence of bias by indication can be difficult to resolve [53,54]. We were especially concerned about confounding from risk factors that independently could promote the development of cirrhosis among patients with HCV and also influence the decision whether or not to initiate antiviral therapy. We carefully assessed an array of clinical and psychosocial risk factors and, not unexpectedly, found that never treated patients were older, more likely to engage in ongoing alcohol or other substance abuse, and to experience social instability compared with treatment nonresponders. We speculated that differing biobehavioral risk profiles were unlikely to account for the reduced incidence of cirrhosis in untreated patients since many of these would be predicted to increase, rather than reduce fibrosis progression. We used two alternative strategies to statistically adjust for these potential confounders in our Cox proportional hazards models [27]. Using either adjustment method, treatment nonresponders were found to have a significantly greater hazard of developing cirrhosis than the never treated group–a finding that was observed in the both the SFVA and UCSF cohorts. Some differences between treated and never treated patients were identified that could not be completely corrected in our statistical models. Treated patients were followed for approximately 1.5 years longer than never treated patients and had, on average, one additional diagnostic procedure. Both the duration of follow-up and the number of diagnostic procedures were entered into predictive models, but were not found to be confounders for either outcome (time-to-cirrhosis or time-to-death). It is still possible that unmeasured confounding factors linked to treatment failure may have biased the results, but rigorous data collection, robust statistical methods, and the stability of a significant hazard ratio for cirrhosis among nonresponders in both cohorts make a compelling case for the validity of these findings. Furthermore the congruence of the findings from two diverse patient populations–the SFVA cohort comprised of comparably aged veterans with similar risk behavior histories and the more demographically diverse UCSF cohort–suggest that these results may be generalizable.

Our results suggest the possibility that treatment with IFNα-based regimens without viral clearance may be associated with progressive liver disease. Although these data reflect the long-term outcomes for two entire patient cohorts at independent institutions, they should be interpreted with caution as they are derived from retrospective chart reviews. If confirmed, these results make a compelling case for the enhanced use of sensitive diagnostic and predictive tools, including recently described genetic tests, to identify patients most likely to benefit from IFNα-based treatment

[36,55]. Moreover, the potential for adverse outcomes should be considered in current and future studies examining HCV treatment using pegylated-IFNα/RBV in combination with newer agents such as HCV protease inhibitors, as a substantial proportion of null or partial responders with advanced fibrosis will emerge from these treatment groups. In particular, it may be advisable not to retreat these patients with IFNα, but to keep them under observation until IFNα-free regimens are available.

Supporting Information

Figure S1 Cumulative incidence of cirrhosis among UCSF patients with baseline fibrosis stages 2 and 3. Age adjusted proportional hazards curves indicate that there were no differences in the incidence of cirrhosis among treatment groups, unadjusted for other risk factors.

Figure S2 Proportion remaining alive among UCSF patients with baseline liver fibrosis stage 0–1 (panel A) and stage 2–4 (panel B). Age adjusted proportional hazards curves indicate that there were no deaths among treated patients with baseline fibrosis stage 0–1 (panel A). Amongst patients with baseline fibrosis stage 2–4, relapsers and never treated a greater proportion died during follow-up than among SVR and nonresponders patients, but these differences were not statistically significant.

Table S1 Demographic and Clinical Characteristics of the UCSF Cohort.

Table S2 Risk Factors of Treated and Untreated Patient Groups (UCSF Cohort).

Table S3 Predictors of Development of Cirrhosis Stratified by Fibrosis Stage (UCSF Cohort).

Table S4 Predictors of Death or Liver Transplant Stratified by Fibrosis Stage (UCSF Cohort).

Statistical Methods S1 Details of Construction and Reduction of Statistical Models.

Replication Cohort S1 UCSF Medical Center Liver Clinic.

Acknowledgments

Sally George, RN, and Amit Arunkumar, BS, for assistance with data collection. Teresa Wright, MD, for her expert care and treatment of patients in this study. Peter Bacchetti, PhD, for consultation on biostatistical methods, and Kenneth R. McQuaid, MD, for his encouragement and intellectual guidance.

Author Contributions

Conceived and designed the experiments: MLC JCR AM. Performed the experiments: MLC JCR HS ES RMY RL RW AM. Analyzed the data: HS MLC JCR RL AM. Contributed reagents/materials/analysis tools: HS MLC. Wrote the paper: MLC JCR AM.

References

1. Armstrong GL, Wasley A, Simard EP, McQuillan GM, Kuhnert WL, et al. (2006) The prevalence of hepatitis C virus infection in the United States, 1999 through 2002. Ann Intern Med 144: 705–714.
2. Bialek SR, Terrault NA (2006) The changing epidemiology and natural history of hepatitis C virus infection. Clin Liver Dis 10: 697–715.
3. Hoofnagle JH, Seeff LB (2006) Peginterferon and ribavirin for chronic hepatitis C. N Engl J Med 355: 2444–2451.
4. McHutchison JG, Gordon SC, Schiff ER, Shiffman ML, Lee WM, et al. (1998) Interferon alfa-2b alone or in combination with ribavirin as initial treatment for chronic hepatitis C. Hepatitis Interventional Therapy Group. N Engl J Med 339: 1485–1492.
5. McHutchison JG, Manns M, Patel K, Poynard T, Lindsay KL, et al. (2002) Adherence to combination therapy enhances sustained response in genotype-1-infected patients with chronic hepatitis C. Gastroenterology 123: 1061–1069.
6. Yee HS, Chang MF, Pocha C, Lim J, Ross D, et al. (2012) Update on the management and treatment of hepatitis C virus infection: recommendations from the Department of Veterans Affairs Hepatitis C Resource Center Program and the National Hepatitis C Program Office. Am J Gastroenterol 107: 669–689; quiz 690.
7. Jacobson IM, McHutchison JG, Dusheiko G, Di Bisceglie AM, Reddy KR, et al. (2011) Telaprevir for previously untreated chronic hepatitis C virus infection. N Engl J Med 364: 2405–2416.
8. Pawlotsky JM (2011) The results of Phase III clinical trials with telaprevir and boceprevir presented at the Liver Meeting 2010: a new standard of care for hepatitis C virus genotype 1 infection, but with issues still pending. Gastroenterology 140: 746–754.
9. Poordad F, McCone J, Bacon BR, Bruno S, Manns MP, et al. (2011) Boceprevir for untreated chronic HCV genotype 1 infection. N Engl J Med 364: 1195–1206.
10. Heathcote EJ, Shiffman ML, Cooksley WG, Dusheiko GM, Lee SS, et al. (2000) Peginterferon alfa-2a in patients with chronic hepatitis C and cirrhosis. N Engl J Med 343: 1673–1680.
11. Poynard T, McHutchison J, Manns M, Trepo C, Lindsay K, et al. (2002) Impact of pegylated interferon alfa-2b and ribavirin on liver fibrosis in patients with chronic hepatitis C. Gastroenterology 122: 1303–1313.
12. Shiffman ML, Hofmann CM, Thompson EB, Ferreira-Gonzalez A, Contos MJ, et al. (1997) Relationship between biochemical, virological, and histological response during interferon treatment of chronic hepatitis C. Hepatology 26: 780–785.
13. Mallat A, Preaux AM, Blazejewski S, Rosenbaum J, Dhumeaux D, et al. (1995) Interferon alfa and gamma inhibit proliferation and collagen synthesis of human Ito cells in culture. Hepatology 21: 1003–1010.
14. Goodman ZD, Stoddard AM, Bonkovsky HL, Fontana RJ, Ghany MG, et al. (2009) Fibrosis progression in chronic hepatitis C: morphometric image analysis in the HALT-C trial. Hepatology 50: 1738–1749.
15. Pockros PJ, Hamzeh FM, Martin P, Lentz E, Zhou X, et al. (2010) Histologic outcomes in hepatitis C-infected patients with varying degrees of virologic response to interferon-based treatments. Hepatology 52: 1193–1200.
16. Shiffman ML, Hofmann CM, Contos MJ, Luketic VA, Sanyal AJ, et al. (1999) A randomized, controlled trial of maintenance interferon therapy for patients with chronic hepatitis C virus and persistent viremia. Gastroenterology 117: 1164–1172.
17. Poynard T, McHutchison J, Davis GL, Esteban-Mur R, Goodman Z, et al. (2000) Impact of interferon alfa-2b and ribavirin on progression of liver fibrosis in patients with chronic hepatitis C. Hepatology 32: 1131–1137.
18. Shiratori Y, Ito Y, Yokosuka O, Imazeki F, Nakata R, et al. (2005) Antiviral therapy for cirrhotic hepatitis C: association with reduced hepatocellular carcinoma development and improved survival. Ann Intern Med 142: 105–114.
19. Poynard T, Bruix J, Schiff ER, Diago M, Berg T, et al. (2012) Improved inflammatory activity with peginterferon alfa-2b maintenance therapy in non-cirrhotic prior non-responders: A randomized study. J Hepatol.
20. Dienstag JL, Ghany MG, Morgan TR, Di Bisceglie AM, Bonkovsky HL, et al. (2011) A prospective study of the rate of progression in compensated, histologically advanced chronic hepatitis C. Hepatology 54: 396–405.
21. Bruce-Chwatt LJ (1965) Declaration of Helsinki. Recommendations Guiding Doctors in Clinical Research. WHO Chron 19: 31–32.
22. Seeff LB (2002) Natural history of chronic hepatitis C. Hepatology 36: S35–46.
23. Harris DR, Gonin R, Alter HJ, Wright EC, Buskell ZJ, et al. (2001) The relationship of acute transfusion-associated hepatitis to the development of cirrhosis in the presence of alcohol abuse. Ann Intern Med 134: 120–124.
24. Batts KP, Ludwig J (1995) Chronic hepatitis. An update on terminology and reporting. Am J Surg Pathol 19: 1409–1417.
25. Brunt EM (2000) Grading and staging the histopathological lesions of chronic hepatitis: the Knodell histology activity index and beyond. Hepatology 31: 241–246.
26. Sofair AN, Barry V, Manos MM, Thomas A, Zaman A, et al. (2009) The epidemiology and clinical characteristics of patients with newly diagnosed alcohol-related liver disease: results from population-based surveillance. J Clin Gastroenterol 44: 301–307.

27. Bini EJ, Brau N, Currie S, Shen H, Anand BS, et al. (2005) Prospective multicenter study of eligibility for antiviral therapy among 4,084 U.S. veterans with chronic hepatitis C virus infection. Am J Gastroenterol 100: 1772–1779.
28. Ghany MG, Strader DB, Thomas DL, Seeff LB (2009) Diagnosis, management, and treatment of hepatitis C: an update. Hepatology 49: 1335–1374.
29. Allison PD (1995) Survival Analysis Using the SAS® System: A Practical Guide Cary, NC: SAS Institute Inc. 292 p.
30. Etzioni R, Pepe M, Longton G, Hu C, Goodman G (1999) Incorporating the time dimension in receiver operating characteristic curves: a case study of prostate cancer. Med Decis Making 19: 242–251.
31. Luo Z, Gardiner JC, Bradley CJ (2010) Applying propensity score methods in medical research: pitfalls and prospects. Med Care Res Rev 67: 528–554.
32. Shah BR, Laupacis A, Hux JE, Austin PC (2005) Propensity score methods gave similar results to traditional regression modeling in observational studies: a systematic review. J Clin Epidemiol 58: 550–559.
33. Dominitz JA, Boyko EJ, Koepsell TD, Heagerty PJ, Maynard C, et al. (2005) Elevated prevalence of hepatitis C infection in users of United States veterans medical centers. Hepatology 41: 88–96.
34. Kayali Z, Tan S, Shinkunas L, Voigt M, LaBrecque DR, et al. (2007) Risk factors for hepatitis C fibrosis: a prospective study of United States veterans compared with nonveterans. J Viral Hepat 14: 11–21.
35. Conjeevaram HS, Fried MW, Jeffers LJ, Terrault NA, Wiley-Lucas TE, et al. (2006) Peginterferon and ribavirin treatment in African American and Caucasian American patients with hepatitis C genotype 1. Gastroenterology 131: 470–477.
36. Ge D, Fellay J, Thompson AJ, Simon JS, Shianna KV, et al. (2009) Genetic variation in IL28B predicts hepatitis C treatment-induced viral clearance. Nature 461: 399–401.
37. Terrault NA, Im K, Boylan R, Bacchetti P, Kleiner DE, et al. (2008) Fibrosis progression in African Americans and Caucasian Americans with chronic hepatitis C. Clin Gastroenterol Hepatol 6: 1403–1411.
38. Butt AA, Wang X, Moore CG (2009) Effect of hepatitis C virus and its treatment on survival. Hepatology 50: 387–392.
39. Coverdale SA, Khan MH, Byth K, Lin R, Weltman M, et al. (2004) Effects of interferon treatment response on liver complications of chronic hepatitis C: 9-year follow-up study. Am J Gastroenterol 99: 636–644.
40. Singal AG, Volk ML, Jensen D, Di Bisceglie AM, Schoenfeld PS (2010) A sustained viral response is associated with reduced liver-related morbidity and mortality in patients with hepatitis C virus. Clin Gastroenterol Hepatol 8: 280–288, 288 e281.
41. Thomas H, Foster G, Platis D (2003) Mechanisms of action of interferon and nucleoside analogues. J Hepatol 39 Suppl 1: S93–98.
42. Brinkmann V, Geiger T, Alkan S, Heusser CH (1993) Interferon alpha increases the frequency of interferon gamma-producing human CD4+ T cells. J Exp Med 178: 1655–1663.
43. Tam RC, Pai B, Bard J, Lim C, Averett DR, et al. (1999) Ribavirin polarizes human T cell responses towards a Type 1 cytokine profile. J Hepatol 30: 376–382.
44. Kamal SM, Ismail A, Graham CS, He Q, Rasenack JW, et al. (2004) Pegylated interferon alpha therapy in acute hepatitis C: relation to hepatitis C virus-specific T cell response kinetics. Hepatology 39: 1721–1731.
45. Veldt BJ, Heathcote EJ, Wedemeyer H, Reichen J, Hofmann WP, et al. (2007) Sustained virologic response and clinical outcomes in patients with chronic hepatitis C and advanced fibrosis. Ann Intern Med 147: 677–684.
46. Koretz RL, Pleguezuelo M, Arvaniti V, Barrera Baena P, Ciria R, et al. (2013) Interferon for interferon nonresponding and relapsing patients with chronic hepatitis C. Cochrane Database Syst Rev Art. No.: CD003617. DOI: 10.1002/14651858.
47. Singal AG, Waljee AK, Shiffman M, Bacon BR, Schoenfeld PS (2010) Meta-analysis: re-treatment of genotype I hepatitis C nonresponders and relapsers after failing interferon and ribavirin combination therapy. Aliment Pharmacol Ther 32: 969–983.
48. Poynard T, Bruix J, Schiff ER, Diago M, Berg T, et al. (2013) Improved inflammatory activity with peginterferon alfa-2b maintenance therapy in non-cirrhotic prior non-responders: A randomized study. J Hepatol 58: 452–459.
49. Dienstag JL, Ghany MG, Morgan TR, Di Bisceglie AM, Bonkovsky HL, et al. (2011) A prospective study of the rate of progression in compensated, histologically advanced chronic hepatitis C. Hepatology 54: 396–405.
50. Di Bisceglie AM, Stoddard AM, Dienstag JL, Shiffman ML, Seeff LB, et al. (2011) Excess mortality in patients with advanced chronic hepatitis C treated with long-term peginterferon. Hepatology 53: 1100–1108.
51. Shiratori Y, Imazeki F, Moriyama M, Yano M, Arakawa Y, et al. (2000) Histologic improvement of fibrosis in patients with hepatitis C who have sustained response to interferon therapy. Ann Intern Med 132: 517–524.
52. Yoshida H, Arakawa Y, Sata M, Nishiguchi S, Yano M, et al. (2002) Interferon therapy prolonged life expectancy among chronic hepatitis C patients. Gastroenterology 123: 483–491.
53. Bosco JL, Silliman RA, Thwin SS, Geiger AM, Buist DS, et al. (2010) A most stubborn bias: no adjustment method fully resolves confounding by indication in observational studies. J Clin Epidemiol 63: 64–74.
54. Stukel TA, Fisher ES, Wennberg DE, Alter DA, Gottlieb DJ, et al. (2007) Analysis of observational studies in the presence of treatment selection bias: effects of invasive cardiac management on AMI survival using propensity score and instrumental variable methods. JAMA 297: 278–285.
55. Suppiah V, Gaudieri S, Armstrong NJ, O'Connor KS, Berg T, et al. (2011) IL28B, HLA-C, and KIR variants additively predict response to therapy in chronic hepatitis C virus infection in a European Cohort: a cross-sectional study. PLoS Med 8: e1001092.

4

Adrenal Gland Infection by Serotype 5 Adenovirus Requires Coagulation Factors

Lucile Tran[1], Laure-Hélène Ouisse[1], Peggy Richard-Fiardo[2,3], Philippe R. Franken[2,3], Jacques Darcourt[2,3], Gaétan Cornilleau[4], Karim Benihoud[4], Georges Vassaux[2,3]*

1 INSERM U948, Nantes, France, 2 Faculté de Médecine, Université de Nice-Sophia-Antipolis, Nice, France, 3 UMRE4320, CEA, Nice, France, 4 Université Paris-Sud, UMR 8203, Institut Gustave Roussy, Villejuif Cedex, France

Abstract

Recombinant, replication-deficient serotype 5 adenovirus infects the liver upon *in vivo*, systemic injection in rodents. This infection requires the binding of factor X to the capsid of this adenovirus. Another organ, the adrenal gland is also infected upon systemic administration of Ad, however, whether this infection is dependent on the cocksackie adenovirus receptor (CAR) or depends on the binding of factor X to the viral capsid remained to be determined. In the present work, we have used a pharmacological agent (warfarin) as well as recombinant adenoviruses lacking the binding site of Factor X to elucidate this mechanism in mice. We demonstrate that, as observed in the liver, adenovirus infection of the adrenal glands *in vivo* requires Factor X. Considering that the level of transduction of the adrenal glands is well-below that of the liver and that capsid-modified adenoviruses are unlikely to selectively infect the adrenal glands, we have used single-photon emission computed tomography (SPECT) imaging of gene expression to determine whether local virus administration (direct injection in the kidney) could increase gene transfer to the adrenal glands. We demonstrate that direct injection of the virus in the kidney increases gene transfer in the adrenal gland but liver transduction remains important. These observations strongly suggest that serotype 5 adenovirus uses a similar mechanism to infect liver and adrenal gland and that selective transgene expression in the latter is more likely to be achieved through transcriptional targeting.

Editor: Knut Stieger, Justus-Liebig-University Giessen, Germany

Funding: This work is supported by grants from INSERM, la Ligue Nationale Contre le Cancer, Canceropole "Grand Ouest", Vaincre la Mucoviscidose. KB wants to acknowledge for their support the Centre National de la Recherche Scientifique (CNRS), the INCa and the PRES Univer Sud. The funders had no role in study design, data collection and analysis, decision to publish, or preparation of the manuscript.

* E-mail: georges.vassaux@inserm.fr

These authors contributed equally to this work.

Introduction

Recombinant, serotype 5 adenoviruses are probably the most widely used delivery vectors in gene therapy. *In vitro* and *in vivo* upon local injection, they can infect a wide range of cell types such as epithelial cells [1,2,3], cardiomyocytes [4] and cancer cells [5,6,7,8]. *In vivo*, systemic injection of recombinant adenovirus is followed by a rapid disappearance of the virus from the blood stream [9] and leads to a predominant expression in hepatocytes [10,11,12,13,14]. Another organ efficiently infected by adenoviruses upon systemic injections is the adrenal glands [15,16,17,18,19]. Although the infectivity of the adrenal gland is below that of the liver [18], it is equivalent to that of the spleen [17]. In the adrenal gland, the site of synthesis of cortisol and corticosterone, the *zona fasciculata*, has been shown to be particularly prone to infection [18].

Classically, the sequence of *in vitro* infection of an adenovirus serotype 5 is thought to involve the binding of the viral fiber to the coxsackie adenovirus receptor (CAR), followed by internalization mediated by cellular αv-integrins [20,21]. If the sequence of events involved for *in vivo* infection was initially thought to be similar to the *in vitro* one, recent data have changed the overall consensus: Despite a strong expression of CAR in the liver [22], conflicting results using capsid-modified adenoviruses were reported [10,23,24] questioning the role of CAR in adenovirus infection of the liver *in vivo*. Since then, different studies have demonstrated a role of vitamin K-dependent blood factors in liver transduction [25,26,27,28,29]. More precisely, this phenomenon was attributed to factor X (FX) binding to capsid hexon protein, making a bridge between the virus and hepatocyte heparan sulfate glycosaminoglycans [25,26,27,28,29].

Although adrenal glands can be infected through systemic administration of the virus, the level of transgene expression achieved remains low. This modest level of transgene expression is illustrated by the fact that gene transfer in the adrenal glands cannot be visualized by sensitive, whole-body imaging techniques such as PET or even SPECT using the Na/I symporter (NIS) as a reporter gene, while transgene expression in the liver can easily be detected and quantified using either of these methodologies [30,31]. Two strategies could be envisaged to restrict and/or increase transgene expression in the adrenal gland: i) selective transduction of the adrenal glands, but, for this strategy to be efficient, the mechanism of infection of the two organs would have to be different and ii) a more localized type of injection (i.e. direct injection in the kidney) would increase the viral load in the vicinity of the adrenal gland and potentially increase transduction.

In this context, the aim of the present study is to gain a better understanding of the transduction of the adrenal glands by type 5 adenovirus and to assess a new administration routes to improve adrenal gland transduction by this vector.

Materials and Methods

Adenovirus

The replication-incompetent adenovirus, Ad-CMV-rNIS, in which the immediate-early promoter of CMV drives the expression of rat NIS, has been described previously [32]. Ad-CMV-nls-LacZ, is a recombinant, replication deficient adenovirus in which the expression of the β-galactosidase gene containing a nuclear localization signal is driven by the immediate-early CMV promoter. Both viruses were produced and titrated at the "Plateforme de production de vecteurs pré-cliniques du CHU de Nantes", using a standard protocol.

Animals Studies

Animal housing and procedures were conducted according to the guidelines of the French Agriculture Ministry and were approved by the institutional review board (CIEPAL: Comité Institutionnel d'Ethique Pour l'Animal de Laboratoire) (Permit number # A06-088-14). Gene-transfer studies were performed on female Balb/c mice obtained at 8 weeks of age from Janvier (Le Genest Saint Isle, France). Ad-CMV-rNIS (5×10^8 or 1×10^9 PFU/mouse) in sterile saline buffer (final volume, 200 μl) was administered intravenously. For the intra-renal injections, Ad-CMV-rNIS (5×10^8 PFU/mouse) were injected into the parenchyma of the left kidney of anaesthetised, 7-week-old Balb/c mice. For biodistribution studies, mice were also injected subcutaneously (s.c.) with 133 μg of warfarin/mouse 3 and 1 day prior to Ad vector injections as previously described [25].

MicroSPECT/CT Studies

Forty eight hours after adenovirus administration, mice were injected intraperitoneally with 100 MBq ^{99m}Tc pertechnetate ($^{99m}TcO_4^-$) obtained from a freshly eluted ^{99}Mo/^{99m}Tc generator. Precisely 20 min later, mice were imaged under Isofluran anaesthesia (Baxter, Aerane). Localization of the kidney was performed using ^{99m}Tc-Dimercaptosuccinic acid (^{99m}Tc-DMSA) as a probe. Briefly, DMSA (TechneScan DMAS) was labelled using a standard procedure [33]. This tracer (95 MBq) was administered by intraperitoneal injection. Five hours later, the animals were anaesthetized and scanned. In both cases (^{99m}Tc pertechnetate and ^{99m}Tc-DMSA) SPECT/CT scans were performed using a micro-SPECT-CT (eXplore speCZT CT120, General Electric), using a previously published protocol [31]. Image analyses and quantification were performed using the 'AMIDE' software [34].

Enzymatic and PCR Assays

β-galactosidase activity was measured as previously described [29]. Total RNA from the livers or adrenal glands of adenovirus-injected mice were extracted using Nucleospin RNAII (Macherey-Nagel, France) and transcribed into cDNA using the Superscript III enzyme (Invitrogen, France). CAR and 18S expression were determined using primers and experimental conditions described in [35] and [36], respectively. Real-time PCR was performed with the 7900HT Fast Real-Time PCR System and carried out using TaqMan® gene expression assays (Applied Biosystem, France). Primer sets (Rn 00583900-m1 for NIS and Mm-013518-11 for GAPDH) were designed by, and purchased from, Applied Biosystems. Cycle parameters were 95°C for 20 s followed by 40 cycles of 95°C for 1 s and 60°C for 20 s. Relative mRNA expression levels were determined using ΔCt values obtained by subtracting Ct control (mouse GAPDH) from Ct target gene (rat NIS), measured in the same RNA preparation.

Results

Adenovirus Infection of the Adrenal Gland is CAR-independent

We first assessed whether the CAR receptor is expressed in the adrenal glands. For that purpose, mRNA was extracted from dissected adrenal glands or a liver biopsy (as a positive control) and subjected to reverse-transcription and PCR amplification. As expected, CAR is indeed expressed in the liver (Figure 1A). By contrast, in the adrenal glands, CAR is undetectable (Figure 1A).

To exclude completely a CAR-dependent mechanism and provide new insight into the infection of the adrenal glands, we compared transgene expression upon injection of a wild-type, replication-deficient adenovirus (AdHwt, 10^9 PFU) and a replication-deficient adenovirus in which the hexon hypervariable region 5 had been modified (AdH[GA]24, 10^9 PFU). Both viruses encode the LacZ gene driven by the same promoter and both are equally able to infect CAR-positive cells [29]. β-galactosidase staining of the whole liver obtained forty-eight hours after systemic AdHwt injection showed an intense blue colour, characteristic of LacZ gene expression (Fig. 1B), while staining of a liver obtained from an AdH[GA]24-injected animal remained unstained (Fig. 1B). This set of results confirms previous data by Vigant et al [29] and highlights the requirement of functional hexon proteins for adenovirus infection, *in vivo*. In the adrenal glands, systemic administration of AdHwt resulted in a very significant increase in β-galactosidase expression compared to untreated controls, while systemic injection of AdH[GA]24 resulted in levels of β-galactosidase transcripts fifty times lower than those obtained with AdHwt (Fig. 1C; $P<0.001$). Altogether, these results demonstrate that, in contrast to the wild-type AdHwt, AdH[GA]24 is unable to transduce either the liver (Fig. 1B) or the adrenal glands (Fig. 1C). These data strongly suggest that, as in the liver, infection of the adrenal glands involves blood factors that bind to the viral capsid.

Involvement of Blood Factors in Adenovirus Infection of the Adrenal Glands

To determine whether blood factors are indeed involved in the infection of the adrenal glands by type 5 adenovirus, a pharmacological intervention (warfarin pre-treatment) was used. Warfarin inhibits the vitamin K-dependent γ carboxylation of the glutamic acid residues in the N-termini of Factor II, VII, IX and X as well as protein C and results in reduced functional, circulating levels of these coagulation factors. To compare the effect of warfarin on adenovirus-mediated gene transfer in the liver and the adrenal glands, warfarin was administered three and one days before virus administration. Twenty-four hours after the last injection of warfarin, the animals were administered intravenously with 6×10^8 PFU of Ad-CMV-nls-LacZ. As expected, systemic injection of this virus led to strong levels of β-galactosidase activity in the liver (Figure 2A). Pre-treatment of the experimental animals with warfarin reduced dramatically this activity (Figure 2A). In the adrenal glands, systemic administration of Ad-CMV-nls-LacZ resulted in a significant increase in β-galactosidase activity that

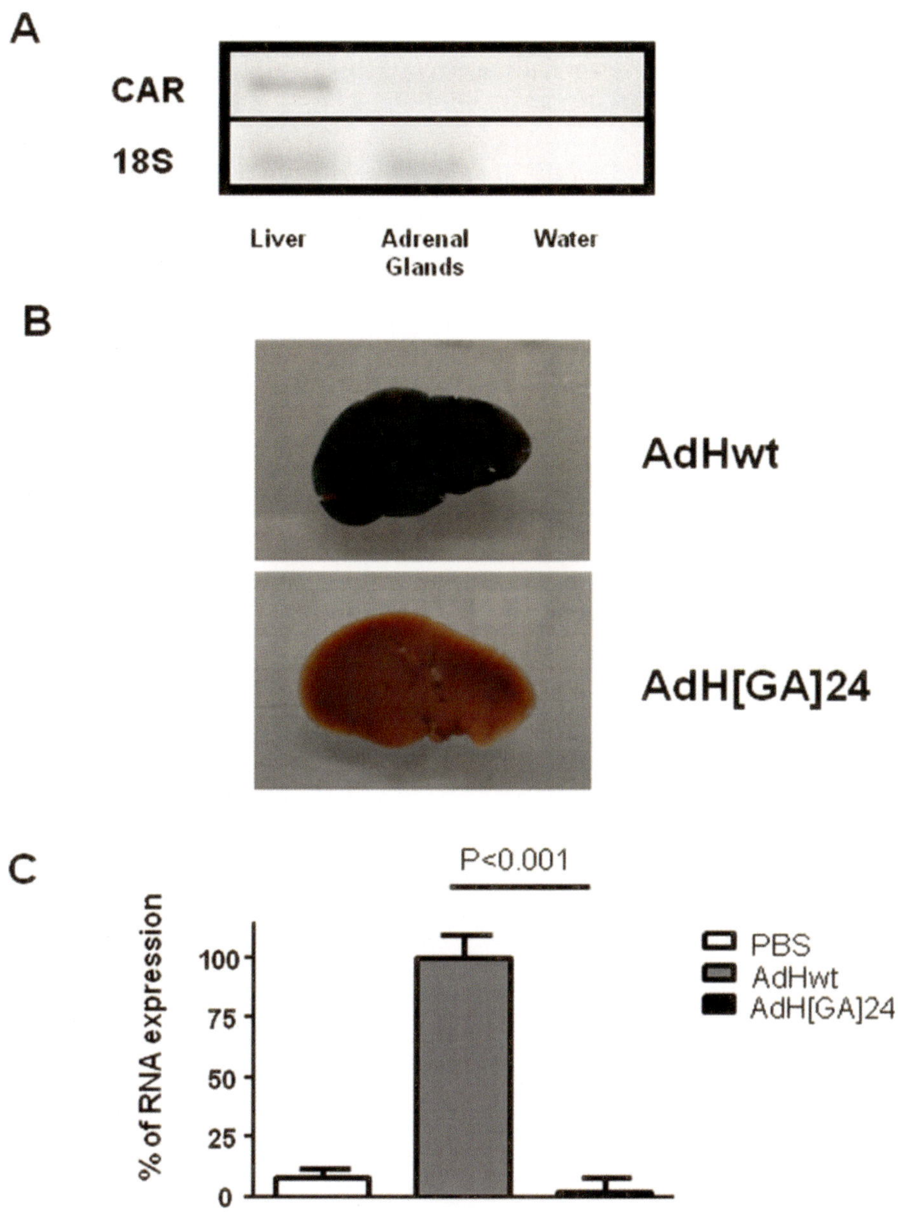

Figure 1. A: CAR expression in the liver and the adrenal glands. Total RNAs were extracted from liver biopsies or total adrenal glands and subjected to reverse transcription and PCR amplification. The PCR products were separated by electrophoresis. B and C: Mice were injected systemically with 10^9 PFU of either AdHwt (n = 7) or AdH[GA]24 (n = 7) or PBS (n = 4). Forty-eight hours later, the animals were culled and the livers and adrenal glands were collected. B: Whole liver were stained for β-galactosidase expression. C: Total RNA were extracted from the adrenal glands (two glands from the same animal were pooled), reversed-transcribed and subjected to quantitative PCR to detect LacZ expression or 18S RNA. The ratio LacZ/18S of adrenal glands collected from animals injected with AdHwt was used as 100%. The data presented are means+SEM. Statistical test: ANOVA (Prism, Graph-Pad softwares).

was significantly reduced ($p<0.05$) by warfarin pre-treatment (Figure 2A). RT-qPCR to measure β-galactosidase transcripts levels on mRNA extracted from the liver or the adrenal glands of warfarin-treated or non-treated animals confirmed these data (Figure 2B). In both cases, warfarin pre-treatment reduced β-galactosidase-specific mRNA expression by more than a factor 10 (Figure 2B). These results suggest that blood factors are required not only for efficient transduction of liver but also for adrenal glands transduction by adenovirus type 5.

Involvement of Factor X

To determine whether factor X can restore gene transfer abolished by warfarin, 6×10^8 PFU of Ad-CMV-nls-LacZ were injected systemically in warfarin-treated mice or warfarin-treated mice supplemented with 33 µg of recombinant factor X (Haematologic Technologies, Essex Junction, VT, USA) (intravenous injection) prior to adenovirus administration. Forty-eight hours later, experimental animals were culled and livers and adrenal glands were collected. Figure 3A shows that factor X administration restores the transduction of the liver, measured by β-galactosidase staining of the whole organ. The

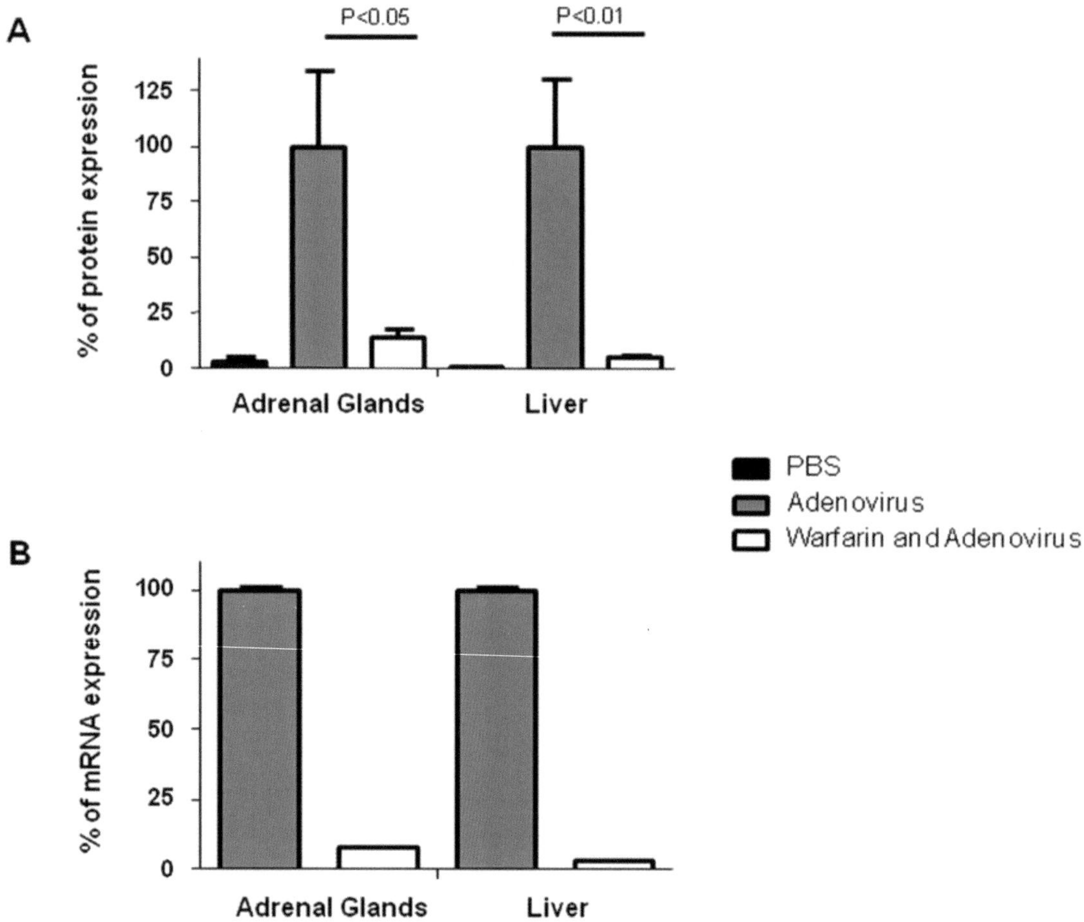

Figure 2. Effect of warfarin pre-treatment on adenoviral transgene expression. A replication-deficient recombinant adenovirus encoding the Lac-Z gene (6×10^8 PFU) was injected in control- (Adenovirus) or warfarin-pretreated animals (Warfarin and Adenovirus). Twenty-four hours later, liver biopsies or adrenal glands were collected. A: Measurement of the β-galactosidase protein in the samples was performed. The data presented are percentages of mean +/− SEM from untreated animals (n = 2), adenovirus-injected animals (n = 10) and adenovirus-injected animals, pre-treated with warfarin (n = 10). 100% represents the average of β-galactosidase activity in the adrenal glands (100% = 7584 β-gal units/mg of protein) or liver (100% = 24805 β-gal units/mg of protein) of adenovirus-injected animals. Statistical test: ANOVA (Prism, Graph-Pad softwares). B) Total RNA were collected from individual adrenal glands or liver biopsies, reversed-transcribed and subjected to quantitative PCR to detect LacZ or 18S RNA. The ratio LacZ/18S of liver or adrenal glands collected from animals injected with adenovirus was set at 100%. Data presented are duplicate determinations from a single adrenal gland and liver biopsy and is representative of 4 independent experiments.

same phenomenon can be observed in the adrenal gland of these animals, as the levels of LacZ transcripts are nearly ten times higher in the adrenal glands of factor X-complemented animals than in the adrenal glands of warfarin control animals (Fig. 3B). These results demonstrate that the mechanism of infection of the adrenal glands by adenovirus requires, as observed for the liver, a complex between factor X and the viral particle.

Visualization of the Kidneys by SPECT/CT

The SPECT tracer ^{99m}Tc-dimercaptosuccinic acid (^{99m}Tc-DMSA) is used in nuclear medicine to visualize the renal cortex [33]. This tracer was injected to mice. Five hours later, the animals were anaesthetized and subjected to a SPECT/CT scan. Figure 4A show transverse, coronal and sagittal views of the accumulation of ^{99m}Tc-DMSA in the kidneys. A three-dimensional reconstruction of the images is also presented (Figure 4B). Altogether, the information obtained allow a localization of the kidneys in the SPECT/CT images which can in turn be use for an accurate localization of the adrenal glands.

Adrenal Glands Transduction Upon Intra-renal Injection of Adenovirus Type 5 is Detectable by SPECT/CT Imaging and is Warfarin-dependent

To investigate whether intra-renal administration of adenovirus could lead to improved transduction, mice were injected with 5×10^8 PFU of Ad-CMV-rNIS in the left kidney. Forty-eight hours later, the animals were administered intra-peritoneally with the tracer $^{99m}TcO_4^-$. This tracer accumulates selectively in organs expressing the Na/I symporter (NIS) [31], i.e the thyroid, stomach and salivary glands that express NIS endogenously as well as the organs/tissues transduced by the adenovector. The animals were then anaesthetized and positioned into a SPECT/CT scanner.

The SPECT/CT images, analyzed in the light of the images obtained using the kidney specific probe ^{99m}Tc-DMSA (Figure 4), revealed a strong, discrete signal just above the kidney, in an area expected to encompass the adrenal gland (Figure 5A). As such a signal is absent in SPECT/CT images of mice administered intravenously with the same adenovirus [31] or in the contra-lateral kidney (not shown), this set of data suggests that the intra-renal route of administration of adenovirus is more efficient than

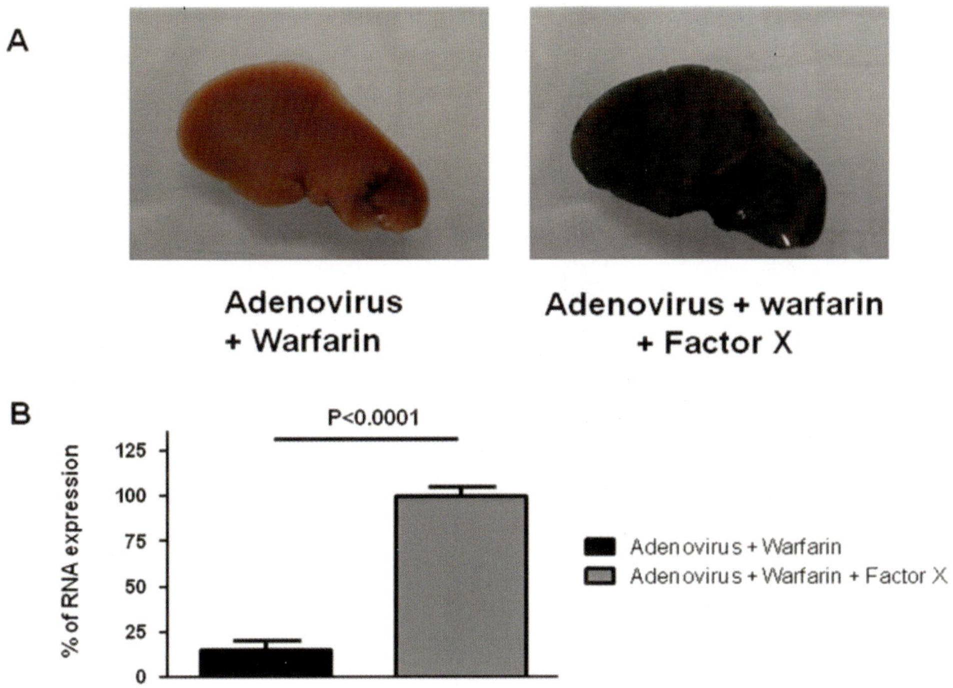

Figure 3. Influence of Factor X on adenovirus transduction in warfarin-treated mice. A replication-deficient recombinant adenovirus encoding the Lac-Z gene (6×10^8 PFU) was injected in warfarin-pretreated animals (n = 7) or warfarin-pre-treated, factor X-complemented animals (n = 5). Forty-eight hours later, liver biopsies or adrenal glands were collected. A) Whole liver were stained for β-galactosidase expression. B: Total RNA were extracted from the adrenal glands (two glands from the same animal were pooled), reversed-transcribed and subjected to quantitative PCR to detect LacZ expression or 18S RNA. The ratio LacZ/18S of adrenal glands collected from warfarin-pre-treated, factor X-complemented animals injected with adenovirus was set at 100%. The data presented are means+SEM. Statistical analysis: Student t test (Prism, Graph-Pad softwares).

the intravenous one to transduce this organ. A similar imaging protocol involving intra-renal administration of 5×10^8 PFU of Ad-CMV-rNIS in mice pre-treated with warfarin resulted in a lack of signal in the adrenal glands area (Figure 5B), confirming that adrenal gland infection depends on blood factors. Images focusing on the liver showed that intra-renal administration of Ad-CMV-rNIS led to an important transduction of this organ (Fig. 6A). Quantitative analysis of liver adenoviral transduction in animals administered using the intra-venous or intra-renal route failed to show any statistically-significant difference. In addition, SPECT/CT analysis of the liver of animals administered intra-renal with Ad-CMV-rNIS confirmed that liver transduction is warfarin dependent (Fig. 6B). To verify the data obtained through imaging, analysis of transgene expression was performed using quantitative RT-PCR on liver and adrenal gland biopsies. The data presented in Figure 7 confirm the imaging data and demonstrate that the intra-renal route of administration results in the transduction of the adrenal glands and that both liver and adrenal gland transduction are warfarin-dependent.

Discussion

Although adenovirus infection has been thought, for more than a decade, to require the binding of the virus to the cellular CAR, recent data have demonstrated that, *in vivo*, when the virus is administered systemically, CAR is not required for infection. The current consensus describes the formation of a complex between the adenovirus and a blood factor (factor X) and this complex is taken up by cells in a CAR-independent mechanism. This concept has been elucidated in the liver but has also been demonstrated in the spleen [26], lung and heart [37,38] and human epithelial cells [39] and involves heparan sulfate proteoglycans [40]. In the adrenal glands, CAR mRNA is undetectable (Figure 1A). This result is in agreement with previous work describing the lack of CAR-specific immuno-reactivity in mouse adrenal glands [41] and suggests strongly that the infection of the adrenal glands by adenovirus type 5 is CAR-independent. Subsequent experiments using both capsid-modified adenoviruses and pharmacologic interventions confirmed this hypothesis and demonstrated that adenovirus infection in this tissue depends on Factor X. Therefore, our data demonstrate that the adrenal glands are infected in a way similar to that described for infection of the liver, spleen, lung, heart and human epithelial cells. In this context, our data strengthen the point of view suggesting the general nature of this mechanism.

To our knowledge, this is the first time that the warfarin-sensitive nature of adenovirus infection *in vivo* as well as transduction of the adrenal glands by any gene delivery vector was demonstrated using imaging of gene expression. In this context, monitoring of gene transfer using NIS as a reporter gene by SPECT/CT offers many advantage. This methodology allows repetitive, longitudinal studies of transgene expression [31] and has also been used and validated to monitor the spread of oncolytic virus [7,42]. Humans and clinical trials have validated the utilization of the NIS reporter gene to monitor cancer gene therapy [43] and to adjust treatment [44]. The data presented in the present work demonstrates that the detection of NIS expression can benefit from the utilization of well-established SPECT probes in nuclear medicine such as ^{99m}Tc-DMSA to help to locate transgene expression.

Local delivery of adenovector, through intra-renal injection, results in an increased transduction of the adrenal gland.

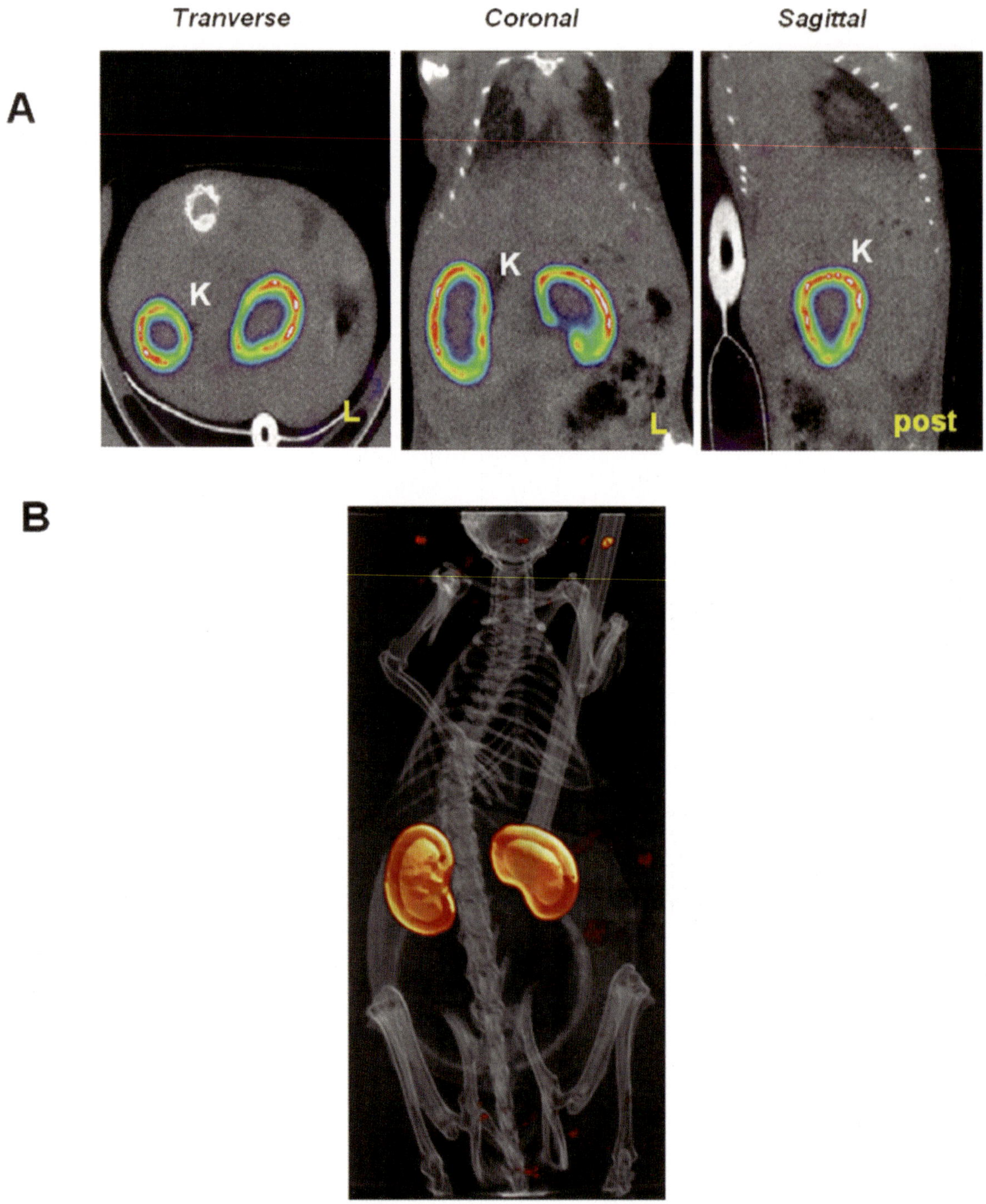

Figure 4. Localization of the kidneys using ^{99m}Tc-DMSA. Mice were injected intra-peritoneally with 95 MBq of ^{99m}Tc-DMSA. Five hours later, the animals were anaesthetized and SPECT/CT scans performed. A) Transverse, coronal and sagittal sections centered on the kidneys. B) Volume rendering of the whole animal in which the kidneys appear in yellow. Legend: K: kidney, L: left, post: posterior side of the animal.

SPECT/CT imaging of gene expression using this route to administer a replication-deficient adenovirus encoding the Na/I symporter led to a clear, discrete signal in the kidney area. The transduction of the adrenal glands was verified by RT-PCR on biopsies and RT-PCR on mRNAs extracted from the kidneys failed to provide any signal. Quantitative analysis of the images suggested that transgene expression was increased by a factor varying from two to five with the intra-renal route of administration. Considering the short half-life of adenoviruses in the circulation [9], the difference of transduction observed with the two modes of injection is likely to be due to the increased availability of the vector in the adrenal glands. More specifically, upon intra-renal administration, the adenovector probably ends up in the circulation and that the first "transduceable" organ that it encounters is the adrenal glands, followed by the liver. Consistent with this hypothesis and

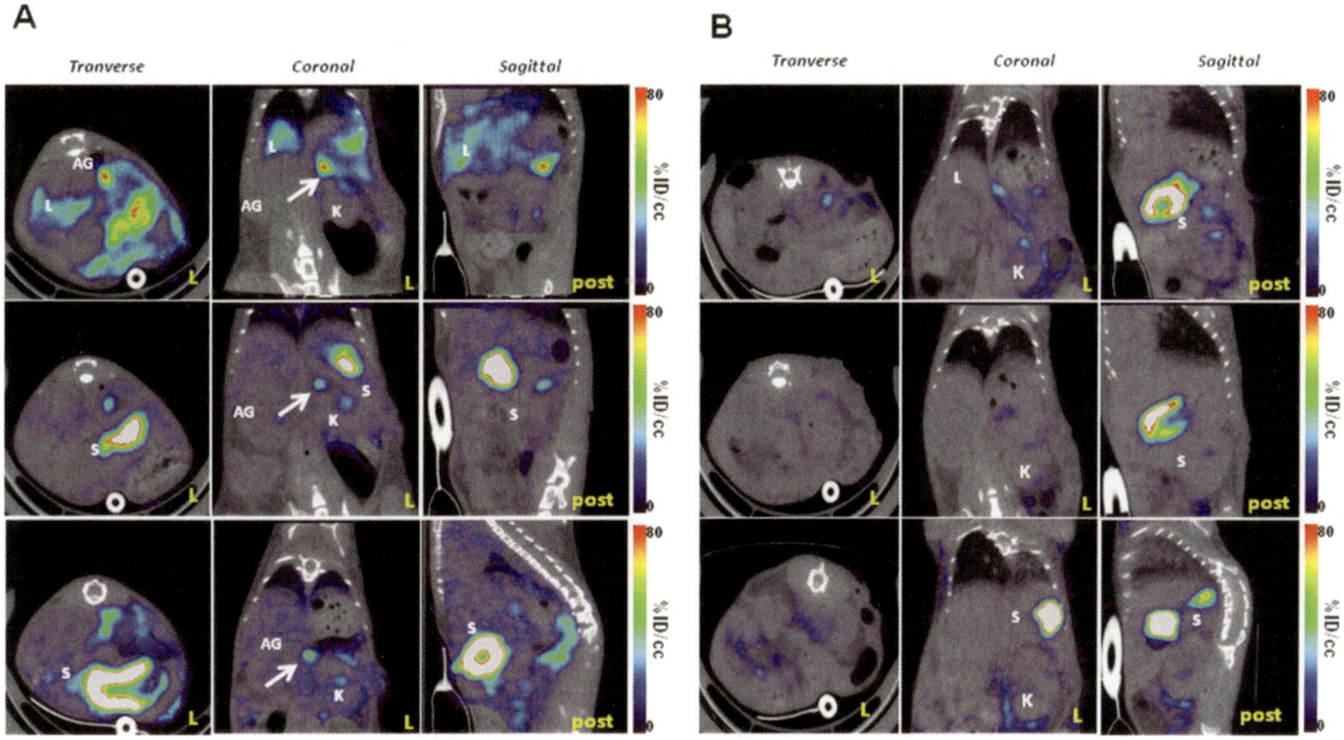

Figure 5. Visualization of gene transfer in the adrenal gland upon intra-renal injection: Effect of warfarin. Direct injection of 5×10^8 PFU Ad-CMV-rNIS in the left kidney was performed on control (A) or warfarin-treated mice (B). Forty-eight hours later, the mice were anaesthetized and SPECT/CT scans performed. The transverse, coronal and sagittal sections presented are centered on the adrenal glands. Legend: AG: adrenal glands, L: liver, K: kidneys, S: stomach, post: posterior side of the animal.

considering the dramatic difference in size of the liver versus the adrenal glands, it is not surprising that the intra-renal or intravenous mode of administration led to a level of transduction that was not statistically different (not shown). Therefore, the intra-renal route is relevant to increase adrenal gland transduction but is inefficient at reducing liver transduction.

Adenoviral infection of the adrenal glands has been exploited in pre-clinical gene therapy protocols for diseases related to adrenal

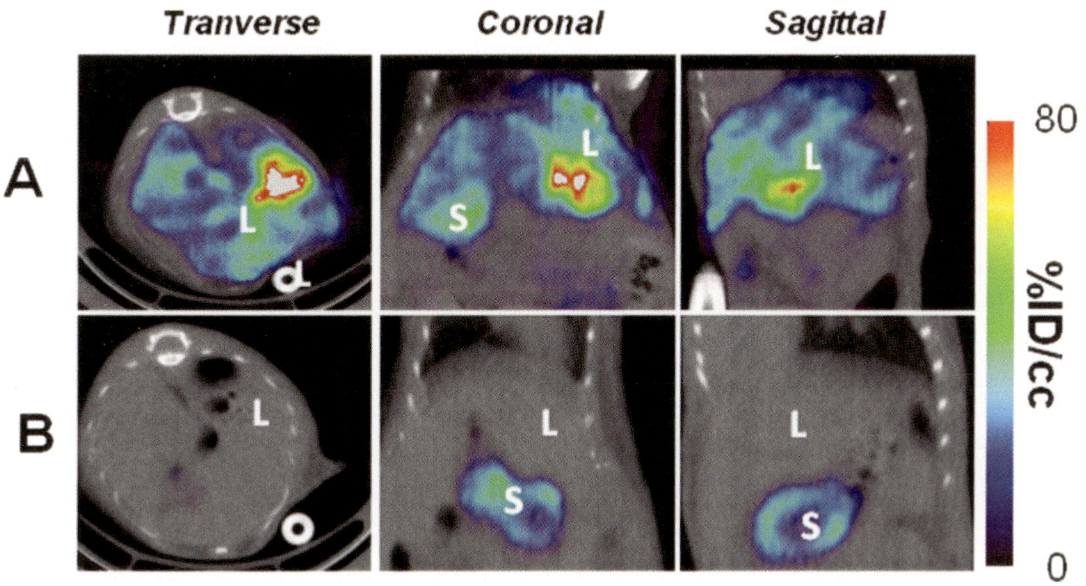

Figure 6. Visualization of gene transfer in the liver upon intra-renal injection: Effect of warfarin. Direct injection of 5×10^8 PFU Ad-CMV-rNIS in the left kidney was performed on control (A) or warfarin-treated mice (B). Forty-eight hours later, the mice were anaesthetized and SPECT/CT scans performed. The transverse, coronal and sagittal sections presented are centered on the liver. Legend: L: liver, S: Stomach.

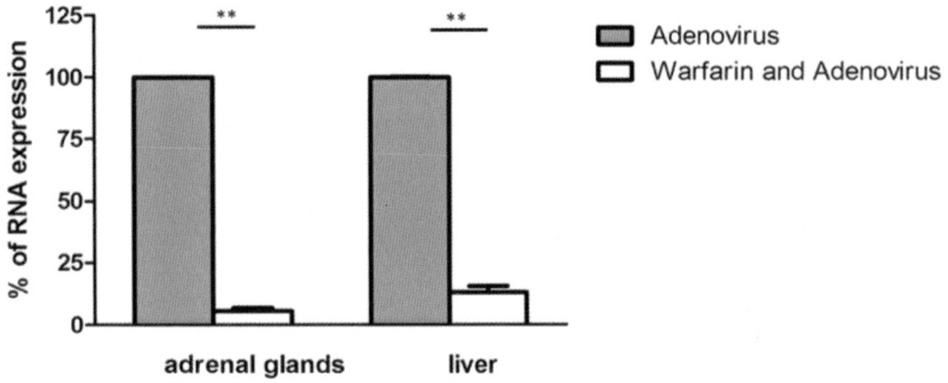

Figure 7. Effect of warfarin pre-treatment on adenoviral transgene expression following intra-renal administration. Ad-CMV-rNIS, a replication-deficient recombinant adenovirus encoding the NIS gene (5×10^8 PFU) was injected into the left kidney of control- (Adenovirus) or warfarin-pretreated animals (Warfarin and Adenovirus). Fourty-eight hours later, liver biopsies and adrenal glands were collected. Total RNA were collected from individual adrenal glands (on the left kidney) or liver biopsies, reversed-transcribed and subjected to quantitative PCR to detect rNIS expression or GAPDH RNA. The ratio rNIS/GAPDH of liver or adrenal glands collected from animals injected with adenovirus was set at 100%. Data presented are triplicate determinations from three adrenal gland and liver biopsies. The data presented are means+SEM. Statistical analysis: Student t test (Prizm, Graph-Pad softwares). $^{**}p\leq0{,}01$.

dysfunctions [45,46]. Alternatively, infection of the adrenal glands can also be seen as a source of side-effect of an adenoviral gene therapy approach targeting another organ: Adenoviral infection of cells from the adrenal glands has been shown to induce inflammatory cytokines [47], as well as affecting steroid hormone production [47,48]. In the latter context, the availability of an adenovector that would avoid selectively the transduction of the adrenal glands would prevent potential undesired effects. Reciprocally, an adenovector capable of selective transduction of the adrenal glands would be a useful tool. However, considering that the mechanism of infection appears to be the identical in all tissues infectable in vivo, the best strategy to restrict transgene expression to the adrenal glands is transcriptional targeting rather that targeted transduction. For this purpose, liver-specific [49] or adrenal specific [50] promoter fragments have already been described and may be envisaged.

Acknowledgments

The authors would like to thank Dr Jamila Faivre (Inserm U785, Villejuif, France) for providing the recombinant adenovirus encoding rat NIS and and the radiopharmaceutical team of the Centre Antoine Lacassagne (Nadine Sapin, Guy Martinico, Stéphane Espitallier, Didier Alberato) for their help with radioisotope production and handling.

Author Contributions

Conceived and designed the experiments: GV. Performed the experiments: LT LHO PRF. Analyzed the data: PRF JD KB GV. Contributed reagents/materials/analysis tools: GC KB. Wrote the paper: GV KB.

References

1. Cohen CJ, Shieh JT, Pickles RJ, Okegawa T, Hsieh JT, et al. (2001) The coxsackievirus and adenovirus receptor is a transmembrane component of the tight junction. Proc Natl Acad Sci U S A 98: 15191–15196.
2. Merron A, Peerlinck I, Martin-Duque P, Burnet J, Quintanilla M, et al. (2007) SPECT/CT imaging of oncolytic adenovirus propagation in tumours in vivo using the Na/I symporter as a reporter gene. Gene Ther 14: 1731–1738.
3. Walters RW, Freimuth P, Moninger TO, Ganske I, Zabner J, et al. (2002) Adenovirus fiber disrupts CAR-mediated intercellular adhesion allowing virus escape. Cell 110: 789–799.
4. Li L, Okada H, Takemura G, Kosai K, Kanamori H, et al. (2009) Postinfarction gene therapy with adenoviral vector expressing decorin mitigates cardiac remodeling and dysfunction. Am J Physiol Heart Circ Physiol 297: H1504–1513.
5. Wang Y, Thorne S, Hannock J, Francis J, Au T, et al. (2005) A novel assay to assess primary human cancer infectibility by replication-selective oncolytic adenoviruses. Clin Cancer Res 11: 351–360.
6. Peerlinck I, Amini-Nik S, Phillips RK, Iggo R, Lemoine NR, et al. (2008) Therapeutic potential of replication-selective oncolytic adenoviruses on cells from familial and sporadic desmoid tumors. Clin Cancer Res 14: 6187–6192.
7. Merron A, Baril P, Martin-Duque P, de la Vieja A, Tran L, et al. (2010) Assessment of the Na/I symporter as a reporter gene to visualize oncolytic adenovirus propagation in peritoneal tumours. Eur J Nucl Med Mol Imaging 37: 1377–1385.
8. Martinico SC, Jezzard S, Sturt NJ, Michils G, Tejpar S, et al. (2006) Assessment of endostatin gene therapy for familial adenomatous polyposis-related desmoid tumors. Cancer Res 66: 8233–8240.
9. Alemany R, Suzuki K, Curiel DT (2000) Blood clearance rates of adenovirus type 5 in mice. J Gen Virol 81: 2605–2609.
10. Alemany R, Curiel DT (2001) CAR-binding ablation does not change biodistribution and toxicity of adenoviral vectors. Gene Ther 8: 1347–1353.
11. Groot-Wassink T, Aboagye EO, Wang Y, Lemoine NR, Keith WN, et al. (2004) Noninvasive imaging of the transcriptional activities of human telomerase promoter fragments in mice. Cancer Res 64: 4906–4911.
12. Peerlinck I, Merron A, Baril P, Conchon S, Martin-Duque P, et al. (2009) Targeted radionuclide therapy using a Wnt-targeted replicating adenovirus encoding the Na/I symporter. Clin Cancer Res 15: 6595–6601.
13. Coughlan L, Vallath S, Saha A, Flak M, McNeish IA, et al. (2009) In vivo retargeting of adenovirus type 5 to alphavbeta6 integrin results in reduced hepatotoxicity and improved tumor uptake following systemic delivery. J Virol 83: 6416–6428.
14. Descamps D, Benihoud K (2009) Two key challenges for effective adenovirus-mediated liver gene therapy: innate immune responses and hepatocyte-specific transduction. Curr Gene Ther 9: 115–127.
15. Chao J, Zhang JJ, Lin KF, Chao L (1998) Human kallikrein gene delivery attenuates hypertension, cardiac hypertrophy, and renal injury in Dahl salt-sensitive rats. Hum Gene Ther 9: 21–31.
16. Themis M, Schneider H, Kiserud T, Cook T, Adebakin S, et al. (1999) Successful expression of beta-galactosidase and factor IX transgenes in fetal and neonatal sheep after ultrasound-guided percutaneous adenovirus vector administration into the umbilical vein. Gene Ther 6: 1239–1248.
17. Groot-Wassink T, Aboagye EO, Glaser M, Lemoine NR, Vassaux G (2002) Adenovirus biodistribution and noninvasive imaging of gene expression in vivo by positron emission tomography using human sodium/iodide symporter as reporter gene. Hum Gene Ther 13: 1723–1735.
18. Wang Y, Groot-Wassink T, Lemoine NR, Vassaux G (2003) Cellular characterization of the tropism of recombinant adenovirus for the adrenal glands. Eur J Clin Invest 33: 794–798.
19. Barzon L, Boscaro M, Palu G (2004) Endocrine aspects of cancer gene therapy. Endocr Rev 25: 1–44.

20. Wickham TJ, Mathias P, Cheresh DA, Nemerow GR (1993) Integrins alpha v beta 3 and alpha v beta 5 promote adenovirus internalization but not virus attachment. Cell 73: 309–319.
21. Bergelson JM, Cunningham JA, Droguett G, Kurt-Jones EA, Krithivas A, et al. (1997) Isolation of a common receptor for Coxsackie B viruses and adenoviruses 2 and 5. Science 275: 1320–1323.
22. Fechner H, Haack A, Wang H, Wang X, Eizema K, et al. (1999) Expression of coxsackie adenovirus receptor and alphav-integrin does not correlate with adenovector targeting in vivo indicating anatomical vector barriers. Gene Ther 6: 1520–1535.
23. Mizuguchi H, Koizumi N, Hosono T, Ishii-Watabe A, Uchida E, et al. (2002) CAR- or alphav integrin-binding ablated adenovirus vectors, but not fiber-modified vectors containing RGD peptide, do not change the systemic gene transfer properties in mice. Gene Ther 9: 769–776.
24. Yun CO, Yoon AR, Yoo JY, Kim H, Kim M, et al. (2005) Coxsackie and adenovirus receptor binding ablation reduces adenovirus liver tropism and toxicity. Hum Gene Ther 16: 248–261.
25. Parker AL, Waddington SN, Nicol CG, Shayakhmetov DM, Buckley SM, et al. (2006) Multiple vitamin K-dependent coagulation zymogens promote adenovirus-mediated gene delivery to hepatocytes. Blood 108: 2554–2561.
26. Waddington SN, Parker AL, Havenga M, Nicklin SA, Buckley SM, et al. (2007) Targeting of adenovirus serotype 5 (Ad5) and 5/47 pseudotyped vectors in vivo: fundamental involvement of coagulation factors and redundancy of CAR binding by Ad5. J Virol 81: 9568–9571.
27. Kalyuzhniy O, Di Paolo NC, Silvestry M, Hofherr SE, Barry MA, et al. (2008) Adenovirus serotype 5 hexon is critical for virus infection of hepatocytes in vivo. Proc Natl Acad Sci U S A 105: 5483–5488.
28. Waddington SN, McVey JH, Bhella D, Parker AL, Barker K, et al. (2008) Adenovirus serotype 5 hexon mediates liver gene transfer. Cell 132: 397–409.
29. Vigant F, Descamps D, Jullienne B, Esselin S, Connault E, et al. (2008) Substitution of hexon hypervariable region 5 of adenovirus serotype 5 abrogates blood factor binding and limits gene transfer to liver. Mol Ther 16: 1474–1480.
30. Groot-Wassink T, Aboagye EO, Wang Y, Lemoine NR, Reader AJ, et al. (2004) Quantitative imaging of Na/I symporter transgene expression using positron emission tomography in the living animal. Mol Ther 9: 436–442.
31. Richard-Fiardo P, Franken PR, Lamit A, Marsault R, Guglielmi J, et al. (2012) Normalisation to blood activity is required for the accurate quantification of Na/I symporter ectopic expression by SPECT/CT in individual subjects. PLoS One 7: e34086.
32. Faivre J, Clerc J, Gerolami R, Herve J, Longuet M, et al. (2004) Long-term radioiodine retention and regression of liver cancer after sodium iodide symporter gene transfer in wistar rats. Cancer Res 64: 8045–8051.
33. Jouret F, Walrand S, Parreira KS, Courtoy PJ, Pauwels S, et al. (2010) Single photon emission-computed tomography (SPECT) for functional investigation of the proximal tubule in conscious mice. Am J Physiol Renal Physiol 298: F454–460.
34. Loening AM, Gambhir SS (2003) AMIDE: a free software tool for multimodality medical image analysis. Mol Imaging 2: 131–137.
35. Mirza M, Hreinsson J, Strand ML, Hovatta O, Soder O, et al. (2006) Coxsackievirus and adenovirus receptor (CAR) is expressed in male germ cells and forms a complex with the differentiation factor JAM-C in mouse testis. Exp Cell Res 312: 817–830.
36. Cany J, Avril A, Pichard V, Aubert D, Ferry N, et al. (2007) A transgenic mouse with beta-Galactosidase as a fetal liver self-antigen for immunotherapy studies. J Hepatol 47: 396–403.
37. Alba R, Bradshaw AC, Coughlan L, Denby L, McDonald RA, et al. (2010) Biodistribution and retargeting of FX-binding ablated adenovirus serotype 5 vectors. Blood 116: 2656–2664.
38. Koski A, Rajecki M, Guse K, Kanerva A, Ristimaki A, et al. (2009) Systemic adenoviral gene delivery to orthotopic murine breast tumors with ablation of coagulation factors, thrombocytes and Kupffer cells. J Gene Med 11: 966–977.
39. Jonsson MI, Lenman AE, Frangsmyr L, Nyberg C, Abdullahi M, et al. (2009) Coagulation factors IX and X enhance binding and infection of adenovirus types 5 and 31 in human epithelial cells. J Virol 83: 3816–3825.
40. Bradshaw AC, Parker AL, Duffy MR, Coughlan L, van Rooijen N, et al. (2010) Requirements for receptor engagement during infection by adenovirus complexed with blood coagulation factor X. PLoS Pathog 6: e1001142.
41. Raschperger E, Thyberg J, Pettersson S, Philipson L, Fuxe J, et al. (2006) The coxsackie- and adenovirus receptor (CAR) is an in vivo marker for epithelial tight junctions, with a potential role in regulating permeability and tissue homeostasis. Exp Cell Res 312: 1566–1580.
42. Haddad D, Zanzonico PB, Carlin S, Chen CH, Chen NG, et al. (2012) A vaccinia virus encoding the human sodium iodide symporter facilitates long-term image monitoring of virotherapy and targeted radiotherapy of pancreatic cancer. J Nucl Med 53: 1933–1942.
43. Barton KN, Stricker H, Brown SL, Elshaikh M, Aref I, et al. (2008) Phase I study of noninvasive imaging of adenovirus-mediated gene expression in the human prostate. Mol Ther 16: 1761–1769.
44. Barton KN, Stricker H, Elshaikh MA, Pegg J, Cheng J, et al. (2011) Feasibility of adenovirus-mediated hNIS gene transfer and 131I radioiodine therapy as a definitive treatment for localized prostate cancer. Mol Ther 19: 1353–1359.
45. Tajima T, Okada T, Ma XM, Ramsey W, Bornstein S, et al. (1999) Restoration of adrenal steroidogenesis by adenovirus-mediated transfer of human cytochromeP450 21-hydroxylase into the adrenal gland of21-hydroxylase-deficient mice. Gene Ther 6: 1898–1903.
46. Lymperopoulos A, Rengo G, Zincarelli C, Soltys S, Koch WJ (2008) Modulation of adrenal catecholamine secretion by in vivo gene transfer and manipulation of G protein-coupled receptor kinase-2 activity. Mol Ther 16: 302–307.
47. Matkovic U, Pacenti M, Trevisan M, Palu G, Barzon L (2009) Investigation on human adrenocortical cell response to adenovirus and adenoviral vector infection. J Cell Physiol 220: 45–57.
48. Alesci S, Ramsey WJ, Bornstein SR, Chrousos GP, Hornsby PJ, et al. (2002) Adenoviral vectors can impair adrenocortical steroidogenesis: clinical implications for natural infections and gene therapy. Proc Natl Acad Sci U S A 99: 7484–7489.
49. Willhauck MJ, Sharif Samani BR, Klutz K, Cengic N, Wolf I, et al. (2008) Alpha-fetoprotein promoter-targeted sodium iodide symporter gene therapy of hepatocellular carcinoma. Gene Ther 15: 214–223.
50. Morley SD, Viard I, Parker KL, Mullins JJ (1996) Adrenocortical-specific transgene expression directed by steroid hydroxylase gene promoters. Endocr Res 22: 631–639.

5

Novel Algorithm for Non-Invasive Assessment of Fibrosis in NAFLD

Jan-Peter Sowa[1], Dominik Heider[2], Lars Peter Bechmann[1], Guido Gerken[1], Daniel Hoffmann[2], Ali Canbay[1]*

1 Department of Gastroenterology and Hepatology, University Hospital, University Duisburg-Essen, Essen, Germany, 2 Department of Bioinformatics, Center for Medical Biotechnology, University Duisburg-Essen, Essen, Germany

Abstract

Introduction: Various conditions of liver disease and the downsides of liver biopsy call for a non-invasive option to assess liver fibrosis. A non-invasive score would be especially useful to identify patients with slow advancing fibrotic processes, as in Non-Alcoholic Fatty Liver Disease (NAFLD), which should undergo histological examination for fibrosis.

Patients/Methods: Classic liver serum parameters, hyaluronic acid (HA) and cell death markers of 126 patients undergoing bariatric surgery for morbid obesity were analyzed by machine learning techniques (logistic regression, k-nearest neighbors, linear support vector machines, rule-based systems, decision trees and random forest (RF)). Specificity, sensitivity and accuracy of the evaluated datasets to predict fibrosis were assessed.

Results: None of the single parameters (ALT, AST, M30, M60, HA) did differ significantly between patients with a fibrosis score 1 or 2. However, combining these parameters using RFs reached 79% accuracy in fibrosis prediction with a sensitivity of more than 60% and specificity of 77%. Moreover, RFs identified the cell death markers M30 and M65 as more important for the decision than the classic liver parameters.

Conclusion: On the basis of serum parameters the generation of a fibrosis scoring system seems feasible, even when only marginally fibrotic tissue is available. Prospective evaluation of novel markers, i.e. cell death parameters, should be performed to identify an optimal set of fibrosis predictors.

Editor: Wing-Kin Syn, Institute of Hepatology, Foundation for Liver Research, United Kingdom

Funding: This work was supported by the Deutsche Forschungsgemeinschaft (http://www.dfg.de/, grant CA267/4-1 and CA267/8-1) and the Wilhelm Laupitz Foundation. The funders had no role in study design, data collection and analysis, decision to publish, or preparation of the manuscript.

* E-mail: ali.canbay@uni-due.de

Background

Non-alcoholic fatty liver disease (NAFLD) is an increasingly prevalent disease entity, affecting up to one-third of Europeans [1]. NAFLD may progress to non-alcoholic steatohepatitis (NASH) with or without fibrosis and thus predisposes to liver cirrhosis, end stage liver disease and hepatocellular carcinoma (HCC) [2]. Approximately 33% of patients with NASH develop fibrosis and 15% develop cirrhosis [3]. To date, the diagnosis of NASH is established by histological means, including inflammation, steatosis, hepatocellular injury and ballooning. According to Kleiner *et al.*, fibrosis in NAFLD is assessed in a 7-stage system, which includes detailed evaluation of perisinusoidal and periportal fibrosis [4]. However, liver biopsy is associated with a limited, but significant risk of adverse events (bleeding, infection) and a significant rate of observer- and sampling errors, specifically for assessment of fibrosis [5,6]. Given the high prevalence of NAFLD and the limitations of liver biopsies, biomarkers and surrogate parameters of fibrosis might evolve as important diagnostic means in NAFLD patients.

Hepatocyte cell death in NAFLD is an important predictor of hepatic stellate cell (HSC) activation and thus indirectly of fibrogenesis [7,8]. Recently, assessment of hepatocyte apoptosis by quantification of soluble cytokeratin 18 (CK-18) has been validated in large cohorts of NAFLD patients as a novel biomarker of disease activity [9]. As engulfment of remnants from apoptotic hepatocytes (apoptotic bodies) by non-parenchymal cells directly and indirectly activates HSCs [10,11], fibrosis was also found to correlate with serum CK-18 levels in some studies [12,13]. Another derivate marker with regard to collagen production is hyaluronic acid (HA). HA serum levels increase with progressive fibrosis [14]. In fact, some studies showed a correlation between serum HA and fibrosis stage in chronic liver diseases, including NAFLD [15,16]. However, in validation studies, individual biomarkers failed to accurately predict fibrosis [17]. Thus, diagnostic multi-panel tests, including a variety of individual parameters have recently been implied as non-invasive fibrosis tests. Most tests have been established in HCV patients and might lack validity in NAFLD patients [18,19]. Novel tests that include cell death markers, designed for fibrosis assessment in NAFLD, are emerging, but still require large-cohort validation studies [20].

Limitations of these scoring systems comprise small cohorts [21], comparison of no or low-grade cirrhosis *vs.* high-grade of cirrhosis [21,22], and inclusion of metabolic or biometric parameters increasing the effort needed to generate this score for individual patients [21,23]. To monitor early fibrogenesis and progression of disease it would be imperative to differentiate even low grades of fibrosis. This is of utmost clinical significance, as pre-existing chronic liver diseases – even in early fibrotic stages – predispose to acute-on-chronic liver failure [24]. However, currently available non-invasive tests for fibrosis fail to distinguish early fibrosis stages.

Here, we aim to introduce a novel score of non-invasive fibrosis parameters, designed specifically for NAFLD. To this end, we used machine-learning algorithms, which are widely used for prediction and classification problems in biomedical research [25]. Typically, a supervised learning strategy is used for training a machine learning algorithm with a set of training samples, for which the input parameters and associated target classes are known. In the setting presented here, these algorithms were trained to differentiate between fibrosis stage 1 and fibrosis stage 2 within a cohort of adipose NAFLD patients, utilizing serum derived parameters.

Materials and Methods

Ethics Statement

The study protocol conformed to the ethical guidelines of the 1975 Declaration of Helsinki and was approved by the Institutional Review Board (Ethics Committee) at the University Hospital of Essen. All patients provided written, informed consent before enrollment.

Patients and Sample Acquisition

126 morbidly obese patients (BMI: 52.2±0.7 kg/m^2; age: 45.2±0.96; males/females: 28 (22.2%)/98 (77.8%)) who underwent bariatric surgery at a renowned center for bariatric surgery were included (Tab. 1). Some clinical data on this collective have been published previously in a different approach of analysis [26]. Indication for bariatric surgery was made according to NIH guidelines (BMI ≥40 kg/m2 or ≥35 kg/m2, plus co-morbidities). Subjects reporting excessive alcohol consumption (>20 g/day in males or >10 g/day in females) indicating alcoholic liver disease were excluded. Liver serum parameters (ALT, AST) were determined in the central laboratory unit of the University Hospital Essen by standardized methods. Liver biopsies were obtained during the bariatric surgery as wedge biopsy. Individual specimens were stored in 4% formalin solution (Roth, Karlsruhe, Germany) for histological examination. The fibrosis stage was assessed in a blinded fashion by a single pathologist according to Kleiner *et al.* [4].

ELISA

Sera were collected upon admission and throughout hospitalization and stored within 2 h at −20°C until testing. Individual values of clinical and standard laboratory data, overall cell death and apoptosis markers M65 and M30 (determined by the M30-Apoptosense and M65 ELISAs from Peviva; Bromma, Sweden), as well as hyaluronic acid (Corgenix, Bloomfield, CO, USA) were determined. All procedures were conducted according to the manufacturers' instructions.

Dataset and Statistics

The resulting parameters used for classification were ALT, AST, M30, M65 and HA. Samples with incomplete parameters were discarded prior to analysis. The final dataset consisted of 25 samples of fibrosis status 1 (including stages 1a, 1b, 1c; handled as positive samples) and 101 samples of fibrosis status 2 (representing negative samples). We compared all parameters of fibrosis-status 1 (1a, 1b, 1c) with the corresponding parameters of fibrosis-status 2 using Wilcoxon Signed-Rank tests.

Machine Learning

Several machine learning techniques were evaluated, namely logistic regression (logReg), k-nearest neighbors (knn), linear support vector machines (SVM), rule-based systems (RB), decision trees (DT) and random forest (RF). For the logistic regression, we used the implementation in the *stats* package of R (http://www.r-project.org) with standard settings. The k-nearest neighbor implementation in the R package *class* was used with k = 3. The SVM implementation in the package *kernlab* of R was used with the *vanilladot* kernel. For the rule-based systems we used the *Part* [27] implementation provided in the R package *RWeka*. For the DTs we used the implementation in the *rpart* package and for the RFs [28] we used the implementation in the *randomForest* package of R. In our application each RF consisted of 2000 randomly and independently grown decision trees. When using the trained RF for prediction, an unseen instance was assigned to the positive class voted for by at least 50% of the trees. The importance of each variable for the correct classification can be assessed by determining the decrease in Gini impurity [29].

Cross-validation

All machine learning methods were validated using ten-fold leave-one-out cross-validation [29] to assess for the different machine learning methods the mean prediction sensitivity, specificity, and accuracy (see formulas below) and the ability to generalize to unseen instances.

For each test in the cross-validation, the sensitivity (SN), specificity (SP), and accuracy (AC) were calculated according to:

$$SN = \frac{TP}{TP+FN}$$

$$SP = \frac{TN}{TN+FP}$$

$$AC = \frac{TP+TN}{TP+FP+TN+FN}$$

with true positives TP, false positives FP, false negatives FN and true negatives TN. Furthermore, we calculated the Receiver Operating Characteristics (ROC) curve [30] and the corresponding area under the curve (AUC) with ROCR [31]. The ROC curve is built by plotting sensitivity *vs.* specificity for every possible cut-off between the two classes.

Permutation Test

All machine learning methods were tested for significance using a permutation test. The AUC distribution for each classifier was calculated by ten-fold leave-one-out cross-validation. 1000 (= N) random permutations of the class labels were generated and the classifiers were trained and evaluated again. Each of the resulting AUC distributions of the permutation was compared with the *real* AUC distribution using Wilcoxon Signed-Rank test. The number k of permutations for which the mean AUC had no significant differences compared to the *real* AUC was counted for each classifier. The p-value of the permutation test was calculated by

$$p = \frac{k}{N}$$

Statistical Comparison

All models were compared by applying Wilcoxon Signed-Rank test on the AUC distributions from the ten-fold leave-one-out cross-validation runs. The null hypothesis was that there are no differences between the compared classifiers.

Results

Patient Characteristics

Detailed data of the included patients can be found in table 1, comprising distribution of demographic parameters as well as standard parameters of liver damage (transaminases, bilirubin, gamma-GT and LDH). Serum parameters for liver damage were within normal range and no pathological alterations were detected. As the patient collective consisted of adipose patients, the BMI was significantly above normal ranges. Partial data of this patient cohort has been presented before in a different type of analysis in Kälsch *et al.* [26].

No Prognostic Value of Individual Parameters

We found no significant differences between ALT, AST, M30, M65 and HA of fibrosis status 1 and 2 with regard to Wilcoxon Signed-Rank test ($p = 0.55$, $p = 0.30$, $p = 0.70$, $p = 0.87$ and $p = 0.86$, respectively).

Accuracy of the New Diagnostic Algorithm for Prediction of Fibrosis Stage

Most of the classifiers were not able to accurately predict the fibrosis status (or the results were insignificant according to the permutation test). Neither the logistic regression, nor support vector machines, nor rule-based systems were able to predict the fibrosis status from the given blood parameters. However, random forests and the k-nearest-neighbor algorithms had an accuracy of about 79%. The RFs reached an AUC of 0.6704+/−0.0062 ($p = 0.008$). A cutoff of 0.22 between positive and negative samples led to a sensitivity of over 60% and a specificity of 77% (Figure 1). The knn reached a sensitivity of 30.8% with a specificity of 91.3% ($p = 0.02$), which is slightly worse compared to the RFs (sensitivity of 30.8% with specificity of 92.2%). Decision trees displayed the best performance (sensitivity of 53.9% and specificity of 94.2), but failed to reach a significance level of 5% in the permutation test ($p = 0.099$).

Furthermore, we analyzed the prediction output for each sample. The output of the RFs is shown as boxplots for each of the two classes in Figure 2. Subjects from stage 1 had higher prediction values compared to subjects from stage 2 on average.

As mentioned before, RFs are able to identify the most important parameters for the classification process. The RFs identified M30 and M65 as being slightly more important than the other variables, which is in accordance with the DTs (only M30, M65 and AST are used in the trees, see Figure 3). The estimated importance for each parameter is shown in table 2.

Table 1. Demographic and basic parameters of the investigated patient collective.

Parameter	Fibrosis Stage 1 (1a, 1b, 1c)	Fibrosis Stage 2
Age (y)[1]	45.04±2.54	45.84±0.99
Gender[1]	M 16% (n = 4)/F 84% (n = 21)	M 24% (n = 24)/F 76% (n = 77)
BMI (kg/m^2)[1]	51.96±1.59	52.25±0.81
AST[1]	27.12±2.65	29.98±1.61
ALT[1]	34.44±4.81	37.67±2.59
gamma-GT[1]	34.24±4.48	55.29±12.40
LDH	232.92±9.99	226.47±5.31
bilirubin	0.56±0.08	0.55±0.03

No significant differences were found between stage 1 and stage 2.
[1]These data have been previously shown in a different analysis of this patient cohort in Kälsch *et al.* [28].

Discussion

Diagnosis of liver fibrosis or cirrhosis provides important clinical information. Different etiologies and conditions, affecting liver integrity and function may increase susceptibility to various toxins (e.g. drugs) or viruses and are associated with enhanced morbidity or mortality in acute liver injury [24]. Pre-existing liver disease, though, often persists in presence of marginally or only slightly elevated classic liver parameters, which would not suggest a liver biopsy to test for fibrosis. This is particularly common in obese NAFLD patients, as we have recently shown. Then again even a liver biopsy – comprising only 1/50.000th of the total liver volume – may not lead to an unambiguous judgement by a pathologist [21,32,33]. Moreover, liver biopsy is a painful invasive technique, which also confers a certain health risk, especially for patients with already reduced functional liver mass. Thus non-invasive methods that indicate progression to fibrosis or cirrhosis are needed that more reliably predict which patients should undergo a liver biopsy, or have their fibrosis status estimated if a biopsy is clinically not feasible.

A major concern for all attempts to establish such adequate scoring systems, is that as reference the gold standard has to be applied, which is biopsy and subsequent histological examination. As mentioned above, this technique contains two main sources of error that have to be considered when calculating a score for fibrosis/cirrhosis estimation [32,33].

Previous studies could clearly demonstrate that single serum parameters are not sufficient to reach the sensitivity or specificity of liver histology [19,21]. A scoring system combining different parameters seems to be the most promising approach. Knowing that cell death by apoptosis is a critical step for NASH development, integrating markers of cell death appears reasonable. Subsequent activation of HSC by hepatocyte apoptosis leads to ECM production [11,34]. In our calculations we included an importance analysis, demonstrating the highest importance for cell death parameters and hyaluronic acid, which has been linked to cirrhosis and collagen production [14]. This would fit with current theories discussing hepatocellular death and subsequent activation of non-parenchymal cells as crucial events in fibrogenesis and progression to cirrhosis in chronic, but also in acute liver injury [35].

While there have been previous attempts to establish a non-invasive method to detect fibrosis or cirrhosis, most groups have done their analyses in patients with viral hepatitis, where abundant collagen deposition and progression to cirrhosis is given. Systems which were established in NAFL/NASH cohorts often distinguish only no or low-grade fibrosis from cirrhosis [22]. This obviously does not suffice to monitor fibrosis progression in NAFLD, where

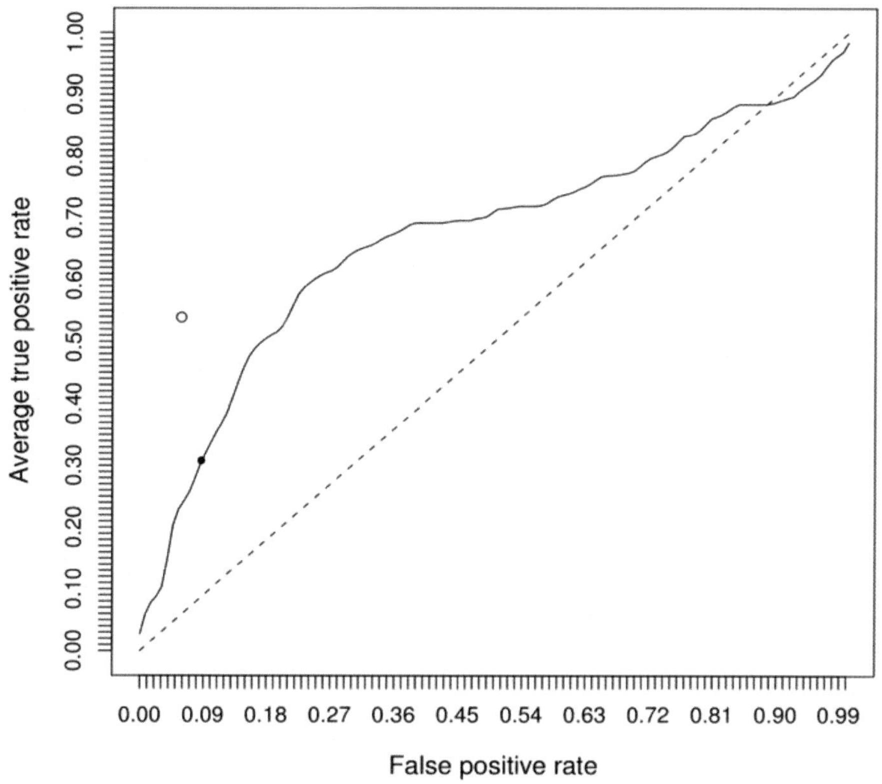

Figure 1. Prediction performance. The ROC curve of the RF is shown (p = 0.008). Black dot: performance of the 3 nn (p = 0.02); white circle: performance of the DT (p value = 0.099). The dashed line marks the performance by chance.

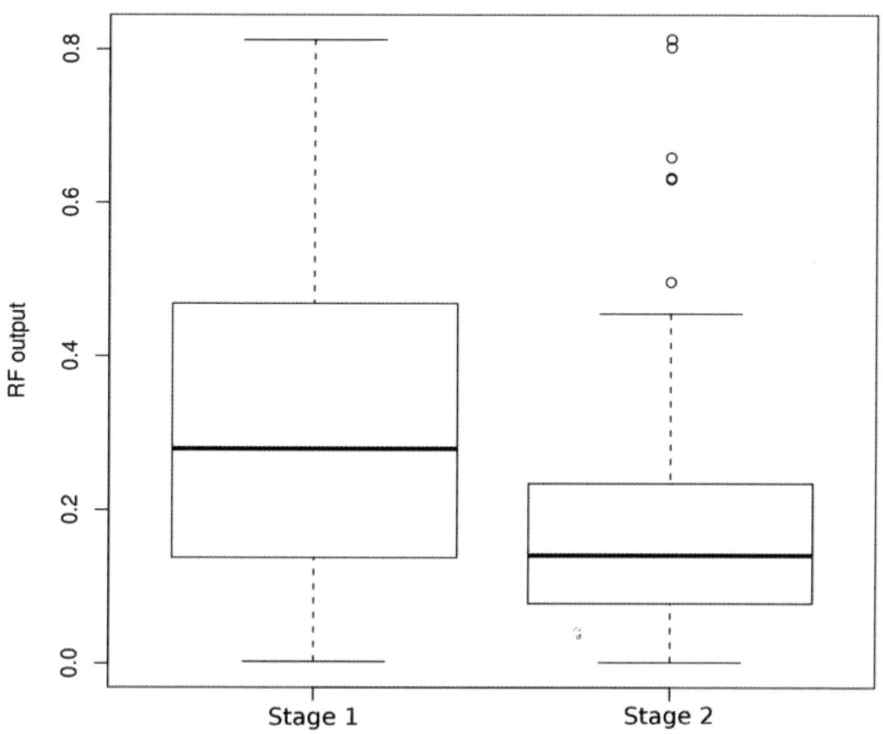

Figure 2. Boxplots of the outputs of the RFs. On the y-axis the predicted class probabilities for stage 1 and stage 2 are plotted. Generally, the RFs give higher prediction values for subjects from stage 1 compared to subjects from stage 2. The upper and the lower quartiles, the median (bold line) as well as outliers (circles) are shown.

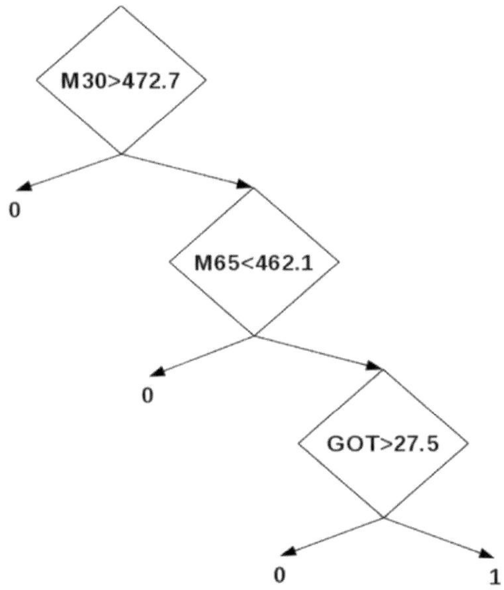

Figure 3. Decision Tree. The decision tree (DT) focuses on the parameters M30, M65 and AST (GOT), which is in partial agreement with the RFs. At the first level, the DT focuses on M30. If the M30 value for a given sample is less than 472.7, it is assigned to the negative class (0). If the M30 value is greater than 472.7, it is transferred to the next level that uses M65. If the M65 value for the given sample is greater than 462.1, it is assigned to the negative class, otherwise it is transferred to the last level. The last level in the DT focuses on GOT. If the GOT value for the given sample is less than 27.5, the sample is assigned as negative, otherwise as a positive sample (1).

progression is rather slow compared to viral or alcoholic hepatitis. Moreover, when at some point a therapeutic intervention against fibrosis is possible, detecting established cirrhosis vs. low fibrosis may not be helpful to identify patients in need of this – hypothetical – medication. Thus, early detection of fibrosis may be crucial for a therapeutic approach to counter fibrosis progression, lowering vulnerability to additional, acute injury. A recent study by Tomeno *et al.* assessed the efficacy of real time transient elastography to detect liver fibrosis [36]. While the calculated liver fibrosis index correlated well with histological scores in chronic hepatitis, no such correlation was found for NAFLD. One could speculate that either overweight or fat deposition within the liver may interfere with elastography measurements in NAFLD. In any case, elastography has to be interpreted with care in the setting of NAFLD. Some NAFLD related fibrosis scores took the distinctiveness of this etiology into account and included biometric data [21,23], which requires additional data for each patient (height, weight). This may not be a limitation for a few individual patients, though it has to be viewed in the light of increasing numbers of overweight or obese individuals in the general population. Constraining the utilized markers to serum derived parameters reduces the clinical course of

Table 2. Importance analysis.

parameter	importance
ALT	6.76
AST	6.53
M30	9.90
M65	9.57
hyaluronic acid	8.28

action to a single blood withdrawal. This would allow a true screening of patients without the need to take additional measurements.

Another major difference to other scoring systems is the employment of non-linear machine learning techniques. For instance, the RFs allow to estimate variable importance and hence can be used to further improve prediction performance. Moreover, some of these methods provide simple rules, which can be applied in clinical settings to predict the fibrosis status of new patients and thus estimate a potential progression of the liver disease.

Limitations of our results are due to the number of patients with a complete dataset and moreover on the limited variability of fibrosis stages. As we did our investigation on a mostly obese collective with a probable NAFLD/NASH type of liver damage, the generation of fibrotic tissue is expected to be rather slow, in contrast to viral etiologies or alcohol abuse. Thus, we decided to differentiate between the two lowest fibrosis stages and trained the models accordingly. Although the dataset has the mentioned limitations, we were able to build a model that is able to discriminate between the two fibrosis classes with a reasonable sensitivity and specificity. Prospective studies recruiting a more diverse group of patients, exhibiting the full range of fibrotic stages (0–4) could increase the quality of the prediction model. Moreover, a broader range of parameters should be included to identify those parameters with the highest importance for diagnosis of fibrosis using machine learning techniques. Another possible option is to combine serum parameters with other non-invasive data, e.g. transient elastography of the liver. Additionally, it might also be possible to accurately predict the NAS status with an enlarged dataset.

Acknowledgments

The authors thank Martin Schlattjan for sample and data collection.

Author Contributions

Sample acquisition and data collection: LPB AC. Obtained funding: GG AC. Conceived and designed the experiments: JPS D. Heider AC. Performed the experiments: JPS D. Heider. Analyzed the data: JPS D. Heider D. Hoffman. Contributed reagents/materials/analysis tools: GG D. Hoffman. Wrote the paper: JPS D. Heider LPB AC.

References

1. Ratziu V, Bellentani S, Cortez-Pinto H, Day C, Marchesini G (2010) A position statement on NAFLD/NASH based on the EASL 2009 special conference. J. Hepatol. 53: 372–384.
2. Feldstein AE (2010) Novel insights into the pathophysiology of nonalcoholic fatty liver disease. Semin. Liver Dis 30: 391–401.
3. Argo CK, Caldwell SH (2009) Epidemiology and natural history of non-alcoholic steatohepatitis. Clin Liver Dis 13: 511–531.
4. Kleiner DE, Brunt EM, Van Natta M, Behling C, Contos MJ, et al. (2005) Design and validation of a histological scoring system for nonalcoholic fatty liver disease. Hepatology 41: 1313–1321.
5. Grønbaek K, Christensen PB, Hamilton-Dutoit S, Federspiel BH, Hage E, et al. (2002) Interobserver variation in interpretation of serial liver biopsies from patients with chronic hepatitis C. J. Viral Hepat. 9: 443–449.
6. Ratziu V, Charlotte F, Heurtier A, Gombert S, Giral P, et al. (2005) Sampling variability of liver biopsy in nonalcoholic fatty liver disease. Gastroenterology 128: 1898–1906.

7. Feldstein AE, Canbay A, Angulo P, Taniai M, Burgart LJ, et al. (2003) Hepatocyte apoptosis and fas expression are prominent features of human nonalcoholic steatohepatitis. Gastroenterology 125: 437–443.
8. Canbay A, Friedman S, Gores GJ (2004) Apoptosis: the nexus of liver injury and fibrosis. Hepatology 39: 273–278.
9. Feldstein AE, Wieckowska A, Lopez AR, Liu Y-C, Zein NN, et al. (2009) Cytokeratin-18 fragment levels as noninvasive biomarkers for nonalcoholic steatohepatitis: a multicenter validation study. Hepatology 50: 1072–1078.
10. Canbay A, Feldstein AE, Higuchi H, Werneburg N, Grambihler A, et al. (2003) Kupffer cell engulfment of apoptotic bodies stimulates death ligand and cytokine expression. Hepatology 38: 1188–98.
11. Gieseler RK, Marquitan G, Schlattjan M, Sowa J-P, Bechmann LP, et al. (2011) Hepatocyte apoptotic bodies encasing nonstructural HCV proteins amplify hepatic stellate cell activation: implications for chronic hepatitis C. J. Viral Hepat. 18: 760–767.
12. Fitzpatrick E, Mitry RR, Quaglia A, Hussain MJ, DeBruyne R, et al. (2010) Serum levels of CK18 M30 and leptin are useful predictors of steatohepatitis and fibrosis in paediatric NAFLD. J. Pediatr. Gastroenterol. Nutr. 51: 500–506.
13. Bechmann LP, Gieseler RK, Sowa J-P, Kahraman A, Erhard J, et al. (2010) Apoptosis is associated with CD36/fatty acid translocase upregulation in non-alcoholic steatohepatitis. Liver Int 30: 850–859.
14. Ramadori G, Zöhrens G, Manns M, Rieder H, Dienes HP, et al. (1991) Serum hyaluronate and type III procollagen aminoterminal propeptide concentration in chronic liver disease. Relationship to cirrhosis and disease activity. Eur. J. Clin. Invest. 21: 323–330.
15. McHutchison JG, Blatt LM, De Medina M, Craig JR, Conrad A, et al. (2000) Measurement of serum hyaluronic acid in patients with chronic hepatitis C and its relationship to liver histology. Consensus Interferon Study Group. J. Gastroenterol. Hepatol. 15: 945–951.
16. Nobili V, Alisi A, Torre G, De Vito R, Pietrobattista A, et al. (2010) Hyaluronic acid predicts hepatic fibrosis in children with nonalcoholic fatty liver disease. Transl Res 156: 229–234.
17. Malik R, Chang M, Bhaskar K, Nasser I, Curry M, et al. (2009) The clinical utility of biomarkers and the nonalcoholic steatohepatitis CRN liver biopsy scoring system in patients with nonalcoholic fatty liver disease. J. Gastroenterol. Hepatol. 24: 564–568.
18. Ratziu V, Massard J, Charlotte F, Messous D, Imbert-Bismut F, et al. (2006) Diagnostic value of biochemical markers (FibroTest-FibroSURE) for the prediction of liver fibrosis in patients with non-alcoholic fatty liver disease. BMC Gastroenterol 6: 6.
19. Guha IN, Parkes J, Roderick P, Chattopadhyay D, Cross R, et al. (2008) Noninvasive markers of fibrosis in nonalcoholic fatty liver disease: Validating the European Liver Fibrosis Panel and exploring simple markers. Hepatology 47: 455–460.
20. Calès P, Lainé F, Boursier J, Deugnier Y, Moal V, et al. (2009) Comparison of blood tests for liver fibrosis specific or not to NAFLD. J. Hepatol 50: 165–173.
21. Vizzutti F, Arena U, Nobili V, Tarquini R, Trappoliere M, et al. (2009) Non-invasive assessment of fibrosis in non-alcoholic fatty liver disease. Ann Hepatol 8: 89–94.
22. Lydatakis H, Hager IP, Kostadelou E, Mpousmpoulas S, Pappas S, et al. (2006) Non-invasive markers to predict the liver fibrosis in non-alcoholic fatty liver disease. Liver Int. 26: 864–871.
23. Younossi ZM, Page S, Rafiq N, Birerdinc A, Stepanova M, et al. (2011) A biomarker panel for non-alcoholic steatohepatitis (NASH) and NASH-related fibrosis. Obes Surg 21: 431–439.
24. Canbay A, Gieseler RK, Gores GJ, Gerken G (2005) The relationship between apoptosis and non-alcoholic fatty liver disease: an evolutionary cornerstone turned pathogenic. Z Gastroenterol 43: 211–217.
25. Sajda P (2006) Machine learning for detection and diagnosis of disease. Annu Rev Biomed Eng 8: 537–565.
26. Kälsch J, Bechmann LP, Kälsch H, Schlattjan M, Erhard J, et al. (2011) Evaluation of Biomarkers of NAFLD in a Cohort of Morbidly Obese Patients. J Nutr Metab 2011: 369168.
27. Frank E, Witten I (1998) Generating Accurate Rule Sets Without Global Optimization. http://www.odysci.com/article/1010112985954253/generating-accurate-rule-sets-without-global-optimization (Accessed December 17, 2012).
28. Breiman L (2001) Random Forests. Machine Learning 45: 5–32.
29. Cawley GC, Talbot NLC (2004) Fast exact leave-one-out cross-validation of sparse least-squares support vector machines. Neural Netw 17: 1467–1475.
30. Fawcett T (2006) An introduction to ROC analysis. Pattern Recognit. Lett. 27: 861–874.
31. Sing T, Sander O, Beerenwinkel N, Lengauer T (2005) ROCR: visualizing classifier performance in R. Bioinformatics 21: 3940–3941.
32. Castera L, Pinzani M (2010) Biopsy and non-invasive methods for the diagnosis of liver fibrosis: does it take two to tango? Gut 59: 861–866.
33. Bacchetti P, Boylan R (2009) Estimating Complex Multi-State Misclassification Rates for Biopsy-Measured Liver Fibrosis in Patients with Hepatitis C. Int J Biostat 5: 5.
34. Canbay A, Higuchi H, Bronk SF, Taniai M, Sebo TJ, et al. (2002) Fas enhances fibrogenesis in the bile duct ligated mouse: a link between apoptosis and fibrosis. Gastroenterology 123: 1323–1330.
35. Dechêne A, Sowa J-P, Gieseler RK, Jochum C, Bechmann LP, et al. (2010) Acute liver failure is associated with elevated liver stiffness and hepatic stellate cell activation. Hepatology 52: 1008–1016.
36. Tomeno W, Yoneda M, Imajo K, Suzuki K, Ogawa Y, et al. (2012) Evaluation of the Liver Fibrosis Index calculated by using real-time tissue elastography for the non-invasive assessment of liver fibrosis in chronic liver diseases. Hepatol. Res.

6

Identification of the Plasma Metabolomics as Early Diagnostic Markers between Biliary Atresia and Neonatal Hepatitis Syndrome

Dongying Zhao[1], Lianshu Han[1], Zhengjuan He[1], Jun Zhang[1,2], Yongjun Zhang[1,2]*

1 XinHua Hospital, Shanghai Jiaotong University School of Medicine, Shanghai, China, 2 MOE and Shanghai Key Laboratory of Children's Environmental Health, Shanghai, China

Abstract

Early detection is the most effective way to improve the clinical outcome of biliary atresia (BA). Emerging metabolomics provides a powerful platform for discovering novel biomarkers and biochemical pathways to improve early diagnosis. The aim of this study is to find the potential biomarkers to distinguish BA from neonatal hepatitis syndrome (NHS) by using a metabolomics method. We comprehensively analyzed the serum metabolites in a total of 124 blood samples from patients with BA or neonatal hepatitis syndrome (NHS) and from normal individuals using advanced metabolomic approaches, and found that the levels of glutarylcarnitine (C5DC) significantly increased in the BA group while the levels of threonine (Thr) significantly rose in the NHS group comparing with the other groups. The levels of glutamic acid (Glu) in the BA group were significantly elevated compared to those in the NHS group, but still lower than the hyperbilirubinemia and normal controls. The levels of propionyl carnitine (C3), isovaleryl carnitine (C5) and glutamine (Gln) were reduced in the BA group compared to those in the NHS group, but still higher than the hyperbilirubinemia and normal controls. This study demonstrates the possibility of metabolomics as non-invasive biomarkers for the early detection of BA and also provides new insight into pathophysiologic mechanisms for BA.

Editor: Jean-Marc A. Lobaccaro, Clermont Université, France

Funding: This work was supported by the Shanghai Natural Science Foundation (No. 11ZR1423800), the Program of "New One Hundred Talented People" of the Shanghai Jiaotong University School of Medicine, Science Foundation for The Excellent Youth Scholars of Xinhua Hospital (to Y. Zhang). The funders had no role in study design, data collection and analysis, decision to publish, or preparation of the manuscript.

* E-mail: zhangyongjun@sjtu.edu.cn

Introduction

Biliary atresia (BA) is one of the most serious hepatobiliary diseases during infantile period, accounting for about 75% of liver transplantations in children younger than 2 years [1]. The reported incidence of BA varies from 5/100,000 to 32/100,000 live births [2]. The etiology and pathogenesis of BA are largely unknown. Virus infection and autoimmune disorders are the two major theoretic mechanisms [3–6]. Since the Kasai procedure and liver transplantation have developed over the years, BA can be treated or cured. However, the better outcomes for infants depend on early diagnosis and timely Kasai portoenterostomy. It is generally known that children operated before day 60 achieve biliary drainage and stabilization in up to 80% of cases, while in patients operated only after day 90, the success rate decreases to 20% [7]. Therefore it is extremely important to differentiate BA from other causes of neonatal cholestatic jaundice promptly and accurately. However, besides BA, neonatal hepatitis syndrome (NHS) is another major cause of cholestatic jaundice in infants. The clinical manifestations and liver function test between the two diseases are too similar to distinguish. Up to date, there is still no accuracy investigation to diagnose BA. For example, the abdominal ultrasound of BA has a high specificity but low sensitivity, while the hepatobiliary scintigraphy (HBS) has a high sensitivity but low specificity [8,9]. The "gold standard" of diagnosing BA is liver biopsy, which is invasive. Therefore, more sensitive and specific biomarkers for the early diagnosis of BA are needed.

Metabonomics is concerned with the measurement of global sets of low molecular weight metabolites, which can be regarded as important indicators of various states of disease. Through analyzing and verifying the specific biomarkers of a disease, metabolomics enables us to better understand pathological processes, and substance metabolic pathways. Compared with traditional diagnostic methods, even small changes of metabolites can help to detect early pathologic changes more sensitively [10,11]. Its utility has been demonstrated by the identification of new biomarkers for Hepatocellular Carcinoma, Kidney Injury, and Alzheimer's disease [11–13].

Today, the improved efficiency and accuracy of metabolomic biomarkers and early diagnostic technologies have been increasingly used in a clinic setting. By applying advanced analytical and statistical tools, the "metabolome" is mined for biomarkers that are associated with the state of BA. It may help to understand the mechanism of BA occurrence and progression on the metabolic level and provide information for the identification of early and differential marker metabolites for BA. Thus, the aim of this study was to evaluate the usefulness of the metabolic alterations as a rapid metabolomics screening technique for BA. As such, the identification of serum biomarkers may provide useful information

Table 1. The scanning mass-to-charge ratio of amino acids and acyl carnitine.

Name	mass-to-charge ratio	Name	mass-to-charge ratio
Ala	m/z 146.1	Cit	m/z 232.1/m/z 113.1
D4-Ala	m/z 150.1	D2-Cit	m/z 234.2/m/z 115.2
Val	m/z 174.2	C0	m/z 218.2
D8-Val	m/z 182.2	D9-C0	m/z 227.2
Met	m/z 206.1	C2	m/z 260.2
D3-Met	m/z 209.1	D3-C2	m/z 263.2
Phe	m/z 222.2	C3	m/z 274.2
D5-Phe	m/z 227.2	D3-C3	m/z 277.2
Tyr	m/z 238.1	C4	m/z 288.2
C6-Tyr	m/z 244.1	D3-C4	m/z 291.2
Asp	m/z 246.2	C5	m/z 302.2
D3-Asp	m/z 249.2	D9-C5	m/z 311.2
Gly	m/z 132.1/m/z 76.1	C8	m/z 344.3
N1-C1-Gly	m/z 134.1/m/z 78.1	D3-C8	m/z 347.3
Orn	m/z 189.2/m/z 70.2	C14	m/z 428.4
D2-Orn	m/z 191.2/m/z 72.2	D9 -C14	m/z 437.4
Arg	m/z 231.2/m/z 70.2	C 16	m/z 456.4
D4-C1-Arg	m/z 236.2/m/z 75.1	D3-C16	m/z 469.4

for early diagnosis of BA, and effectively distinguish BA from other diseases such as NHS and hyperbilirubinemia.

Methods

Ethics and Clinical Populations

This study was a prospectively randomized controlled trial, whose design has been approved by the Ethical Committees of the Xinhua Hospital affiliated to Shanghai Jiaotong University School of Medicine. All parents or legal guardians signed an agreement after being disclosed to necessary information on this study.

From January 2008 to December 2011, a total of 61 cholestasis infants were included in the study and 32 hyperbilirubinemia infants and 31 normal infants as control. For all patients, serum alanine transaminase (ALT), aspartate transaminase (AST), total bilirubin (TB), direct bilirubin (DB), γ-glutamyl transpeptidase (γ-GT), total bile acid (TBA) and alkaline phosphatase (ALP) were measured. Four dried blood spots samples were obtained from infants by heel prick and spotted on filter paper [S&S 903# (CFH)] at the patients' first presentation to hospital and then stored at -20°C.

Cholestasis infants were defined as conjugated bilirubin more than 20% of the total bilirubin when the total bilirubin is 85 μmol/L or more and 17 μmol/L or more when the total bilirubin is 85 μmol/L or less [14]. First, history taking and physical examination of all patients were conducted carefully. And then they underwent differential diagnosis and etiologic work-up of cholestasis, including a complete blood count, virus biomarkers, serum-concentration of α_1-antitrypsin, blood tandem mass spectrometry and urine gas chromatography inspection as well as magnetic resonance cholangiopancreatography, abdominal ultrasound and HBS. In addition, specific biochemical tests were done as needed. For all, there were 45 cases suspicious for BA underwent intraoperative cholangiography and liver biopsy. And all of them had a 3 to 6 month clinical follow-up. Exclusion criteria: 1. Cholestasis infants with any family history such as progressive familial intrahepatic cholestasis, (PFIC), α_1-antitrypsin deficiency; 2. Cholestasis infants with other obvious accompany manifestation like endocrine disorders, chromosomal disorders and Alagille's syndrome. 3. Cholestasis infants with any amino, organic, and fatty acid disorders such as neonatal cholestasis induced by citrin deficiency (NICCD), tyrosinemia. Diagnostic criteria: 1.Hyperbilirubinemia group: Infants had a serum bilirubin up to 221 μmol/L or clinical jaundice appearing greater than 14 days of life with a conjugated bilirubin less than 20% of the total bilirubin. 2. Biliary atresia group: the confirmed diagnosis of BA was based on laparoscopy with surgical cholangiography and liver biopsy. The gallbladders or the remnants of gallbladders were found, but extrahepatic biliary duct could not be detected during the operation. And liver biopsy showed the typical histopathologic features, including bile duct proliferation, bile plugs, giant cell transformation, canalicular and cellular bile stasis and periportal fibrosis [15]. At last, 30 patients were identified as BA. 3. Neonatal hepatitis syndrome group: There were 15 infants who had undergone laparoscopy with surgical cholangiography and liver biopsy. During the operation all of them showed biliary tree and the giant cell transformation, inflammatory cell infiltration, and lobular disorganization on liver biopsy. They were finally diagnosed as NHS. Additionally, 16 patients recovered from jaundice and had the normalization of laboratory values during the clinical follow-up for about 3–6 months. So it was unnecessary to perform an intraoperative cholangiography. We confirmed these patients as idiopathic neonatal hepatitis. Finally, 30 cases of BA and 31 cases of NHS were enrolled in this study.

Samples Preparation

At the time of LC-MS/MS analysis, the frozen blood spots samples were thawed in normal atmospheric temperature. According to the previous report [16], three millimeter discs were punched and incubated in the methanolic internal standard solution (100 μL) for 20 min. The internal standards of amino acids and acylcarnitine were purchased from Cambridge Isotope Labs, USA. The concentrations of the deuterium-labeled internal standards per liter of methanol were as follows: [^{15}N,2-^{13}C$_1$]-glycine ([N1]-[C1]-Gly), 12.5 μmol/L; [^{2}H$_4$]- alanine([D4]-Ala), 2.5 μmol/L; [^{2}H$_8$]- valine ([D8]-Val), 2.5 μmol/L; [^{2}H$_3$]-leucine ([D3]-Leu), 2.5 μmol/L; [^{2}H$_3$]-methionine ([D3]-Met), 2.5 μmol/L; [^{2}H$_5$]-phenylalanine([D5]-Phe),2.5 μmol/L; [^{13}C$_6$]-tyrosine([C6]-Tyr), 2.5 μmol/L; [^{2}H$_3$]-aspartic acid ([D3]-Asp), 2.5 μmol/L; [^{2}H$_3$]-glutamic acid ([D3]-Glu), 2.5 μmol/L; [^{2}H$_2$]-ornithine ([D2]-Orn), 2.5 μmol/L; [^{2}H$_2$]-citrulline ([D2]-Cit), 2.5 μmol/L; [^{2}H$_4$-^{13}C$_1$]-arginine ([D4]-[C1]- Arg), 2.5 μmol/L; [^{2}H$_9$]-carnitine([D9]- C0), 0.76 μmol/L; [^{2}H$_3$]-acetylcarnitine([D3]-C2), 0.19 μmol/L; [^{2}H$_3$]-propionylcarnitine ([D3]-C3), 0.04 μmol/L; [^{2}H$_3$]-butyrylcarnitine([D3]-C4), 0.04 μmol/L; [^{2}H$_9$]-isovalerylcarnitine([D9]-C5), 0.04 μmol/L; [^{2}H$_3$]-octanoylcarnitine ([D3]-C8), 0.19 μmol/L; [^{2}H$_9$]-myristoylcarnitine([D9]-C14), 0.04 μmol/L; [^{2}H$_3$]-palmitoylcarnitine ([D3]-C16), 0.08 μmol/L. The diluted sample was then manually transferred to a 96 well polypropylene microtiter plate (membrane pore size 0.2/0.45 μm, Millipore Corporation, USA) and dried by a hot air blower (Dri-Block DB-30, Techne, Britain) at 55°C. Each diluted sample was placed in 65°C forced air oven for 15 min by the addition of 60 μl of n-butanol hydrochloride (3 mol/L), covered with a thin Teflon sheet. After the plate was removed from the oven, the hot air blower removed the butanol hydrochloride. The

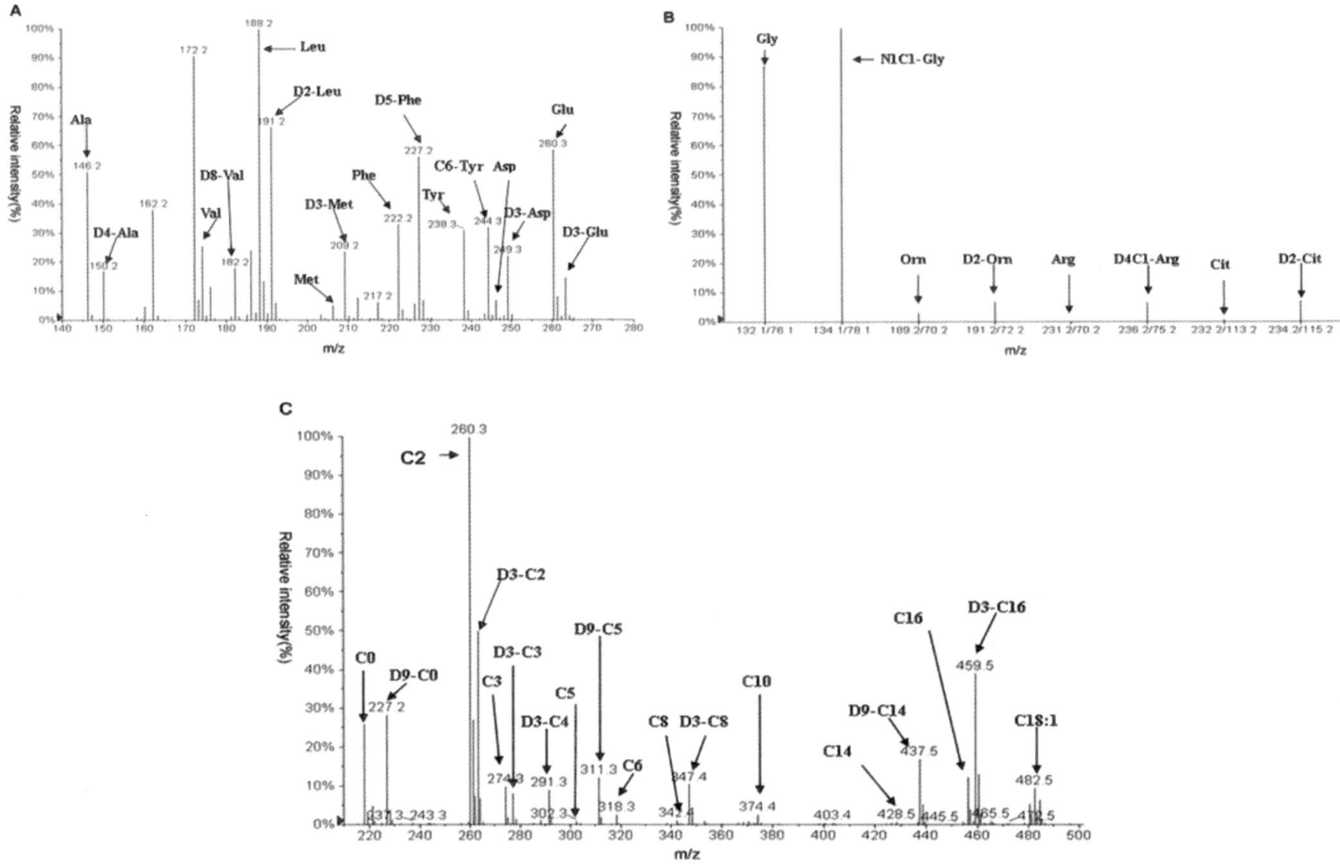

Figure 1. A typical LC-MS/MS spectrum of blood spots from patients. Blood samples were prepared and mass spectrometric analysis of individual sample was performed as described in "Methods" in details. Panel A shows a mass spectrum was acquired in the neutral loss scan mode. The scan was range from m/z 140 to m/z 280. It can detect most of the amino acids. Panel B shows a mass spectrum was acquired in the multiple reaction monitor mode. It was mainly used to detect Gly, Orn, Arg, Cit and its internal standard. Panel C shows a mass spectrum was acquired in precursor ion scanning mode. It used to detect the acylcarnitine in the sample.

butanol-derivatized samples were reconstituted with 100 μL of acetonitrile and water (80:20 by volume), and each plate was covered with aluminum foil. The samples were then ready for MS/MS analysis.

LC-MS/MS Measurements

An API Mass spectrometer 2000 (Applied Biosystems, USA) coupled with a HPLC system of Agilent 1000 (Agilent Technologies, USA) was used to detect amino acids and acylcarnitine in the samples. Twenty microliters of prepared sample and solvent were introduced by autosampler into MS1 of the API Mass spectrometer 2000. Mobile phase used 80% acetonitrile: water and quaternary pump were used to set flow speed: 140 μl/min, 0.2 min→30 μl/min,1 min→300 μl/min, 0.2 min. The obtained spectra of amino acids were analyzed with neutral loss scan (neutral loss fragment butyl formate, m/z102) and multiple reaction monitoring. Neutral loss scan range of m/z 140 to m/z 280 and multiple reaction monitoring were test for Gly, Orn, Arg, Cit and its internal standard. The obtained spectrum of acylcarnitine in every sample was using precursor ion scanning mode. The precursor ion scan range from m/z 210 to m/z 502 and the product ion fragment was m/z 85. Hexanoylcarnitine (C6) has no internal standards. As the mass to charge ratio of butyl-esterified C6 was 316.3, we detected it with D9-C5 quantitatively. The scan time of all the amino acids and acylcarnitine was set to 1.4 minutes and the each test sample would be detected with four minutes. The mass to charge ratio of all the amino acid and acylcarnitine was shown in Table 1 and the spectra were seen in Fig. 1.

Data Processing

The data were analyzed by Chem View b5, (U.S. Applied Biosystems), which was in-house analytical software in API 2000 MS. Based on a variety of amino acid ester and acylcarnitine and its isotopic ion peak intensity of the internal standard, this software enables peak identification and quantification using an in-house metabolite library. The markers were expressed as "concentration" or as a "ratio" and were exported in EXCEL format. The overall resultant data included 17 amino acids (Alanine [Ala], Aspartic acid [Asp], Glutamic acid [Glu], Methionine [Met], Phenylalanine [Phe], Tyrosine [Tyr], Leucine [Leu], Tryptophane [Trp], Valine [Val], Argnine [Arg], Citrulline [Cit], Glycine [Gly], Ornithine [Orn], Glutamine [Gln], Histidine [His], Serine [Ser], Threonine [Thr]) and 30 acylcarnitine concentrations (Free carnitine [C0], Acetyl carnitine [C2], Propionyl carnitine [C3], Malonyl carnitine [C3DC], Butyrylcholinesterase carnitine [C4], 3-hydroxybutyrate acyl carnitine [C4-OH], Succinic acid carnitine [C4DC], Isovaleryl carnitine [C5], Senecioyloxy carnitine [C5:1], 3-hydroxy-isovaleryl-carnitine [C5-OH], Glutaryl carnitine [C5DC], Hexanoyl carnitine [C6], Hexene acyl carnitine

Table 2. Comparison of clinical data among four groups.

Parameters	BA	NHS	Hyperbilirubinemia	Normal	Significance
N	30	31	32	31	
Male	17	21	14	15	N.S.1
Female	13	10	18	16	
Age at presentation(d)					
mean	58.5	54.8	11.1a	46.5	<0.052
sd	27.5	21.8	7.8	14.8	
range	25–120	25–150	3–38	19–81	
Weight at presentation (kg)					
mean	4.6	4.5	3.4 a	4.4	<0.052
sd	1.0	1.3	0.6	0.8	
TB(μmol/l)					
mean	163.0b	137.1b	283.2a	26.6	<0.052
sd	57.5	85.8	54.4	25.9	
DB(μmol/l)					
mean	112.9b	97.5b	19.8	6.4	<0.052
sd	39.0	64.1	16.0	4.8	
ALT(U/L)					
mean	150.8b	205.2b	16.2	23.1	<0.052
sd	87.6	122.9	7.0	9.8	
AST(U/L)					
mean	241.1b	286.0b	50.7	41.3	<0.052
sd	125.5	250.4	30.9	18.9	
γ-GT (U/L)					
mean	552.5c	277.0b	137.6	81.5	<0.052
sd	353.9	185.7	61.9	69.6	
TBA(μmol/l)					
mean	116.4b	139.5b	12.7	16.1	<0.052
sd	43.3	99.1	10.8	11.7	
ALP(U/L)					
mean	507.2b	567.9b	193.9	70.8	<0.052
sd	253. 5	224.5	63.7	12.7	

[1] χ2-test.
[2] one-way ANOVA followed by a LSD Test.
[a] Comparison vs normal group $p<0.05$.
[b] Comparison vs hyperbilirubinemia and normal group $p<0.05$.
[c] Comparison vs NHS group, hyperbilirubinemia and normal group $p<0.05$.

[C6:1], Adipic acid carnitine [C6DC], Octanoyl carnitine [C8], Octene carnitine [C8:1], Sim two acyl carnitine [C8DC], Kwai acyl carnitine [C10], Aoi enoyl-carnitine [C10:1], Lauroylcarnitine [C12], Myrcene carnitine [C12:1], Myristoyl carnitine [C14], Nutmeg enoyl-carnitine [C14:1], 3-hydroxy-myristoyl-carnitine [C14-OH], Palmitoyl carnitine [C16], Palm enoyl-carnitine [C16:1], 3-hydroxy-palmitoyl carnitine [C16-OH], Octadecadienoic acid carnitine [C18], Carnitine octadecene [C18:1], 3-hydroxy-octadecadienoic acid carnitine [C18-OH]) as well as 7 amino acid ratios (Arg/Orn, Cit/Arg, Orn/Cit, Met/Phe, Leu/Phe, Phe/Tyr, Gly/Phe) and 8 acylcarnitine ratios (C3/C0, C3/C2, C4/C2, C5/C2, C5-OH/C2, C5DC/C8, C8/C2, C14:1/C8:1).

Statistical Analysis

Orthogonal partial least squares discriminant analysis (OPLS-DA) was applied to analyze LC-MS spectral data by SIMCA-P+ (v12.0 version, Umetrics, Umeå, Sweden). The number of components for OPLS-DA models was auto-fitted using a cross validation. OPLS-DA, a supervised pattern recognition (PR) method, was conducted to maximize the difference between the BA and other groups. The variable importance for projection (VIP) score for each component was derived from the OPLS-DA analysis and served as an indication of contribution to the OPLS model. The quality of the models was assessed by a 10-fold cross-validation method. The obtained parameters R^2 stands for the total explained variation of the model and describes how well the derived model fit the data, and Q^2 represents the predictability of the model and provides a measure of the model quality. According to a greater-than-one threshold of VIP in the OPLS-DA model, a

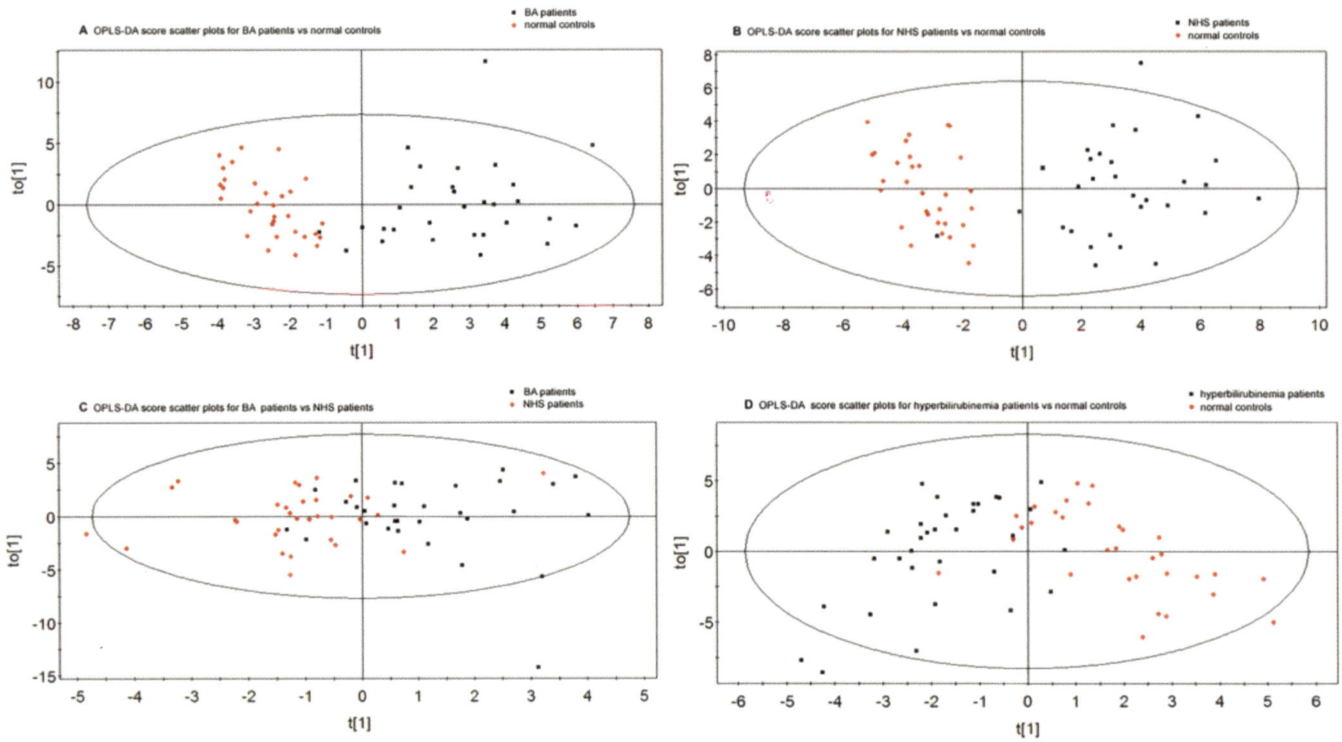

Figure 2. OPLS-DA score scatter plots obtained from of LCMS analysis of samples. A. OPLS-DA score plots of BA and normal; B. OPLS-DA score plots of with NHS and normal; C. OPLS-DA score plots of BA and NHS; D. OPLS-DA score plots of hyperbilirubinemia and normal. The fig. showing that the two populations are well separated respectively.

number of variables are responsible for the differences in the metabolic profiling between BA, INH, hyperbilirubinemia and normal groups. Variables that were normally distributed and had homogeneous variance were then analyzed by one-way ANOVA with a LSD test from SPSS Statistics 12.0 (SPSS, Chicago, IL, USA). We examined if different biomarker candidates obtained from the OPLS-DA models were statistically significant among the four groups at the univariate level. A p-value <0.05 (confidence level 95%) was considered statistically significant. Besides, other distributed data were also analyzed using one-way ANOVA followed by a LSD test by SPSS.

Table 3. Summary of statistical values of OPLS-DA with different scaling methods for data obtained from LC-MS analyses[a].

Comparison model	N	R^2X (cum)	R^2Y (cum)	Q^2 (cum)
BA vs normal group	61	0.486	0.769	0.619
NHS vs normal group	62	0.382	0.787	0.704
BA vs NHS	61	0.269	0.410	0.242
hyperbilirubinemia vs normal group	63	0.321	0.601	0.429

[a]Including the different cumulated modeled variations in X [R^2X(cum)] and Y [R^2Y(cum)] matrix on spectral datasets and predictability of the model [Q^2(cum)].

Results

Demographic Characteristics

There were a total of 124 patients including 67 boys and 57 girls with a mean age of 39.8±26.9 days and a mean weight of 4.3±1.1 kg. These infants were divided into four groups as described above. Table 2 shows clinical data including the patients' demographic information and serum liver function values. There was no apparent difference in the age of presentation, sex distribution and the liver function parameters including TB, DB, ALT, AST, TBA and ALP between NHS and BA groups. However, the γ-glutamyl transpeptidase (γ-GT) value was extremely higher in BA group than other groups.

Discovery and Identification of Metabolic Biomarkers

The LC-MS variables obtained from all subjects were used to construct an OPLS-DA model. In those four groups, we analyzed two sets of pair-wise data to identify the metabolic biomarkers to discriminate the BA and NHS groups. Fig. 2 show a clear separation between BA and normal group, NHS and normal group, BA and NHS group, hyperbilirubinemia and normal group. Table 3 indicates the performance parameters of the four models, suggesting that these models were reliable and highly predictive.

The VIP score for each compared model was generated for each OPLS-DA analysis. A VIP score >1.0 implied that the metabolite contributed significantly towards the differentiation of the two compared groups, shown in Fig. 3.

As shown in Fig. 3, from model A and model B, we obtained the specific metabolites of BA and NHS group, compared with the normal group respectively. From model C, we verified whether

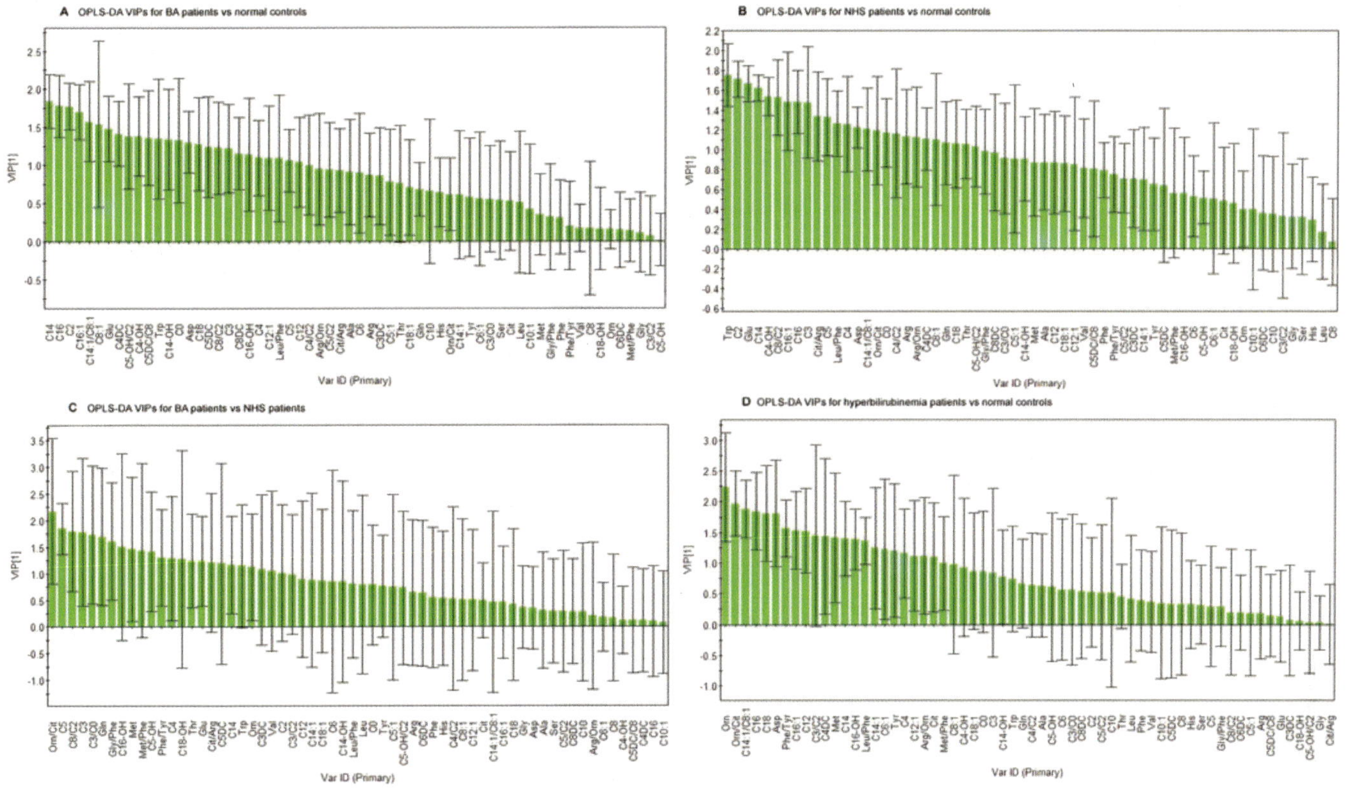

Figure 3. The amino acid and acylcarnitine with a VIP value above 1.0 were identified as markers to discriminate the two comparing group. The Variables were aligned in descending order of their VIP values. From model A and model B, we can obtain the identified metabolites of BA and NHS. From model C, we can verify these metabolites obtained above can distinguish BA from NHS. From model D, we can exclude the interference of metabolites in hyperbilirubinemia infants.

these metabolites obtained above could distinguish BA from NHS. And from model D, we excluded the interference of metabolites in hyperbilirubinemia infants. Finally, according to the criterion for VIP statistics (VIP>1), we obtained a total of nine metabolites for their most contribution in discriminating profiles between BA and NHS cohorts. Their VIPs were shown in Table 4. Then One-way analysis of variance (ANOVA) test by LSD was used to examine the statistical significance of these metabolites among the four groups. At last, six of which were detected with significant differences. (Table 5). The results suggest that the levels of C5DC significantly increased in the BA group, while in the NHS group, the levels of Thr significantly rose. The levels of Glu were significantly elevated in the BA group compared to those in the NHS group, but still lower than the hyperbilirubinemia and normal controls. The levels of C3, C5 and Gln in BA were significantly reduced compared to those in the NHS group, but still higher than those in the hyperbilirubinemia and normal controls.

Table 4. VIP value of the potential metabolites in the differences of NHS and BA[a].

Metabolites	BA vs normal group	NHS vs normal group
	VIP	VIP
C5DC	1.3	<1.0
Cit/Arg	<1.0	1.4
Gln	<1.0	1.1
Thr	<1.0	1.1
Glu	1.5	1.7
Trp	1.4	1.7
C2	1.7	1.7
C3	1.2	1.5
C5	1.1	1.3

[a]VIP: The variable importance for projection.

Discussion

Since the Kasai hepatoportoenterostomy has been evolving over the years, more and more studies have demonstrated that the earlier age at Kasai was a predictor of improved native liver survival and overall survival of BA [17,18]. But it is still difficult to differentiate BA from other causes of neonatal cholestatic jaundice especially the NHS. Because of limitations in conventional approaches, several noninvasive tests have been developed to facilitate such a diagnosis. With recent advances in metabonomics, serum metabolites could be used as a novel diagnostic indicator for disease [19].

Accruing evidence suggests that metabolic profiles are useful for identification of diagnostic biomarkers in BA. Zhou and Mushtaq have suggested that bile acids elevated in biliary atresia by comparing with other forms of cholestatic hepatobiliary diseases or neonatal jaundice group basing on tandem mass spectrometry [20,21]. In the future, we also intend to further investigate the

Table 5. Comparison of the potential metabolites in different groups by LSD post hoc analysis.

Metabolites	BA	NHS	Hyperbilirubinemia	Normal
C5DC (μmol/l)				
mean	0.06[a]	0.05	0.04	0.04
sd	0.02	0.02	0.01	0.01
C2(μmol/l)				
mean	22.94[b]	26.54[b]	12.70	11.61
sd	10.24	9.14	5.04	4.17
C3 (μmol/l)				
mean	2.68[a]	3.68[b]	1.17	1.49
sd	1.64	1.67	0.66	1.00
C5 (μmol/l)				
mean	0.12[a]	0.17[b]	0.08	0.09
sd	0.06	0.08	0.03	0.03
Cit/Arg				
mean	3.13[b]	2.23[b]	4.66	4.66
sd	2.67	1.20	2.13	2.06
Gln (μmol/l)				
mean	9.50[a]	12.33[b]	5.41	7.10
sd	4.44	3.93	5.61	5.54
Thr (μmol/l)				
mean	59.46	73.07[c]	50.96	46.61
sd	32.22	35.45	17.49	14.95
Glu (μmol/l)				
mean	204.62[a]	171.21[b]	279.32	282.56
sd	83.53	52.35	55.11	52.00
Trp (μmol/l)				
mean	43.47[b]	35.26[b]	68.37	63.93
sd	26.82	14.54	13.71	12.03

[a]Have a significant difference at $P<0.05$ compared to NHS group, hyperbilirubinemia and normal group.
[b]Have a significant difference at $P<0.05$ compared to hyperbilirubinemia and normal group.
[c]Have a significant difference at $P<0.05$ compared to BA group, hyperbilirubinemia and normal group.

metabolomics of amino acids and acylcarnitine profiles of BA. In this study, we attempted to identify sensitive and specific metabolites to distinguish BA form NHS based on LC/MS, which does not require the time-consuming derivatization procedure and is suitable for analysis of the metabolites compounds [22]. Because the symptoms of BA initially are indistinguishable from neonatal hyperbilirubinemia and later other symptoms like clay colored stools, dark urine, and large hardened liver are indistinguishable from NHS. We set both hyperbilirubinemia and NHS as the study groups.

In the previous studies, there were different amino acid and acylcarnitine metabolite profiles corresponding to the different forms of liver disease [11,23–27]. However there were only a few studies on BA using LC-MS-based metabonomic methods to investigate the acylcarnitine profiles. As generally known, carnitine plays an important role in fatty acid oxidation and energy production. It helps long-chain fatty acids to enter into the mitochondria for the purpose of β-oxidation and regulating the proportion and coenzyme A and acylcoenzyme A. The carnitine bound with acyl-CoA to form acylcarnitine, which help the elimination of organic acid. Animal experiments indicate that biliary export was a major route for acylcarnitine clearance and long-chain acyl-carnitine was hardly excreted through bile duct [28,29]. So short-chain carnitine are the mainly excretion of carnitine in the bile duct. Selimoglu MA et al reported that plasma carnitine levels were significantly increased in children with biliary atresia [23]. In this study, we also found that there was a set of short-chain carnitine metabolites elevating in the BA patients. Among them, the C5DC concentrations in BA were higher than the other three groups, and C2, C5 concentrations in BA are statistically lower than NHS group but still higher than hyperbilirubinemia and normal controls. The elevated glutaryl-carnitine (C5DC) suggested the deficient or nonfunctional of glutaryl-CoA dehydrogenase. And this was usually seen in the Glutaric aciduria type I disorder, acting as an important neurological dysfunction resembling an episode of encephalitis with movement disorders such as dystonia and/or dyskinesia [30]. However, in our study, the BA patients did not show such clinical onset, so the further mechanisms that lead to the pathophysiological changes are to be studied.

As the liver plays a central role in amino acid metabolism, it is of great importance to investigate the metabolite profiles in BA and NHS. From the liver function tests, we found that there was no significantly different elevation of serum ALT and AST in BA and NHS patients. However, there was a set of significantly different amino acids concentrations between BA and NHS.

Gln significantly increased while Glu significantly decreased in the serum of NHS patients compared with BA patients in our study. Coincidentally, these amino acids participate in the urea cycle and these changes suggest impairment in the urea cycle. Urea cycle describes the conversion reactions of ammonia into urea, which help the toxic ammonia removed from the body. A lot of reports on proteomic analysis of urea cycle revealed the regulation of urea cycle enzymes had dysfunction in the liver injury such as glutamine synthetase, glutamate dehydrogenase [31,32]. As a result, the decreased levels of Glu and increased levels of Gln were detected in serum of NHS patients. Besides, higher levels of Thr were also found in the NHS infants, presumably because of the activity of threonine-degrading enzymes decreased. Above all, these reactions mainly occur in the liver especially in mitochondria of liver cell. So this change reflects the different degree of liver cell injury. According to the previous study, the patients with hepatitis have oxidative stress, which plays a crucial role in the induction and progression of liver injury [33]. Oxidative stress produced by inflammation in the NHS infants appears to be more active than those in the BA infants and results in a more serious liver damage. Subsequently there was a different amino acids profile between the two groups.

The aim of this study was to discover new noninvasive biomarkers for BA. We quantitatively analyzed the metabolites from patients. Our results indicate that there is a metabolic profile shift of amino acid and acylcarnitine in BA from NHS. The alterations of these metabolites suggest different disturbances in metabolism between BA and NHS. They can be potentially developed into a clinically useful diagnostic tool for contributing towards an improved understanding of a disease mechanism.

Acknowledgments

We are grateful to Dr SL Tong for critical revision of the manuscript.

Author Contributions

Conceived and designed the experiments: YZ. Performed the experiments: DZ LH. Analyzed the data: DZ YZ ZH JZ. Contributed reagents/materials/analysis tools: DZ LH ZH JZ YZ. Wrote the paper: DZ YZ JZ.

References

1. Hartley JL, Davenport M, Kelly DA (2009) Biliary atresia. Lancet 374: 1704–1713.
2. Chardot C (2006) Biliary atresia. Orphanet J Rare Dis 1: 28.
3. Feldman AG, Mack CL (2012) Biliary atresia: cellular dynamics and immune dysregulation. Semin Pediatr Surg 21: 192–200.
4. Moore SW, Zabiegaj-Zwick C, Nel E (2012) Problems related to CMV infection and biliary atresia. S Afr Med J 102: 890–892.
5. Szavay PO, Leonhardt J, Czech-Schmidt G, Petersen C (2002) The role of reovirus type 3 infection in an established murine model for biliary atresia. Eur J Pediatr Surg 12: 248–250.
6. Mack CL, Feldman AG, Sokol RJ (2012) Clues to the etiology of bile duct injury in biliary atresia. Semin Liver Dis 32: 307–316.
7. Baumann U, Ure B (2012) Biliary atresia. Clin Res Hepatol Gastroenterol 36: 257–259.
8. Kianifar HR, Tehranian S, Shojaei P, Adinehpoor Z, Sadeghi R, et al. (2013) Accuracy of hepatobiliary scintigraphy for differentiation of neonatal hepatitis from biliary atresia: systematic review and meta-analysis of the literature. Pediatr Radiol.43: 905–919.
9. Yang JG, Ma DQ, Peng Y, Song L, Li CL (2009) Comparison of different diagnostic methods for differentiating biliary atresia from idiopathic neonatal hepatitis. Clin Imaging 33: 439–446.
10. Dutta M, Joshi M, Srivastava S, Lodh I, Chakravarty B, et al. (2012) A metabonomics approach as a means for identification of potential biomarkers for early diagnosis of endometriosis. Mol Biosyst 8: 3281–3287.
11. Wang X, Zhang A, Sun H (2013) Power of metabolomics in diagnosis and biomarker discovery of hepatocellular carcinoma. Hepatology 57: 2072–2077.
12. Han X, Rozen S, Boyle SH, Hellegers C, Cheng H, et al. (2011) Metabolomics in early Alzheimer's disease: identification of altered plasma sphingolipidome using shotgun lipidomics. PLoS One 6: e21643.
13. Noto A, Cibecchini F, Fanos V, Mussap M (2013) NGAL and metabolomics: the single biomarker to reveal the metabolome alterations in kidney injury. Biomed Res Int 2013: 612032.
14. Moyer V, Freese DK, Whitington PF, Olson AD, Brewer F, et al. (2004) Guideline for the evaluation of cholestatic jaundice in infants: recommendations of the North American Society for Pediatric Gastroenterology, Hepatology and Nutrition. J Pediatr Gastroenterol Nutr 39: 115–128.
15. Esmaili J, Izadyar S, Karegar I, Gholamrezanezhad A (2007) Biliary atresia in infants with prolonged cholestatic jaundice: diagnostic accuracy of hepatobiliary scintigraphy. Abdom Imaging 32: 243–247.
16. Zytkovicz TH, Fitzgerald EF, Marsden D, Larson CA, Shih VE, et al. (2001) Tandem mass spectrometric analysis for amino, organic, and fatty acid disorders in newborn dried blood spots: a two-year summary from the New England Newborn Screening Program. Clin Chem 47: 1945–1955.
17. Jimenez-Rivera C, Jolin-Dahel KS, Fortinsky KJ, Gozdyra P, Benchimol EI (2013) International incidence and outcomes of biliary atresia. J Pediatr Gastroenterol Nutr 56: 344–354.
18. Shneider BL, Brown MB, Haber B, Whitington PF, Schwarz K, et al. (2006) A multicenter study of the outcome of biliary atresia in the United States, 1997 to 2000. J Pediatr 148: 467–474.
19. Zhang A, Sun H, Wang X (2012) Serum metabolomics as a novel diagnostic approach for disease: a systematic review. Anal Bioanal Chem 404: 1239–1245.
20. Zhou K, Lin N, Xiao Y, Wang Y, Wen J, et al. (2012) Elevated bile acids in newborns with Biliary Atresia (BA). PLoS One 7: e49270.
21. Mushtaq I, Logan S, Morris M, Johnson AW, Wade AM, et al. (1999) Screening of newborn infants for cholestatic hepatobiliary disease with tandem mass spectrometry. BMJ 319: 471–477.
22. Xu F, Zou L, Liu Y, Zhang Z, Ong CN (2011) Enhancement of the capabilities of liquid chromatography-mass spectrometry with derivatization: general principles and applications. Mass Spectrom Rev 30: 1143–1172.
23. Selimoglu MA, Aydogdu S, Yagci RV, Huseyinov A (2001) Plasma and liver carnitine status of children with chronic liver disease and cirrhosis. Pediatr Int 43: 391–395.
24. Kalhan SC, Guo L, Edmison J, Dasarathy S, McCullough AJ, et al. (2011) Plasma metabolomic profile in nonalcoholic fatty liver disease. Metabolism 60: 404–413.
25. Zhang A, Sun H, Han Y, Yan G, Wang X (2013) Urinary metabolic biomarker and pathway study of hepatitis B virus infected patients based on UPLC-MS system. PLoS One 8: e64381.
26. Ressom HW, Xiao JF, Tuli L, Varghese RS, Zhou B, et al. (2012) Utilization of metabolomics to identify serum biomarkers for hepatocellular carcinoma in patients with liver cirrhosis. Anal Chim Acta 743: 90–100.
27. Byrd DJ, Wiltfang A, Rodeck B, Latta A, Burdelski M, et al. (1993) The plasma amino acid profile and its relationships to standard quantities of liver function in infants and children with extrahepatic biliary atresia and preterminal liver cirrhosis. Eur J Clin Chem Clin Biochem 31: 197–204.
28. Krahenbuhl S, Brass EP, Hoppel CL (2000) Decreased carnitine biosynthesis in rats with secondary biliary cirrhosis. Hepatology 31: 1217–1223.
29. Ramsay RR, Gandour RD, van der Leij FR (2001) Molecular enzymology of carnitine transfer and transport. Biochim Biophys Acta 1546: 21–43.
30. Couce ML, Lopez-Suarez O, Boveda MD, Castineiras DE, Cocho JA, et al. (2013) Glutaric aciduria type I: outcome of patients with early- versus late-diagnosis. Eur J Paediatr Neurol 17: 383–389.
31. Fleming KE, Wanless IR (2013) Glutamine synthetase expression in activated hepatocyte progenitor cells and loss of hepatocellular expression in congestion and cirrhosis. Liver Int 33: 525–534.
32. Antoine DJ, Dear JW, Starkey-Lewis P, Platt V, Coyle J, et al. (2013) Mechanistic biomarkers provide early and sensitive detection of acetaminophen-induced acute liver injury at first presentation to hospital. Hepatology. 58: 777–787.
33. Soga T, Sugimoto M, Honma M, Mori M, Igarashi K, et al. (2011) Serum metabolomics reveals gamma-glutamyl dipeptides as biomarkers for discrimination among different forms of liver disease. J Hepatol 55: 896–905.

7

Role of Docosahexaenoic Acid Treatment in Improving Liver Histology in Pediatric Nonalcoholic Fatty Liver Disease

Valerio Nobili[1]¶, Guido Carpino[2]¶, Anna Alisi[1], Rita De Vito[3], Antonio Franchitto[4,5], Gianfranco Alpini[6], Paolo Onori[4], Eugenio Gaudio[4]*

1 Unit of Liver Research, Bambino Gesù Children's Hospital, Rome, Italy, **2** Department of Movement, Human and Health Sciences, University of Rome "Foro Italico", Rome, Italy, **3** Unit of Pathology, Bambino Gesù Children's Hospital, Rome, Italy, **4** Department of Anatomical, Histological, Forensic Medicine and Orthopedics Sciences, Sapienza University of Rome, Rome, Italy, **5** Eleonora Lorillard Spencer-Cenci Foundation, Rome, Italy, **6** Department of Medicine, Scott & White and Texas A&M Health Science Center College of Medicine, Temple, Texas, United States of America

Abstract

Introduction: Nonalcoholic fatty liver disease (NAFLD) is one of the most important causes of liver-related morbidity and mortality in children. Recently, we have reported the effects of docosahexaenoic acid (DHA), the major dietary long-chain polyunsaturated fatty acids, in children with NAFLD. DHA exerts a potent anti-inflammatory activity through the G protein-coupled receptor (GPR)120. Our aim was to investigate in pediatric NAFLD the mechanisms underlying the effects of DHA administration on histo-pathological aspects, GPR120 expression, hepatic progenitor cell activation and macrophage pool.

Patients and Methods: 20 children with untreated NAFLD were included. Children were treated with DHA for 18 months. Liver biopsies before and after the treatment were analyzed. Hepatic progenitor cell activation, macrophage pool and GPR120 expression were evaluated and correlated with clinical and histo-pathological parameters.

Results: GPR120 was expressed by hepatocytes, liver macrophages, and hepatic progenitor cells. After DHA treatment, the following modifications were present: i) the improvement of histo-pathological parameters such as NAFLD activity score, ballooning, and steatosis; ii) the reduction of hepatic progenitor cell activation in correlation with histo-pathological parameters; iii) the reduction of the number of inflammatory macrophages; iv) the increase of GPR120 expression in hepatocytes; v) the reduction of serine-311-phosphorylated nuclear factor kappa B (NF-κB) nuclear translocation in hepatocytes and macrophages in correlation with serum inflammatory cytokines.

Conclusions: DHA could modulate hepatic progenitor cell activation, hepatocyte survival and macrophage polarization through the interaction with GPR120 and NF-κB repression. In this scenario, the modulation of GPR120 exploits a novel crucial role in the regulation of the cell-to-cell cross-talk that drives inflammatory response, hepatic progenitor cell activation and hepatocyte survival.

Editor: Frances M. Sladek, Univeristy of California Riverside, United States of America

Funding: Grant support: E. Gaudio was supported by research project grant from the University "Sapienza" of Rome, FIRB grant # RBAP10Z7FS_001 and by PRIN grant # 2009X84L84_001. The funders had no role in study design, data collection and analysis, decision to publish, or preparation of the manuscript.

* E-mail: eugenio.gaudio@uniroma1.it

¶ These authors contributed equally to this work.

Introduction

Nonalcoholic fatty liver disease (NAFLD) is one of the most important causes of liver-related morbidity and mortality in children [1]. NAFLD includes a spectrum of diseases ranging from simple fatty liver to nonalcoholic steatohepatitis (NASH). NASH development in children is characterized by intricate interactions between resident and recruited cells that enable liver damage progression [1,2]. Interestingly, we demonstrated that hepatic stem/progenitor cells (HPCs) may be involved in the response of the liver to oxidative stress in pediatric NAFLD, and their activation was correlated with fibrosis and NASH [3].

Recently, there has been growing interest in N-3 long-chain polyunsaturated fatty acids (LC-PUFA) supplementation as potential treatment for liver steatosis [4,5]. The problems of adherence to lifestyle interventions to achieve sustainable weight loss especially in children, and side-effects with pharmacological agents make of dietary fish oil supplementation a simple and practical alternative therapy. Fish oil provides a convenient source of essential N-3 LC-PUFA with few side effects and may directly reduce hepatic lipogenesis and steatosis [5–7]. We have recently reported the short-term (6 months) and long-term (up to 24 months) effects of docosahexaenoic acid (DHA), the major dietary N-3 LC-PUFA, after 6, 12, 18 and 24 months of treatment with different concentrations (DHA 250 mg/day and DHA 500 mg/day) combined with diet and exercise [8,9]. In these studies, algae DHA supplementation improved liver steatosis in children with NAFLD and was able to reduce the levels of serum ALT and triglycerides [8,9].

DHA exerts a potent anti-inflammatory activity through the G protein-coupled receptor GPR120 [10]; dietary DHA suppresses hepatic markers of oxidative stress, inflammation and fibrosis [11]. However, its effects on histo-pathological features, as well as its cellular and molecular mechanisms in pediatric NAFLD remain to be established.

The aim of this study was to investigate the mechanisms underlying the effects of DHA administration in pediatric NAFLD (pNAFLD) on histo-pathological aspects, GPR120 expression, Macrophage (MΦ)/Kupffer cell(KC) polarization and HPC activation.

Patients and Methods

Ethics Statement

The study protocol conformed to the ethical guidelines of the 1975 Declaration of Helsinki. The study was approved by the local ethics committee (Bambino Gesù Children's Hospital IRCCS, Rome, Italy). A written informed consent was obtained from the next of kin, caretakers, or guardians on behalf of the children enrolled in this study.

Patients, Anthropometrics and Laboratory Data

The study was performed on 20 patients from the randomised controlled clinical trial registered on http://www.clinicaltrials.gov (Trial identifier NCT00885313) conducted at the Liver Unit of the Bambino Gesù Pediatric Hospital (Rome, Italy). For the patients enrolment the entry criteria were: persistently elevated serum alanine transaminase (ALT ≥40 U/l), diffusely hyperechogenic liver at ultrasonography and liver biopsy consistent with NAFLD. Furthermore, patients with secondary causes of steatosis, including alcohol abuse (≥140 g/week), total parenteral nutrition, drugs, hepatitis A, B, C, cytomegalovirus, Epstein-Barr virus infections, autoimmune liver disease, metabolic liver diseases, Wilson's disease, and alpha-1-antitrypsin deficiency were excluded from the trial. The children included in our analyses showed clinical and pathological features resembling those seen in our general pediatric population with NAFLD [12].

These patients were diagnosed with NAFLD through liver biopsy recommended because of persistently (>6 months) elevated ALT levels and the presence of an echogenic texture of the liver on ultrasonography. Furthermore, the patients received no dietary or other therapeutic treatment regimens before diagnosis.

The clinical indication for biopsy was either to assess the presence of NASH and the degree of fibrosis or to diagnose other likely independent or competing liver diseases. Liver biopsy was performed after an overnight fast by using an automatic core biopsy 18-gauge needle under general anesthesia and ultrasound guidance. Two biopsies passing within different liver segments were performed for each subject.

Patients were treated with DHA 250 mg/day (39% DHA oil obtained from Schyzochitrium, Martek Biosciences Corporation, Columbia, MD, USA). Liver biopsy was performed after 18 months of treatment.

Liver specimens from 6 lean, non-diabetic children (boys, 4; girls, 2; median age: 13 years, range, 12–16 years) without liver disease were used as controls. Control liver fragments were obtained from patients who underwent laparotomy or laparoscopic procedures (for cholecystectomy), from liver donors (orthotopic liver transplantation) or incidental "normal" liver biopsies (children exhibiting persistent/intermittent elevations of liver enzymes for >6 months).

Weight, height, and body mass index (BMI) were measured [12]. Alanine and aspartate aminotransferase, gamma-glutamyl-transpeptidase, total triglycerides and total cholesterol were evaluated using standard laboratory methods. Insulin was measured using a radio-immunoassay (Myria Technogenetics, Milan, Italy). Glucose and insulin were measured at 0, 30, 60, 90 and 120 minutes of an oral glucose tolerance test performed with 1.75 grams of glucose per kilogram of body weight (up to 75 g). The degree of insulin resistance and sensitivity was determined by the homeostatic model assessment insulin resistance (HOMA-IR), and the insulin sensitivity index (ISI) derived from an oral glucose tolerance test (OGGT), respectively. Data at baseline and after 18 month of treatment were acquired.

Liver Ultrasonography

Liver ultrasonography was performed by an experienced radiologist using an Acuson Sequoia C512 scanner equipped with a 15L8 transducer (Universal Diagnostic Solutions, Oceanside, CA). Steatosis has been graded by a validated score [13]. Absent steatosis (grade 0) was defined as normal liver echo-texture; mild steatosis (grade 1) as slight and diffuse increase in fine parenchymal echoes with normal visualization of diaphragm and portal vein borders; moderate steatosis (grade 2) as moderate and diffuse increase in fine echoes with slightly impaired visualization of diaphragm and portal vein borders; and severe steatosis (grade 3) as fine echoes with poor or no visualization of diaphragm, portal vein borders and posterior portion of the right lobe.

Histopathology, Immunohistochemistry (IHC) and Immunofluorescence (IF)

Steatosis, inflammation, hepatocyte ballooning and fibrosis were scored using the NAFLD Clinical Research Network (CNR) criteria [14]. Steatosis, lobular inflammation, and hepatocyte ballooning were combined to obtain the NAFLD activity score (NAS). A microscopic diagnosis based on overall injury pattern (steatosis, hepatocyte ballooning, inflammation) as well as the presence of additional lesions (e.g. zonality of lesions, portal inflammation and fibrosis) has been assigned to each case [15]. Accordingly, biopsies were classified into: not steatohepatitis (not-SH), definite steatohepatitis (definite-SH), borderline zone 1 pattern or borderline zone 3 pattern subcategories [15]. PNHS, a more adequate score for pNAFLD [16], was also calculated. Histological analysis was performed by a single pathologist blinded to clinical and laboratory data.

For IHC and IF, sections were incubated overnight at 4°C with primary antibodies against cytokeratin (CK)7 (Dako, mouse monoclonal, code: M7018, dilution: 1:100), EpCAM (Dako, mouse monoclonal, code: M3525, dilution: 1:100), CD68 (Dako, mouse monoclonal, code: M0876, dilution: 1:100), GPR120 (Sigma-Aldrich, rabbit polyclonal, code: HPA-042563, dilution: 1:30), and serine-311-phosphorylated NF-κB (p-65NF-κB) purchased from Santa Cruz Biotechnology (goat polyclonal, code: sc-33039-R, dilution 1:50). For IHC, samples were than incubated for 20 minutes at room temperature with secondary biotinylated antibody and, successively, with streptavidin-Horse radish peroxidase (LSAB+, Dako, code K0690). Diaminobenzidine (Dako, code K3468) was used as the substrate and the sections were counterstained with hematoxylin. For double IF staining, non-specific protein binding was blocked with 5% normal goat serum. After the incubation with primary antibodies, specimens were washed and incubated for 1 h with labeled isotype-specific secondary antibodies (anti-mouse AlexaFluor-488 and anti-rabbit Alexafluor-564, Invitrogen) and counterstained with 4,6-diamidino-2-phenylindole (DAPI) for visualization of cell nuclei. For all immunoreactions, negative controls (the primary antibody was replaced with pre-immune serum) were also included [17].

Sections were examined with a Leica Microsystems DM 4500 B Microscopy (Weltzlar, Germany) equipped with a Jenoptik Prog Res C10 Plus Videocam (Jena, Germany). Only biopsies containing at least 5 portal spaces were considered [18].

The ductular reaction (DR) extension was evaluated on liver section stained for CK7. Slides were scanned and processed by a digital scanner (Aperio Scanscope CS System, Aperio Technologies, Inc). The virtual slide have been visualized and processed by the software included in the Aperio Scanscope CS System (ImageScope). An image analysis algorithm, that automatically analyzes, the digital slides has been used to quantify the area occupied by CK7 positive cells. The algorithm was applied on the entire sections. The extent of DR was expressed as the percentage of the parenchymal area occupied by reactive ductules [19]. Solitary CK7-positive HPCs or those in small clumps that were localized in the parenchyma or at the portal interface were included in these counts because they should be considered as a histological sectioning of bile/reactive ductules through a transverse plane without any unique immunohistochemical markers to distinguish them from cells within bile/reactive ductules [19]. Cholangiocytes lining the interlobular bile ducts were excluded from the counts.

The activation of HPC compartment was evaluated by counting the number of EpCAM-positive cells within the bile/reactive ductules and expressed as number of positive cells per high power field (HPF: at 40×) [20].

Intermediate hepatocytes (IHs) were defined as cells with sizes between those of hepatocytes and HPCs (<40 but >6 μm in diameter), with faint CK-7 immunoreactivity in the cytoplasm and reinforcement at the plasma membrane7. The presence of IHs was scored as reported elsewhere: 0 = no IH, 1 = single occasional IHs and 2 = clusters of His [21].

GPR120 expression by EpCAM-positive HPCs or CD68-positive macrophages was evaluated in serial sections and by double IF. The number of positive macrophages per HPF was calculated. GPR120 expression by hepatocytes and HPCs was semi-quantitatively scored [22]. The nuclear expression of p-65NF-κB was calculated counting the number of MΦ/KC or hepatocytes with positive nuclei. Data were expressed as a percentage of positive cells. At least 30 lobular fields at 40× magnification were analyzed for each section [3].

Cytokine Assay

Serum levels of pro-inflammatory cytokines were determined using cytokine-specific ELISA assays. Concentrations were evaluated by manufacturing protocols from RayBiotech Inc (Norcross GA, USA) for IL-1β and IL-6 and from Immundiagnostik (AG, Bensheim, Germany) for tumour necrosis factor (TNF)-α.

Statistical Methods

Data are indicated as mean±standard deviation (SD). The Student t test or Mann–Whitney U test was used to determine differences between groups for normally or not normally distributed data, respectively. To evaluate the modification of variables after DHA treatment, the paired-samples T Test was applied. The Pearson correlation coefficient or the Spearman nonparametric correlation were used. A p-value of <0.05 was considered statistically significant. Analyses were performed using SPSS software.

Results

Clinical and Histological Data

We evaluated 20 patients enrolled in the aforementioned trial before and after DHA-250 treatment (18 months) [8]. With regard to anthropometric and laboratory data (**Table 1**), total triglycerides, ALT, AST and ISI were significantly reduced after DHA treatment while no differences were found in BMI, GGT, total cholesterol, basal glycemia and insulinemia and HOMA-IR. Finally, the steatosis grade assessed by liver ultrasonography was strongly ameliorated after DHA treatment (p<0.001). Serum levels of pro-inflammatory cytokines (IL-1β, IL-6 and TNF-α) were significantly reduced after DHA treatment.

Before the treatment, the biopsies were classified in accordance to the NASH CNR criteria [14,23], into 4 distinct groups (**Supplementary Figure 1**): not-SH (N = 3), definite-SH or NASH (N = 12), borderline zone1 pattern (N = 1), and borderline zone3 pattern (N = 4). NAS scores ranged from 1 to 7. PNHS scores ranged from 1.60 to 100. Fibrosis of some degree was seen in all biopsy samples: stage 1c in 9 samples, stage 2 in 10, and stage 3 in 1. Control biopsy samples had normal histological features.

After the treatment with DHA, the classification of biopsies indicated a decrease of definite-SH or NASH diagnosis (N = 3) and an increase of not-SH diagnosis (N = 15).

Moreover, NAS (t = 5.69; p<0.001), PNHS score (t = 2.61; p<0.05), steatosis (t = 4.86; p<0.001), ballooning (t = 5.34; p<0.001) and lobular inflammation (t = 2.35; p<0.05) were significantly reduced (**Table 2**), while no differences were found in fibrosis.

Table 1. Anthropometric and laboratory parameters of the study-population.

	Before DHA Treatment	After DHA treatment	Paired-samples T Test (p-value)
Sex (M/F)	11/9	11/9	–
Age (years)	10.1±2.0	12.3±2.0	<0.001*
Weight (kg)	57.1±9.9	59.8±9.9	<0.001*
Height (cm)	151±17	165±16	<0.001*
BMI (kg/m2)	26.1±2.5	25.63±2.2	0.072
Cholesterol (mg/dL)	172.1±11.2	169.6±12.9	0.729
Triglycerides (mg/dL)	91.9±30.1	78.8±17.7	0.048*
ALT (U/L)	65.4±21.3	38.9±6.2	0.001*
AST (U/L)	50.0±15.7	35.4±5.8	0.007*
GGT (U/L)	21.3±5.6	19.1±3.1	0.204
Glucose (mg/dL)	84.9±6.7	86.6±3.7	0.328
Insulin (μU/mL)	14.7±8.1	12.0±4.8	0.057
HOMA-IR	3.1±1.8	2.5±1.0	0.089
ISI	3.0±0.5	3.4±0.5	0.038*
TNF-alpha (pg/mL)	19.85±3.32	5.89±2.09	<0.001*
IL-6 (pg/mL)	12.55±1.32	5.85±2.23	<0.001*
IL-1B (pg/mL)	25.10±1.46	8.87±2.86	<0.001*
US	2.6±0.5	1.3±0.6	<0.001*

Data are reported as Means ± SD * = p<0.05.

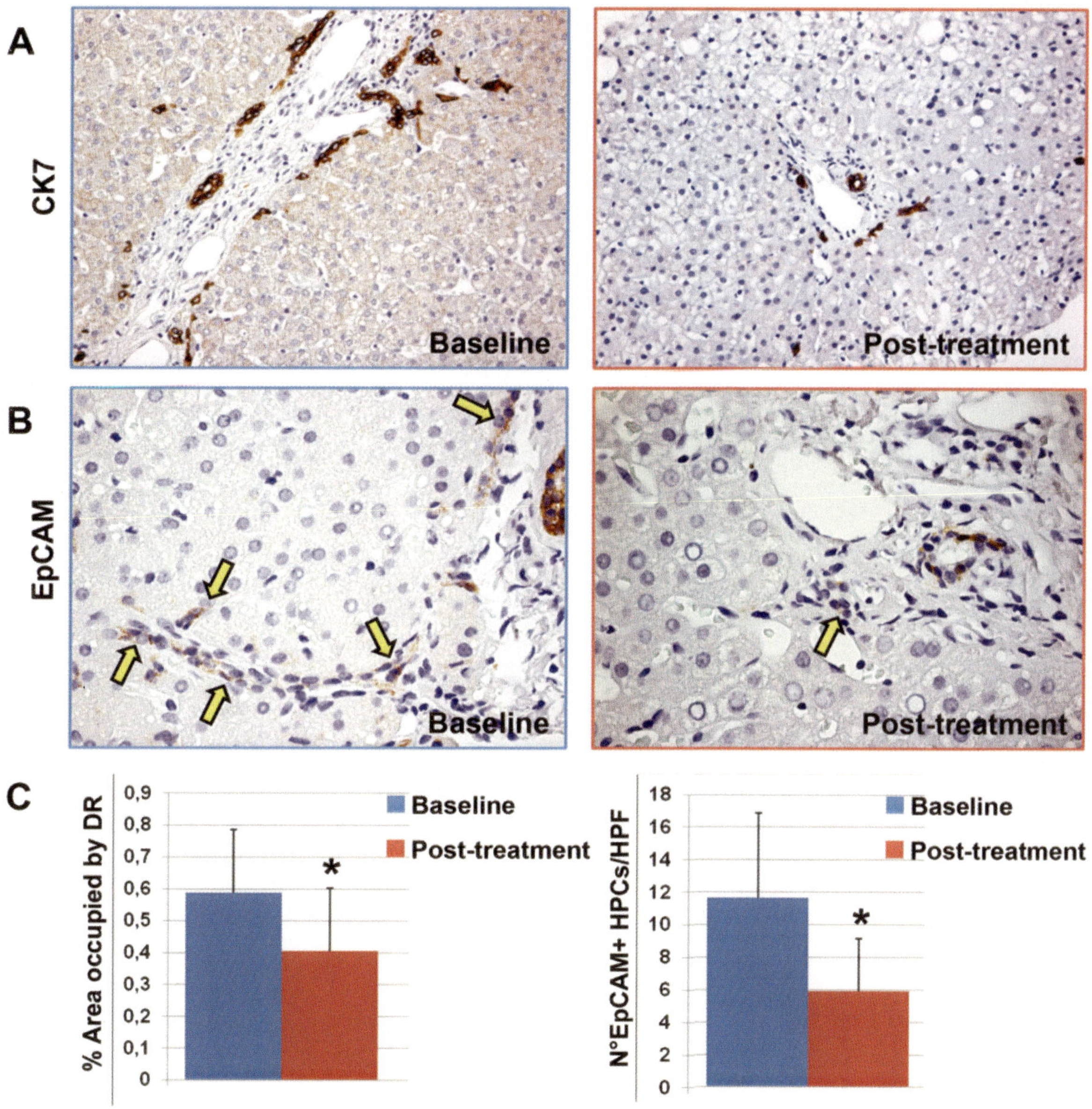

Figure 1. Immunohistochemistry for Cytokeratin(CK) 7 and EpCAM in liver biopsies of pediatric NAFLD patients. A) at the beasline, pediatric NAFLD biopsies were characterized by a prominent expansion of hepatic progenitor cell (HPC) pool and the presence of reactive ductules at the periphery of portal spaces. After DHA treatment, a minimal involvement of the HPC compartment was present. Original magnification 20×. B) EpCAM-positive HPCs (arrows) were significant reduced by DHA treatment in comparison with the biopsies at the baseline. Original magnification 40×. C) Histograms show the reduction of HPC expansion (ductular reaction extension) and activation (number of EpCAM+ cells) after DHA treatment. Data are shown as Means ± Standard Deviation. * = $p<0.05$.

Effect of DHA Treatment on HPCs in pNAFLD Biopsy Samples

Before treatment, the pNAFLD biopsy samples showed an expanded DR (0.59±0.20) compared with those of normal livers (0.21±0.07, $p<0.01$). After DHA treatment, the DR expansion was reduced when a test for paired samples was applied ($t = 3.521$, $p<0.01$; **Figure 1A/C**). Moreover, DR was correlated with NAS ($r = 0.458$; $p<0.05$) and PNHS scores ($r = 0.478$; $p<0.05$) and with ballooning ($r = 0.526$; $p<0.05$) but not with fibrosis, hepatic steatosis or lobular inflammation.

Then, we evaluated the number of EpCAM-positive cells per HPF (**Figure 1B/C**). EpCAM is considered a specific marker of activated HPCs and several lines of evidence indicated that EpCAM expression is tightly regulated and only occurs in case of a temporary need for proliferation and is immediately down-regulated upon terminal differentiation [24,25]. Before treatment, pNAFLD biopsy samples showed an expanded number of EpCAM-positive HPCs (11.64±5.24) compared with those of normal livers (3.54±1.15; $p<0.01$). After DHA treatment, the number of EpCAM-positive HPCs was statistically reduced when a test for paired samples was applied ($t = 4.102$, $p<0.01$). Consistently, the number of EpCAM-positive HPCs was strictly correlated with the extension of DR ($r = 0.625$; $p<0.01$). Moreover, the number of EpCAM-positive HPCs was strictly correlated with NAS ($r = 0.606$; $p<0.01$) and PNHS scores ($r = 0.595$; $p<0.01$), with hepatic steatosis ($r = 0.499$; $p<0.05$)

Table 2. Histo-pathologic evaluation of the study-population.

	Before DHA Treatment	After DHA treatment	Paired-samples T Test (p-value)
Steatosis	1.70±1.08	0.50±0.61	<0.001
Ballooning	0.85±0.67	0.25±0.44	<0.001
Lobular inflammation	1.15±0.59	0.85±0.37	<0.05
NAS	3.70±1.78	1.60±1.05	<0.01
PNHS	71.31±40.84	5.8±8.3	<0.05
Fibrosis	1.60±0.60	1.45±0.76	=0.481

Data are reported as Means ± SD.

and ballooning ($r = 0.683$; $p = 0.01$) but not with fibrosis or lobular inflammation. Taking in account the diagnostic categories, the number of EpCAM-positive HPCs was significantly lower in not-SH in comparison with biopsies with definite-SH diagnosis ($t = 2.704$; $p<0.02$).

As regard clinical parameters, DR extension and the number of EpCAM-positive HPCs were correlated with ALT ($r = 0.467$; $p< 0.05$ and $r = 0.657$; $p<0.01$, respectively) and with the steatosis grade assessed by liver ultrasonography ($r = 0.490$; $p<0.05$ and $r = 0.632$; $p<0.01$, respectively).

GPR120 Expression and its Correlation with Histo-pathological Parameters

In liver biopsies, GPR120 was expressed by hepatocytes, cholangiocytes, HPCs and MΦ/KC pool as seen both in IHC sections and through double IF with specific cell markers (**Figures 2, 3**).

GPR120 was also expressed by HPCs as shown in serial sections and in double IF staining (**Figure 2A/B**). No significant differences were found comparing pNAFLD biopsies before and after DHA treatment. However, considering all pNAFLD biopsy samples, the overall GPR120 expression by HPCs was inversely correlated with the presence of intermediate hepatocytes ($r = -0.496$, $p<0.05$), NAS score ($r = -0.501$, $p<0.05$) and steatosis ($r = -0.575$, $p = 0.01$).

With regard GPR120 expression in hepatocytes (**Figure 2C**), a higher expression of GPR120 was observable (2.33±0.88) in biopsies after DHA treatment when compared with pre-treatment biopsies (1.58±1.08; $t = -3.00$; $p<0.05$). Moreover, when the diagnostic categories were taken in account, the number of GPR120 expression in hepatocytes was significantly higher in not-SH in comparison with biopsies with definite-SH diagnosis ($t = -2.223$; $p<0.05$). In addition, the expression of GPR120 by hepatocytes was correlated with basal glycemia ($r = -0.505$, $p< 0.05$).

The number of GPR120-positive MΦ/KC has been evaluated in IHC sections and by double IF with the specific marker, CD68 (**Figure 3**). CD68 clearly and specifically recognized MΦ/KC in liver sinusoids but was consistently negative in other liver cells.

Evaluation of GPR120 expression showed that the number of MΦ/KC expressing GPR120 per HPF was increased in pNAFLD patients (8.25±3.47) in comparison with normal livers (2.83±1.47, $p<0.01$). Moreover, a significant reduction (**Figure 3**) in the number of GPR120-positive MΦ/KC (4.08±2.97) within the liver ($t = 4.20$; $p<0.01$) was observable after the treatment with DHA.

Interestingly, the number of GPR120-positive MΦ/KC per HPF was directly correlated with serum levels of pro-inflammatory cytokines (TNF-alpha $r = 0.519$, $p<0.01$; IL-6: $r = 0.670$, $p<0.001$ and IL-1B: $r = 0.569$, $p<0.04$: **Figure 4C**). In addition, the number of GPR120-positive MΦ/KC per HPF was inversely correlated with the presence of intermediate hepatocytes ($r = -0.512$, $p<0.05$).

Phosphorylated(p) NF-κB Expression in Macrophages and Hepatocytes

As phosphorylation of NF-κB at serine 311 is important for its TNF-dependent binding to p300 coactivator and recruitment to target promoters after nuclear translocation, we evaluated p-NF-κB expression in our patients. We found that p-NF-κB was expressed by hepatocytes and MΦ/KCs at cytoplasmic and nuclear levels (**Figures 4A–5A**). The percentage of cells, which displayed a nuclear translocation of p-NF-κB, has been determined. The percentages of hepatocytes and MΦ/KCs expressing p-NF-κB was reduced in pNAFLD patients after the treatment with DHA (**Figure 4B–5B**) when the paired-samples T Test was applied ($t = 2.21$ and $t = 2.94$, respectively $p<0.05$). In addition, the percentage of p-NF-κB-positive hepatocytes was directly correlated with NAS, ductular reaction and activation of HPCs ($p<0.05$), whereas the macrophage expression of p-NF-κB was correlated with NAS and ductular reaction extension ($p<0.05$). Interestingly, the nuclear expression of p-NF-κB in macrophages was strongly correlated with serum levels of pro-inflammatory cytokines (TNF-α: $r = 0.585$; $p<0.001$; IL-6: $r = 0.467$, $p<0.01$; IL-1B: $r = 0.547$, $p<0.001$, **Figure 4D**). Finally, the number of GPR120-positive macrophages was correlated with the expression of p-NF-κB ($r = 0.384$; $p<0.05$).

Discussion

This is the first follow-up study demonstrating the liver specific effects of 18-months treatment with DHA in pNAFLD which (i) improves hepatic steatosis, ballooning, inflammation NAS and PNHS scores but was ineffective on fibrosis; (ii) causes a remarkable reduction of DR and HPC activation strongly associated with NAS and PNHS scores; (iii) induces a reduction of GPR120-positive inflammatory MΦ/KCs and an increase of GPR120-positive hepatocytes; and (iv) downregulates nuclear translocation rate of phosphorylated form of p65NF-κB in hepatocytes and liver macrophages.

In a recently completed randomized clinical trial, we found that a 24-months supplementation with DHA was able to determine a decrease in liver fat [9]. Clinically speaking, in pediatric cohort of this study, decreases at 18-months in total triglycerides, ALT, AST and ISI were observed in DHA-supplemented children but their estimates were imprecise and larger sample sizes are needed to adequately estimate these effects. In the present study, DHA

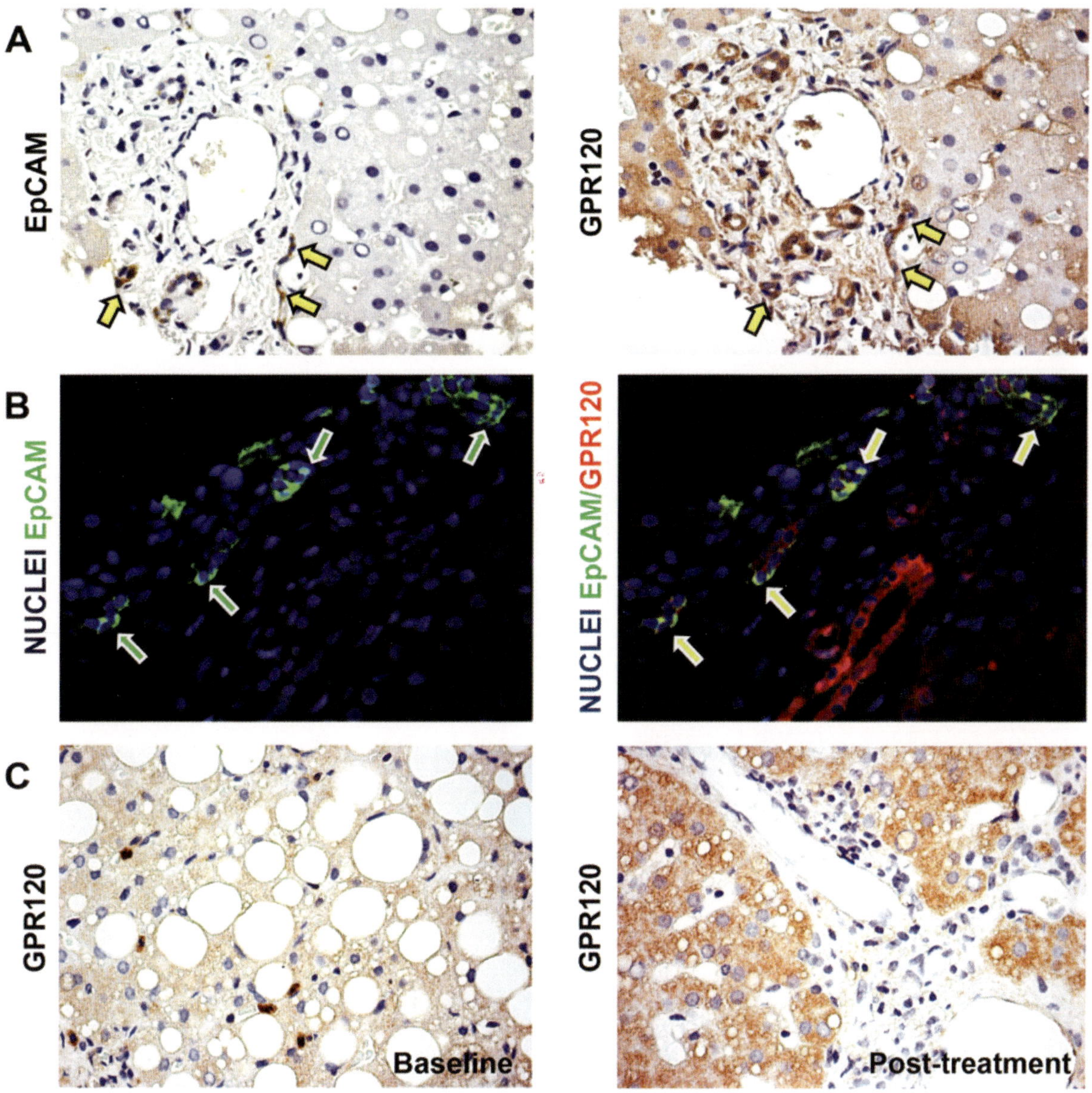

Figure 2. GPR120 expression by HPC and Hepatocytes in pediatric NAFLD patients. A) Immunohistochemistry for EpCAM and GPR120 in serial sections of pediatric NAFLD biopsies. CK-7-positive HPCs highly express GPR120 (arrows). B) Double immunofluorescence for EpCAM (green) and GPR120 (red) in NAFLD biopsies. Nuclei are shown in blue. Numerous EpCAM-positive progenitor cells co-express GPR120 (yellow cells: yellow arrows) confirming the findings obtained through immunohistochemistry in serial sections. C) Immunohistochemistry for GPR120 in sections of pediatric NAFLD biopsies before and after DHA treatment. A significant increase of GPR120-positive hepatocytes was clearly seen after DHA treatment. Original magnification: 40×.

treatment ameliorated hepatocyte steatosis, ballooning, NAS and PNHS scores. Taking in account the diagnostic category, no treated patient had a progression of the histo-pathological damaging and a worse diagnosis at the biopsy after the 18-months therapy. Moreover, 13/17 patients, which were classified as definite SH or borderline before the treatment, presented a more positive diagnosis after the treatment.

A limitation of the present study could be represented by the lack of biopsies from a placebo group. In the completed randomized clinical trial, clinical, laboratory and liver ultrasound data were used to discriminate effects between DHA treated and placebo groups [26]. Indeed, considering that patients were children, the placebo group did not receive liver biopsy at 18 months.

LC-PUFAs exert their actions by the modulation of GPR120 [10,27]. Here, we showed that GPR120 was expressed by several cell types in human liver as MΦs/KCs within sinusoids, hepatocytes and HPCs. Accordingly, the clinical effects and the histo-pathological changes after DHA treatment in pNAFLD patients could be determined through the DHA action on all these different cells.

GPR120 has been indicated as a lipid-sensing receptor highly expressed in proinflammatory macrophages [10]. By signaling through GPR120, DHA mediates potent anti-inflammatory effects by inhibiting both Toll-Like Receptor (TLR) and Tumor Necorsis Factor(TNF)-α signaling pathways [10,27]. Moreover, GPR120 seems to have a key role in counter-inflammation representing a feedback signal that blocks NF-κB phosphorylation [27,28]. Our

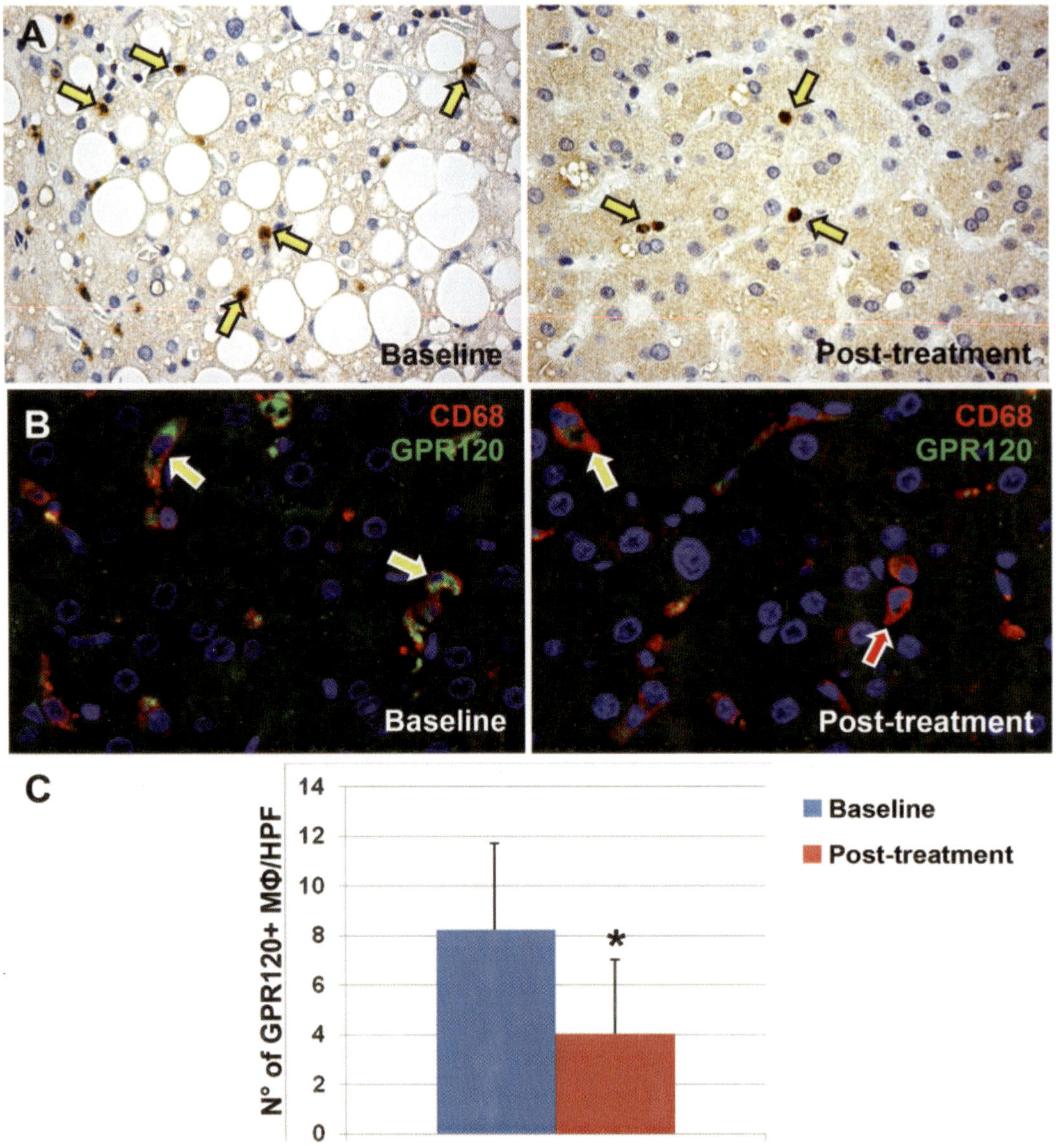

Figure 3. GPR120 expressions by Macrophages in pediatric NAFLD patients. A) Immunohistochemistry for GPR120 in sections of pediatric NAFLD biopsies. B) Double immunofluorescence for CD68 (red) and GPR120 (green) in NAFLD biopsies. Nuclei are shown in blue. CD68-positive macrophages express GPR120 (yellow arrows). Original magnification: 40×. C) The histogram shows the number of GPR120-positive macrophages per high power field (HPF) at the baseline and after DHA treatment. A significant reduction of GPR120-positive macrophages was seen after DHA treatment. * = $p<0.05$.

results were in accordance with this scenario. In pNAFLD, the number of GPR120-positive (inflammatory) MΦ/KCs was increased in comparison with normal. Interestingly, DHA treatment induced a significant reduction of GPR120-positive MΦ/KC pool that matched with a strong decrease of macrophages expressing serine 311 phosphorylated form of NF-κB at nuclear level. These results suggested that, in pNAFLD, DHA treatment was able to reduce the inflammatory macrophage pool and induce an anti-inflammatory macrophage polarization. Two distinct modes of macrophage activation were proposed to differentiate between M1 and M2 macrophages [29]. M1-macrophages produce pro-inflammatory cytokines such as Interleukin (IL)-1β, IL-6, IL- 8, IL-12, and TNF-α. Macrophage can be polarized toward alternative activation phenotype (M2) which has a role in promoting wound healing through the releasing of anti-inflammatory cytokines and the promotion of a efficient clearance of apoptotic cells [30].

In keeping, GPR120 macrophage expression was strongly correlated with the serum levels of pro-inflammatory cytokines (TNF-α, IL-6 and IL-1β). These data seem to confirm that, in pNAFLD, GPR120-positive macrophages within the liver are responsible of pro-inflammatory cytokine production and the treatment with DHA could switch the macrophage polarization via the modulation of NF-κB pathway.

DHA treatment caused a decrease of DR and HPC activation that was strongly correlated with the improvement of clinical and imaging parameters, hepatocyte steatosis and ballooning, NAS and PNHS. Noteworthy, the activation of HPC compartment was higher in definite steatohepatitis compared with not steatohepatitis biopsies. Taken together, these results highlight the pivotal role of

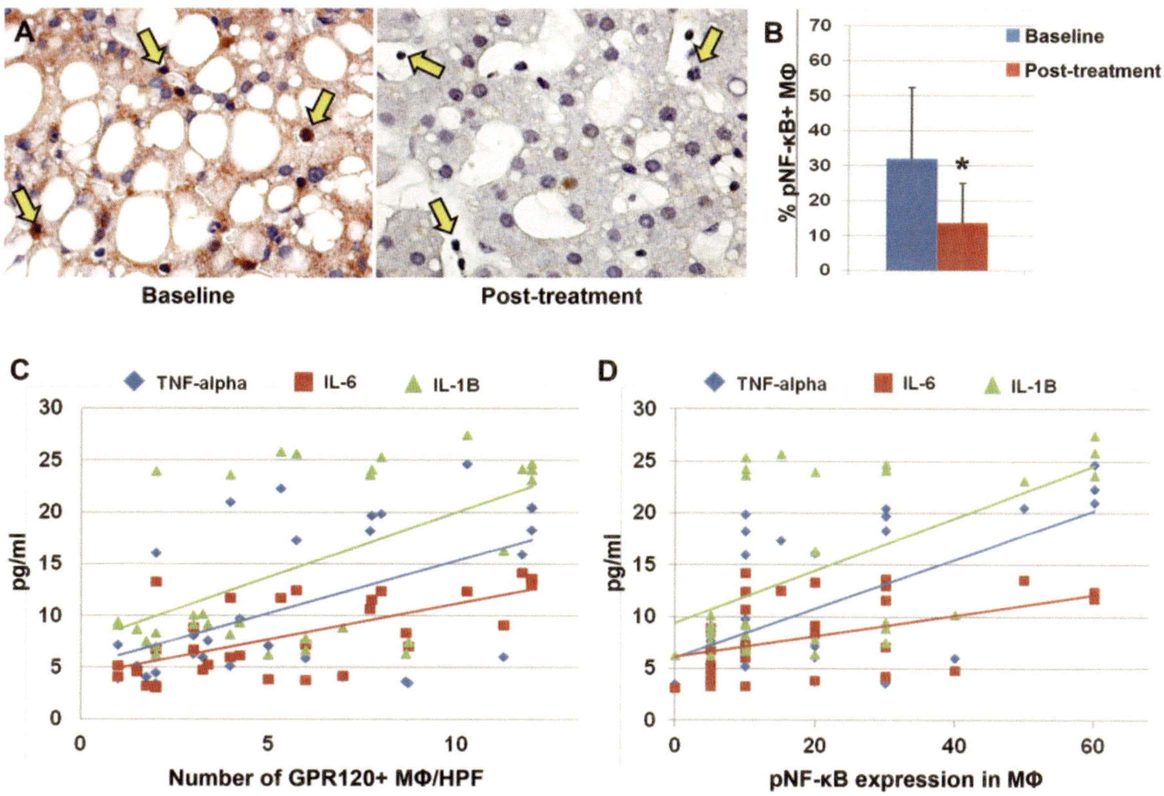

Figure 4. Nuclear expression of phosphorylated (p) NF-κB by Macrophages in pediatric NAFLD patients. A) Immunohistochemistry for serine-311-phosphorylated NF-κB (pNF-κB) in pediatric NAFLD biopsies before and after DHA treatment. In parallel with GPR120 expression, the DHA treatment determined a reduction of pNF-κB expression and its nuclear translocation in macrophages (A, yellow arrows). Original magnification: 40×. B) Histogram shows the significant reduction of pNF-κB nuclear translocation in macrophages after DHA treatment. Data are shown as Means ± Standard Deviation. * = $p<0.05$. C–D) The number of GPR120-positive macrophages (C) and the pNF-κB nuclear expression in macrophages. (D) were correlated with serum level of inflammatory cytokines.

HPC activation in pNAFLD and its potential impact on the progression towards NASH.

Recently, we demonstrated that HPC expansion, especially in children with NASH, is associated with the degree of liver injury, hepatocyte apoptosis, and cell-cycle arrest [3]. In general, the local microenvironment has a key role in achieving a defined progenitor specification in response to diverse injuries [20,31]. Recently, macrophages have been indicated as a key component of HPC niche [31]; during hepatocyte regeneration, an inefficient efferocytosis of hepatocyte debris could be able to induced Wnt3a expression by macrophages; this resulted in canonical Wnt signaling in nearby HPCs, thus promoting their specification to hepatocytes [31]. Interestingly, in the present study, the presence of intermediate hepatocytes, a sign of HPC differentiation towards hepatocyte fate, was correlated with the number of GPR120-positive macrophages. In this context, DHA could exert a dual effect on HPC niche acting directly on HPCs by GPR120 modulation or indirectly on macrophage polarization [20,32].

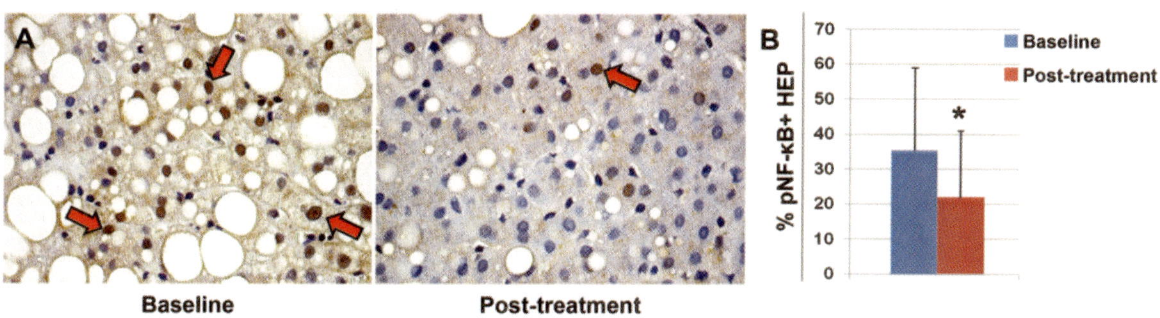

Figure 5. Nuclear expression of phosphorylated (p) NF-κB by hepatocytes in pediatric NAFLD patients. A) Immunohistochemistry for pNF-κB in pediatric NAFLD biopsies demonstrates the reduction of pNF-κB in hepatocyte nuclei (red arrows) after DHA treatment. B) DHA treatment determined a significant reduction of pNF-κB expression and its nuclear translocation in hepatocytes. Data are shown as Means ± Standard Deviation. * = $p<0.05$.

Our results indicated that GPR120 hepatocyte expression was highly enhanced by treatment with DHA and was higher in not steatohepatitis in comparison with definite SH biopsies. Parallel, DHA determined a reduction of pNF-kB in hepatocyte nuclei. The activation of TLR4 signaling in hepatocytes, accompanied with the relocation of NF-κB into the nucleus, was proven to play an important role during the initiation of NAFLD [33,34]. Our data showed that the nuclear expression of pNF-κB in hepatocytes was correlated with the serum levels of pro-inflammatory cytokines, thus suggesting that NF-kB activation and its modulation in hepatocytes could have a role in liver and systemic inflammatory status.

In conclusion, our results highlight the anti-inflammatory effects of DHA administration in pNAFLD and the liver-resident cells which could be stimulated through the interaction with GPR120-mediated NF-κB pathway. Furthermore, in this scenario, LC-PUFA-mediated modulation of GPR120 exploits a novel crucial role in the regulation of the cell-to-cell cross-talk that controls lipid homeostasis, insulin sensitivity, danger recognition and immune tolerance response.

Supporting Information

Figure S1 Histopathological aspects of pediatric NAFLD biopsies. A) The different diagnostic categories in which biopsies were characterized were showed: definite steatohepatitis (Nash: NAS Score ≥5); Nash Borderline (NAS Score = 3–4); Not-steatohepatitis (Not Nash: NAS score = 1–2); B) liver biopsies at baseline and after DHA treatment. Steatosis and ballooning were significantly reduced after the DHA treatment. Hematoxylin-Eosin. Original Magnification: 10X. C) Histo-pathological evaluation: NAS, steatosis, ballooning, and lobular inflammation were significantly reduced after the DHA treatment while no differences were found in fibrosis. * = $p<0.05$.

Author Contributions

Conceived and designed the experiments: VN GC EG. Performed the experiments: VN GC RDV. Analyzed the data: VN GC AA RDV AF PO. Contributed reagents/materials/analysis tools: VN EG. Wrote the paper: VN GC AA GA EG.

References

1. Alisi A, Feldstein AE, Villani A, Raponi M, Nobili V (2012) Pediatric nonalcoholic fatty liver disease: a multidisciplinary approach. Nat Rev Gastroenterol Hepatol 9: 152–161.
2. Carpino G, Renzi A, Onori P, Gaudio E (2013) Role of Hepatic Progenitor Cells in Nonalcoholic Fatty Liver Disease Development: Cellular Cross-Talks and Molecular Networks. Int J Mol Sci 14: 20112–20130.
3. Nobili V, Carpino G, Alisi A, Franchitto A, Alpini G, et al. (2012) Hepatic progenitor cells activation, fibrosis and adipokines production in pediatric nonalcoholic fatty liver disease. Hepatology 56: 2142–2153.
4. Masterton GS, Plevris JN, Hayes PC (2010) Review article: omega-3 fatty acids - a promising novel therapy for non-alcoholic fatty liver disease. Aliment Pharmacol Ther 31: 679–692.
5. Parker HM, Johnson NA, Burdon CA, Cohn JS, O'Connor HT, et al. (2012) Omega-3 supplementation and non-alcoholic fatty liver disease: a systematic review and meta-analysis. J Hepatol 56: 944–951.
6. Capanni M, Calella F, Biagini MR, Genise S, Raimondi L, et al. (2006) Prolonged n-3 polyunsaturated fatty acid supplementation ameliorates hepatic steatosis in patients with non-alcoholic fatty liver disease: a pilot study. Aliment Pharmacol Ther 23: 1143–1151.
7. Pettinelli P, Del Pozo T, Araya J, Rodrigo R, Araya AV, et al. (2009) Enhancement in liver SREBP-1c/PPAR-alpha ratio and steatosis in obese patients: correlations with insulin resistance and n-3 long-chain polyunsaturated fatty acid depletion. Biochim Biophys Acta 1792: 1080–1086.
8. Nobili V, Alisi A, Della Corte C, Rise P, Galli C, et al. (2012) Docosahexaenoic acid for the treatment of fatty liver: Randomised controlled trial in children. Nutr Metab Cardiovasc Dis.
9. Nobili V, Bedogni G, Alisi A, Pietrobattista A, Rise P, et al. (2011) Docosahexaenoic acid supplementation decreases liver fat content in children with non-alcoholic fatty liver disease: double-blind randomised controlled clinical trial. Arch Dis Child 96: 350–353.
10. Oh DY, Talukdar S, Bae EJ, Imamura T, Morinaga H, et al. (2010) GPR120 is an omega-3 fatty acid receptor mediating potent anti-inflammatory and insulin-sensitizing effects. Cell 142: 687–698.
11. Depner CM, Philbrick KA, Jump DB (2013) Docosahexaenoic Acid Attenuates Hepatic Inflammation, Oxidative Stress, and Fibrosis without Decreasing Hepatosteatosis in a Ldlr−/− Mouse Model of Western Diet-Induced Nonalcoholic Steatohepatitis. J Nutr.
12. Nobili V, Manco M, Devito R, Di Ciommo V, Comparcola D, et al. (2008) Lifestyle intervention and antioxidant therapy in children with nonalcoholic fatty liver disease: a randomized, controlled trial. Hepatology 48: 119–128.
13. Shannon A, Alkhouri N, Carter-Kent C, Monti L, Devito R, et al. (2011) Ultrasonographic quantitative estimation of hepatic steatosis in children With NAFLD. J Pediatr Gastroenterol Nutr 53: 190–195.
14. Kleiner DE, Brunt EM, Van Natta M, Behling C, Contos MJ, et al. (2005) Design and validation of a histological scoring system for nonalcoholic fatty liver disease. Hepatology 41: 1313–1321.
15. Brunt EM (2001) Nonalcoholic steatohepatitis: definition and pathology. Semin Liver Dis 21: 3–16.
16. Alkhouri N, De Vito R, Alisi A, Yerian L, Lopez R, et al. (2012) Development and validation of a new histological score for pediatric non-alcoholic fatty liver disease. J Hepatol 57: 1312–1318.
17. Glaser S, Lam IP, Franchitto A, Gaudio E, Onori P, et al. (2010) Knockout of secretin receptor reduces large cholangiocyte hyperplasia in mice with extrahepatic cholestasis induced by bile duct ligation. Hepatology 52: 204–214.
18. Glaser SS, Gaudio E, Rao A, Pierce LM, Onori P, et al. (2009) Morphological and functional heterogeneity of the mouse intrahepatic biliary epithelium. Lab Invest 89: 456–469.
19. Roskams TA, Theise ND, Balabaud C, Bhagat G, Bhathal PS, et al. (2004) Nomenclature of the finer branches of the biliary tree: canals, ductules, and ductular reactions in human livers. Hepatology 39: 1739–1745.
20. Spee B, Carpino G, Schotanus BA, Katoonizadeh A, Vander Borght S, et al. (2010) Characterisation of the liver progenitor cell niche in liver diseases: potential involvement of Wnt and Notch signalling. Gut 59: 247–257.
21. Katoonizadeh A, Nevens F, Verslype C, Pirenne J, Roskams T (2006) Liver regeneration in acute severe liver impairment: a clinicopathological correlation study. Liver Int 26: 1225–1233.
22. Carpino G, Cardinale V, Onori P, Franchitto A, Berloco PB, et al. (2012) Biliary tree stem/progenitor cells in glands of extrahepatic and intraheptic bile ducts: an anatomical in situ study yielding evidence of maturational lineages. J Anat 220: 186–199.
23. Brunt EM, Kleiner DE, Wilson LA, Belt P, Neuschwander-Tetri BA (2011) Nonalcoholic fatty liver disease (NAFLD) activity score and the histopathologic diagnosis in NAFLD: distinct clinicopathologic meanings. Hepatology 53: 810–820.
24. Yoon SM, Gerasimidou D, Kuwahara R, Hytiroglou P, Yoo JE, et al. (2011) Epithelial cell adhesion molecule (EpCAM) marks hepatocytes newly derived from stem/progenitor cells in humans. Hepatology 53: 964–973.
25. Trzpis M, McLaughlin PM, de Leij LM, Harmsen MC (2007) Epithelial cell adhesion molecule: more than a carcinoma marker and adhesion molecule. Am J Pathol 171: 386–395.
26. Nobili V, Alisi A, Della Corte C, Rise P, Galli C, et al. (2012) Docosahexaenoic acid for the treatment of fatty liver: Randomised controlled trial in children. Nutr Metab Cardiovasc Dis 23: 1066–1070.
27. Ichimura A, Hirasawa A, Poulain-Godefroy O, Bonnefond A, Hara T, et al. (2012) Dysfunction of lipid sensor GPR120 leads to obesity in both mouse and human. Nature 483: 350–354.
28. Talukdar S, Olefsky JM, Osborn O (2011) Targeting GPR120 and other fatty acid-sensing GPCRs ameliorates insulin resistance and inflammatory diseases. Trends Pharmacol Sci 32: 543–550.
29. Gordon S, Taylor PR (2005) Monocyte and macrophage heterogeneity. Nat Rev Immunol 5: 953–964.
30. Lumeng CN, Saltiel AR (2011) Inflammatory links between obesity and metabolic disease. J Clin Invest 121: 2111–2117.
31. Boulter L, Govaere O, Bird TG, Radulescu S, Ramachandran P, et al. (2012) Macrophage-derived Wnt opposes Notch signaling to specify hepatic progenitor cell fate in chronic liver disease. Nat Med 18: 572–579.
32. Gaudio E, Carpino G, Cardinale V, Franchitto A, Onori P, et al. (2009) New insights into liver stem cells. Dig Liver Dis 41: 455–462.
33. Dela Pena A, Leclercq I, Field J, George J, Jones B, et al. (2005) NF-kappaB activation, rather than TNF, mediates hepatic inflammation in a murine dietary model of steatohepatitis. Gastroenterology 129: 1663–1674.
34. Li L, Chen L, Hu L, Liu Y, Sun HY, et al. (2011) Nuclear factor high-mobility group box1 mediating the activation of Toll-like receptor 4 signaling in hepatocytes in the early stage of nonalcoholic fatty liver disease in mice. Hepatology 54: 1620–1630.

8

Analysis of Hepatitis B Virus Intrahepatic Covalently Closed Circular DNA and Serum Viral Markers in Treatment-Naive Patients with Acute and Chronic HBV Infection

Weijie Li[1,2]❡, Jingmin Zhao[3]❡, Zhengsheng Zou[2], Yan Liu[2], Baosen Li[2], Ying Sun[2], Xiaodong Li[2], Shuhong Liu[3], Shaoping Cai[2], Weimin Yao[2], Shaojie Xin[2], Fengmin Lu[1]*, Dongping Xu[1,2]*

1 Department of Microbiology, Peking University Health Science Center, Beijing, China, **2** Institute of Infectious Diseases and Medical Center for Liver Failure, Beijing 302 Hospital, Beijing, China, **3** Department of Pathology, Beijing 302 Hospital, Beijing, China

Abstract

Background: This study aimed to investigate the relationships of intrahepatic cccDNA with serum HBsAg and with HBV DNA in treatment-naive patients throughout acute and chronic HBV infection.

Methods: A total of 120 patients who had a liver biopsy were enrolled, including 19 with acute hepatitis B (AHB), and 101 patients with chronic HBV infection (CHB) of whom were 10 in immune-tolerant (IT) phase, 59 in immune-clearance (IC) phase, 8 in low-replicative (LR) phase, and 24 in HBeAg-negative hepatitis (ENH) phase. Intrahepatic cccDNA, serum HBsAg and serum HBV DNA levels were comparatively analyzed.

Results: The median intrahepatic cccDNA levels were 0.18 4.80, 3.81, 0.22 and 0.97 copies/cell for patients with AHB, CHB-IT, CHB-IC, CHB-LR, and CHB-ENH, respectively. In AHB patients, intrahepatic cccDNA was positively correlated with serum HBsAg ($r=0.665$, $P=0.003$), as well as serum HBV DNA ($r=0.536$, $P=0.022$). In CHB patients, intrahepatic cccDNA was positively correlated with serum HBsAg in the IC phase ($r=0.392$, $P=0.005$), and with serum HBV DNA in the IC phase ($r=0.301$, $P=0.036$) and ENH phase ($r=0.588$, $P=0.013$). HBV replicative efficiency, defined as the ratio of serum HBV DNA to intrahepatic cccDNA, was obviously lower in AHB and CHB-LR patients than in CHB-IT, CHB-IC and CHB-ENH patients (0.70 and 0.53 vs. 1.12, 1.09 and 0.99, $P<0.001$, values were logarithmic transformed for analysis). In CHB-IC patients, HBV replicative efficiency was positively correlated with histological activity index of liver inflammation ($r=0.308$, $P=0.009$).

Conclusion: Serum HBsAg and HBV DNA levels may reflect the amount of active intrahepatic cccDNA in treatment-naive AHB and CHB-IC patients. Reduced intrahepatic cccDNA and HBV replicative efficiency may imply effective immune control of HBV infection.

Editor: Haitao Guo, Drexel University College of Medicine, United States of America

Funding: This work was supported by the National Natural Science Foundation of China (81171617), and 12th Five-Year High-Tech Grand (2010gxjs009), and 12th Five-Year Special Grand project for Infectious Diseases (2012ZX10004503). The funders had no role in study design, data collection and analysis, decision to publish, or preparation of the manuscript. The funders had no role in study design, data collection and analysis, decision to publish, or preparation of the manuscript.

* E-mail: xudongping302@sina.com (DX); lu.fengmin@hsc.pku.edu.cn (FL)

❡ These authors contributed equally to this work.

Introduction

Chronic hepatitis B virus (HBV) infection remains a serious health problem. Around 350–400 million people worldwide and 93 million in China are chronic HBV surface antigen (HBsAg) carriers [1,2]. Chronic HBV infection is associated with high risk of developing liver cirrhosis and hepatocellular carcinoma [3]. One crucial step in HBV life cycle is the formation of covalently closed circular DNA (cccDNA), which serves as original template for viral replication and plays an important role in the persistence of HBV infection [4,5,6]. Quantitation of intrahepatic HBV cccDNA is suggested to be valuable in evaluating anti-HBV therapeutic efficacy and estimating treatment endpoint [7,8,9,10,11,12]. In addition, HBV cccDNA level is considered to be a valuable marker for HBV recurrence after liver transplantation and extrahepatic HBV infection [13,14].

The major obstacle for quantitation of cccDNA in clinic is the requirement for invasive liver biopsy. Therefore, finding serum surrogate maker of intrahepatic cccDNA is clinically meaningful. Recently, correlation between serum HBsAg and HBV DNA levels with intrahepatic cccDNA level has been actively investigated for patients with chronic hepatitis B infection (CHB) [15,16,17]. Serum HBsAg and HBV DNA levels were suggested

Table 1. Definitions of phases of persistent HBV infection.

Phase	HBeAg status	HBV DNA (IU/ml)	ALT* (U/L)
immune tolerance (IT)	(+)	>107	<ULN
immune clearance (IC)	(+)	>2000	>2× ULN
low-replicative (LR)	(−)	<2000	<ULN
HBeAg(-) hepatitis (ENH)	(−)	>2000	>2× ULN

*In IT and LR groups patients with ALT activity of <1.5 ULN were accepted if no inflammation in liver biopsy was observed. In IC and ENH groups patients with ALT activity of >ULN were accepted if significant inflammation.

to serve as a surrogate markers of intrahepatic cccDNA for evaluating effectiveness and endpoint of anti-HBV treatment for patients with chronic hepatitis B, particularly for HBeAg-positive patients. However, controversial conclusion existed. For examples, patients on treatment with nucleos(t)ide analogs with greater reductions in levels of cccDNA had greater reductions in HBsAg, but these reductions were not statistically significant [11]; serum HBV DNA, but not HBsAg, reflected the amount of cccDNA and the replicatvive efficiency of HBV in patients with HBeAg-negative hepatitis B [12]. Similarly, inconsistent results were documented on the relationship between intrahepatic cccDNA and serum HBV DNA among HBeAg-positive patients prior to antiviral treatment [7,16].

The dynamic processes of intrahepatic and serum HBV replication markers and histopathological damage are suggested to be complex in CHB patients [18,19]. The production of HBsAg by the cccDNA can be independent of the replication of the virus [16], and study results could be influenced by disease stages, antiviral treatments, sample resource and size, and cccDNA quantitative assays. There is still a paucity of data presenting the correlation of intrahepatic cccDNA with serum viral markers in patients with acute hepatitis B (AHB) and treatment-naive CHB patients at different natural phases. This study aimed to investigate the relationship between intrahepatic cccDNA and serum viral markers including HBsAg and HBV DNA throughout natural phases of acute and chronic HBV infection.

Materials and Methods

Study Subjects

The study population consisted of 19 AHB and 101 CHB Chinese patients who were admitted to Beijing 302 Hospital from January 2008 to December 2012. CHB patients comprised of 10 in immune-tolerant (IT) phase, 59 in immune-clearance (IC) phase, 8 in low-replicative (LR) phase, and 24 in HBeAg-negative (ENH) phase. The diagnosis criteria for acute and chronic hepatitis B were according to the 2000 Xi'an Viral Hepatitis Management Scheme issued by the Chinese Society of Infectious Diseases and Parasitology and the Chinese Society of Hepatology, of the Chinese Medical Association [20], and had been described in details in our previous studies [21,22]. The definitions of phases of persistent HBV-infection were shown in Table 1 according to previous definitions [23]. The clinical backgrounds of patients were summarized in Table 2. In the 32 HBeAg-negative patients, 27 harbored G1896A and (or) A1762T+G1764A mutations (19 with G1896A, 18 with A1762T+G1764A, and 10 with the both). HBeAb was positive for 29 of the 32 HBeAg-negative patients. Patients co-infected with hepatitis A, C, D, E, and F virus, or patients with autoimmune or metabolic liver disease were excluded. The study was approved by ethics committee of Beijing 302 Hospital and the written informed consents were obtained from all patients.

Sample Collection, Quantitation of Serum HBsAg and HBV DNA

Liver biopsy was obtained from all patients. Sera were collected on the same day of liver biopsy for biochemical, virological and serological analyses. The titer of serum HBsAg was quantitated by a chemiluminescence assay using the Architect i2000SR platform and Abbott Architect HBsAg reagents (Abbott Laboratories, Chicago, IL), according to the manufacture's instruction. The lower limit of detection was 0.05 IU/mL. If the initial test value was higher than the upper limit of detection (250 IU/mL), the samples were diluted (1:500) and reassessed. Serum HBV DNA was quantitated by Taqman real-time polymerase chain reaction using commercially available HBV-DNA real-time quantitative PCR kit (Fosun Pharmaceutical Co., Ltd., Shanghai, China) with a lower detection limit of 100 IU/mL, or COBAS AmpliPrep/ COBAS TaqMan (Roche Diagnostics, Mannheim, Germany) with a lower detection limit of 12 IU/mL if needed.

Table 2. Clinical details of the studied patients.

	AHB (n = 19)	CHB-IT (n = 10)	CHB-IC (n = 59)	CHB-LR (n = 8)	CHB-ENG (n = 24)	*P* value
Gender (M/F)	15/4	7/3	49/10	4/4	17/7	0.257
Age (years)	32 (24–41)	18 (10–34)	30 (14–43)	30 (15–42)	35 (23–41)	0.332
TBil (μmol/L)	122 (33.9–171.5)	8.4 (5.7–13.1)	12.2 (8.6–24.6)	10.7 (7.8–12.8)	15.0 (8.8–20.4)	<0.001
Albumin (g/L)	39 (36–41)	40 (38–41)	40 (37–43)	39 (38–42.3)	41 (38–46)	0.330
Albumin/globulin	1.4 (1.2–1.8)	1.7 (1.4–1.9)	1.6 (1.3–1.9)	1.5 (1.4–1.8)	1.6 (1.3–1.9)	0.871
Cholinesterase (IU/L)	5661(4270–7225)	7662 (6091–8634)	5899 (4827–7364)	7920 (5788–9544)	6332 (5127–7851)	0.210
ALT (IU/L)	1571(1014–2142)	33 (17–39)	132 (62–398)	20 (17–32)	138 (63–346)	<0.001
HBV DNA (log_{10} IU/mL)	3.88 (2.87–4.80)	7.95 (7.35–8.32)	6.43 (4.86–7.84)	3.08 (2.44–3.14)	6.1 (5.21–8.01)	<0.001
HBeAg	Positive	Positive	Positive	Negative	Negative	
HBV genotype (B/C)	7/12	2/8	11/48	1/7	4/20	

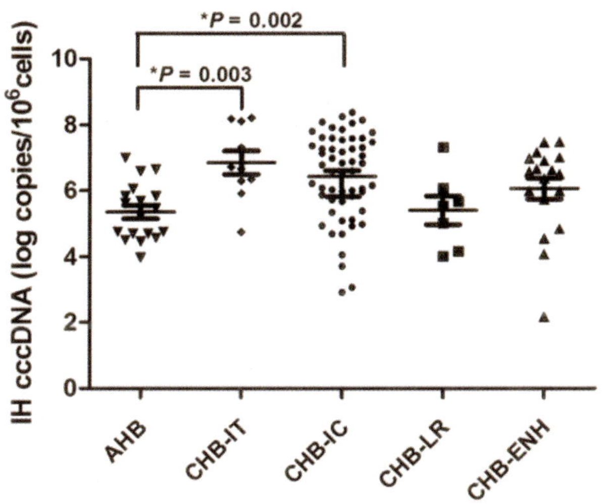

Figure 1. Comparison of intrahepatic (IH) HBV cccDNA levels among patients with different clinical presentations. The horizontal lines illustrate the 25th, 50th, and 75th percentiles of the cccDNA levels. Symbols * and ** represent *P* value less than 0.01 and 0.05, respectively. AHB, acute hepatitis B; CHB, chronic HBV infection; IT, immune-tolerant; IC, immune-clearance; LR, low-replicative; ENH, HBeAg-negative hepatitis.

HBV Genotype Classification

HBV genotype assignment as based on phylogenetic analysis of the 1,225-bp-long S/Pol gene sequence (nucleotides 54 to 1278) as we described previously [24]. Phylogenetic and molecular evolutionary analyses were performed in MEGA version 4. Phylogenetic trees were constructed using neighbor-joining (NJ) analysis with bootstrap test confirmation performed on 1,000 resampling standard reference sequences acquired from the online Hepatitis Virus Database (http://www.ncbi.nlm.nih.gov/projects/genotyping/formpage.cgi).

Histological Examination of Liver Tissues

Histological sections of liver biopsy specimens were stained with hematoxylin-eosin. Histologic grading of necroinflammation and staging of fibrosis were performed using Knodell histological activity index (HAI) (range 0 to 18) and the Ishak fibrosis score (range 0 to 6) respectively, as previously described [18,25,26]. The degree of necroinflammation was classified into score 0–3, 4–8, 9–12, and >score 12 groups. The stage of fibrosis was classified into 4 groups based on the Ishak fibrosis scores.

Quantitation of Intrahepatic HBV cccDNA

Intrahepatic HBV cccDNA was extracted and quantitated by the assay as we described previously [27]. Briefly, about 30 µm formalin fixed paraffin-embedded (FFPE) liver biopsy tissue was sectioned to 6 µm each for DNA extraction. To prevent contamination, disposable tweezers, brush and interleaver were used and sectioning blades were carefully cleaned with 70% ethanol after every sampling. The DNA was extracted using QIAamp FFPE DNA Mini Kit (QIAGEN, GmbH, Hilden, Germany) according to the instructions of the manufacturer. PSAD (Epicentre, Madison, WI, USA) was used to digest HBV rcDNA, replicative dsDNA and ssDNA. Afterwards, rolling Circle Amplification (RCA) was conducted to selectively amplify circle DNA. Using the RCA products as template, HBV cccDNA was further amplified and quantified with TaqMan real-time PCR mediated by a pair of cccDNA-selective primers and a probe that targets the gap region between the two direct repeat regions (DR1 and DR2) of the viral genome. To quantitate cell numbers, a set of primers and a probe for reference control DNA segment of human beta-actin were used in the real-time PCR process. Cell numbers were calculated based on an estimation of 6.667 pg/hgDNA per cell.

Statistical Analysis

Data were presented as median and inter-quartile range. Differences between variables was tested by Student's *t*-test or one-way ANOVA test where it is appropriate. Regression and

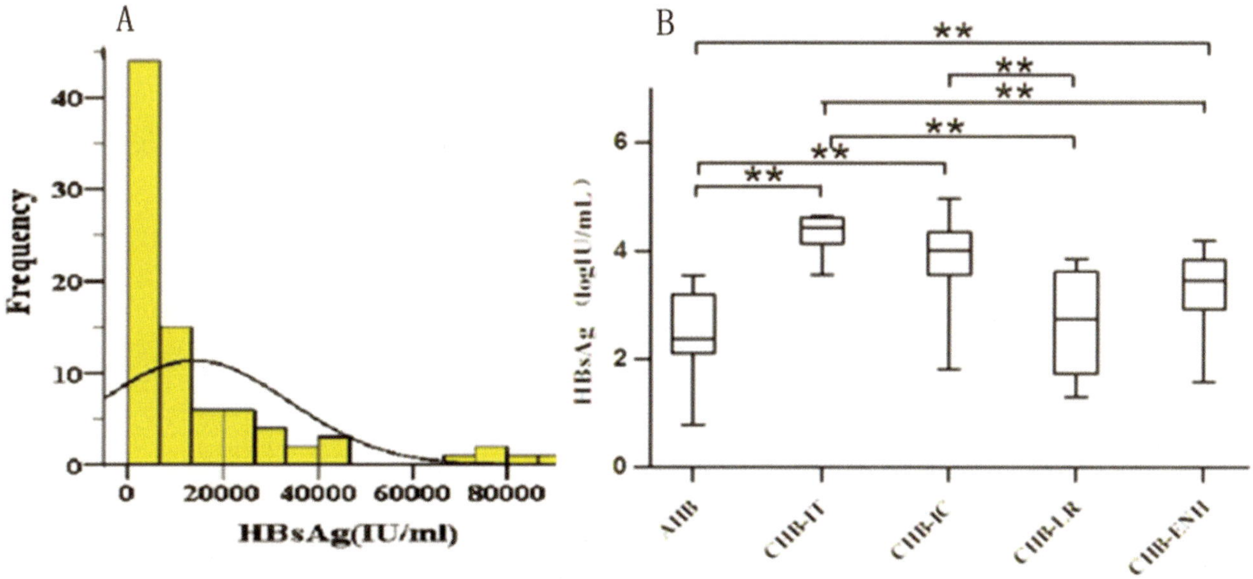

Figure 2. Quantitation of serum HBsAg for 120 HBV-infected patients with different clinical presentations. The distribution of serum HBsAg level across the study population (A). Comparison of serum HBsAg levels among patients with different clinical presentations (B). Symbol ** represent *P* value less than 0.01.

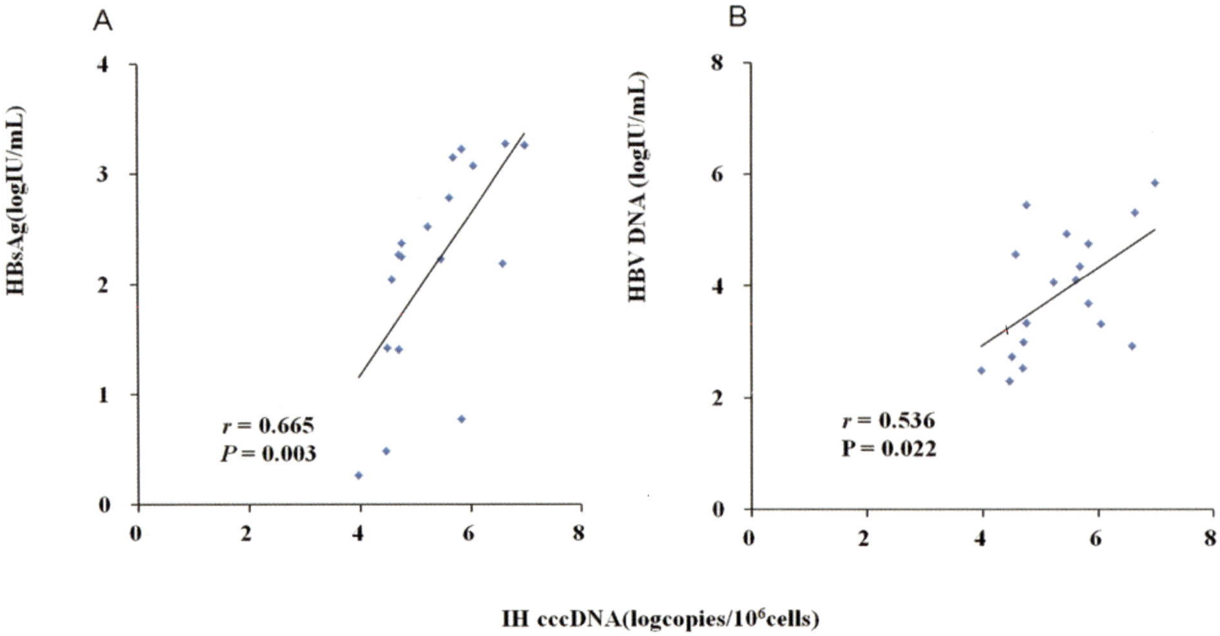

Figure 3. Analysis of correlation between intrahepatic (IH) HBV cccDNA and serum HBV markers for 19 patients with acute hepatitis B. Correlation between intrahepatic HBV cccDNA level and serum HBsAg level (A). Correlation between intrahepatic HBV cccDNA level and serum HBV DNA level (B).

Pearson's correlation analysis were applied to compare the data obtained by real-time PCR methods. A *P*-value (2-tailed) of <0.05 was considered statistically significant. All statistical analyses were carried out in Statistical Program for Social Sciences (SPSS 18.0 for Windows; SPSS Inc., Chicago, IL).

Results

Intrahepatic HBV cccDNA Levels in Different Groups of Patients

The median (25th–75th centile) intrahepatic cccDNA levels were 0.17 (0.04–0.68), 4.80 (1.66–136.97), 3.81 (0.23–29.43), 0.22 (0.11–1.02) and 0.97 (0–7.09) copies/cell in patients with AHB, CHB-IT, CHB-IC, CHB-LR, and CHB-ENH, respectively. HBV cccDNA level was significantly lower in patient with AHB than in

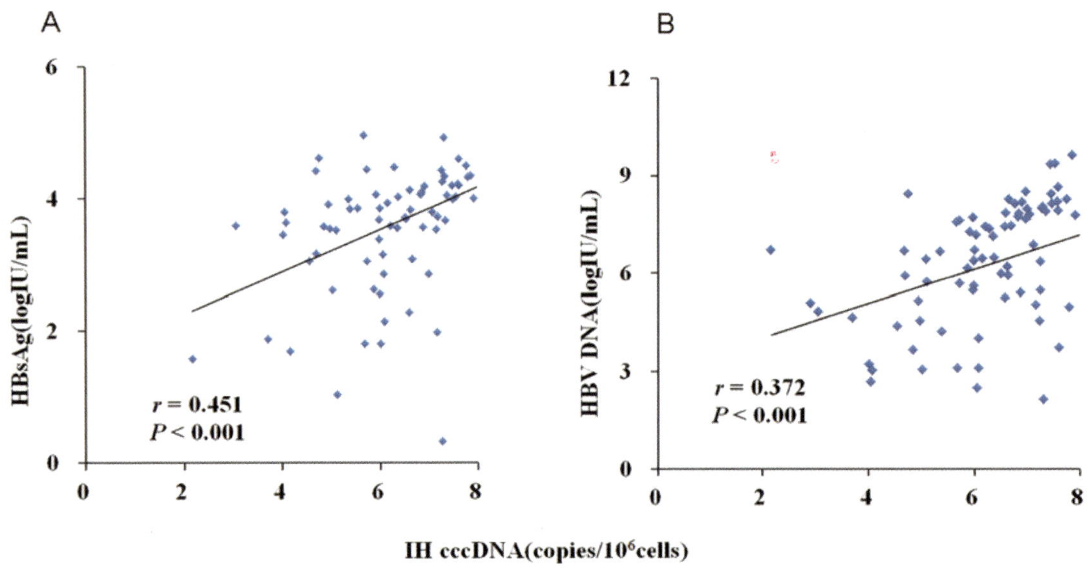

Figure 4. Overall analysis of correlation between intrahepatic (IH) HBV cccDNA and serum HBV markers across 101 patients with chronic HBV infection. Correlation between IH cccDNA level and serum HBsAg level (A). Correlation between IH cccDNA level and serum HBV DNA level (B).

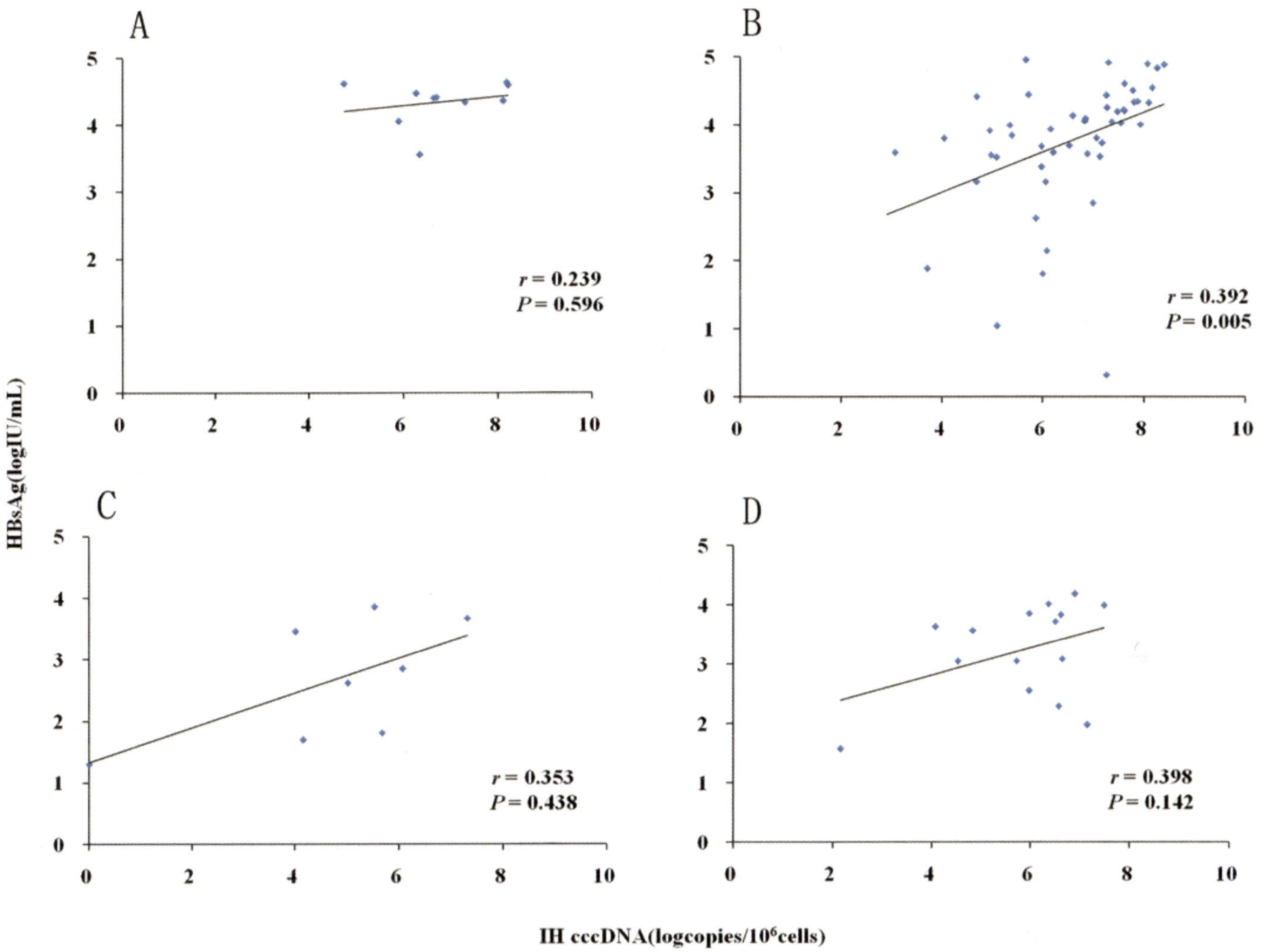

Figure 5. Phase-categorized analysis of correlation between intrahepatic (IH) HBV cccDNA level and serum HBsAg level for patients with chronic HBV infection. Analysis for 10 patients in immune-tolerant phase (A). Analysis for 59 patients in immune-clearance phase (B). Analysis for 8 patients in low-replicative phase (C). Analysis for 24 patients in HBeAg-negative hepatitis phase (D).

patients with CHB-IT and CHB-IC patients; CHB-IT and CHB-IC patients had a significantly higher cccDNA level than CHB-LR patients (Figure 1).

Serum HBsAg Levels in Different Groups of Patients

As shown in Figure 2A, the distribution of serum HBsAg level across the study population was skewed (median 3850, range 1.9–91 000 IU/ml in studied population). AHB patients had a significantly lower median serum HBsAg level than CHB patients (186 IU/ml vs. 6,330 IU/ml, $P<0.001$). Specifically, HBsAg level was different between AHB patients and CHB-IT/CHB-IC/CHB-ENH but not CHB-LR patients. The median serum HBsAg levels for CHB patients in different phases were 22 550 IU/ml (range 3 610–43 900 IU/ml) in CHB-IT patients, 8 680 IU/ml (range 2.1–91 000 IU/ml) in CHB-IC, 563 IU/ml (range 2.1–7 210 IU/ml) in CHB-LR patients, and 2 895 IU/ml (range 38–15 400 IU/ml) in ENH patients, respectively. CHB-IT patients had a significantly higher HBsAg level than CHB-LR and CHB-ENH patients. CHB-IC patients had a significantly higher HBsAg level than CHB-LR patients (Figure 2B).

Correlation of Intrahepatic cccDNA with Serum HBsAg and Serum HBV DNA

In AHB patients, positive correlation was observed between intrahepatic cccDNA and serum HBV DNA ($r = 0.536$, $P = 0.022$), as well as HBsAg level ($r = 0.665$, $P = 0.003$) (Figure 3).

In the entire cohort of CHB patients, positive correlation was observed between intrahepatic cccDNA level and serum HBsAg level ($r = 0.451$, $P<0.001$), as well as serum HBV DNA level ($r = 0.372$, $P<0.001$) (Figure 4). When analyzing the different phases of patients separately, the significant correlation between intrahepatic cccDNA level and serum HBsAg level was only observed in the IC phase rather than in other three phases (Figure 5); and significant correlation between intrahepatic cccDNA level and serum HBV DNA level was observed in the IC and ENH phases rather than in the IT and LR phases (Figure 6).

Dynamics of Serum HBsAg and HBV DNA Levels

In AHB patients, a progressive reduction of serum HBsAg level was observed, which was closely associated with a rapid decline of serum HBV DNA level (Figure 7). The reduction medians (25th–

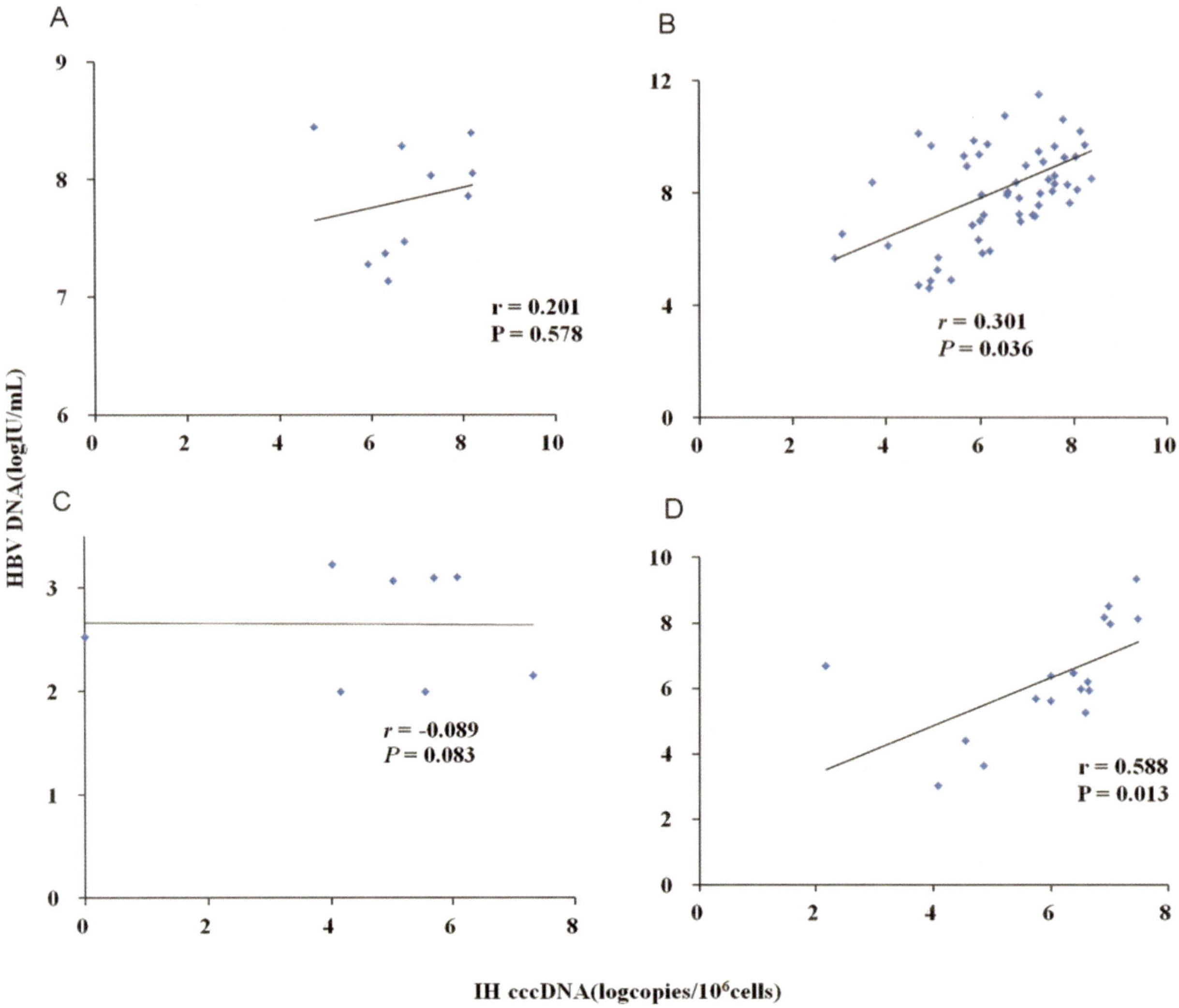

Figure 6. Phase-categorized analysis of correlation between intrahepatic (IH) HBV cccDNA level and serum HBV DNA level for patients with chronic HBV infection in different phases. Analysis for 10 patients in immune-tolerant phase (A). Analysis for 59 patients in immune-clearance phase (B). Analysis for 8 patients in low-replicative phase (C). Analysis for 24 patients in HBeAg-negative hepatitis phase (D).

75th centile) were 0.62 (0.20–2.07) and 2.54 (2.30–2.99) $\log_{10}$ IU/mL for serum HBsAg and HBV DNA 14 days post patient admission, respectively. By contrast, in CHB patients. serum HBsAg level changed much slower and its associations with HBV DNA level was weak or missing.

Comparison of HBV Replicative Efficiency among Different Groups of Patients

HBV replicative efficiency, defined as the ratio of serum HBV DNA to intrahepatic cccDNA ($\log_{10}$ serum HBV DNA/$\log_{10}$ cccDNA (copies/10^6 cells) [12], was analyzed. The replicative efficiency medians (25th–75th centile) were 0.70 (0.55–0.81) in AHB patients, 1.12 (1.01–1.24) in CHB-IT patients, 1.09 (0.78–1.20) in CHB-IC patients, 0.53 (0.22–0.66) in CHB-LR patients, and 0.99 (0.91–1.06) CHB-ENH patients. AHB and CHB-LR patients had significantly lower replicative efficiency than CHB-IT, CHB-IC and CHB-ENH patients ($P<0.001$). The values of HBV replicative efficiency were not statistically different among CHB-IT, CHB-IC, and CHB-ENH patients.

In CHB patients, HBV replicative efficiency was positively associated with alanine aminotransferase (ALT) level ($r=0.390$, $P<0.001$). Further analysis showed that replicative efficiency was correlated with ALT level only in CHB-IC patients ($r=0.515$, $P<0.001$), but not in CHB-IT patients ($r=0.333$, $P=0.347$), CHB-LR patients ($r=0.653$, $P=0.180$), or CHB-ENH patients ($r=0.221$, $P=0.393$).

In CHB-IC patients, HBV replicative efficiency had a correlation with the histological grade of active inflammation ($r=0.348$, $P=0.030$). The replicative efficiency medians (25th–75th centile) were 0.97 (0.64–1.14), 1.07 (0.91–1.23), and 1.13 (1.05–1.20) in score 0–3, 4–8 and 9–12 groups, exhibiting a stepwise elevation with the increase of the inflammation grade. By contrast, HBV replicative efficiency was not correlated with stage of fibrosis ($r=0.189$, $P=0.248$) (Figure 8). In the other 3 phases of CHB patients, no significant correlation was observed between HBV replicative efficiency and the liver histological activities (data not shown).

Discussion

This study for the first time revealed the comprehensive relationship of intrahepatic cccDNA with serum HBsAg and

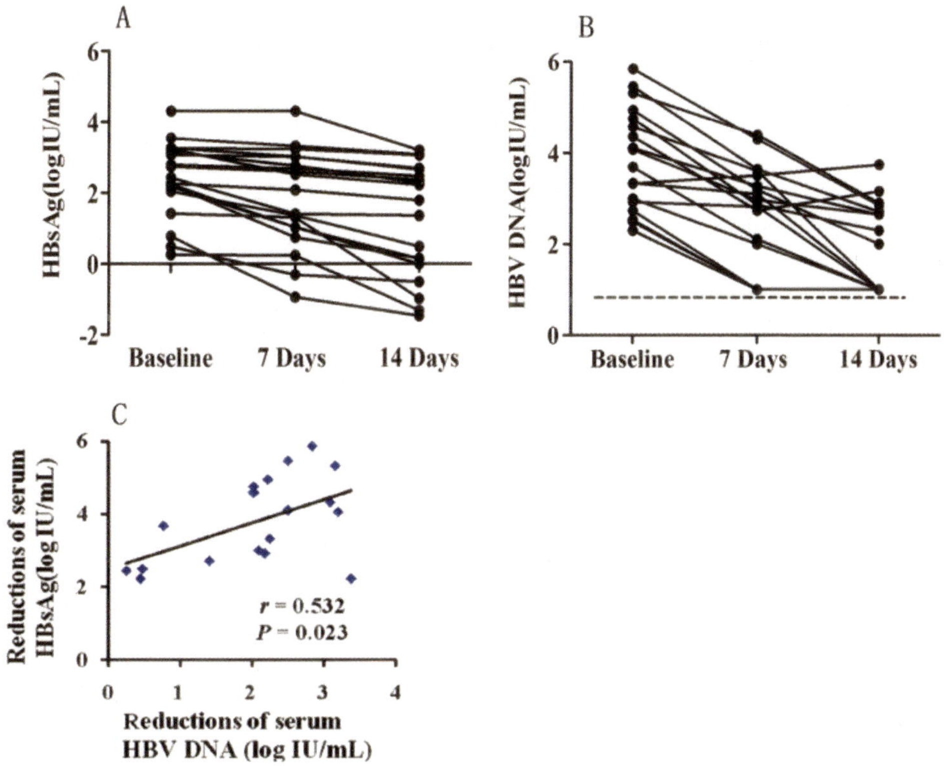

Figure 7. Monitoring of serum HBsAg and HBV DNA levels in patients with acute hepatitis B. Dynamical change of serum HBsAg level (A). Dynamical change of serum HBV DNA level (B). Association of reductions between serum HBsAg level and HBV DNA level 14 days post patient admission (C).

HBV DNA throughout the natural phases of both acute and chronic HBV infections. Previous studies have not described intrahepatic cccDNA with serum markers in AHB patients, nor CHB patients in the LR phase, owing to the particular difficulty in obtaining liver biopsy from these patients in clinical practice. The current study made a great effort to fill up the knowledge gap.

Intrahepatic cccDNA level was significantly lower in AHB patients than that in CHB patients in this study. Dynamical observation showed that both serum HBsAg and HBV DNA levels

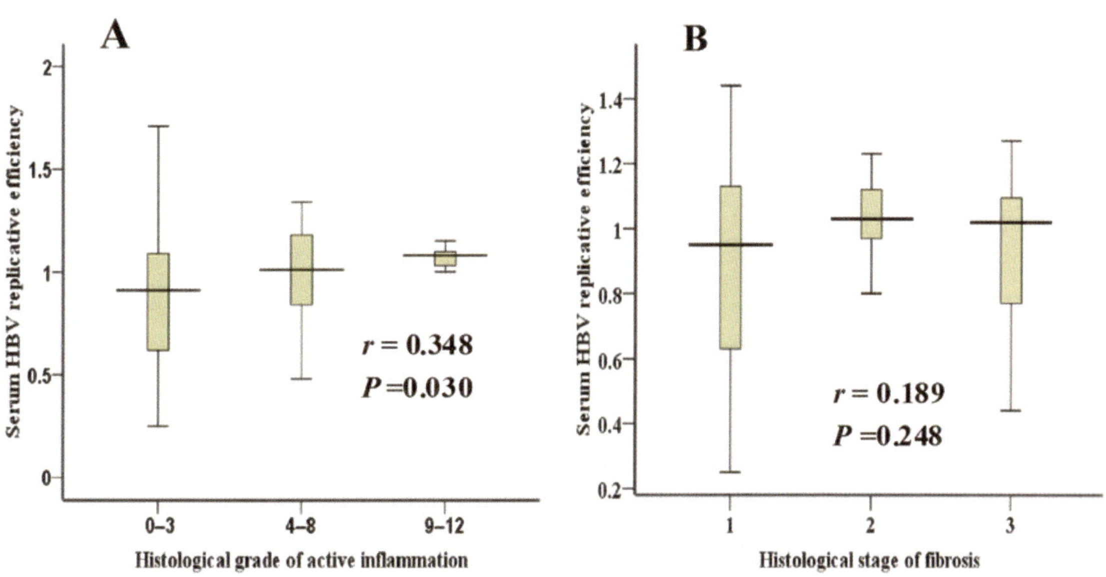

Figure 8. Relationship of HBV replicative efficiency with histological activitiesin CHB-IC patients. Correlation between HBV replicative efficiency and histological grade of active inflammation (A). Correlation between HBV replicative efficiency and histological stage of fibrosis(B).

progressively declined in a short period of time with a good correlation to each other. These evidence suggested that active anti-HBV immune response in AHB patients could effectively eliminate intrahepatic cccDNA and the effect was reflected well in peripheral. Thus, serum HBsAg and HBV DNA levels could serve as surrogate markers for intrahepatic cccDNA level in AHB patients.

In this study, HBV replicative efficiency was significantly lower in AHB patients than in CHB patients in overall, but CHB-LR patients had a low HBV replicative efficiency value similarly as in AHB patients. Consistently, patients with inactive HBeAg-negative chronic hepatitis B was observed to have a lower cccDNA level and a lower viral replicative efficiency than patients with active HBeAg-negative chronic hepatitis B [12]. This suggested that rate of active cccDNA loss was faster than the rate of total cccDNA loss when HBV activity is well checked by host immunity, such that reduced replicative efficiency may imply effective immune control of HBV infection.

Discrepancy in the relationship between intrahepatic HBV cccDNA level and histological activities has been described from previous studies [12,18,28,29]. In this study, intrahepatic cccDNA level was not correlated with histological activities of liver inflammation or fibrosis. Our results are consistent with that by Lin et al [12] and by Guner et al [18]. The reason for the lack of correlation may be that histopathological damage was developed over time or that damage was mainly caused by differences in immune response [18]. Interestingly, we found that HBV replicative efficiency (ratio of $\log_{10}$ serum HBV DNA to $\log_{10}$ intrahepatic cccDNA) was correlated with the histological index of inflammation activity and ALT level in CHB-IC patients, suggesting that HBV replicative efficiency was a valuable indicator associated with liver damage in the IC phase.

One limitation of the study is the relatively small sample size for CHB-LR and CHB-IT groups. In addition, HBV cccDNA activity could be influenced by epigenetic regulation, including DNA methylation, histoneacetylation, and microRNAs [30,31]. Whether these factors influence the association between intrahepatic cccDNA and serum viral markers needs further clarification.

In summary, the major findings of this study are that (i) Intrahepatic cccDNA levels were significantly lower in patients with AHB and CHB-LR than patients with CHB-IT, CHB-IC, and CHB-ENH. (ii) intrahepatic cccDNA level is positively correlated with serum HBsAg level in untreated AHB and CHB-IC patients, and with serum HBV DNA level in the AHB, CHB-IC, and CHB-ENH patients. (iii) Reduced HBV replicative efficiency may imply effective immune control of HBV infection. (iv) In CHB-IC patients, HBV replicative efficiency is positively correlated with inflammation in the liver. These findings provided new insights on the clinical implications of intrahepatic cccDNA and the serum viral markers in different stages of HBV infection.

Author Contributions

Conceived and designed the experiments: DX FL JZ. Performed the experiments: WL XL SL SC WY. Analyzed the data: WL YL YS. Contributed reagents/materials/analysis tools: JZ ZZ BL SX. Wrote the paper: WL DX.

References

1. European Association For The Study Of The Liver (2012) EASL clinical practice guidelines: Management of chronic hepatitis B virus infection. J Hepatol, 57: 167–185. doi: 10.1016/j.jhep.2012.02. 010.
2. Chinese Society of Hepatology and Chinese Society of Infectious Diseases (2011) Chinese Medical Association, The guideline of prevention and treatment for chronic hepatitis B (2010 version). Zhonghua Gan Zang Bing Za Zhi (Chinese J Hepatol) 19: 13–24. doi:10.3760/cma.j.issn.1007-3418.2011.01.007.
3. Papatheodoridis GV, Manolakopoulos S, Dusheiko G, Archimandritis AJ (2008) Therapeutic strategies in the management of patients with chronic hepatitis B virus infection. Lancet Infect Dis 8: 167–178. doi:10.1016/S1473-3099(07)70264-5.
4. Zoulim F (2005) New insight on hepatitis B virus persistence from the study of intrahepatic viral cccDNA. J Hepatol 42: 302–308. doi:10.1016/j.jhep.2004.12.015.
5. Laras A, Koskinas J, Dimou E, Kostamena A, Hadziyannis SJ (2006) Intrahepatic levels and replicative activity of covalently closed circular hepatitis B virus DNA in chronically infected patients. Hepatology 44: 694–702. doi:10.1002/hep.21299.
6. Levrero M, Pollicino T, Petersen J, Belloni L, Raimondo G, et al. (2009) Control of cccDNA function in hepatitis B virus infection. J Hepatol 51: 581–592. doi:10.1016/j.jhep.2009.05.022.
7. Werle-Lapostolle B, Bowden S, Locarnini S, Wursthorn K, Petersen J, et al. (2004) Persistence of cccDNA during the natural history of chronic hepatitis B and decline during adefovir dipivoxil therapy. Gastroenterology 126: 1750–1758. doi:10.1053/j.gastro.2004.03.018.
8. Sung JJ, Wong ML, Bowden S, Liew CT, Hui AY, et al. (2005) Intrahepatic hepatitis B virus covalently closed circular DNA can be a predictor of sustained response to therapy. Gastroenterology 128: 1890–1897. doi:10.1053/j.gastro.2005.03.009.
9. Bourne EJ, Dienstag JL, Lopez VA, Kostamena A, Hadziyannis SJ (2007) Quantitative analysis of HBV cccDNA from clinical specimens: correlation with clinical and virological response during antiviral therapy. J Viral Hepat 14: 55–63. doi:10.1111/j.1365-2893.2006.00775.x.
10. Takkenberg B, Terpstra V, Zaaijer H, Weegink C, Dijkgraaf M, et al. (2011) Intrahepatic response markers in chronic hepatitis B patients treated with peginterferon alpha-2a and adefovir. J Gastroenterol Hepatol 26: 1527–1535. doi: 10.1111/j.1440–1746.2011.06766.x.
11. Wong DK, Seto WK, Fung J, Ip P, Huang FY, et al. (2013) Reduction of hepatitis B surface antigen and covalently closed circular DNA by nucleos(t)ide analogues of different potency. Clin Gastroenterol Hepatol 11: 1004–10.e1. doi: 10.1016/j.cgh.2013.01.026.
12. Lin LY, Wong VW, Zhou HJ, Chan HY, Gui HL, et al. (2010) Relationship between serum hepatitis B virus DNA and surface antigen with covalently closed circular DNA in HBeAg-negative patients. J Med Virol, 82: 1494–1500. doi:10.1002/jmv.21863.
13. Lenci I, Marcuccilli F, Tisone G, Di Paolo D, Tariciotti L, et al. (2010) Total and covalently closed circular DNA detection in liver tissue of long-term survivors transplanted for HBV-related cirrhosis. Dig Liver Dis 42: 578–584. doi:10.1016/j.dld.2009.12.003.
14. Lu L, Zhang HY, Yueng YH, Cheung KF, Luk JM, et al. (2009) Intracellular levels of hepatitis B virus DNA and pregenomic RNA in peripheral blood mononuclear cells of chronically infected patients. J Viral Hepat 16: 104–112.doi: 10.1111/j.1365–2893.
15. Wursthorn K, Lutgehetmann M, Dandri M, Volz T, Buggisch P, et al. (2006) Peginterferon alpha-2b plus adefovir induce strong cccDNA decline and HBsAg reduction in patients with chronic hepatitis B. Hepatology 44: 675–684. doi:10.1002/hep.21282.
16. Chan HL, Wong VW, Tse AM, Tse CH, Chim AM, et al. (2007) Serum hepatitis B surface antigen quantitation can reflect hepatitis B virus in the liver and predict treatment response. Clin Gastroenterol Hepatol 5: 1462–1468. doi:10.1016/j.cgh.2007.09.005.
17. Wang M, Qiu N, Lu S, Xiu D, Yu J, et al. (2013) Serum hepatitis B surface antigen is correlated with intrahepatic total HBV DNA and cccDNA in treatment-naïve patients with chronic hepatitis B but not in patients with HBV related hepatocellular carcinoma. J Med Virol 85: 219–227. doi: 10.1002/jmv.23461.
18. Guner R, Karahocagil M, Buyukberber M, Kandemir O, Ural O, et al. (2011) Correlation between intrahepatic hepatitis B virus cccDNA levels and other activity markers in patients with HBeAg-negative chronic hepatitis B infection. Eur J Gastroenterol Hepatol 23: 1185–1191. doi:10.1097/MEG.0b013e32834ba13a.
19. Chan HL, Wong VW, Wong GL, Tse CH, Chan HY, et al. (2010) A longitudinal study on the natural history of serum hepatitis B surface antigen changes in chronic hepatitis B. Hepatology 52: 1232–1241. doi:10.1002/hep.23803.
20. Chinese Society of Infectious Diseases and Parasitology, Chinese Society of Hepatology. (2000) Management scheme of diagnostic and therapy criteria of viral hepatitis. Zhonghua Gan Zang Bing Za Zhi (Chinese J Hepatol) 6: 324–329.
21. Liu Y, Zhong Y, Zou Z, Xu Z, Li B, et al. (2010) Features and clinical implications of hepatitis B virus genotypes and mutations in basal core promoter/precore region in 507 Chinese patients with acute and chronic hepatitis B. J Clin Virol 47: 243–247. doi:10.1016/j.jcv.2009.12.013.

22. Xu Z, Liu Y, Liu L, Li X, Bai S, et al. (2013) Association of Interferon-gamma induced protein 10 promoter polymorphisms with the disease progression of hepatitis B virus infection in Chinese Han population. PLOS ONE 8: e72799. doi:10.1371/journal.pone.0072799.
23. Jaroszewicz J, Serrano BC, Wursthorn K, Deterding K, Schlue J, et al. (2010) Hepatitis B surface antigen (HBsAg) levels in the natural history of hepatitis B virus (HBV)-infection: A European perspective. J Hepatol 52: 514–522. doi:10.1016/j.jhep.2010.01.014.
24. Li X, Wang L, Zhong Y, Wong VW, Xu Z, et al. (2010) Hepatitis B virus (HBV) subgenotypes C2 and B2 differ in lamivudine- and adefovir-resistance-associated mutational patterns in HBV-infected Chinese patients. J Clin Microbiol 48: 4363–4369. doi: 10.1128/JCM.01518-10.
25. Seto WK, Wong DK, Fung J, Ip PP, Yuen JC, et al. (2012) High hepatitis B surface antigen levels predict insignificant fibrosis in hepatitis B e antigen positive chronic hepatitis B. PLoS One 7: e43087. doi:10.1371/journal.pone.0043087.
26. Wong DK, Yuen MF, Yuan H, Sum SS, Hui CK, et al. (2004) Quantitation of covalently closed circular hepatitis B virus DNA in chronic hepatitis B patients. Hepatology 40: 727–737. doi: 10.1002/hep.20353.
27. Zhong Y, Han J, Zou Z, Liu S, Ren X, et al. (2011) Quantitation of HBV covalently closed circular DNA in micro formalin fixed paraffin-embedded liver tissue using rolling circle amplification in combination with real-time PCR. Clin Chim Acta 412: 1905–1911. doi:10.1016/j.cca.2011.06.031.
28. Takkenberg RB, Zaaijer HL, Menting S, Kandemir O, Ural O, et al. (2010) Detection of hepatitis B virus covalently closed circular DNA in paraffin-embedded and cryo-preserved liver biopsies of chronic hepatitis B patients. Eur J Gastroenterol Hepatol 22: 952–960. doi:10.1097/MEG.0b013e32834-ba13a.
29. Larsson SB, Eilard A, Malmström S, Hannoun C, Dhillon AP, et al. (2013) HBsAg quantification for identification of liver disease in chronic hepatitis B virus carriers. Liver Int doi: 10.1111/liv.12345. [Epub ahead of print].
30. Kim JW, Lee SH, Park YS, Hwang JH, Jeong SH, et al. (2011) Replicative activity of hepatitis B virus is negatively associated with methylation of covalently closed circular DNA in advanced hepatitis B virus infection. Inter virology 54, 316–325. doi:10.1159/000321450.
31. Zhang X, Hou J, Lu M (2013) Regulation of hepatitis B virus replication by epigenetic mechanisms and micro RNAs. Front Genet 14: 202. doi:10.3389/fgene.2013.00202.

9

Non-Invasive Assessment of Hepatic Steatosis in Patients with NAFLD Using Controlled Attenuation Parameter and ^{1}H-MR Spectroscopy

Thomas Karlas[1,2], David Petroff[1,3], Nikita Garnov[1,4], Stephan Böhm[5], Hannelore Tenckhoff[5], Christian Wittekind[6], Manfred Wiese[5], Ingolf Schiefke[7], Nicolas Linder[1,4], Alexander Schaudinn[1,4], Harald Busse[4], Thomas Kahn[4], Joachim Mössner[2], Thomas Berg[5], Michael Tröltzsch[2], Volker Keim[2], Johannes Wiegand[1,2,5]*

1 IFB AdiposityDiseases, Leipzig University Medical Center, Leipzig, Germany, **2** Department of Medicine, Neurology and Dermatology, Division of Gastroenterology and Rheumatology, University Hospital Leipzig, Leipzig, Germany, **3** Clinical Trial Center, University of Leipzig, Leipzig, Germany, **4** Department of Diagnostics and Interventional Radiology, University Hospital Leipzig, Leipzig, Germany, **5** Department of Medicine, Neurology and Dermatology, Division of Gastroenterology and Rheumatology, Section of Hepatology, University Hospital Leipzig, Leipzig, Germany, **6** Institute of Pathology, University Hospital Leipzig, Leipzig, Germany, **7** Clinic for Gastroenterology and Hepatology, Klinikum St. Georg, Leipzig, Germany

Abstract

Introduction: Non-invasive assessment of steatosis and fibrosis is of growing relevance in non-alcoholic fatty liver disease (NAFLD). ^{1}H-Magnetic resonance spectroscopy (^{1}H-MRS) and the ultrasound-based controlled attenuation parameter (CAP) correlate with biopsy proven steatosis, but have not been correlated with each other so far. We therefore performed a head-to-head comparison between both methods.

Methods: Fifty patients with biopsy-proven NAFLD and 15 healthy volunteers were evaluated with ^{1}H-MRS and transient elastography (TE) including CAP. Steatosis was defined according to the percentage of affected hepatocytes: S1 5-33%, S2 34–66%, S3 ≥67%.

Results: Steatosis grade in patients with NAFLD was S1 36%, S2 40% and S3 24%. CAP and ^{1}H-MRS significantly correlated with histopathology and showed comparable accuracy for the detection of hepatic steatosis: areas under the receiver-operating characteristics curves were 0.93 vs. 0.88 for steatosis ≥S1 and 0.94 vs. 0.88 for ≥S2, respectively. Boot-strapping analysis revealed a CAP cut-off of 300 dB/m for detection of S2-3 steatosis, while retaining the lower cut-off of 215 dB/m for the definition of healthy individuals. Direct comparison between CAP and ^{1}H-MRS revealed only modest correlation (total cohort: r = 0.63 [0.44, 0.76]; NAFLD cases: r = 0.56 [0.32, 0.74]). For detection of F2–4 fibrosis TE had sensitivity and specificity of 100% and 98.1% at a cut-off value of 8.85 kPa.

Conclusion: Our data suggest a comparable diagnostic value of CAP and ^{1}H-MRS for hepatic steatosis quantification. Combined with the simultaneous TE fibrosis assessment, CAP represents an efficient method for non-invasive characterization of NAFLD. Limited correlation between CAP and ^{1}H-MRS may be explained by different technical aspects, anthropometry, and presence of advanced liver fibrosis.

Editor: Kostas Pantopoulos, Lady Davis Institute for Medical Research/McGill University, Canada

Funding: This work was supported by the Federal Ministry of Education and Research (BMBF), Germany, FKZ: 01EO1001 (Project No. K7-40). The funders had no role in study design, data collection and analysis, decision to publish, or preparation of the manuscript.

Competing Interests: The authors have read the journal's policy and have the following conflicts: TK received travel grants from Echosens/France. All other authors have declared that no competing interests exist.

* E-mail: johannes.wiegand@medizin.uni-leipzig.de

Introduction

Hepatic steatosis is commonly observed upon histopathological evaluation of patients with different chronic liver diseases like alcoholic or non-alcoholic fatty liver disease (NAFLD), chronic hepatitis B or C or drug induced liver injuries (e.g. by long-term corticosteroid or amiodarone exposure) [1,2]. NAFLD is the most prevalent chronic liver disease in the Western world and affects up to 30% of the population [3]. Its spectrum ranges from simple steatosis and steatohepatitis to fibrosis and long-term complications like liver cirrhosis and hepatocellular carcinoma [4,5]. The reliable quantification of hepatic steatosis is of growing clinical relevance, because increasing steatosis may favor progression of fibrosis [3,6] and limit treatment response, e.g. in patients with viral hepatitis [7,8]. Moreover, detailed quantification of steatosis is important in estimating the therapeutic success of different pharmaceutical treatment options in NAFLD [9,10].

The current gold standard for the assessment of hepatic steatosis and associated necroinflammatory activity is liver biopsy. However, results can be limited by sampling errors, intra- and inter-observer variability and difficulties in acquiring repetitive and longitudinal data due to the invasiveness of the procedure [11,12]. Therefore, a number of imaging or laboratory based methods (e.g. SteatoTest [13], Fatty Liver Index [14]) have been developed in the last years to quantify hepatic steatosis non-invasively. Imaging modalities include ultrasound, computed tomography (CT), and magnetic resonance imaging (MRI) [15]. Recently, an additional ultrasound based method named Controlled Attenuation Parameter (CAP) has been developed to investigate hepatic steatosis [16]. CAP is included in the transient elastography system (TE), which uses vibration induced elastic shear-waves for assessment of liver stiffness. For the 3.5 MHz TE M probe, the CAP algorithm calculates the attenuation of ultrasonic signals used for characterization of the shear-wave propagation. In contrast to conventional B-mode ultrasound, which is impaired by low sensitivity and difficulties in differentiating different grades of hepatic steatosis, CAP has shown adequate performance for the detection and semi-quantification of steatosis in several biopsy-controlled clinical studies [17–22].

1H-magnetic res°nance spectroscopy (^{1}H-MRS) is a safe and non-invasive alternative for quantification of hepatic fat content which offers good reproducibility and detailed investigation of different liver lobes and has been studied in various clinical studies [23–26]. Although potential limitations are high costs and availability of the method, it seems especially helpful in clinical scenarios in which quantitative data of hepatic steatosis are of relevance [15].

Both the CAP technology and ^{1}H-MRS reliably estimate the hepatic fat content and correlate with the histopathological evaluation of hepatic steatosis [27,28]. However, a direct comparison between both non-invasive methods has not been performed yet. These data can be important to determine which non-invasive imaging method may be used in future clinical studies to investigate the clinical course of patients with NAFLD. We therefore performed a cross-sectional trial with head-to-head comparison between CAP and ^{1}H-MRS.

Patients and Methods

Patients and controls

Between March and December 2012 outpatients with biopsy-proven NAFLD or NASH and absence of concomitant liver diseases were invited to participate in the study. Healthy volunteers without any known liver disease, diabetes mellitus, or metabolic syndrome were enrolled as control group. Weekly alcohol consumption above 210 g for men and 140 g for woman was ruled out for all study participants by a thorough clinical interview prior to inclusion [1]. In healthy controls, signs of hepatic steatosis in conventional ultrasound (increased echogenicity pattern of liver parenchyma compared to the right renal cortex using a conventional convex ultrasound probe) were regarded as exclusion criterion.

All patients underwent clinical examination, abdominal ultrasound, liver stiffness measurement with transient elastography combined with measurement of controlled attenuation parameter and laboratory assessment on the same day of presentation. In addition, ^{1}H-MRS was performed within a time period of three weeks, in the majority of cases on the day of ultrasound assessment. Fasting for at least three hours was required prior to the ultrasound and elastography examinations.

Ethics statement

The study was performed in accordance with the ethical guidelines of the Helsinki Declaration and was approved by the local ethics committee (University of Leipzig, register no. 283-11-22082011). All participants provided written informed consent.

Liver histology

Diagnosis of NAFLD or NASH was based on liver biopsy. The NAFLD activity score (NAS) was assessed by a single expert pathologist blinded to the clinical data. Steatosis was defined according to the number of affected hepatocytes: S1 (5–33%, "mild"), S2 (33–66%, "moderate"), S3 (>66%, "severe"). Fibrosis was classified according the NAS staging [1,29].

A time interval between liver biopsy and study inclusion of up to 48 months was arbitrary accepted for enrolment in the study (median interval between biopsy and study inclusion 8.5 months, range 0–40 months).

Elastography, CAP, and ultrasound

All subjects underwent liver stiffness measurement using the M probe of transient elastography (Echosens, Paris, France; Software Version 2.01.4_1889). In brief, the device transmits a mechanical vibration to the tissue and induces elastical shear-wave propagation which is tracked by pulse-echo ultrasound signals at a measuring depth of 2.5 to 6.5 cm [30]. The shear-wave velocity is directly related to the tissue stiffness and expressed in kPa. TE was performed in supine position in a right intercostal space. Ten valid measurements were taken with the M probe according to the manufacturer's recommendation. A success rate of >60% was required for a valid measurement. Examinations with an interquartile range (IQR) >30% of the median liver stiffness value were classified as unreliable and excluded from further analysis [31]. The controlled attenuation parameter (CAP) represents the ultrasonic attenuation coefficient of the ultrasonic signals used during the TE examination and is expressed in dB/m. The technical background has been recently described in detail [16]. The algorithm is included in the TE software and data are automatically calculated simultaneously with the liver stiffness measurement. CAP was only appraised in case of a valid and reliable TE measurement [16,19].

The distance between skin and liver capsule at the site of TE measurement was measured using a conventional linear ultrasound transducer.

Magnetic resonance spectroscopy and volumetry

MR examinations were performed on a 1.5-T scanner (Achieva XR, Philips Healthcare, Best, Netherlands) with the patient in supine position. Single-voxel MR spectra were acquired with the integrated body coil using a point-resolved spectroscopy (PRESS) technique and local shimming. Voxels (size $20 \times 20 \times 20$ mm^3) were placed in the right liver lobe (segment VII) trying to avoid bile ducts and larger vessels. Scans were acquired during free breathing (using breath triggering) with the following sequence parameters: repetition time, TR = 3,500 ms, echo time, TE = 25 ms, 512 data points, bandwidth, BW = 1,000 Hz/pixel, 40 averages, total acquisition time, TA = 140 s, and without water suppression.

MR spectra were analyzed with a commercial tool that uses an optimized set of basis functions to determine the relative concentrations of hepatic lipids (LCModel 6.3, Oakville, Canada). Calculated peak areas of water and fat were corrected for T2 relaxation applying previously published literature values [32] and were used to calculate the liver fat content (hepatic fat fraction; given in %) according to the ratio LFC = Sfat/(Sfat + Swater) with Sfat as the sum of the areas under the methyl (0.9 ppm), methylene (1.3 ppm) and allylic (2.1 ppm) peaks and Swater as the area under the water peak (4.7 ppm).

The liver volume calculation was performed using a custom-made software tool (Matlab, MathWorks, Natick, MA, USA). The liver was manually segmented on the images acquired with an in-phase/opposed-phase sequence described in Thörmer et al. 2013 [33] trying to avoid bile ducts and larger vessels. The volume of the visceral adipose tissue (VAT) and subcutaneous adipose tissue (SAT) was determined using software for automated abdominal fat quantification [34] in a single slice (10 mm thick) at the level of the lower end of L3 which represents the best association to the abdominal fat volume [34–36].

Laboratory assessment, NAFLD fibrosis score, and PNPLA3 genotyping

Blood samples were collected from all study participants after the ultrasound examinations. Blood count and serum levels of aminotransferases (ALT and AST), glycohemoglobin (HbA1c), ferritin, albumin, and lipids (triglycerides, low density lipoprotein LDL, and high density lipoprotein HDL) were determined after fasting > 3 h (43/65 cases fasting > 12 h).

The non-alcoholic fatty liver disease fibrosis score was calculated as follows Score = −1.675 + 0.037× age (years) + 0.094× body mass index (kg/m^2) + 1.13× diabetes (yes 1, no 0) + 0.99× AST/ALT ratio − 0.013× platelet (Gpt/l) − 0.66× albumin (g/dl) [37].

Genotyping of PNPLA3 variant p.I148M (rs738409, allele C/G) was performed according to a previously described protocol with some modifications [38]. Briefly, we extracted genomic DNA from peripheral blood leukocytes and performed polymerase chain reaction (PCR) with subsequent melting curve analysis. PNPLA3 genotypes were determined by analytical melting using a pair of fluorescent resonance energy transfer (FRET) hybridization probes complementary to the mutated sequence. Primers and probes were synthesized according to the published nucleotide sequence (GenBank: NG_008631): Forward primer 5′-CTTATGAAG-GATCAGGAAAATTAAA-3′, Reverse primer 5′-GGGACA-GACCCTGAGGT-3′, Anchor probe 5′-ACCACGCCTCT-GAAGGAAGGAGGGATAAG-FL-3′, Sensor probe 5′-LC610-CCACTGTAGAACGGCATGAAGC-PH-3′.

Statistical analysis

Ordinal and nominal data were collected in a Microsoft® Excel file. Statistical analyses were conducted by using MedCalc 12.7 (MedCalc Software, Belgium) and the R statistical package (Version 2.14.0) and the pROC sub-package for receiver operating characteristics [39]. Clinical and laboratory data were expressed as median and range or mean ± standard deviation (SD), as appropriate. Elastography, CAP and ^{1}H-MRS results are presented as boxplots and strip charts.

Fisher's exact test and chi-square test were used to test for association of variables. Nonparametric tests were chosen to compare pseudo-median values of two independent samples (Mann-Whitney U test) or groups (Kruskal-Wallis test) or expected trends (one-sided Jonckheere-Terpstra test). The t-test was used for comparison of mean values of independent samples. For trends in the mean, an ANOVA with polynomial contrasts was performed, where the p-value for the linear term was used after verifying that higher order terms did not contribute significantly. Post-hoc analyses after finding a group effect looked at all combinations of pairs or contiguous pairs if a trend test was performed and corrected for multiple testing using Bonferroni-Holm correction. If such a correction was employed, the corresponding p-value is denoted a "corrected p-value". Correlations between variables were examined using Pearson's correlation coefficients and the comparison of two sub-groups used the Fisher z-transform [40]. A p-value < 0.05 was considered significant.

The potential influence of biopsy age was investigated by including it both as a continuous and categorial variable in linear/logistic regressions.

Diagnostic performance of the non-invasive methods was evaluated using receiver operating characteristic curves. The probabilities of a true-positive (sensitivity, sens.) and a true-negative (specificity, spec.) were estimated as the proportions in the cohort (i.e. maximum likelihood) and Wilson confidence intervals were constructed. The area under the receiver operating characteristics curve (AUC) was calculated using the trapezoidal rule, where confidence intervals were found according to [41].

Cut-off calculation

For the ROC curve analysis, cut-off values optimizing the Youden index were calculated for comparison with previous results, some of which implicitly stressed high sensitivity and others high specificity. In addition, we applied published cut-off-values for TE and CAP to our study cohort: For TE, a cut-off of 7.9 kPa has been described for sensitive identification of patients at risk of advanced NAFLD associated fibrosis in a large biopsy controlled cohort [42]. More recently, CAP had a sensitivity > 90% for the detection of hepatic steatosis ≥ S1 and ≥ S2 in patients with chronic liver disease at a cut-off value of 215 and 252 dB/m, respectively [19].

For the CAP procedure an additional cut-off value considering the specific clinical diagnostic requirements was determined by introducing a score to be optimized and estimating the associated confidence interval with bootstrapping procedures.

Results

Clinical characteristics of the study cohort

We recruited 53 patients with NAFLD and 17 healthy volunteers. However, three patients had histological and clinical features of concomitant autoimmune or cholestatic liver disease. Two control cases showed signs of liver disease (one with steatotic liver ultrasound pattern, one with elevated aminotransferases) and were excluded. Therefore, 50 patients with NAFLD and 15 healthy controls were included in the final analysis.

Patients with NAFLD were classified by a single expert pathologist according to the histological degree of steatosis: 18, 20, and 12 cases had mild (S1), moderate (S2), and severe (S3) steatosis, respectively [1,29]. Fibrosis staging revealed F0, F1, F2, F3, and F4 fibrosis in 10, 32, 2, 3, and 3 cases. The associations between CAP, ^{1}H-MRS and histology were essentially unaffected by the age of the biopsy (all p-values > 0.3).

Clinical characteristics of the study cohort are presented in table 1. Gender distribution did not differ significantly between the three NAFLD subgroups and only slight differences in age were observed. Time span since liver biopsy did not differ significantly. NAFLD cases with mild steatosis (S1) had a lower prevalence of hepatocellular inflammation (NASH) (n = 4/18 vs. 22/32, p = 0.003), arterial hypertension (n = 4/18 vs. 20/32, p = 0.008), and a trend towards a lower prevalence of diabetes mellitus type 2 (n = 2/18 vs. 12/32, p = 0.056) compared to patients with more advanced steatosis (S2 and S3). Moreover, S2 and S3 patients had a higher frequency of the non-CC *PNPLA3* genotype (n = 22/32 vs. 4/18, p = 0.003) and a trend towards a higher risk profile according to the NAFLD score (intermediate/high risk n = 16/32 vs. 4/18, p = 0.074) (table 1).

Table 1. Baseline characteristics of the study cohort.

		Healthy Controls	Patients with NAFLD		
Degree of steatosis	**NAS**	**(S0)**	**S1**	**S2**	**S3**
Anthropometry					
sex	male/female	6/9	11/7	9/11	5/7
age*	years	38.5 ± 11.8	50.4 ± 12.9	60.0 ± 7.5	54.7 ± 9.1
BMI*	kg/m^2	22.9 ± 2.4	25.9 ± 4.1	29.0 ± 4.0	33.0 ± 4.9
waist-to-hip*	ratio	0.86 ± 0.13	0.90 ± 0.09	0.96 ± 0.08	0.96 ± 0.06
Comorbidities					
diabetes mell. type 2	n	0	2 (11%)	6 (30%)	6 (50%)
arterial hypertension	n	0	4 (22%)	12 (60%)	8 (67%)
Histology					
time since biopsy*	months	-	14.8 ± 14.4	13.3 ± 12.9	17.6 ± 14.6
fibrosis	F0	(15)	8	1	1
	F1	-	9	14	9
	F2	-	0	1	1
	F3	-	0	2	1
	F4	-	1	2	0
inflammation	absent/present	(15/0)	14/4	6/14	4/8
PNPLA3 genotyping					
rs738409 CC/CG/GG	n	8/6/1	14/4/0	7/10/3	3/8/1
NAFLD Score					
low risk	n	14	14	11	5
indeterminate risk	n	1	3	7	7
high risk	n	0	1	2	0
Laboratory values					
ALT/ULN*	ratio	0.43 ± 0.09	1.20 ± 1.13	1.32 ± 1.06	1.04 ± 0.31
AST/ULN*	ratio	0.53 ± 0.10	0.89 ± 0.44	1.07 ± 0.63	0.98 ± 0.40
GGT/ULN*	ratio	0.41 ± 0.24	2.51 ± 3.43	2.05 ± 1.82	1.98 ± 2.13
HbA1c*	(%)	4.98 ± 0.21	5.14 ± 0.50	5.56 ± 0.71	6.04 ± 0.96
ferritin/ULN*,**	ratio	0.50 ± 0.56	0.82 ± 0.70	1.08 ± 0.77	0.88 ± 0.85
triglycerides*	(μmol/l)	0.97 ± 0.49	1.17 ± 0.51	1.77 ± 0.89	2.18 ± 1.19
LDL cholesterol*	(mmol/l)	2.74 ± 0.80	3.48 ± 0.82	3.49 ± 1.08	3.59 ± 1.19
HDL cholesterol*	(mmol/l)	1.90 ± 0.43	1.77 ± 0.62	1.39 ± 0.44	1.41 ± 0.39

* values presented as mean and standard deviation.
** values missing in three individuals (2x S1, 2x S3).
Abbreviations: BMI – body mass index, ULN – upper limit of normal.

Transient elastography and performance of CAP

Valid and reliable TE and CAP results could be obtained in all control cases (100%) and 46/50 patients with NAFLD (92%). Patients with fibrosis stage F2–4 (n = 8) had higher median TE values (18.0 kPa) compared to NAFLD cases with stage F0–1 and controls (4.8 kPa, n = 53), 95% CI for increase in median [9.0, 22.4] kPa, $p<0.0001$. The ROC curve analysis for differentiation between F0–1 and F2–4 fibrosis revealed a high accuracy (sensitivity 100% [67.6, 100]%, specificity 98.1% [90.1, 99.9]%, AUC 0.991 [0.971, 1]) at a cut-off value of 8.85 kPa.

Median CAP values increased significantly with the degree of hepatic steatosis ($p < 0.0001$) and differed by an estimated 52 dB/m ([19, 80] dB/m, corrected $p = 0.002$) between the controls and S1 and by 67 dB/m ([40, 80] dB/m, corrected $p = 0.0001$) between S1 and S2 (table 2, figure 1A). ROC curve analysis revealed a high accuracy for differentiation between absence vs. any degree of steatosis (S0 vs. S1–3, AUC 0.930 [0.865, 0.996]) and mild vs. moderate/severe (S0–1 vs. S2–3, AUC 0.934 [0.883, 0.994]) hepatic steatosis, whereas the area under the curve for differentiation between S0–2 and S3 steatosis was 0.816 [0.701, 0.932] (table 3).

MR imaging and performance of MR spectroscopy

All healthy subjects and 48 patients with NAFLD (96%) underwent MRI examinations. One patient was excluded from MRI due to a contraindication (pacemaker), one patient refused examination because of claustrophobia. In addition, ^{1}H-MRS data from one healthy volunteer were lost due to a technical error during data acquisition.

Liver volume and visceral fat volume showed a stepwise increase compared to the degree of hepatic steatosis. A similar trend was

Table 2. Elastography, Controlled attenuation parameter (CAP) and magnetic resonance imaging.

		Healthy Controls	NAFLD Patients – degree of steatosis			p-value
		(S0)	S1	S2	S3	
Transient Elastography	valid/all	15/15	16/18	19/20	11/12	0.6
skin-to-liver-capsule distance*	mm	16.3 ± 2.7	19.7 ± 3.7	23.5 ± 6.4	26.2 ± 5.3	p < 0.0001
liver stiffness**	kPa	4.4 [2.3–5.9]	4.8 [1.9–59.3]	5.3 [2.7–70.6]	5.4 [3.5–21.8]	p = 0.003
CAP*	dB/m	201 ± 44	253 ± 43	321 ± 42	335 ± 43	p < 0.0001
Magnetic resonance imaging	available (n)	15	18	19	11	-
liver volume*	ml	1346 ± 223	1435 ± 353	1746 ± 394	2067 ± 390	p < 0.0001
subcutaneous fat volume (L3)*	ml	240 ± 116	283 ± 81	318 ± 99	384 ± 109	p = 0.002
visceral fat volume (L3)*	ml	75 ± 106	113 ± 59	194 ± 103	247 ± 137	p < 0.00001
^{1}H-MRS (segment VII)**	rel. lipid signal	0.8 [0–8.6]#	5.2 [0.9–33.7]	15.4 [1.6–32.3]	22 [8.2–34.9]	p < 0.00001

* values presented as mean and standard deviation
** values presented as median and range
#available in 14 cases of the control cohort
Abbreviations: MRS – magnetic resonance spectroscopy

observed for the subcutaneous fat volume (post-hoc analyses could verify only that it was significant for S0 vs. S3 however) (table 2).

The median hepatic fat fraction measured by ^{1}H-MRS also increased significantly with the degree of hepatic steatosis ($p < 0.001$) with an estimated change of 3 percentage points ([1,6], corrected $p = 0.01$) between the control group and S1, of 9 percentage points ([2,14], corrected $p = 0.01$) between S1 and S2 and an estimated 6 percentage points ([−1, 13], $p = 0.1$) between S2 and S3 (table 2, figure 2). All degrees (S1–3), moderate/severe (S2–3), and severe (S3) hepatic steatosis were detected with good accuracy (AUC > 0.85, lower end of 95% CI > 0.75) (table 3, figure 1B).

Comparison of CAP and MR spectroscopy

Correlation of CAP and ^{1}H-MRS was analyzed using Pearson's correlation coefficient. Both methods correlated modestly in the total study cohort ($n = 58$ with available valid CAP and ^{1}H-MRS results, $r = 0.63$ [0.44, 0.76], $p<0.001$), while analysis of NAFLD cases only resulted in an even weaker correlation ($n = 44$; $r = 0.56$, [0.32, 0.74], $p<0.001$). We therefore further analyzed the influence of liver fibrosis on correlation between CAP and ^{1}H-MRS: the correlation in patients with biopsy proven liver fibrosis F2–4 ($n = 8$, $r = -0.2$, [−0.8, 0.6]) differed significantly from the correlation for those with no or mild fibrosis (F0–1) ($r = 0.7$, [0.5, 0.8]), in whom the comparison of these correlations resulted in $p < 0.0001$ (figure 2). The individuals with F2–4 fibrosis showed higher ferritin levels compared to cases with F0–1 fibrosis (median 113%ULN vs. 59%ULN, difference in pseudo-median 70 percentage points [11, 207], $p = 0.02$).

Cut-off values for clinical use

Applying a TE cut-off value of 7.9 kPa [42] to our cohort resulted in 100% [68, 100]% sensitivity for the detection of F2–4 fibrosis with a specificity of 94% [85, 98]%. Similarly, a CAP cut-off of 252 dB/m resulted in a 100% [89%, 100%] sensitivity for detecting and S2–3 steatosis, but a specificity of only 71% [53%, 84%] (figure 3A). At the 252 dB/m threshold, steatosis quantification was accurate for controls and patients with steatosis S2 and S3, while 8/16 (50%) of S1 patients with valid CAP results were misclassified. These eight patients had a trend toward a higher BMI (27.0±4.1 vs. 23.6±2.3 kg/m^2, $p = 0.06$), NAFLD score (−1.4±1.6 vs. −3.0±1.2, $p = 0.04$) and skin-to-liver-capsule distances (20.8±3.3 vs. 17.5±2.1, $p = 0.03$) compared to correctly classified S1 patients. Only one of the misclassified patients had a skin-to-liver-capsule distance above 25 mm (27.2 mm).

In clinical practice diagnostic tests with high specificity are required [43]. This requirement cannot be met with a single cut-off and we thus chose to employ a second, higher one, which will permit us to improve specificity at the price of introducing the category of "unclassified" patients requiring further testing.

We did so by determining the CAP value for the detection of steatosis ≥ S2 that maximizes the score

score = (true positives + 0.5 true negatives −3 false positives − false negatives −0.25 unclassified)/(n_patients + 0.5 n_control)

which has the value 1 for a perfect test. While the choice of four coefficients may seem to permit a large amount of arbitrariness, we point out that other methods, such as optimizing a ROC curve or the sensitivity, make similar choices implicitly. They lack however the freedom to provide a weight to each item as appropriate to the diagnosis under scrutiny.

This calculation revealed a cut-off of 301 dB/m. Bootstrapping (5000 times repetition) with a random selection of half the data points results in a median cut-off of 294 dB/m with 95% of the values in the interval [257, 345] dB/m. We therefore used a cut-off of 300 dB/m for the detection of S2–3 steatosis to obtain high specificity, while retaining the lower cut of 215 dB/m for the definition of healthy individuals (figure 3B). Applying these cut-offs to the 61 patients/controls with valid CAP measurements results in 20 true positive and one false negative diagnosis, 9 true negative and no false negative cases and 31 who are unclassified and require further testing. The implications regarding positive and negative predictive values and the proportion of unclassified cases can be found in figure 4. There, one can see that predictive values are above 80% for prevalences roughly between 0.25 and 0.7, but with 40 to 60% of the patients remaining uncharacterized.

Discussion

Non-invasive hepatic fat quantification has a growing importance for the diagnosis and monitoring of hepatic steatosis [15,16]. To our knowledge, this is the first study that provides a head-to-head comparison of the ultrasound based CAP technology and MR spectroscopy for hepatic steatosis quantification. CAP is

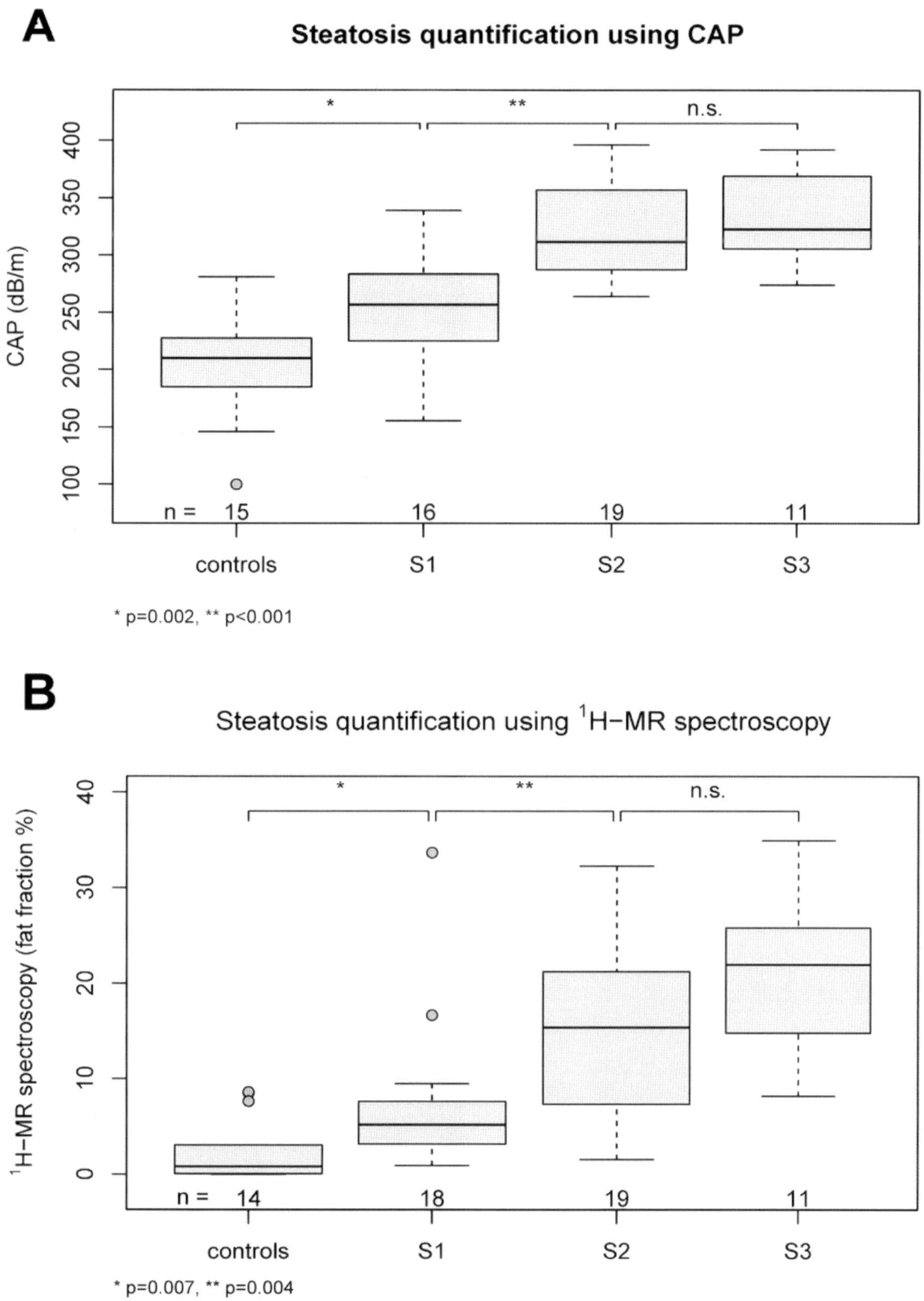

Figure 1. CAP (A) and ^{1}H-MRS (B) correlate with hepatic steatosis. CAP and ^{1}H-MRS values correlate with the amount of hepatic fat and show a stepwise increase compared to the NAS staging (61 and 62 valid measurements available, respectively).

calculated from the TE ultrasound signal attenuation and can therefore only be acquired given a successful TE measurement [27]. Thus, limitations of TE – mainly obesity – likewise impair CAP feasibility [27,31,44]. In addition, influencing factors on CAP accuracy and quality standards (e.g. exclusion of results with high IQR values) are not yet defined [18,19]. In our study cohort, although CAP results were only considered when TE fulfilled the commonly accepted quality criteria [19], a high success rate was

Table 3. Diagnostic performance for detection of hepatic steatosis at optimal cut-off (optimizing the Youden Index).

		CAP	^{1}H-MRS
S0 (controls) vs. S1–3	cases (n)#	15/46	14/48
	Sensitivity	93% [80, 100]%	79% [57, 100]%
	Specificity	87% [76, 96]%	88% [77, 96]%
	AUC*	0.93 [0.86, 1.00]	0.88 [0.78, 0.99]
	cut-off	233.5 dB/m	3.12% fat fraction
S0–1 vs. S2–3	cases (n)#	31/30	32/30
	Sensitivity	97% [90, 100]%	91% [81, 100]%
	Specificity	81% [64, 94]%	77% [60, 90]%
	AUC*	0.94 [0.88, 0.99]	0.88 [0.79, 0.97]
	cut-off	268.5 dB/m	8.77% fat fraction
S0–2 vs. S3	cases (n)#	50/11	51/11
	Sensitivity	82% [55, 100]%	91% [73, 100]
	Specificity	76% [64, 88]%	75% [63, 86]
	AUC*	0.82 [0.70, 0.93]	0.85 [0.75, 0.95]
	cut-off	301.2 dB/m	13.69% fat fraction

#Only patients with valid measurements were considered for this analysis.
* Comparison of CAP and ^{1}H-MRS ROC curves did not reveal significant differences of AUC.

observed for both healthy individuals (100%) and patients with NAFLD (92%).

1H-MRS techniques expl°it the difference in resonance frequencies between water and fat signals for estimation of hepatic fat concentration and usually have a high feasibility (>90% in our cohort) [28]. Their application is limited by implanted medical devices and claustrophobia, and can also be impaired by severe obesity [45].

CAP and ^{1}H-MRS each correlated fairly well with biopsy proven steatosis and significantly differentiated between S0, S1 and S2 patients (figure 1). However, a significant difference could not be detected in subjects with advanced disease (S2–S3), which is in line with the CAP data of Myers et al. [18] and de Ledinghen et

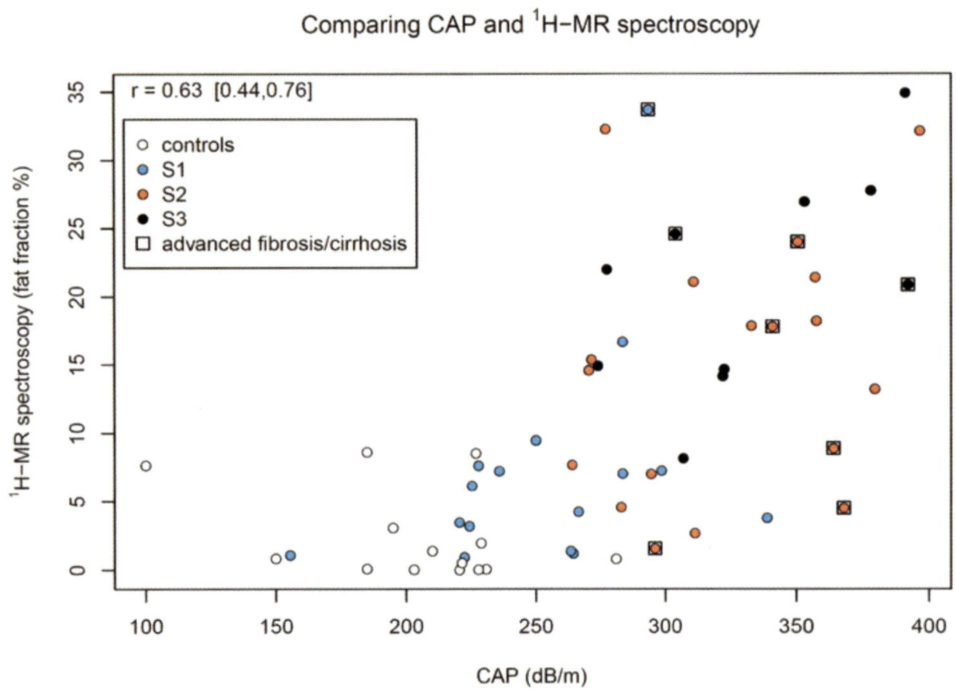

Figure 2. Correlation of CAP and ^{1}H-MRS. CAP and ^{1}H-MRS achieved only a modest correlation, especially in patients with concomitant fibrosis (labeled with squares). A total of 61 valid measurements were available.

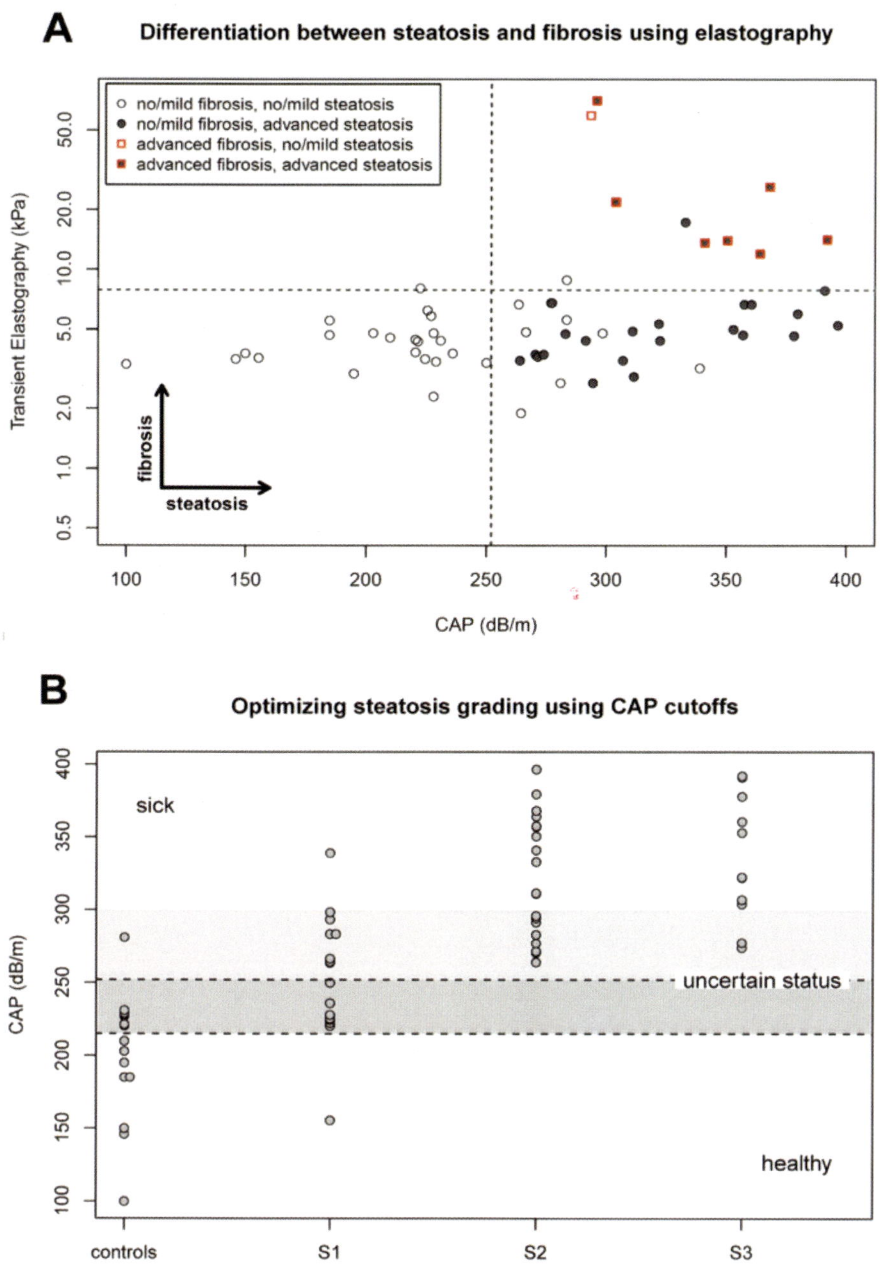

Figure 3. CAP and TE cut-off values for clinical use. Application of published cut-off values for TE (7.9 kPa) and CAP (252 dB/m^2) results in high sensitivity for detection of distinct fibrosis and steatosis (A) [19,43]. CAP values between 215 dB/m [19] and 300 dB/m require further diagnostic procedures for differentiation of the degree of steatosis ("grey area") (B).

al. [19] and may limit adequate monitoring of steatosis changes in these patients.

In the head-to-head comparison between both methods, CAP and ^{1}H-MRS achieved only a modest correlation, especially in patients with concomitant fibrosis (figure 2). In these individuals increased serum ferritin levels suggest NASH associated hepatic iron deposition [46] which can interfere with MR-based steatosis assessment and thus may have contributed to imprecise liver fat quantification [47,48]. Correlation may be further impaired by anthropometrical characteristics like high BMI or large skin to liver capsule distance, which can affect accuracy of transient elastography and hence CAP [22,49,50] and cannot be assessed without the additional use of ultrasound.

Anthropometrically related limitations of the TE and CAP technology may be overcome by further development of the TE XL probe. At present, CAP is only available for the M probe of the transient elastography system which reduces feasibility and reliability in patients with BMI values > 28 kg/m^2 and high skin-to-liver capsule distances [51]. Implementation of CAP in the TE XL probe, which is designed for liver stiffness assessment in obese patients, may overcome this limitation in the future [27,51].

Considering non-invasive methods as an alternative to liver biopsy, cut-off values for steatosis grading are required. Our ^{1}H-MRS cut-off value for the detection of any steatosis grade (3.12% fat fraction) corresponds to data from Szczepaniak et al. who determined a hepatic fat fraction signal of 5.56% as upper 95th

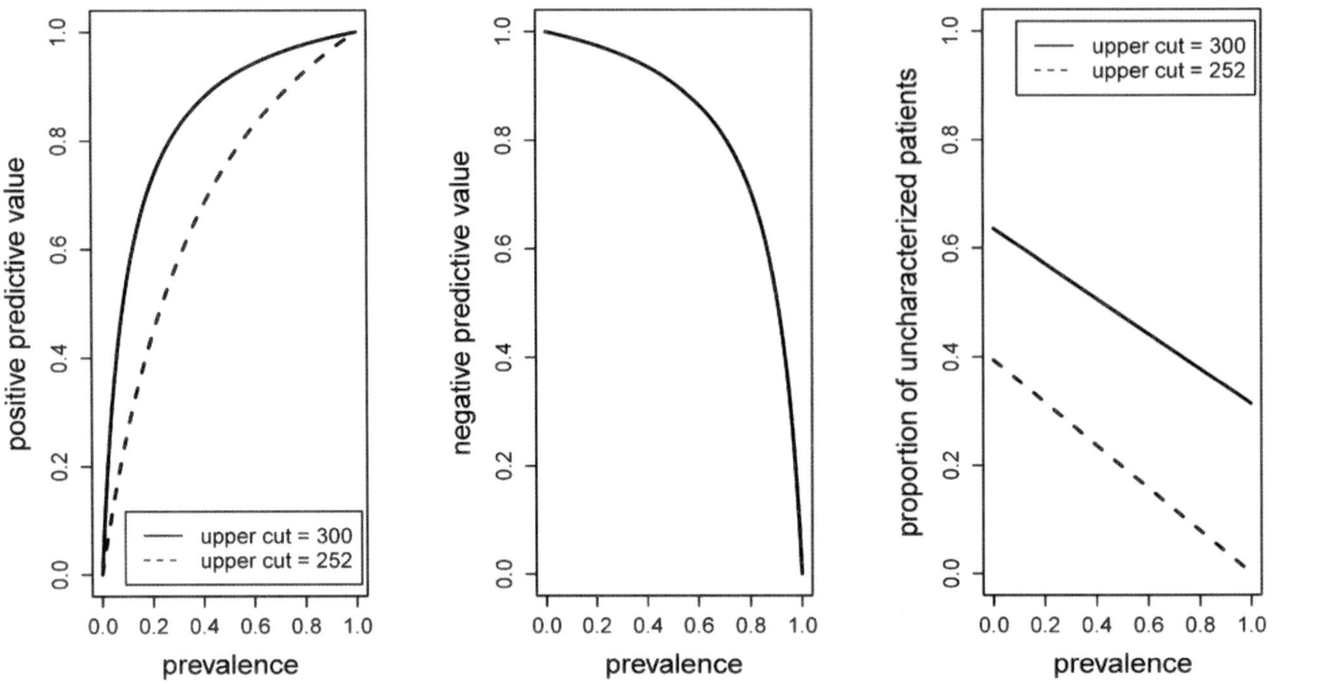

Figure 4. Positive and negative predictive values as well as proportion of uncharacterized cases as they depend upon prevalence. S0–1 patients and controls were classified as healthy and S2–3 as sick. The diagnostic procedure made use of CAP where those with values below 215 dB/m were diagnosed as healthy, those with values above 300 dB/m (or 252 dB/m, dashed lines) were diagnosed as sick and those in between were not diagnosed. A total of 61 valid measurements were available.

percentile in healthy individuals [23]. However, further biopsy controlled studies applying ^{1}H-MRS did not provide cut-off values thus rendering a comparison difficult [17,52,53].

Our CAP cut-off values for different grades of hepatic steatosis are in line with data from previous biopsy controlled studies evaluating CAP in various chronic liver diseases [17–21]. To date, CAP and ^{1}H-MRS results show a distinct overlap between NAFLD subgroups (figure 1) which affects correct classification in a considerable proportion of patients: depending on the applied cut-off value and the estimated prevalence of steatosis in the population of interest, CAP correctly classifies 50% of individuals with absent/mild (S0–1) or moderate/severe (S2–3) steatosis (figure 3b, figure 4). The introduction of two cut-offs is important for dealing with this issue and improving the predictive value of the technique. We point out that one cannot expect, or even strive for very high predictive values so long as the gold standard itself contains a considerable amount of error. As described above, this is the case with biopsies, meaning that the "correct" diagnosis itself may be erroneous in a considerable fraction of cases [11,12].

However, care for patients with NAFLD in clinical practice requires not only grading of hepatic steatosis, but precise cut-off values for identification of "healthy" and "sick" individuals. Therefore, a clear diagnostic and therapeutic concept is necessary when non-invasive methods of steatosis grading are implemented in clinical routine or as diagnostic tools in clinical studies with special regard to patients assigned to the "grey area": Careful patient selection, consideration of interfering factors (e.g. body mass index, skin to liver capsule distance, fibrosis) and combination of different methods may improve the diagnostic accuracy of non-invasive liver assessment and underline its potential as a guidance to liver biopsy [54]. Longitudinal studies are required to define the value of CAP as a monitoring tool for hepatic steatosis in interventional studies.

In addition to the steatosis evaluation with the CAP technology, transient elastography could simultaneously diagnose hepatic fibrosis. Applying the cut-off value of 7.9 kPa, which has been proposed for patients with NAFLD with F3-4 fibrosis by Wong et al. [42], fibrosis could be detected in all individuals at risk for disease progression (cases with F2–F4 fibrosis) in our cohort (figure 3A). Differences in the classification of F2 patients in our study compared to Wong et al. may be related to the baseline characteristics of the study cohorts, as Wong et al. included 48% individuals with Chinese ethnicity [42] and the low case numbers. Thus, transient elastography with the M probe and simultaneous CAP measurement are promising tools to non-invasively characterize major histopathological aspects of patients with NAFLD. In the future, these methods have to prove recent data for the NAFLD fibrosis score which could show that non-invasive characterization of NAFLD better predicts long-term outcome than histology [55].

Our study has some limitations:

i) We used liver histology as a reference standard for steatosis grading and fibrosis staging. Histology classifies steatosis according to the number of affected hepatocytes without assessing the hepatic triglyceride concentration [29]. This limits its comparability with hepatic fat fraction measurement by ^{1}H-MRS and ultrasound signal attenuation calculation by CAP. In this regard, further biopsy controlled longitudinal studies are required to determine whether the proportion of affected hepatocytes, the type of steatosis (micro- or macrovesicular), or the hepatic lipid concentration are the best marker for disease severity and risk of progression.

ii) We cannot exclude alteration of histological NAFLD features during the time interval from biopsy to study inclusion. Although unlikely for simple steatosis [56], significant disease progression may have contributed to the finding of narrow differences of CAP and ^{1}H-MRS results in patients with S2 and S3 steatosis. Our analyses could not detect any such effect however. In addition, liver biopsies were not performed as part of our study examinations for ethical reasons as this invasive procedure would not have influenced the clinical management in our NAFLD patients.

iii) Our results were acquired in a NAFLD population with a limited prevalence of advanced liver damage (16% of cases with ≥F2 fibrosis). Therefore, further studies are required to investigate the correlation of CAP and ^{1}H-MRS in cohorts with advanced NAFLD stages.

In conclusion, our pilot data suggest a comparable diagnostic accuracy of CAP and ^{1}H-MRS for non-invasive characterization of hepatic steatosis. Together with the simultaneous fibrosis assessment by transient elastography, it represents a fast and easy to use method to characterize patients with NAFLD non-invasively. Considering the increasing NAFLD prevalence, its growing medical impact, and the need for easy, repetitive, and reliable diagnostic tools, it is encouraging that CAP can already correctly classify 50% of individuals with values <215 dB/m excluding hepatic steatosis and results >300 dB/m identifying > 33% steatosis.

Acknowledgments

We thank Katrin Moritz and Sieglinde Erdmann for their dedicated support in coordinating the study as well as Claudia Taubert and Lars Selig for technical support. We further thank Cornelia Borchers and Michael Stumvoll for their support of the research grant application.

Author Contributions

Conceived and designed the experiments: T. Karlas NG HT CW HB T. Kahn JM TB MT VK JW. Performed the experiments: T. Karlas NG SB CW NL AS HB MT VK JW. Analyzed the data: T. Karlas DP NG SB CW MW IS NL AS HB T. Kahn JM TB MT VK JW. Contributed reagents/materials/analysis tools: T. Karlas DP NG SB HT CW MW IS NL AS HB T. Kahn JM TB MT VK JW. Wrote the paper: T. Karlas DP NG SB HT CW HB JM TB MT VK JW. Figure preparation: DP. Study Logistics: HT. Reference Pathology: CW. Revision of manuscript: MW IS NL AS T. Kahn.

References

1. Chalasani N, Younossi Z, Lavine JE, Diehl AM, Brunt EM, et al. (2012) The diagnosis and management of non-alcoholic fatty liver disease: practice Guideline by the American Association for the Study of Liver Diseases, American College of Gastroenterology, and the American Gastroenterological Association. Hepatology 55: 2005–2023.
2. O'Shea RS, Dasarathy S, McCullough AJ (2010) Alcoholic liver disease. Hepatology 51: 307–328.
3. Ratziu V, Bellentani S, Cortez-Pinto H, Day C, Marchesini G (2010) A position statement on NAFLD/NASH based on the EASL 2009 special conference. J Hepatol 53: 372–384.
4. Musso G, Gambino R, Cassader M, Pagano G (2011) Meta-analysis: natural history of non-alcoholic fatty liver disease (NAFLD) and diagnostic accuracy of non-invasive tests for liver disease severity. Ann Med 43: 617–649.
5. Karlas T, Wiegand J, Berg T (2013) Gastrointestinal complications of obesity: non-alcoholic fatty liver disease (NAFLD) and its sequelae. Best Pract Res Clin Endocrinol Metab 27: 195–208.
6. Tilg H, Moschen AR (2010) Evolution of inflammation in nonalcoholic fatty liver disease: the multiple parallel hits hypothesis. Hepatology 52: 1836–1846.
7. Adinolfi LE, Restivo L, Marrone A (2013) The predictive value of steatosis in hepatitis C virus infection. Expert Rev Gastroenterol Hepatol 7: 205–213.
8. Jin X, Chen Y, Yang Y, Li Y, Zheng L, Xu C (2012) Association between hepatic steatosis and entecavir treatment failure in Chinese patients with chronic hepatitis B. PLoS ONE 7: e34198.
9. Musso G, Cassader M, Rosina F, Gambino R (2012) Impact of current treatments on liver disease, glucose metabolism and cardiovascular risk in non-alcoholic fatty liver disease (NAFLD): a systematic review and meta-analysis of randomised trials. Diabetologia 55: 885–904.
10. Iwasaki T, Yoneda M, Inamori M, Shirakawa J, Higurashi T, et al. (2011) Sitagliptin as a novel treatment agent for non-alcoholic Fatty liver disease patients with type 2 diabetes mellitus. Hepatogastroenterology 58: 2103–2105.
11. Bedossa P, Carrat F (2009) Liver biopsy: the best, not the gold standard. J Hepatol 50: 1–3.
12. Castera L, Pinzani M (2010) Biopsy and non-invasive methods for the diagnosis of liver fibrosis: does it take two to tango? Gut 59: 861–866.
13. Poynard T, Ratziu V, Naveau S, Thabut D, Charlotte F, et al. (2005) The diagnostic value of biomarkers (SteatoTest) for the prediction of liver steatosis. Comp Hepatol 4: 10.
14. Bedogni G, Bellentani S, Miglioli L, Masutti F, Passalacqua M, et al. (2006) The Fatty Liver Index: a simple and accurate predictor of hepatic steatosis in the general population. BMC Gastroenterol 6: 33.
15. Schwenzer NF, Springer F, Schraml C, Stefan N, Machann J, Schick F (2009) Non-invasive assessment and quantification of liver steatosis by ultrasound, computed tomography and magnetic resonance. J Hepatol 51: 433–445.
16. Sasso M, Miette V, Sandrin L, Beaugrand M (2012) The controlled attenuation parameter (CAP): a novel tool for the non-invasive evaluation of steatosis using Fibroscan. Clin Res Hepatol Gastroenterol 36: 13–20.
17. Friedrich-Rust M, Romen D, Vermehren J, Kriener S, Sadet D, et al. (2012) Acoustic radiation force impulse-imaging and transient elastography for non-invasive assessment of liver fibrosis and steatosis in NAFLD. Eur J Radiol 81: e325–331.
18. Myers RP, Pollett A, Kirsch R, Pomier-Layrargues G, Beaton M, et al. (2012) Controlled Attenuation Parameter (CAP): a noninvasive method for the detection of hepatic steatosis based on transient elastography. Liver Int 32: 902–910.
19. Lédinghen V de, Vergniol J, Foucher J, Merrouche W, Le Bail B (2012) Non-invasive diagnosis of liver steatosis using controlled attenuation parameter (CAP) and transient elastography. Liver Int 32: 911–918.
20. Sasso M, Tengher-Barna I, Ziol M, Miette V, Fournier C, et al. (2012) Novel controlled attenuation parameter for noninvasive assessment of steatosis using Fibroscan(®): validation in chronic hepatitis C. J Viral Hepat 19: 244–253.
21. Kumar M, Rastogi A, Singh T, Behari C, Gupta E, et al. (2013) Controlled attenuation parameter for non-invasive assessment of hepatic steatosis: Does etiology affect performance? J Gastroenterol Hepatol 28: 1194–1201.
22. Chon YE, Jung KS, Kim SU, Park JY, Park YN, et al. (2014) Controlled attenuation parameter (CAP) for detection of hepatic steatosis in patients with chronic liver diseases: a prospective study of a native Korean population. Liver Int 34: 102–109.
23. Szczepaniak LS, Nurenberg P, Leonard D, Browning JD, Reingold JS, et al. (2005) Magnetic resonance spectroscopy to measure hepatic triglyceride content: prevalence of hepatic steatosis in the general population. Am J Physiol Endocrinol Metab 288: e462–468.
24. Belfort R, Harrison SA, Brown K, Darland C, Finch J, et al. (2006) A placebo-controlled trial of pioglitazone in subjects with nonalcoholic steatohepatitis. N Engl J Med 355: 2297–2307.
25. Thomas EL, Potter E, Tosi I, Fitzpatrick J, Hamilton G, et al. (2007) Pioglitazone added to conventional lipid-lowering treatment in familial combined hyperlipidaemia improves parameters of metabolic control: relation to liver, muscle and regional body fat content. Atherosclerosis 195: e181–190.
26. Le T, Chen J, Changchien C, Peterson MR, Kono Y, et al. (2012) Effect of colesevelam on liver fat quantified by magnetic resonance in nonalcoholic steatohepatitis: a randomized controlled trial. Hepatology 56: 922–932.
27. Wong GL (2013) Transient elastography: Kill two birds with one stone? World J Hepatol 5: 264–274.
28. Reeder SB, Cruite I, Hamilton G, Sirlin CB (2011) Quantitative assessment of liver fat with magnetic resonance imaging and spectroscopy. J Magn Reson Imaging 34: 729–749.
29. Kleiner DE, Brunt EM, van Natta M, Behling C, Contos MJ, et al. (2005) Design and validation of a histological scoring system for nonalcoholic fatty liver disease. Hepatology 41: 1313–1321.
30. Sandrin L, Fourquet B, Hasquenoph J, Yon S, Fournier C, et al. (2003) Transient elastography: a new noninvasive method for assessment of hepatic fibrosis. Ultrasound Med Biol 29: 1705–1713.
31. Castéra L, Foucher J, Bernard PH, Carvalho F, Allaix D, et al. (2010) Pitfalls of liver stiffness measurement: a 5-year prospective study of 13,369 examinations. Hepatology 51: 828–835.
32. Hamilton G, Middleton MS, Bydder M, Yokoo T, Schwimmer JB, et al. (2009) Effect of PRESS and STEAM sequences on magnetic resonance spectroscopic liver fat quantification. J Magn Reson Imaging 30: 145–152.
33. Thörmer G, Bertram HH, Garnov N, Peter V, Schütz T, et al. (2013) Software for automated MRI-based quantification of abdominal fat and preliminary evaluation in morbidly obese patients. J Magn Reson Imaging 37: 1144–1450.
34. So R, Matsuo T, Sasai H, Eto M, Tsujimoto T, et al. (2012) Best single-slice measurement site for estimating visceral adipose tissue volume after weight loss in obese, Japanese men. Nutr Metab (Lond) 9: 56.

10

Lymphocytes as Liver Damage Mirror of HCV Related Adipogenesis Deregulation

Antonella Minutolo[1]¶, Beatrice Conti[1]¶, Sandro Grelli[3], Carmela Viscomi[1], Giancarlo Labbadia[4], Clara Balsano[1,2]*

1 Laboratory of Molecular Virology and Oncology, Francesco Balsano Foundation, ex A. Cesalpino Foundation, Rome, Italy, **2** Institute of Biology and Molecular Pathology (IBPM) – CNR (National Research Council), Rome, Italy, **3** U.O.C. Clinical Microbiology, Tor Vergata Hospital, Rome, Italy, **4** Department of Clinical and Medical Therapy, "Sapienza" University of Rome - Umberto I Hospital, Rome, Italy

Abstract

Hepatitis C virus infection leads to a wide spectrum of liver diseases ranging from mild chronic hepatitis to end-stage cirrhosis and hepatocellular carcinoma. An intriguing aspect of the HCV infection is its close connection with lipid metabolism playing an important role in the HCV life cycle and in its pathogenesis. HCV is known to be a hepatotropic virus; however, it can also infect peripheral blood mononuclear cells (PBMCs). The goal of the current investigation is to compare the adipogenesis profile of liver tissues to lymphocytes of HCV infected patients, in order to understand if PBMCs may reflect the alterations of intracellular pathways occurring during HCV-related liver steatosis. Using the Human Adipogenesis PCR Array, gene expression was analyzed in liver samples and PBMCs of chronic HCV+, HBV+ and Healthy Donors (HDs) patients. We observed a similar modulation of lipid metabolism in HCV+ and HBV+liver tissues and lymphoid, cells suggesting that PBMCs reflect the liver adipogenesis deregulation related to infection, even if the two viruses have a different impact in the regulation of the adipogenesis mechanisms. In particular, some genes involved in lipid metabolism and inflammation, as well as in cell transformation, were up-regulated, in a similar way, in both HCV models analyzed. Interestingly, these genes were positively correlated to virological and hepatic functional parameters of HCV+ patients. On the contrary, HBV+ patients displayed a completely different profile. PBMCs of HCV+ patients seem to be useful model to study how HCV-related lipid metabolism deregulation occurs in liver. The obtained data suggest some molecules as new possible biomarkers of HCV-related liver damage progression.

Editor: Gian Maria Fimia, Istituto Nazionale per le Malattie Infettive, Italy

Funding: This work was supported by FIRB-Programma "Futuro in Ricerca" (prot. RBAP10MY35) and MIUR-Programma di ricerca di Rilevante Interesse Nazionale (PRIN) 2009 (prot. 2009YNERCE) grants. The funders had no role in study design, data collection and analysis, decision to publish, or preparation of the manuscript.

* E-mail: clara.balsano@cnr.it

¶ These authors contributed equally to this work.

Introduction

The Hepatitis C virus (HCV) infection affects, approximately, 170 million individuals, about 3% of the world's population [1]. The severity grade and the speed of liver damage progression are defined by several cofactors such as age, gender, the host's genetic background, alcohol and drugs consumption, immune status, co-infections and the metabolic status [2,3]. HCV infects both hepatocytes and peripheral blood mononuclear cells (PBMCs) [4,5,6].

The HCV infection is characterized by specific clinical abnormalities of lipid metabolism, such as hypo-beta-lipoproteinaemia and liver steatosis [7]. The presence of steatosis and the progression throughout fibrosis are some of the main histological features of HCV infected patients [8,9]. The viral deregulation of lipid metabolism affects liver disease progression and the response to antiviral therapies [10]. The density of circulating HCV particles in the blood of chronically infected patients is very heterogeneous. The very low density of some particles has been attributed to an association of the virus with apolipoprotein-beta (apoB) positive and triglyceride rich lipoproteins (TRL) likely, resulting in hybrid lipoproteins, known as lipo-viro-particles (LVP). LVPs contain the viral envelope glycoproteins E1 and E2, capsid and viral HCV-RNA. The specific infectivity of these particles has been shown to be higher than the infectivity of particles of higher density [11,12]. Moreover, lipids play an important role in HCV life cycle: the viral entry is partly mediated by lipoprotein receptors (LDLR) [13]; the maturation and secretion of viral particles are mediated by the Apolipoprotein A–I [14] and the Very Low Density Lipoprotein (VLDL).

Currently, it is clear that HCV affects more than one aspect of the lipoprotein metabolism and the associated liver damage. The HCV-related lipid deregulation causes overexpression of different hepatic enzymes: hormone sensitive Lipase (LIPE), lipoprotein lipase (LPL) and Leptin [15]. Accordingly, patients exhibit serum lipid abnormalities, such as low levels of: LDL [16,17], Resistin (RETN) [18], Adiponectin (ADIPOQ) [19] and Adipogenin (ADIG) [20]. The genes involved in the lipid *de novo* synthesis and beta oxidation, such as the nuclear receptor Liver X Receptor alpha (LXR alpha), the Sterol regulatory element binding transcription factor 1 (SREBP1c), the Fatty acid synthase (FASN) and the Acetyl CoA carboxylase Beta (ACACB) respectively, are associated with HCV infection, too [21], as well as Fatty acid binding protein 4 (FABP4) that modulates inflammatory and metabolic response that is mainly expressed in adipocytes and macrophages [22].

We asked if PBMCs might be the mirror of the adipogenic deregulation occurring in the liver tissue, during HCV infection. Thus, we compared the adipogenesis profile of liver tissues to lymphocytes of HCV infected patients.

Experimental Procedures

Patients recruitment and biological samples collection

This research is born as a descriptive and observational study aimed to characterize adipogenesis profile in HCV+, HBV+ patients and healthy donors. The study protocol was approved by the Ethics Committee of Sapienza University, and written informed consent was obtained from each subject at the time of enrollment. "(Rif. 2534/26.07.2012 n. prot.717/12)". 40 HCV, 20 HBV-infected patients and 20 healthy donors (HDs) were enrolled in an open study by the Department of Public Health and Infectious Disease, University of Rome "La Sapienza" and UOC Clinical Microbiology, "Tor Vergata" Hospital of Rome. Exclusion criteria for HCV and HBV patients were: 1) previous treatment with antiviral therapy, immunosuppressive drugs, and/or regular use of drugs influencing lipid metabolism and/or oxidative stress; 2) advanced cirrhosis; 3) hepatocellular carcinoma; 4) other causes of liver disease or mixed etiologies; 5) human immunodeficiency virus infection; 6) active intravenous drug addiction, 7) alcohol consumption. The current study was performed in accordance with the principles of Good Clinical Practice, the principles of the Declaration of Helsinki, and its appendices, and local and national laws. Liver and Blood samples were collected at the same time and blood samples were used to isolate PBMCs through a density gradient according to the standard Ficoll-Hypaque (Pharmacia) technique. Separate scores for steatosis, lobular inflammation, and hepatocellular ballooning and to stage fibrosis from 0 to 4 [23]. Biopsies of HCV patients were classified for grade and stage according to the Scheuer system [24].

Table 1. Biochemical data of HCV+ and Healthy Donors (HDs).

	HCV (40)	HDs (20)	P^1
Sex (F/M)	25/15	9/11	
Age (years)	53.7±15.3	48.3±6.0	NS
Body weight (kg)	64.6±11.6	64.7±5	NS
BMI (kg/m2) (≤25)	24.6±4	24.7±0.6	NS
HOMA-IR (<2)	2.6±2.0	1.0±1.2	<0.05
cholesterol (81.1–235.5 mg/dL)	172.3±9.7	185.7±26.2	NS
HDL (34.7–56 mg/dL)	62.4±22.6	56.7±4.2	NS
LDL (54.8–120 mg/dL)	89.9±33.8	101.3±13.4	NS
Triglycerides (45.1–235 mg/dL)	91.7±12.9	90.7±15	NS
Ferritin (30–400 μg/L)	209.6±17	201.0±15.5	NS
AST (9–45 IU/mL)	50.6±14.1	29.7±10.2	<0.05
ALT (10–40 IU/mL)	71.6±9.7	26.3±2.3	<0.05
GGT (8–61 IU/mL)	55.1±4.2	50.1±1.0	NS
AP (40–129 IU/mL)	86.7±8.4	65.3±13.6	<0.05
Total bilirubin (<1.20 mg/dL)	0.7±0.3	0.55±0.1	NS
hsCRP (0.1–0.6 g/L)	1.8±0.3	0.4±0.2	<0.05
VES (0–25 mm/h)	13.8±1.5	10.0±0.5	NS
Glucose (73.9–109.9 mg/dL)	102.6±53.1	88.3±10.1	<0.05
Insulin (2.6–24.90 μU/mL)	9.3±3.8	4±1.6	<0.05
Hyaluronic acid (ng/ml)	106.3±45.3	51,7±18.3	NS

Footnotes: P^1 t-test HCV *vs* HDs.

Table 2. Biochemical data of HBV+ patients.

	HBV pts (20)		P^2
Sex (F/M)	12-ago		
Age (years)	51,5±6.35		NS
Body weight (kg)	63,5±10.56		NS
Body mass index (kg/m2) (≤25)	24,86±5		NS
HOMA-IR (<2)	1,71±0.36		NS
Total cholesterol (81.1–235.5 mg/dL)	187±0.63		NS
HDL cholesterol (34.7–56 mg/dL)	60±23.55		NS
LDL cholesterol (54.8–120 mg/dL)	115,5±23.6		NS
Triglycerides (45.1–235 mg/dL)	106,6±15.9		NS
Ferritin (30–400 μg/L)	210,45±13		NS
AST (9–45 IU/mL)	46±5.7	HBeAg −	NS
	49±3.7	HBeAg +	NS
ALT (10–40 IU/mL)	38±9.7	HBeAg −	NS
	78±5.63	HBeAg +	<0.05
GGT (8–61 IU/mL)	53.1±6		NS
AP (40–129 IU/mL)	78,8±7.3		<0.05
Total bilirubin (<1.20 mg/dL)	0,56±0.12		NS
hsCRP (0.1–0.6 g/L)	1,69±0.2		<0.05
VES (0–25 mm/h)	15±1.9		NS
Glucose (73.9–109.9 mg/dL)	90,2±12		NS
Insulin (2.6–24.90 μU/mL)	1,11±2.6		NS
Hyaluronic acid (ng/ml)	86,36		NS

Footnotes: P^2 t-test HBV *vs* HDs.

Table 3. Virological data of HCV+ and HBV+.

HCV pts	HCV-RNA PCR 10^6 (UI/mL)	2,11±27	<0.05*	P^3
	HCV genotype	1a: 42% (19)		
		1b: 30% (13)		
		2c: 17% (5)		
		2a/2c: 11% (3)		
HBV pts	Log10 IU/mL	HBV DNA	HBsAg	
	HBeAg −	4,6±0.36	1,642±0,15	
	HBeAg +	7,3±0.25	9,459±0,85	
		<0.05*	<0.05*	P^4

Footnotes: P^3 HCV *vs* HDsP^4 Anti HBeAg + *vs* Anti HBeAg -.

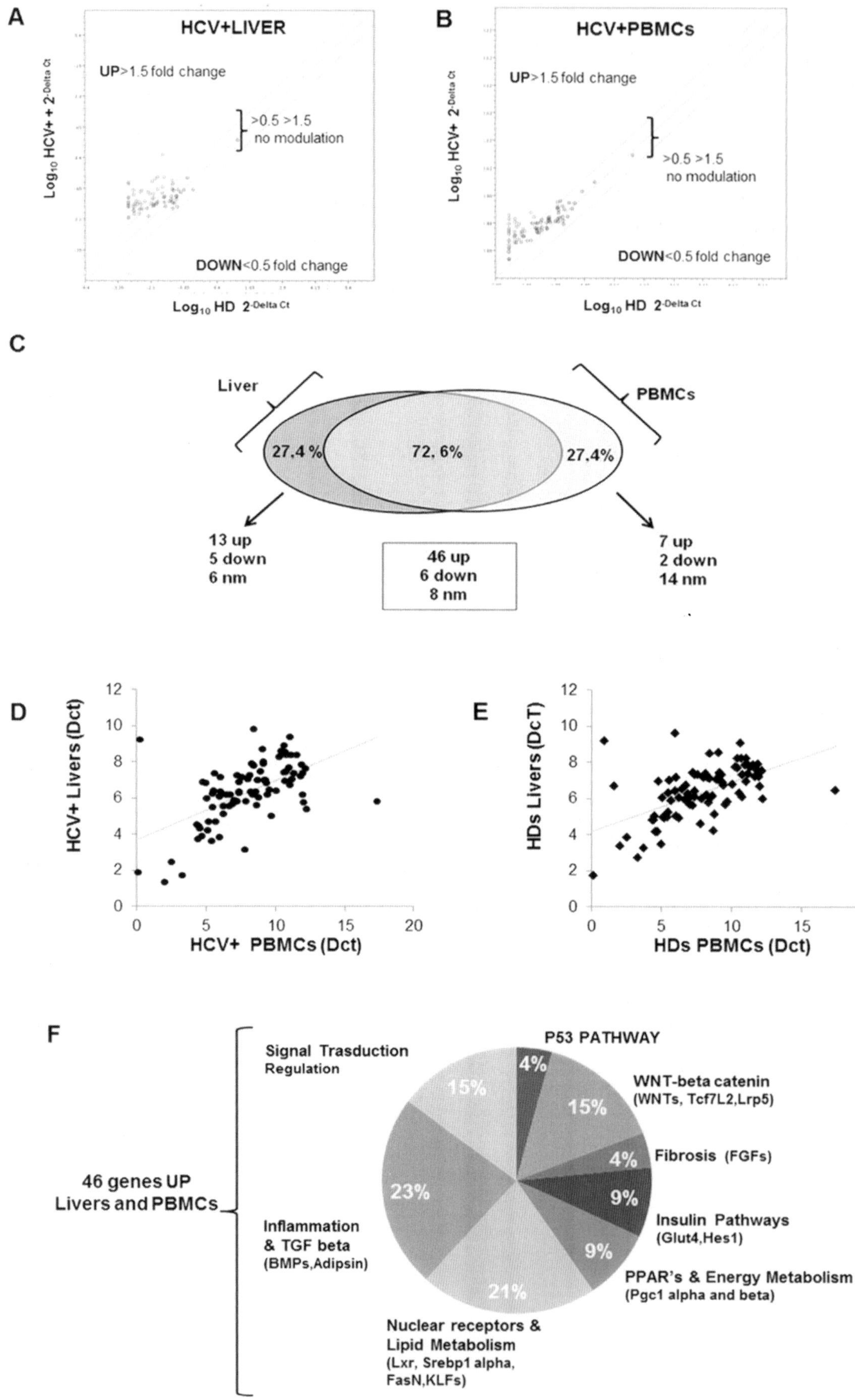
A
HCV+LIVER
UP>1.5 fold change
>0.5 >1.5
no modulation
DOWN<0.5 fold change
Log10 HCV+ + 2-Delta Ct
Log10 HD 2-Delta Ct
B
HCV+PBMCs
UP>1.5 fold change
>0.5 >1.5
no modulation
DOWN<0.5 fold change
Log10 HCV+ 2-Delta Ct
Log10 HD 2-Delta Ct
C
Liver
PBMCs
27.4 %
72, 6%
27.4%
13 up
5 down
6 nm
46 up
6 down
8 nm
7 up
2 down
14 nm
D
HCV+ Livers (Dct)
HCV+ PBMCs (Dct)
E
HDs Livers (DcT)
HDs PBMCs (Dct)
F
46 genes UP
Livers and PBMCs
Signal Trasduction
Regulation
15%
P53 PATHWAY
4%
WNT-beta catenin
(WNTs, Tcf7L2,Lrp5)
15%
Fibrosis (FGFs)
4%
9%
Insulin Pathways
(Glut4,Hes1)
9%
PPAR's & Energy Metabolism
(Pgc1 alpha and beta)
21%
Nuclear receptors &
Lipid Metabolism
(Lxr, Srebp1 alpha,
FasN,KLFs)
23%
Inflammation
& TGF beta
(BMPs,Adipsin)

Figure 1. HCV affects lipid metabolism in livers and PBMCs of chronic HCV + patients. A) Dot Plot Array profile in HCV+ *vs* HDs liver biopsies and PBMCs (B). Transcriptional levels of genes are shown as fold change (HCV+ *vs* HDs). Values >1.50 or <0.5 were considered significantly modified. C) Percentage of the total adipogenesis gene transcripts modulated in chronic HCV+ patients (livers and PBMCs). D, E) Significant positive correlation between all genes in HCV+ livers and PBMCs (rho values 0.688 and 0.889 respectively, p<0.005). F) Percentage of functional genes groups UP modulated in HCV+ livers and PBMCs.

Viral Load and Qualitative detection of antibodies to the Hepatitis C virus

HCV RNA viral load (VL) levels were determined using a quantitative ultrasensitive reverse transcription-polymerase chain reaction assay (Roche Diagnostics).

To detect anti-HCV antibodies in human sera (recombinant proteins NS3-NS4 and anti-capsid antibody) was used The Access (Beckman Coulter) HCV Ab PLUS assay immunoenzymatic method (Biorad).

HBV viral load, HBeAg and HBsAg detection

Qualitative HBeAg and Quantitative HBsAg levels were determined by using the Roche Cobas reagent kits (Roche Diagnostics). The HBV DNA viral load (IU/mL) was determined by using Cobas AmpliPrep/Cobas TaqMan HBV Test (Roche Diagnostics).

Cell culture, Constructs and Reagents

The human hepatoma-derived cell line Huh7.5 were grown in Dulbecco's modified Eagle's medium (DMEM) supplemented with 10% fetal bovine serum, 100 U/ml penicillin and 100 mg/ml streptomycin and 2 mM L-glutamine (Lonza).

J6/JFH1 cDNA (kindly provided by C. Rice, Rockefeller University) was used to generate the HCV cell model. Antibodies anti human KLF15, KLF3, TCF7L2 (Abcam), Adipsin, Adipogenin, Twist 1, beta Actin (Santa Cruz Biotechnology, Santa Cruz, CA), HCV NS5a (Austral Biologicals) were used for immunofluorescence assay. Detection was achieved using horseradish peroxidase–conjugate secondary antibody (Jackson ImmunoResearch Laboratories, West Grove, PA). ECL Plus Western and ECL-Hyperfilm (GE Healthcare Life Sciences) were used. Specific neutral lipids were stained with BODIPY (Invitrogen).

Replication and infection assays

The chimeric J6/JFH1 virus was generated and used according to Lindenbach BD and collegues [25]. Huh7.5 cells were infected (MOI = 0.1) 1 day after seeding. After 3 days cells were harvested and processed for RNA and protein extractions.

The lipid accumulation was evaluated through the fluorescent probe BODIPY used as a stain for neutral and non-polar lipids in immunofluorescent assay.

Immunofluorescence

Cells were grown on coverslips and fixed with 4% paraformaldehyde followed by permeabilization with 0.1% Triton X-100 in phosphate-buffered saline (PBS). Primary antibodies were incubated for 1 h at room temperature and visualized by conjugated secondary antibodies (invitrogen). Coverslips were mounted in SlowFade-Anti-Fade (Invitrogen) and examined under a confocal microscope (Leica TCS SP2)

Samples for mRNA expression analysis

Frozen liver biopsies tissues RNA were prepared with Trizol reagent (Invitrogen). Complementary DNA synthesis was generated from 2 µg of total RNA using the reverse transcription kit (Promega).

Human Adipogenesis PCR Array

To investigate a wide spectrum of genes involved in lipid metabolism the Human Adipogenesis RT^2 Profiler PCR Array (Qiagen) was used. 84 "metabolic" genes were analyzed in addition to positive control genes (beta actin and Ribosomal protein). Real-time PCR was performed with 7500 Fast Real-Time (Applied Biosystems) using Sybr green detection. Results were analyzed by RT^2 Profiler PCR Array Data Analysis. Transcriptional levels of genes were shown as fold change *vs* Healthy Donors, values >1.50 or <0.5 were considered significantly modified. All dataset was submitted in Geo Repository http://www.ncbi.nlm.nih.gov/geo. Accession number: GSE54432

Western blot analysis

For protein extraction, liver biopsies were homogenized and maintained on ice. Cells were collected and lysed and the proteins extracted were analyzed through SDS–PAGE and probed with different antibodies followed by detection with ECL plus (GE Healthcare).

Statistical Analysis

Statistical analysis of data was performed using the SPSS statistical software system (17.0 Windows). The independent samples t-test analysis was performed; for non-parametric correlation, Spearman's rho correlation coefficient was calculated by Bonferroni's correction.

Results

Patients' characteristics

For this pilot study, 40 naïve chronic HCV+ (72% genotype 1; 28% genotype 2), 20 HBV+ patients and 20 Healthy Donors (HDs) matched by age and gender, have been consecutively enrolled. Neither infected patients nor HDs were under any treatment at the moment of the enrollment. **Table 1, 2 and 3** highlight the clinical features of all patients studied. 27.3 % of HCV+ patients had a F2/F3 liver fibrosis, the remaining had F0-F1 liver fibrosis. Regarding the liver state of HBV+ patients, more than 80% had a F0/F1 grade of fibrosis (81,7%), the remaining had F2 status. Moreover 55% HBV population resulted HBeAg positive and 45% HBeAg negative. No steatosis was ecographically detectable in HD patients.

The adipogenesis of chronic HCV infected patients

First of all, we performed the RT-PCR array to investigate the adipogenesis profile on HCV+ liver biopsies. The liver of HCV+ patients was characterized by a deep deregulation of genes involved in the control of glucose and lipid metabolism (**Figure 1A**). Interestingly, we obtained a similar gene expression profile in the HCV+ PBMCs (**Figure 1B**). It is intriguing to note the two experimental models have a similar behavior: the larger part of the analyzed genes was modulated in a similar way (**Figure 1C**). All the details of adipogenesis profile in chronic HCV+ PBMCs and liver tissues were shown in **Table S1**.

In particular, the analysis of the HCV+ biopsies and PBMCs compared to HDs profile, revealed that 72,6 % of the analyzed genes were modulated in the same manner: 46 (77%) genes were

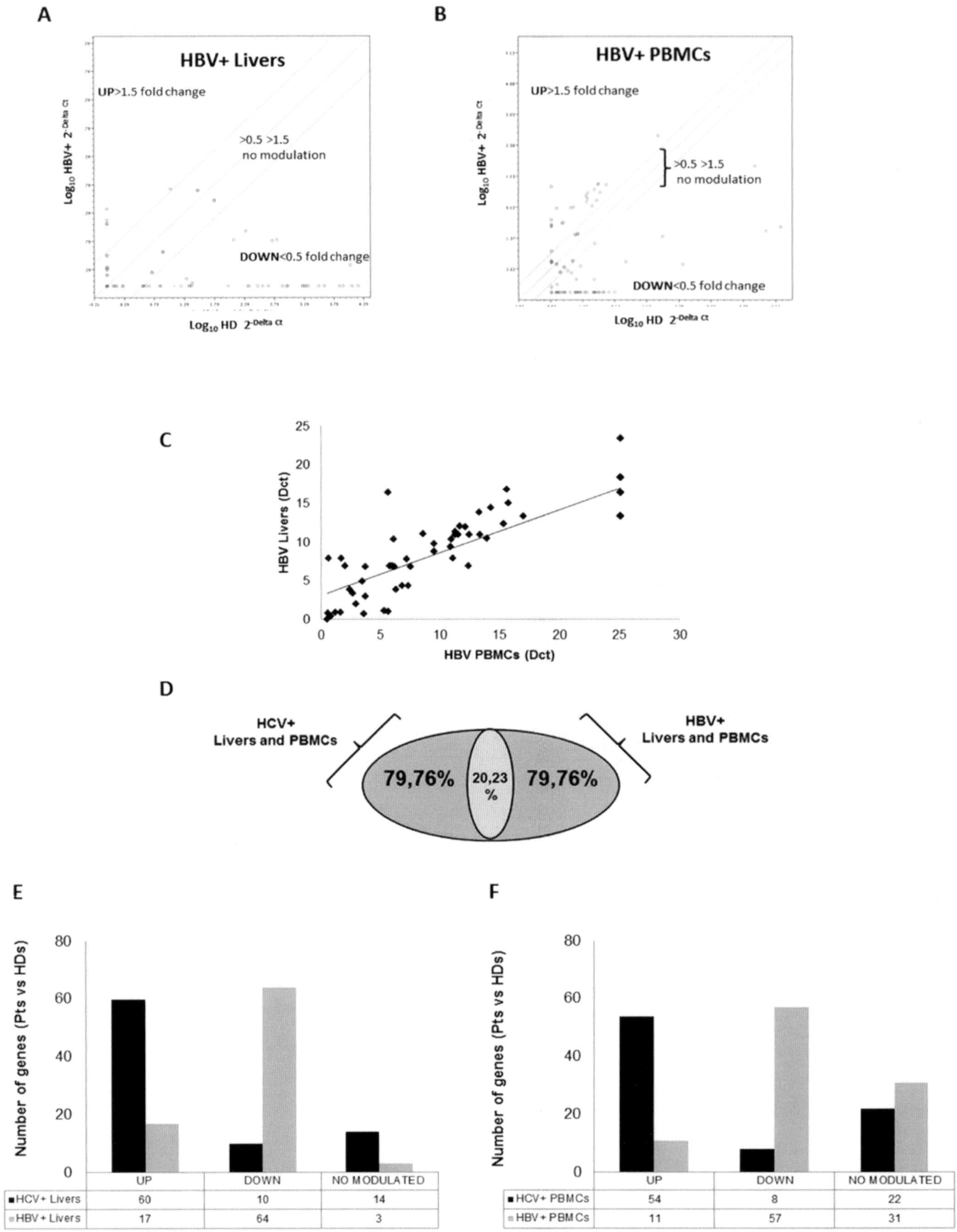

	UP	DOWN	NO MODULATED
HCV+ Livers	60	10	14
HBV+ Livers	17	64	3

	UP	DOWN	NO MODULATED
HCV+ PBMCs	54	8	22
HBV+ PBMCs	11	57	31

Figure 2. HCV and HBV infection adipogenesis profile. A, B) Dot Plot Array profile in HBV+ livers and PBMCs *vs* HDs. C) Significant positive correlation between all genes in HBV+ livers and PBMCs (rho values 0.759, $p<0.05$). D) Percentage of the total adipogenesis gene transcripts modulated in chronic HCV+ *vs* HBV+ patients' livers and PBMCs. E, F). Histogram plot comparing different number of genes modulation in HCV+ and HBV+ livers and PBMCs.

up-regulated, 6 (10%) down-regulated and 8 (13%) were unaffected by the virus. 27,4% of the studied genes were modulated in a different way (**Figure 1C and Table S1D**).

Spearman's rho statistical investigation showed a significant positive correlation (rho $=0.688$, $p<0.001$) among the genes analyzed, in both HCV+ liver biopsies and PBMCs (**Figure 1D**).

The same statistical evaluation was performed in HDs liver tissues and PBMCs, and gave us similar results (**Figure 1E**, rho $=0.889$, $p<0.001$).

Moreover, here we want to underline that HCV *in vitro* model is characterized by a similar transcriptional modulation of some genes (Adig, Adipsin, KLF15, KLF3, TCF7L2, TWIST1) already analyzed in HCV+ liver tissues and PBMCs, supporting the belief that PBMCs might be a good substitute of liver tissues for the investigation of HCV-dependent metabolic derangement (see below).

At this point, we considered interesting to focus our attention on HCV+ up-regulated genes, because in the other two groups (down-regulated and no modulated genes) there weren't genes involved in the control of adipogenic pathways. Among the up regulated genes, 41% of them were transcriptional factors involved in glucose and lipid metabolism (9.5% insulin pathway, 9.5% energy metabolism and 22% nuclear receptors) and 59% in cell transformation (4% p53 pathways, 15% Wnt/beta catenin, 9% fibrosis, 8% signal transduction and regulation and 23% inflammation) (**Figure 1F**).

Moreover we have noticed that the 25% of modulated genes were significantly more expressed in the HCV + patients with elevated liver damage (F2/F3) in comparison to HCV+ F0/F1. (**Figure S1** and **Table S3**, $p<0.05$).

The deregulation of adipogenesis is specifically due to HCV-infection

Since HCV infection causes a similar deregulation of adipogenesis in liver tissues and PBMCs, we wondered whether such alterations were specifically mediated by HCV. To this purpose, we performed the adipogenesis array in HBV+ Livers and PBMCS (**Figure 2A, B**). Also in this case we have appreciated a similar expression in livers and PBMCs (**Table S2**) and a direct significant correlation between gene expression in liver and lymphocytes. Spearman's rho statistical investigation showed a significant positive correlation (** rho $=0.745$) among the genes

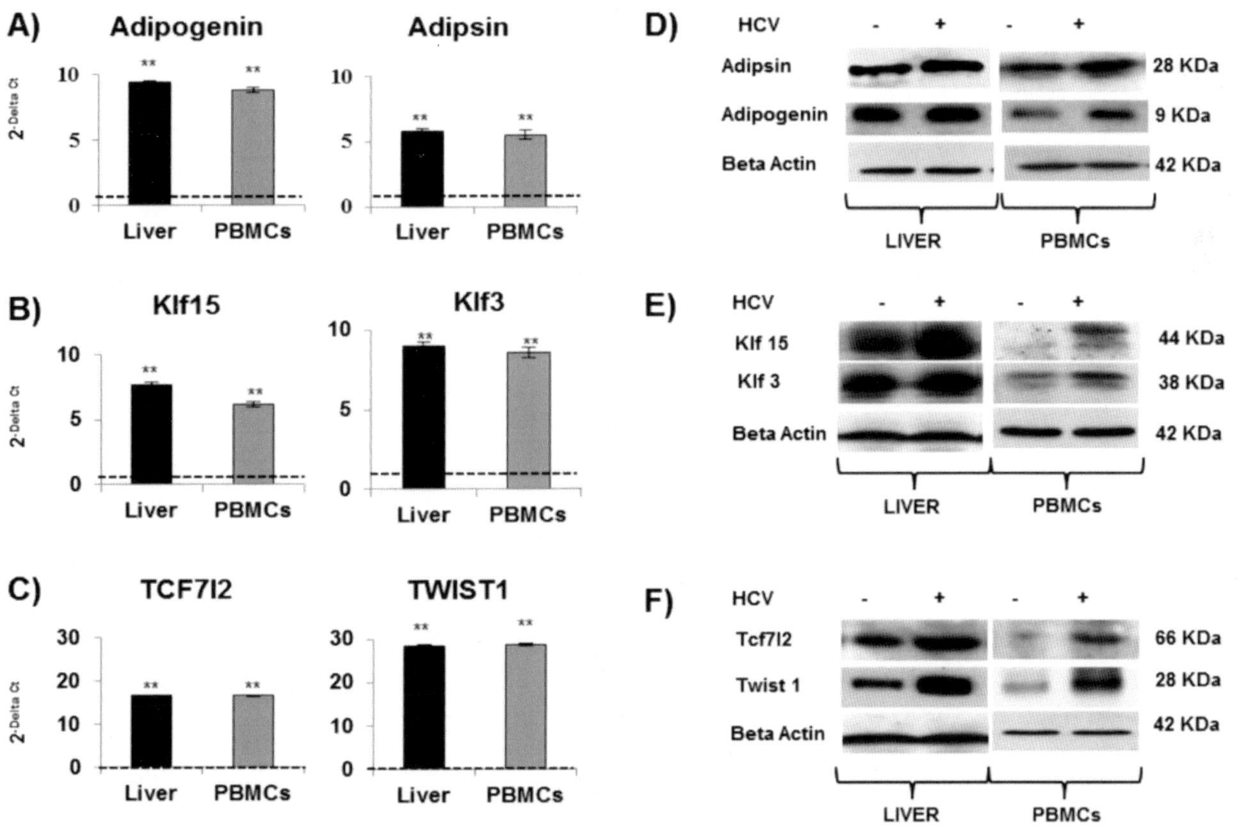

Figure 3. HCV up-regulates genes involved in lipid metabolism but with addictional role in inflammation, proliferation and transformation. Real-time analysis (mean values± S.D) of ADIG and Adipsin (A), KLF15 and KLF3 (B), TCF7L2 and TWIST 1 (C) are expressed as fold change, and normalized with an housekeeping gene. Asterisks indicate significant difference between HCV+ vs HDs (*$p<0,05$; **$p<0.001$) Adipogenin and Adipsin (D); KLF15 and KLF3 (E); TCF7L2 and TWIST 1 (F) protein levels in HCV+/HDs Liver and PBMCs. One experiment representative of all the independent experiments performed is shown. Beta-actin indicates the equal amount of protein loaded for each sample.

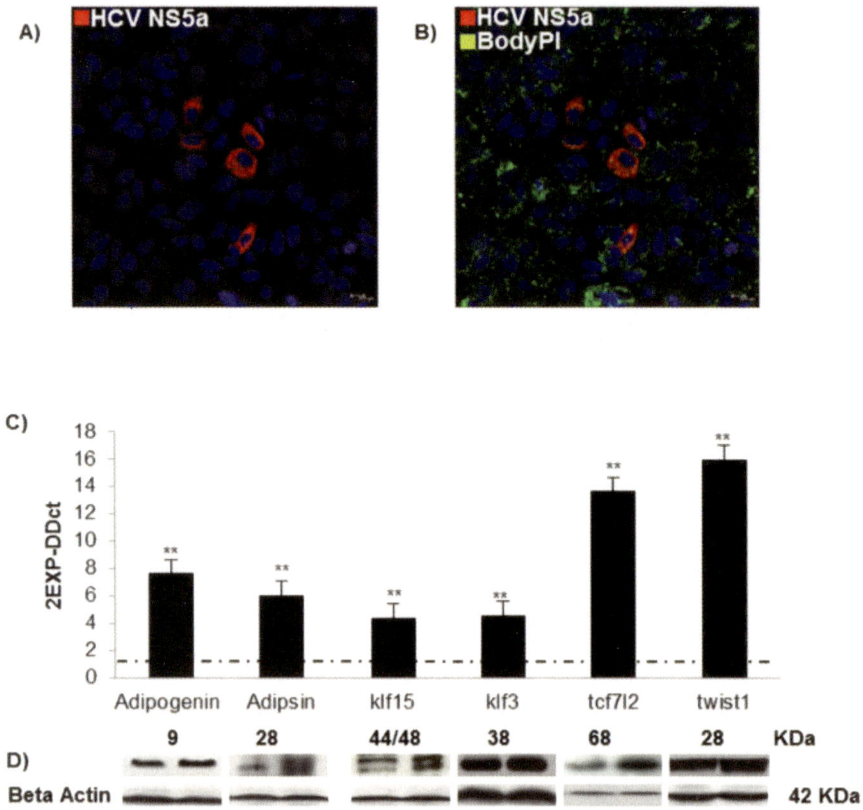

Figure 4. In *in vitro* HCV model up-regulates genes involved in lipid metabolism. Immunofluorescence assay HCV NS5A (red) (A) and lipid accumulation (green) (B). C) Real-time analysis (mean values± S.D) of ADIG, Adipsin, KLF15, KLF3, TCF7L2 and TWIST 1 are expressed as fold change and normalized with a housekeeping gene. Asterisks indicate significant difference between J6/JFH1 HuH7.5 vs HuH7.5 (*p<0,05; **p <0.001). D) protein levels in HCV+/HDs Adipogenin and Adipsin, KLF15, KLF3, TCF7L2, TWIST 1in HuH7.5 and J6/JFH1 HuH7.5. One experiment representative of 5 independent experiments performed is shown. Beta-actin indicates the amount of protein loaded for each sample.

analyzed, in both HBV+ liver biopsies and PBMCs (**Figure 2C**). The HBV+ gene expression was greatly different from the profile displayed by HCV+.(**Figure 2D**) in fact 80% of genes showed a different expression in the two infection groups. (**Figure 2E, F**). Such data highlight the specificity of the adipogenesis profile of HCV infected patients.

Possible novel biomarkers of HCV-dependent liver damage

Some of the analyzed genes struck our attention because had never been directly associated with HCV infection. All the results, obtained the RT PCR-array approach, were confirmed by the relative mRNAs and protein expression levels (** $p<0.001$), (**Figure 3A and B**), and highlighted a strong up-regulation of two important transcription factors: Adipogenin (ADIG), Adipsin (CFD), Krüppel-like transcription factors 15 and 13 (KLF15 and KLF3) (**Figure 3C and D**) and TCF7L2 and Twist1 (**Figure 3E and F**).

Deregulation of metabolic profile in *in vitro* system model of HCV infection

To confirm that the expression of modulated genes in PBMCs reflected what happens in hepatocytes during HCV infection, we used an HCV *in vitro* model. 72 hrs post infection we revealed the presence of HCV-protein NS5A (**Figure 4A**) and a high intracellular fat accumulation in infected hepatocytes (**Figure 4B**).

The HCV *in vitro* model had a similar modulation of the previously analyzed genes (**Figure 4C**, ** $p<0.001$), supporting the idea that PBMCs may possibly be used as a substitute of liver tissues for metabolic investigation, in HCV+ patients.

HCV up-regulated genes are closely related to virological and biochemical liver damage parameters, as well as to the severity of steatosis and fibrosis

Statistical analysis statistically positively correlated the HCV viremia plasma levels (VL) and antibody titer (AbT) to Adipogenin (ADIG), Adipsin (CFD), KLF15, KLF3, TCF7L2 and Twist1, either in HCV+ PBMCs or in liver tissues (**Table 4**,*$p<0.05$). All genes were positively correlated to liver enzymes (ALT and AST) levels, too (*$p<0.05$) Even more interesting was the positive correlation of all these genes with the severity of liver steatosis and Fibroscan parameters (**Table 4**).

The deregulated adipogenetic genes of HBV+ patients do not display any correlation with virological parameters (data not shown).

Discussion

Vital processes regulated by the liver including metabolism, lipid homeostasis, cellular proliferation and immune response are known to be systematically deregulated as result of persistent HCV infection [26,27].

Table 4. *Correlation between mRNA expression levels and virological, biochemical parameters and steatosis.

		HCV+ Liver		HCV+ PBMCs	
mRNA	IU/ml	Spearman's Rho	p	Spearman's Rho	p
Adipogenin	VL	0,2458	*0.04	0,1826	*0.046
	AbT	0,2534	*0.032	0,3430	*0.03
	AST	0,1645	*0.048	0,2598	*0.042
	ALT	0,2673	*0.023	0,2736	*0.032
	Fibro	4,5263	*0.023	0,5944	*0.031
Adipsin	VL	0,3229	*0.012	0,3909	*0.018
	AbT	0,4986	**<0.001	0,6215	**<0.001
	AST	0,2743	*0.035	0,3395	*0.026
	ALT	0,2902	*0.012	0,2472	*0.028
	Fibro	0,5868	**<0.001	0,5152	**<0.001
KLF15	VL	0,2458	*0.025	0,1826	*0.015
	AbT	0,2534	*0.04	0,3430	*0.014
	AST	0,1645	*0.021	0,2566	*0.023
	ALT	0,2673	*0.036	0,2736	*0.032
	Fibro	0,6840	**<0.001	0,5479167	**<0.001
KLF15	VL	0,31875	*0.021	0,390	*0.015
	AbT	0,3229	*0.032	0,3430	*0.011
	AST	0,2340	*0.04	0,2638	*0.014
	ALT	0,3319	*0.031	0,3368	*0.016
	Fibro	0,4569	**<0.001	0,4826	**<0.001
TCF7L2	VL	0,3805	*0.012	0,3909	*0.014
	AbT	0,3229	*0.015	0,3180	*0.023
	AST	0,2472	*0.013	0,316	*0.036
	ALT	0,4090	*0.014	0,4430	*0.021
	Fibro	0,5541	**0.001	0,594	**0.001
TWIST1	VL	0,2701	*0.018	0,2430	*0.04
	AbT	0,31666	*0.014	0,270	*0.013
	AST	0,3034	*0.016	0,3194	*0.025
	ALT	0,2604	*0.045	0,2638	*0.028
	Fibro	0,6701	**<0.001	0,5638	**<0.001

*The Spearman's rho was evaluated (84 genes and 22 biochemical data) with a Bonferroni's correction of 0.000472.

Our data suggest that PBMCs reflect liver adipogenesis deregulation during HCV infection. In fact, we observed a similar modulation of HCV-related lipid metabolism either in HCV+ liver tissues or lymphoid cells, highlighting the function of PBMCs as a surrogate tool of HCV steatotic liver tissues. Hepatitis C virus (HCV) is not only an hepatotropic virus, but it is also able to infect the immune system cells [28,29], and its replication in liver are strictly related to HCV infection status in PBMCs [30]. Through the Human Adipogenesis RT^2 Profiler PCR Array, we analyzed 84 genes involved in adipogenesis mechanism; among these 23 resulted different modulated in liver tissues and PBMCs, emphasizing the genes specificity expression in the two compartments matched. Thus, the main result was that in our HCV+ patients more than the 70% of genes, involved in the control of lipid metabolism, resulted similarly deregulated in HCV+ liver tissues and PBMCs. We confirmed the HCV-related lipid deregulation causing over-expression of: hormone sensitive Lipase (LIPE), lipoprotein lipase (LPL) and Leptin [15], as well as the modulation of genes involved in the lipid *de novo* synthesis and beta oxidation (LXR alpha, SREBP1c, FASN and ACACB) [21]. The specificity of the HCV-related adipogenic deregulated genes was supported by the fact that the adipogenic profile of HBV+ infected livers and PBMCs was deeply different from what observed in HCV+. Accordingly, the J6/JFH1 in *in vitro* HCV infection system displayed a similar adipogenesis profile, suggesting that the PBMCs modulation could really mimic what occur in the hepatocytes and was not an artifact due to lymphocyte infiltrating in the liver during HCV infection.

Some interesting molecules, involved in the control of lipid metabolism, were over-expressed. Among these, Adipogenin (ADIG) [17] that was not previously reported to be up-regulated in HCV infected patients and has an opposite behavior respect to HBV infected patients. ADIG is known to be involved not only in the adipogenesis, but also in the onset of inflammation [20].On the other end the up-regulation of the Krüppel-like transcription factors family (KLFs), in HCV infected patients, was noteworthy. KLFs are expressed in multiple tissues and regulate the expression of genes involved in glucose uptake and adipogenesis [31,32]. KLF3 is an important regulator of several biological processes, including adipogenesis, erythropoiesis, and B cell development [33]; while, KLF15 was proposed for the regulation of the HBV gene expression and replication [34]. The role of KLF15 on HBV replication was confirmed by our experimental data. Interestingly, KLF 3 and 15 are not only implicated in adipogenesis, but also in hepatocarcinogenesis modulation [33,35].

Finally, we appreciated the up-regulation of several genes involved in the transformation: Adipsin or complement factor D (CFD), Transcription Factor 7-like 2 (TCF7L2) and TWIST1. Adipsin is a serine protease secreted by adipocytes into the bloodstream and regulates the activation of the alternative complement pathway [36]. It could be involved in adipogenic transformation of hepatocytes [37]. Interestingly Adipsin was differently regulated in our HCV+ patients respect to HBV+ patients.

TCF7L2 has a key role in the Wnt/beta Catenin signaling [38] that is known to have an important function in the induction of HCV-related HCC and represents a critical process for the invasiveness and metastatic development of several human cancers [39]. This gene resulted positively modulated in the adipogenesis profile of HCV+ patients, while was no modulated in HBV+.

Lastly, another significant gene resulting positively modulated in the adipogenesis profile during the HCV infection is Twist1, which is able to induce the Epithelial-Mesenchymal Transition (EMT) HCV-related neoplastic transformation [40] and tumor progression [41,42,43].

Of noteworthy, all the molecules reported above to be deregulated, in HCV+ patients, displayed an intriguing positive correlation to virological (VL and AbT) and hepatic (ALT and AST) parameters, as well as to the severity of steatosis and fibrosis

In conclusion, the HCV+ PBMCs are able to reflect the behavior of the adipogenesis pathways of liver tissues. PBMCs might be considered a real valid support to investigate the HCV-related pathogenetic mechanisms of lipid metabolism deregulation, and to explore new therapeutical targets to overcome the HCV-related transformation.

Supporting Information

Figure S1 Evaluation of gene expression difference between HCV patients with different grade of fibrosis

(group: F0/F1 vs group F2/F3). Real-time analysis (mean values± S.D) of genes are expressed as fold change, and normalized with an housekeeping gene. Asterisks indicate significant difference between F0/F1 vs F2/F3 in HCV+ livers and PBMCs(*p<0,05; **p <0.001).

Table S1 Microarray analysis of chronic HCV + Liver tand PBMC compared to HDs.

Table S2 Microarray analysis of chronic HBV + Livers and PBMCs compared to HDs.

Table S3 Differences in gene expression between HCV patients with different grade of fibrosis. Real-time analysis (mean values± S.D) of genes are expressed as Ct and normalized with an housekeeping gene. Asterisks indicate significant difference between F0/F1 vs F2/F3 in HCV+ livers and PBMCs.

Acknowledgments

The authors would like to thank Professor Vittorio Colizzi and Doctor Carla Montesano for their intellectual support. We thank Doctor Iuvara Alessandra for her technical contribution to this work and Ms. Giulia Falangola and PhD Chiara Falangola for the english review of our work.

Author Contributions

Conceived and designed the experiments: AM BC CB. Performed the experiments: AM BC CV. Analyzed the data: AM BC. Contributed reagents/materials/analysis tools: SG GL. Wrote the paper: AM BC CB.

References

1. Kensicki E, Mohney R, Hall WW (2011) Metabolomic Profile of Hepatitis C Virus-Infected Hepatocytes. PLoS One 6(8):e23641.
2. Negro F, Sanyal AJ (2009) Hepatitis C virus, steatosis and lipid abnormalities: clinical and pathogenic data. Liver Int 29 Suppl2:26–37.
3. Ploen D, Hafirassou ML, Himmelsbach K, Sauter D, Biniossek ML, et al. (2013) TIP47 plays a crucial role in the life cycle of hepatitis C virus. J Hepatol S0168-8278(13)00066-4.
4. Roque-Cuéllar MC, Sánchez B, García-Lozano JR, Garrido-Serrano A, Sayago M, et al. (2012) Expression of CD81, SR-BI and LDLR in lymphocytes and monocytes from patients with classic and occult hepatitis C virus infection. Journal of Medical Virology 84(11):1727–36.
5. Alisi A, Giannini C, Spaziani A, Anticoli S, Caini P, et al. (2007) Hepatitis C virus core protein enhances B lymphocyte proliferation. Digestive and Liver Disease 39 Suppl 1:S72–5.
6. Alisi A, Giannini C, Spaziani A, Caini P, Zignego AL, et al. (2008) Involvement of PI3K in HCV-related lymphoproliferative disorders. Journal of Cellular Physiology 214(2):396–404.
7. Mancone C, Steindler C, Santangelo L, Simonte G, Vlassi C, et al. (2011) Hepatitis C virus production requires apolipoprotein A-I and affects its association with nascent low-density lipoproteins. Gut 60(3):378–86.
8. Negro F (2010) Abnormalities of lipid metabolism in hepatitis C virus infection. Gut 59(9):1279–1287.
9. Wu C, Gilroy R, Taylor R, Olyaee M, Abdulkarim B, et al. (2011) Alteration of hepatic nuclear receptor-mediated signaling pathways in hepatitis C virus patients with and without a history of alcohol drinking. Hepatology 54(6):1966–74.
10. Negro F (2012) Steatosis and insulin resistance in response to treatment of chronic hepatitis C. Journal of Viral Hepatitis 19 Suppl 1:42–7.
11. Albecka A, Belouzard S, Op de Beeck A, Descamps V, Goueslain L, et al. (2012) Role of low-density lipoprotein receptor in the hepatitis C virus life cycle. Hepatology 55(4):998–1007.
12. Mazumdar B, Banerjee A, Meyer K, Ray R (2011) Hepatitis c virus e1 envelope glycoprotein interacts with apolipoproteins in facilitating entry into hepatocytes. Hepatology 54(4):1149–56.
13. Nielsen SU, Bassendine MF, Burt AD, Martin C, Pumeechockchai W, et al. (2006) Association between hepatitis C virus and very-low-density lipoprotein (VLDL)/LDL analyzed in iodixanol density gradients. Journal of Virology 80(5): 2418–28.
14. Scholtes C, Ramière C, Rainteau D, Perrin-Cocon L, Wolf C, et al. (2012) High plasma level of nucleocapsid-free envelope glycoprotein-positive lipoproteins in hepatitis C patients. Hepatology 56(1): 39–48.
15. Nkontchou G, Bastard JP, Ziol M, Aout M, Cosson E, et al. (2010) Insulin resistance, serum leptin, and adiponectin levels and outcomes of viral hepatitis C cirrhosis. Journal of Hepatology 53(5):827–33.
16. Corey KE, Kane E, Munroe C, Barlow LL, Zheng H, et al. (2009) Hepatitis C virus infection and its clearance alter circulating lipids: implications for long-term follow-up. Hepatology 50:1030–1037.
17. Lambert JE, Bain VG, Ryan EA, Thomson AB, Clandinin MT (2013) Elevated lipogenesis and diminished cholesterol synthesis in patients with hepatitis C viral infection compared to healthy humans. Hepatology 57(5):1697–704.
18. Durazzo M, Belci P, Niro G, Collo A, Grisoglio E, et al. (2013) Variations of serum levels of adiponectin and resistin in chronic viral hepatitis. Journal of Endocrinological Investigation 36(8):600–5.
19. Khattab MA, Eslam M, Shatat M, Abd-Aalhalim H, Mousa YI, et al. (2012) Changes in adipocytokines and insulin sensitivity during and after antiviral therapy for hepatitis C genotype 4. Journal of Gastrointestinal and Liver Diseases 21(1):59–65.
20. Hong YH, Hishikawa D, Miyahara H, Tsuzuki H, Nishimura Y, et al. (2005) Up-regulation of adipogenin, an adipocyte plasma transmembrane protein, during adipogenesis. Molecular and Cellular Biochemistry 276(1–2):133–41.
21. Diamond DL, Syder AJ, Jacobs JM, Sorensen CM, Walters KA, et al. (2010) Temporal proteome and lipidome profiles reveal hepatitis C virus-associated reprogramming of hepatocellular metabolism and bioenergetics. PLoS Pathogen 6(1):e1000719.
22. Zhang M, Zhu W, Li Y (2013) Small Molecule Inhibitors of Human Adipocyte Fatty Acid Binding Protein (FABP4). Medicinal Chemistry Sep 12.
23. Baranova A, Lal P, Birerdinc A, Younossi ZM (2011) Non-invasive markers for hepatic fibrosis. BMC Gastroenterology 11:91.
24. Scheuer PJ (1991) Classification of chronic viral hepatitis: a need for reassessment Journal of Hepatology 13:372–374.
25. Lindenbach BD, Evans MJ, Syder AJ, Wölk B, Tellinghuisen TL, et al. (2005) Complete replication of hepatitis C virus in cell culture. Science 309(5734):623.
26. Mankouri J,Tedbury PR, Gretton S, Hughes ME, Griffin SD, et al. (2010) Enhanced hepatitis C virus genome replication and lipid accumulation mediated by inhibition of AMP-activated protein kinase. Proc Natl Acad Sci U S A. 107(25): 11549–11554.
27. Hartling HJ, Gaardbo JC, Ronit A, Salem M, Laye M, et al. (2013) Impaired thymic output in patients with chronic hepatitis C virus infection. Scand J Immunol. 378–86.
28. Sarhan MA, Chen AY, Russell RS, Michalak TI (2012) Patient-derived hepatitis C virus and JFH-1 clones differ in their ability to infect human hepatoma cells and lymphocytes. The Journal of General Virology 93(Pt 11):2399–407.
29. Sarhan MA, Chen AY, Michalak TI (2013) Differential expression of candidate virus receptors in human T lymphocytes prone or resistant to infection with patient-derived hepatitis C virus. PLoS One 8(4):e62159.
30. Pham TN, Lin DM, Mulrooney-Cousins PM, Churchill ND, Kowala-Piaskowska A, et al. (2013) Hepatitis C virus load and expression of a unique subset of cellular genes in circulating lymphoid cells differentiate non-responders from responders to pegylated interferon alpha-ribavirin treatment. Journal of Medical Virology. 85(3):441–8.
31. Wu Z, Wang S (2013) Role of kruppel-like transcription factors in adipogenesis. Developmental Biological 373(2):235–43.
32. Gray S, Wang B, Orihuela Y, Hong EG, Fisch S, et al. (2007) Regulation of gluconeogenesis by Krüppel-like factor 15. Cell Metababolism 5(4):305–12.
33. McConnell BB, Yang VW (2010) Mammalian Krüppel-like factors in health and diseases. Physiological Review 90(4):1337–81.
34. Zhou J, Tan T, Tian Y, Zheng B, Ou JH, et al. (2011) Krüppel-like factor 15 activates hepatitis B virus gene expression and replication. Hepatology 54(1):109–21.
35. Cao Z, Sun X, Icli B, Wara AK, Feinberg MW (2010) Role of Kruppel-like factors in leukocyte development, function, and disease. Blood 116(22):4404–14.
36. Katschke KJ Jr, Wu P, Ganesan R, Kelley RF, Mathieu MA, et al. (2012) Inhibiting alternative pathway complement activation by targeting the factor D exosite. Journal of Biological Chemistry 287(16):12886–92.
37. Yu S, Matsusue K, Kashireddy P, Cao WQ, Yeldandi V, et al. (2003) Adipocyte-specific gene expression and adipogenic steatosis in the mouse liver due to peroxisome proliferator-activated receptor gamma1 (PPARgamma1) overexpression. Journal of Biological Chemistry 278(1):498–505.
38. Tsedensodnom O, Koga H, Rosenberg SA, Nambotin SB, Carroll JJ, et al. (2011) Identification of T-cell factor-4 isoforms that contribute to the malignant phenotype of hepatocellular carcinoma cells. Experimental Cell Research 317(7):920–31.
39. Koga H, Tsedensodnom O, Tomimaru Y, Walker EJ, Lee HC, et al. (2012) Loss of the SxxSS motif in a human T-cell factor-4 isoform confers hypoxia resistance to liver cancer: an oncogenic switch in Wnt signaling. PLoS One 7(6):e39981.

40. Yang J, Mani S-A, Donaher J-L, Ramaswamy S, Itzykson R-A, et al. (2004). Twist, a master regulator of morphogenesis, plays an essential role in tumor metastasis. Cell 117:927–939
41. Kwok W-K, Ling MT, Lee TW, Lau TC, Zhou C, et al. (2005) Up-regulation of TWIST in prostate cancer and its implication as a therapeutic target. Cancer Research 65(12):5153–5162.
42. Yang M-H, Chen CL, Chau GY, Chiou SH, Su CW, et al. (2009) Comprehensive analysis of the independent effect of twist and snail in promoting metastasis of hepatocellular carcinoma. Hepatology 50(5):1464–74.
43. Conti B, Minutolo A, Arciello M, Balsano C (2013) Are Hedgehog and Wnt/β-catenin pathways involved in hepatitis C virus-mediated EMT? Journal of Hepatology 58(3):636–7.

11

Functions of Liver Natural Killer Cells Are Dependent on the Severity of Liver Inflammation and Fibrosis in Chronic Hepatitis C

Emilie Fugier[1,2¶], Hélène Marche[1,2¶], Marie-Ange Thélu[1,2,3¶], Zuzana Macek Jílková[1,2], Nicolas Van Campenhout[1,2], Tania Dufeu-Duchesne[1,2,3], Vincent Leroy[1,2,3], Jean-Pierre Zarski[1,2,3], Nathalie Sturm[1,2,4], Patrice N. Marche[1,2,3*], Evelyne Jouvin-Marche[1,2]

1 INSERM, U823, Grenoble, France, **2** Université Joseph Fourier, UMR-S823, Grenoble, France, **3** CHU-Grenoble, Clinique Universitaire d'Hépato-Gastroentérologie, Grenoble, France, **4** CHU-Grenoble, Département d'Anatomie et de Cytologie Pathologiques, Grenoble, France

Abstract

During chronic hepatitis C virus (HCV) infection, the role of intra-hepatic (IH) natural killer (NK) cells is still controversial. To clarify their functions, we investigated anti-viral and cytotoxic activity of NK cells in human fresh liver biopsies. We compared the functions of IH-NK cells in HCV-infected and NASH patients in physiological conditions as well as after stimulation using flow cytometric and immunohistochemical analyses. Interestingly, few IH-NK cells produced anti-viral cytokine IFN-γ in HCV-infected patients similarly as in non-infected individuals. Spontaneous degranulation activity was extremely low in peripheral NK cells compared to IH-NK cells, and was significantly higher in IH-NK cells from HCV-infected patients compared to non-infected individuals. Immunohistochemical analysis revealed that perforin granules were polarized at the apical pole of IH-NK cells. The presence of CD107a and perforin in IH-NK cells demonstrated that NK cells exerted a cytolytic activity at the site of infection. Importantly, IH-NK cell functions from HCV-infected patients were inducible by specific exogenous stimulations. Upon *ex vivo* K562 target cell stimulations, the number of degranulating NK cells was significantly increased in the pool of IH-NK cells compared to circulating NK cells. Interestingly, after stimulation, the frequency of IFN-γ-producing IH-NK cells in HCV-infected patients was significantly higher at early stage of inflammation whereas the spontaneous IH-NK cell degranulation activity was significantly impaired in patients with highest inflammation and fibrosis Metavir scores. Our study highlights that some IH-NK cells in HCV-infected patients are able to produce INF-γ and degranulate and that those two activities depend on liver environment including the severity of liver injury. Thus, we conclude that critical roles of IH-NK cells have to be taken into account in the course of the liver pathogenesis associated to chronic HCV infection.

Editor: Birke Bartosch, Inserm, U1052, UMR 5286, France

Funding: This work was supported by grants from Institut National de la Santé et de la Recherche Médicale (INSERM), the Agence Nationale pour la Recherche sur le Sida (ANRS) n°AO 2009 - 2, CSS7. EF and ZMJ received financial support from Centre National de la Recherche Scientifique (CNRS) and Fundation Finovi; AD from ALPHA VAC of the "Pôle de Compétitivité Lyon Biopole", and NVC was the recipient of a grant from the Rhône- Alpes Region Cluster 10 "Infectiologie". The funders had no role in study design, data collection and analysis, decision to publish, or preparation of the manuscript.

* E-mail: patrice.marche@ujf-grenoble.fr

¶ These authors contributed equally to this work.

Introduction

A large majority of hepatitis C virus (HCV)-infected patients develops a chronic disease with increasing hepatic injury over time [1,2]. Despite intensive investigations, the phenomenon of persistent infection and parameters involved in tissue damage are not fully understood. Not surprisingly, NK cells, as one of the major components of the innate immune system, have been known to play an important role in the control of viral hepatitis for many years. Importantly, NK cells do not require priming to recognize infected cells and in addition, they contribute to T cell activation. Functional mechanisms of NK cells include: i) secretion of interferon-γ (IFN-γ), which has an antiviral effect and participates in the induction of the adaptive immune response; ii) a direct cytotoxicity to target cells via the degranulation of cytotoxic granules (perforin, granzyme); iii) and the induction of target cells apoptosis via the up-regulation of Fas ligand and tumor necrosis-related apoptosis-inducing ligand on the surface of NK cells [3,4]. NK cell regulation depends on a fine balance between inhibitory and activating receptors which belong either to Immunoglobulin-like superfamily (Killer cell Immunoglobulin-like receptor or KIR), or to natural cytotoxicity receptors [4,5] that are described as activating receptor able to recognize viral determinants [6,7].

Intra-hepatic (IH)-NK cell functions are strongly influenced by liver microenvironment and are therefore modified depending on liver disease pathogenesis. In HCV-infected patients, IH-NK cells interact with the virus and the pool of these cells decrease with the severity of liver damages [8–10]. It has been reported that phenotypical features of NK cell subset correlate with clinical

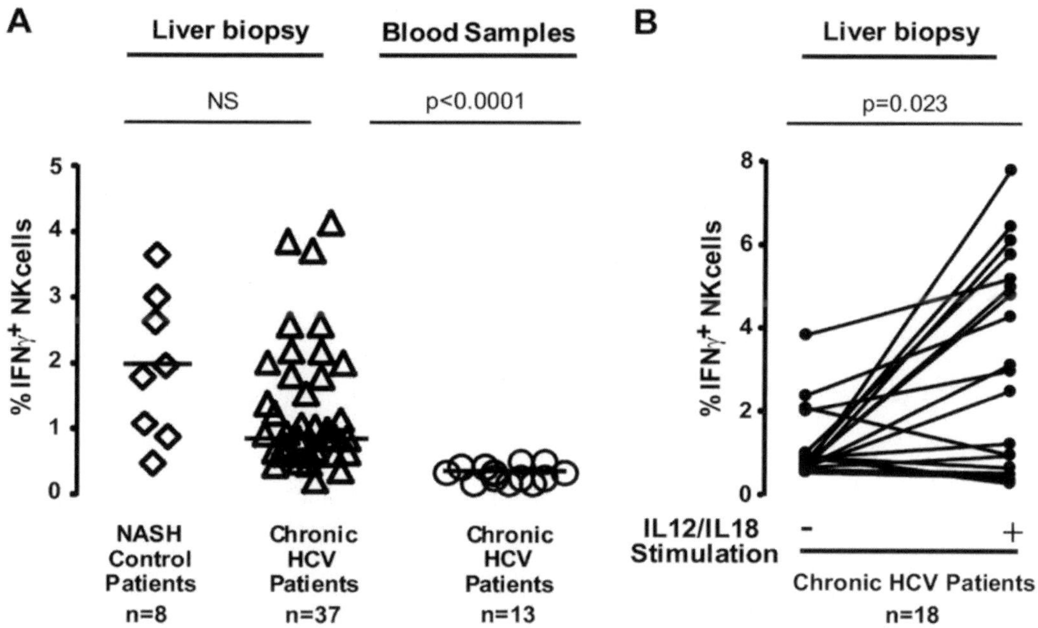

Figure 1. IFN-γ production by NK cells from chronic HCV-infected patients and NASH individuals. A) Flow cytometric analysis of spontaneous intracellular IFN-γ production by IH-NK cells, from NASH individuals (n = 8) and HCV-infected patients (n = 37) and by peripheral NK cells from HCV-infected patients (n = 13). **B**) Analysis of IFN-γ-producing IH-NK cells from HCV patients (n = 18) −/+ 12 h of IL12 and IL18 stimulation. Each symbol represented a patient and median values are indicated by dark lines.

parameters scoring the evolution of HCV infection disease. Bonorino et al. [11] found a positive correlation between NKG2A$^+$NK cells and the necro-inflammatory activity or fibrosis stage according to the Metavir scoring system. The study by Kramer et al. [12] demonstrated that NKp46$^+$high IH-NK cell subset was inversely correlated with fibrosis stage, supporting the hypothesis that NK cells can play an important anti-fibrotic role due to the NK killing activity of hepatic stellate cells [13]. Nevertheless, a recent study suggests that IH-NK cell cytotoxic function is impaired in patients with chronic HCV infection [14] whereas another study provides evidence that IH-NK cells can be further activated by IFN-α antiviral therapy during HCV infection [15]. Thus, further studies are required to clarify the functions of IH-NK cells during chronic HCV infection.

In general, due to difficulties to obtain fresh liver biopsies, most of the previous analyses were performed either in small cohorts or on frozen liver biopsies. Unfortunately, these approaches may lead to biased results or misinterpreted data because of i) the wide heterogeneity among limited number of patients, or ii) the possibility of unspecific activations and modifications as consequences of defrost tissue.

The aim of this study was to determine the IH-NK cell functions immediately after liver biopsies and to clarify if the functions of IH-NK cells from HCV-infected patients are impaired or not. We investigated the capacity of fresh *ex vivo* IH-NK cells to secrete antiviral cytokines and to exert cytotoxic functions. In parallel, we performed similar experiments using the IH-NK cells from Non-Alcoholic Steato-Hepatitis (NASH) individuals with a NAS score ≥3 (non-infected controls) [16,17] to clarify how the HCV itself affects the threshold of degranulation activity of IH-NK cells during viral infection. In addition, we analyzed the ability of IH-NK cells to be activated after the addition of appropriate cytokine or specific target cell stimulation. These data are described herein in the context of clinical parameters of infected patients. Our study demonstrates that IH-NK cells in HCV-infected patients are potentially functional and that their functions depend on the microenvironment of liver.

Results

Analysis of intracellular IFN-γ production in IH-NK cells from HCV-infected and NASH patients

NK cells from fresh liver biopsies were analyzed by flow cytometry (Figure S1). Among IH- CD45$^+$ population, NK cells were identified by CD56$^+$CD3$^-$ cellular expression and intracellular IFN-γ production was directly determined. The spontaneous production of IFN-γ cytokine by IH-NK cells was quantified only when liver biopsy contains more than 1500 IH-NK cells. In liver biopsies from HCV-infected individuals (n = 37), the mean frequency of IH-NK cells was 16.1±8.6% and frequencies of IFN-γ$^+$IH-NK cells varied from 0.3% to 4.1% (Figure 1A). We also monitored IFN-γ production from peripheral lymphocytes in paired liver biopsies and blood samples (n = 13). However, the frequency of IFN-γ$^+$NK cells in blood samples was close to 0.3%. In liver biopsies from NASH individuals (n = 8), the mean frequency of IH-NK cells was 20.1±9.4% and frequencies of IFN-γ producing IH-NK cells varied from 0% to 3.6%. These values were not significantly different from results of IFN-γ production obtained in HCV-infected patients (Figure 1A).

Next, we performed a stimulation assay by adding IL12 and IL18 cytokines to determine if the production of IFN-γ by IH-NK cells from HCV patients could be further activated. To optimize this method, we quantified the amount of IFN-γ released into supernatants of IH-NK cells stimulated with IL12/IL18 cytokines using CBA assays. As shown in Figure S2, IFN-γ was first detectable after 10 h post stimulation. This information allowed us to determine the shortest period of stimulation to precisely study initial population of IH-NK cells at the time of biopsy, i.e. before the expansion of cells, and to avoid the loss of NK cells with time. Thus, we stimulated cytokines over a period of 12 h. Under these

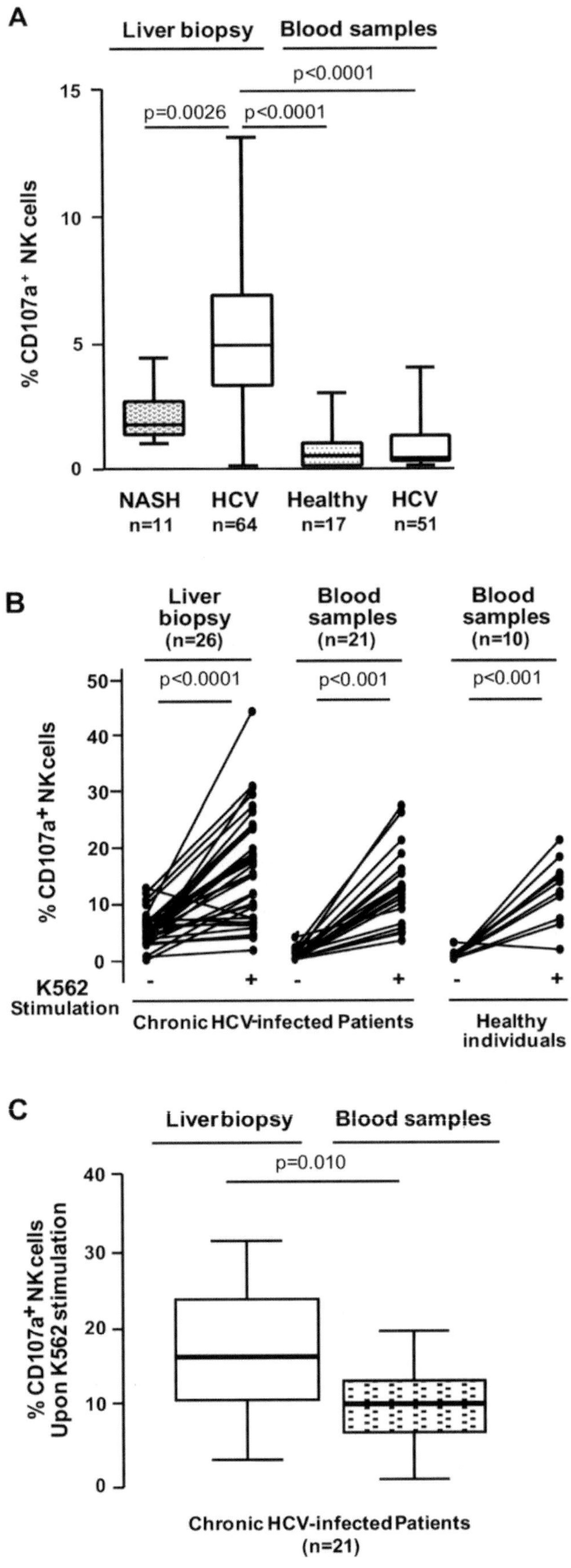

Figure 2. Degranulation activity of NK cells from NASH patients, chronic HCV-infected patients and healthy individuals. A) Flow cytometric analysis of CD107a expression by IH-NK cells from NASH individuals (n = 11) and HCV-infected patients (n = 64) directly after the recovery of liver biopsies and by circulating NK cells from healthy donors (n = 17) and HCV-infected patients (n = 51). **B**) Frequencies of degranulating NK cells −/+ 3 h of K562 target cells activation in the liver and the PBMC from HCV-infected patients (n = 36 and n = 21, respectively) and in the blood from healthy donors (n = 10). Each symbol represented a patient. **C**) Simulated degranulation activity of NK cells in the liver and in the blood from HCV-infected patients (n = 21).

conditions, IFN-γ-producing IH-NK cells were detected in 90% of HCV-infected patients (range from 0.3% to 7.8%, n = 18) and the number of IFN-γ$^+$IH-NK cells after stimulation was significantly increased (~ 3.75 fold, p = 0.023) (Figure 1B).

Altogether, these results indicate that at baseline, the frequency of IFN-γ producing IH-NK cells in HCV-infected patients was low, similar to non-infected individuals (Figure 1A) and independent of HCV viral genotypes (Figure S3A). However, the frequency of IFN-γ$^+$IH-NK cells can be enhanced by a short exposure of appropriate exogenous stimuli, indicating that a significant number of IH-NK cells are functional in HCV-infected patients and can be recruited after stimulation.

Analysis of degranulation activity of IH-NK cells from HCV-infected patients

To further investigate the cytolytic properties of IH-NK cells, we determined the CD107a expression, which is considered as a marker of degranulation [12,14,15]. In 64 HCV-infected samples, IH-NK cells exhibited a spontaneous degranulation activity that varied from 0.1 to 11.2% and was independent of viral genotypes (Figure S3B). The number of CD107a$^+$IH-NK cells in HCV-infected patients was significantly higher compared to the 11 non-infected NASH individuals (median 4.8% versus 1.7% respectively, p = 0.0026) as shown in Figure 2A.

When paired liver biopsies and blood samples were available (n = 51), we also monitored degranulation activity from peripheral blood mononuclear cells (PBMC). Very few NK cells were engaged in the degranulation process in blood samples of HCV-infected individuals as well as in the blood (n = 17) of healthy donors (0.3% and 0.4% respectively) (Figure 2A), meaning that the degranulation process of NK cells occurs mainly in the liver organ. It has to be noticed that in this study, degranulation activity monitored via CD107a$^+$ expression was assessed at a given time without the use of drugs such as monensin, an inhibitor of cell trafficking. Therefore, our results likely reflect the existence of a permanent "pool" of degranulating IH-NK cells.

We next asked whether the cytolytic activity of IH-NK cells within HCV-infected liver was already maximal or if it could be further increased through stimulation. To answer this question, suspensions of liver NK cells (n = 36) were divided in two parts, and immune cells of one part were incubated during 3 hours with specific K562 target cells deficient in CMH-I (HLA-E) molecule. Upon stimulation, we observed a threefold increase of CD107$^+$IH-NK cells (5.4% *vs* 16.4%, p<0.0001) (Figure 2B). Similar increases were observed in peripheral CD107a$^+$NK cells from HCV-infected patients (0.2% vs 11.4%, p<0.0001) and from healthy individuals (0.3% vs 12.6%, p<0.0001). Interestingly, the increase of 21 paired CD107a$^+$NK cells upon K562 stimulation was statistically higher in the liver than in the blood of HCV-infected patients (17.8% *vs* 11.4%, p = 0.010) (Figure 2C). Taken together,

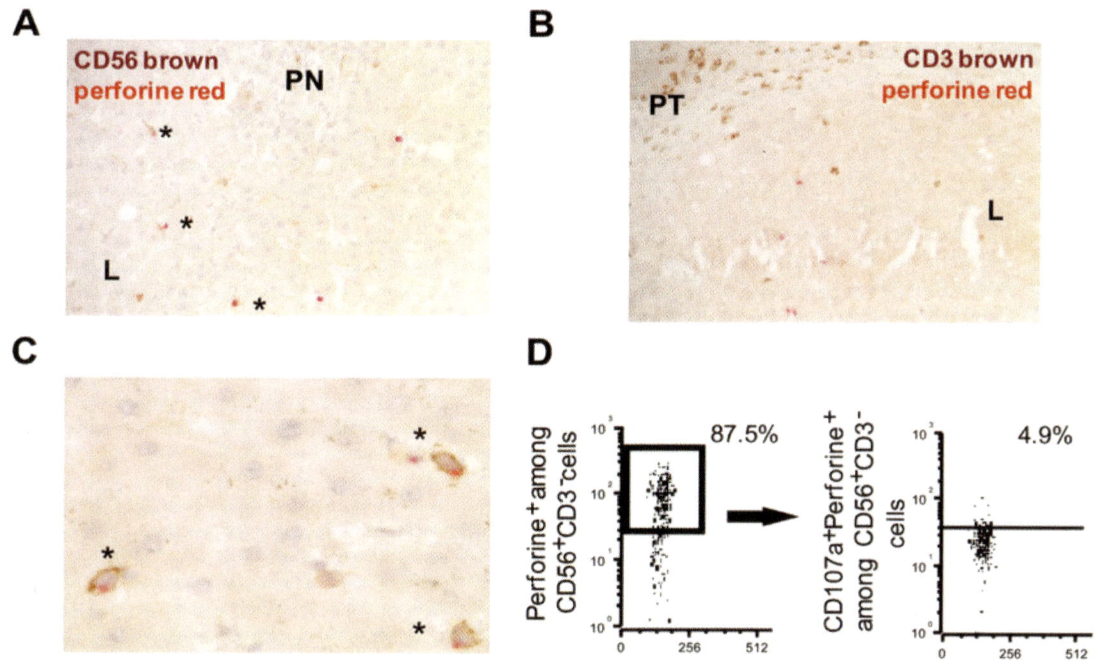

Figure 3. Immunohistochemical detection of perforin$^+$CD56$^+$ and perforin$^+$CD3$^+$ IH cells from HCV-infected patients and flow cytometric analysis. Representative pictures from immunohistochemical staining of HCV-infected liver (n = 4) with double perforin/CD56 labeling (A) showing perforin$^+$CD56$^+$ cells characterized by brown CD56$^+$ staining and red cytoplasmic perforin$^+$ staining in HCV-infected liver with septal fibrosis and low A1 Metavir activity (magnification ×20). Many double positive CD56$^+$perforin$^+$ cells (asterisk) were detected, mainly localized in lobules (L), far away frpm piecemeal necrosis (PN). B) Detection of brown CD3$^+$ cells and red perforin$^+$ cells in HCV-infected liver with septal fibrosis. Rare double positive CD3$^+$perforin$^+$ cells were detected in lobules. C) High magnification (x40) showing that perforin granules were polarized at the apical pole of IH-CD56$^+$ cells. D) Flow cytometric analysis depicting perforin$^+$cells gated on CD56$^+$CD3$^-$ cells and CD107a$^+$ gated on perforin$^+$NK cells.

these results indicate that the frequency of cytotoxic IH-NK cells of HCV-infected patients may be further enhanced upon stimulation with specific target cells.

Analysis of intracellular content of cytotoxic granules in IH-NK cells from HCV-infected patients

As already mentioned in our previous study [11], intracellular content analysis of IH-NK cells indicated that more than 60% of these cells were loaded with perforin granules whereas only on average of 10% of IH-NKT lymphocytes (CD3$^+$CD56$^+$cells) were perforin positive. However, no information was available on the localization of immunopositive perforin$^+$cells in liver tissue. To investigate this point, we performed double immunohistochemical analyses using anti-CD3 or anti-CD56 combined with anti-perforin antibodies on liver tissue sections on four HCV-infected patients. We observed that double CD56$^+$perforin$^+$cells were much more frequent (Figure 3A-3B) than double CD3$^+$perforin$^+$cells. This finding strengthens the fact that most of CD56$^+$cells, which contained intra-cytoplasmic perforin$^+$ granules, were NK cells. Interestingly, we found that double positive CD56$^+$perforin$^+$cells were detected mainly in lobular areas far away from parcellar necrosis, whereas CD3$^+$perforin$^+$cells were detected in fibrotic portal tracts. In addition, as depicted in Figure 3C, perforin granules were observed to be polarized at the apical pole of IH-CD56$^+$ cells, indicating that these cells were probably engaged in the specific target cell lysis through degranulation process. Finally, we checked by flow cytometric analysis using a combination of anti-CD3, anti-CD56, anti-perforin, and anti-CD107a antibodies, the presence of CD107a$^+$perforine$^+$IH-NK cells in the fresh biopsy of 13 HCV-infected patients. We detected CD107a$^+$perforin$^+$IH-NK cells with a frequency varying from 0.3% to 15.7% among the perforin$^+$IH-NK cells (median of 5.6%). This data underline the fact that IH-NK cells of HCV-infected patients exerted a cytolytic activity.

Relationship between the number of IH-NK cells producing IFN-γ and clinical parameters in HCV-infected patients

Then, we investigated the relationship between the frequencies of IH-NK cells producing IFN-γ and the intensity of necro-inflammatory lesions of HCV-infected patients. The liver samples of 37 HCV-infected patients were stratified into two groups based on Metavir activity score: A1 and A2/A3. We observed that in not-stimulated cells, the frequency of IFN-γ-producing IH-NK cells is similar for patients with Metavir activity A1 compared to A2/A3. Interestingly, after stimulation, the frequency of IFN-γ-producing IH-NK cells in patients with A1 Metavir activity (n = 13) was 5 fold higher and statistically different ($p = 0.0019$) compared to patients with A2/3 Metavir activity (n = 5) (Figure 4A).

Relationship between degranulation activity of NK cells and clinical parameters in HCV-infected patients

We next studied the correlation between the frequency of CD107a$^+$IH-NK cells and the clinical parameters. We found that the number of CD107a+ IH-NK cells was slightly higher in patients with A1 compared to A2/A3 Metavir Activity ($p = 0{,}042$) (Figure 4B). Metavir fibrosis stage inversely correlates with the degranulation activity of IH-NK cells (Figure 4C); this is supported by the observation of 5.7% of IH-NK cells from HCV-infected patients were involved in the degranulation process at F0/1 stage

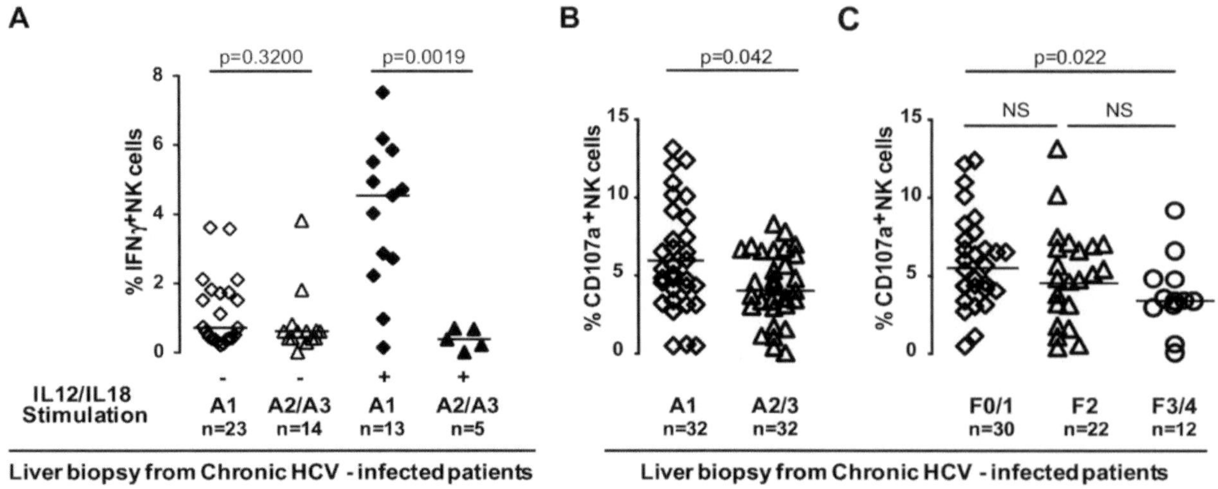

Figure 4. Relationship between intra-hepatic NK cells functions and clinical parameters of HCV-infected patients. A) The number of IFN-γ^+IH-NK cells with and without IL12/IL18 stimulation in patients stratified according to stage of Metavir activity score (A1; A2/A3). The spontaneous degranulation activity in patients with different Metavir activity grade (**B**) and in patients distributed according to the severity of fibrosis (**C**). Each patient is represented by a symbol and median values are indicated by dark lines.

while only 3.4% of CD107a$^+$IH-NK cells were detected at F3/4 stage ($p=0.022$). These results suggest that IH-NK cells from HCV-infected patients display a sustaining spontaneous degranulation activity that is partially reduced with the progression of liver inflammation and fibrosis.

Discussion

Recent observations have shown that NK cell functions in mice are strongly influenced by their environment and that these cells display a greater capacity to adapt to their local context than was previously expected [18]. In addition, the activation of NK cells is dependent on the engagement of activating and inhibitory receptors that determines the reactivity of NK cells [18]. The functions of peripheral blood NK cells in HCV-infected patients have been extensively studied in the last decades and are still debated. During acute HCV infection, the cytotoxic functions of peripheral NK cells and their production of IFN-γ, that can directly inhibit viral replication and prime the adaptive immune response, are higher compared to healthy individuals [19]. In contrast, during chronic HCV infection, the production of IFN-γ decreases and contributes to viral persistence (see reviews [20,21]).

A large number of studies have focused on the functions of peripheral NK cells however analyses of IH-NK cells are very limited. In addition, most of the available data were obtained on frozen liver tissues and cells cultured with cytokines (i.e. IL2), therefore modifying the experimental environment of NK cells present in infected liver can lead to biased conclusions about their functions. Some works provide evidence that IH-NK cell degranulation activity is higher compared to peripheral NK cells [12,22] and can be further activated by IFN-α antiviral therapy of HCV infection [15]. On the other hand, another study suggests that IH-NK cell cytotoxic function is impaired in patients with chronic HCV infection while peripheral NK cells are activated [14].

Here, *ex-vivo* analysis of fresh liver biopsies and blood samples indicates that IH-NK cells have higher degranulation activity and secrete more IFN-γ than peripheral NK cells in HCV-infected patients. Moreover, our data provide evidence that IH-NK cells from HCV-infected patients display higher cytotoxic activity but produce similar amount of IFN-γ as IH-NK cells from non-infected patients. In addition, immunohistochemical approaches show that some IH-NK cells of HCV infected individuals display perforin-containing granules polarized at the apical pole of the cells and that some perforin$^+$ IH-NK cells are CD107$^+$, indicating they are engaged in a degranulation process. By focusing our analysis on the functional responsiveness of IH-NK cells in chronically HCV-infected patients rather than a phenotypic analysis of their activating and inhibitor receptors, we observe that only a limited number of NK cells are reactive whereas it has been previously reported that the majority of those cells express activating receptors such as NKG2D and NKp46 [7,15,22]. This limited pool of active IH-NK cells in chronic HCV infection might be the result of a failure of the signalling network such as the decrease of IFN-α production that is required to activate immune cells including NK cells [20,21,23–25]. Another reason may be that HCV directly inhibits immune cells by contact with HCV-infected hepatocytes as demonstrated *in vitro* [26]. Furthermore, as described in other viral infections, one may propose that IH-NK cells reduce the number of infected antigen presenting cells, thereby facilitating the presence of the virus in the liver tissue [27] or that the NKp46$^+$ IH-NK cells tune their threshold of responsiveness and become tolerant that is similar to the phenotypic behaviour described in neutropenic mice [28]. With respect to the fact that the activity of NK cells is critically affected by a variety of other factors, including dendritic cells, monocytes or CD4$^+$ T cells [4], it is difficult to assess precisely what factors actually limit NK cell activity in the liver of HCV infected patients. However, we show that the frequencies of NK cells producing IFN-γ or degranulating increase after in vitro stimulation by either IL-12 and IL-18 cytokines or by target cells. This supports the fact that some NK cells, even though they remain capable of reactivation, are partially inhibited because either they are not triggered by the right signals to fully exert their functions or they modulate themselves the level of their reactivity in the liver tissue. Furthermore, the frequency of IFN-γ producing NK cells and to a lesser extent the frequency of degranulating NK cells, decrease as the liver inflammation status increases (Metavir Activity Grade and Fibrosis Stage). Therefore, as the inflammatory status remains low, a fraction of NK cells exert their functions, whereas these functions are altered when the inflammatory status of the liver increases. Two hypotheses may account for this observation: either part of NK cells become non reactive because the inflammatory context prevents their activation, or NK cells adapt themselves to their environment by reducing the cytokines production and the release of cytotoxic granules in the aim of limiting tissue damage. We privilege this latter hypothesis that converges with conclusions of animal model studies showing that NK cells reactivity is tuned by the microenvironment and depends on the time of exposure to this environment [28]. In addition, it is also possible that a decline in NK cell activity itself further favours development of liver fibrosis. This is in agreement with the assumption that IH-NK cells during long-lasting chronic infection are hyporesponsible and enable to ensure their role in immunosurveillance, as suggested by Mondelli and others [6,29]. Taken together, IH-NK cells, although activated, are unable to clear the HCV-infection on their own when the infection is chronic, which seems to be a general feature of IH-NK cells rather than the result of viral escape strategy.

In our study, we took the advantage of combining at the same time the reactivity of IH-NK cells with the evaluation/diagnostic of histological damage. Thus, our observations indicated that after stimulation, IH-NK cells were producing IFN-γ at early phases of the liver inflammation disease. This may explain the controversy in current literature that was focusing on IH-NK cell functions during chronic HCV infection (see review [20,21]). More importantly, this finding should be taken into consideration for novel therapeutic strategies that intend to involve direct activation of IH-NK cells or to block IH-NK cell inhibitory receptors in order to enhance the induction of anti-viral cytotoxic activities [24]. Our results also suggest that for successful management of chronic-HCV infection treatment is necessary to focus on the first stage of the liver disease when the tissue damage is not yet significantly developed.

Overall, our study provides clear evidence that some IH-NK cells in HCV-infected patients exert degranulation activity and produce IFN-γ and can be further activated, opening new issues in the follow up of the patients.

Materials and Methods

Patients

One hundred twenty patients included in this study were prospectively selected prior any treatment and separated into 2 groups according to the aetiology of chronic liver disease: Group 1, including 101 patients, chronic HCV (Department of Gastro-enterology and Hepatology, Grenoble University Hospital). All patients were anti-HCV antibody positive (ELISA 3, Ortho Diagnostic Systems, Raritan, NJ, USA) and serum HCV-RNA positive by RT-qPCR (Amplicor HCV, Roche Diagnostic Systems, Meylan, France). HCV genotype was determined by Inno-Lipa technology (Innogenetics, Zwijnaarde, Belgium).; Group 2, including 19 patients with histologically proven Non Alcoholic Fatty Liver Disease (NAFLD), considered as non-infected control group with NAFLD Activity Score (NAS) $\geq$ 3, corresponding to borderline NASH with low necroinflammatory activity (NAS 3 or 4) and definite NASH (NAS$\geq$5). Histological examination was assessed by experienced liver pathologist according to Metavir scoring system for HCV patients and according to Brunt's [16] and Kleiner's [17] scoring system for NASH patients. However, necroinflammatory activity and fibrosis stage of NASH patients were also expressed according Metavir classification, allowing the comparison between HCV and NASH patients. Patients were negative for HIV and HBV infection, without biochemical markers of autoimmune hepatitis, and their alcohol consumption was lower than 30 g/day in male and 20 g/day in women. The main characteristics of all patients are described in Table S1.

Liver biopsies were divided into two parts: one part for histological examination and the other part for immunological analyses [30]. Patients were divided in two cohorts, the first one for IFN-γ-study (37 HCV-infected biopsies and 8 NASH biopsies), and the second cohort for CD107-study (64 HCV-infected biopsies and 11 NASH biopsies). When the length of HCV-infected biopsy was more than 1 cm, the liver specimen was divided in two parts to perform analyses at baseline and after stimulation. Paired blood and liver simple were obtained in 13 HCV-infected patients for IFN-γ study and 51 HCV-infected patients for CD107 study, among this blood samples 21 were stimulated (Figure S4).

PBMC from 17 healthy individuals were collected from EFS (Etablissement Français du Sang). The study was performed in accordance with the Declaration of Helsinki and French legislation, and received approval of the Grenoble University Hospital ethical committee (03/APTF/1). All study participants provided written informed consent.

Flow cytometric analysis

Immediately after the liver biopsy, cells were recovered by mechanical disruption, and immunostained for flow cytometric analysis. The leucocytes of blood sample were extracted with Filcool and the same protocol for immunostaining as for liver samples was used. Immuno-phenotyping was performed on fresh PBMC and liver samples with the following anti-human antibodies: CD3-PE-Cy7, CD56-PE from Beckman Coulter, CD56-FITC, IFN-γ-PE, Perforin-FITC and CD107a-APC from Becton-Dickinson Biosciences, CD3-APC-Cy7, CD45-APC-Cy7, uncoupled CD107a and CD107a Pacific Blue from Biolegend analyses were done as previously described [7,30]. Data were acquired on BD LSRII flow cytometer (BD Biosciences) and analyzed using FCS Express V3 software.

IFN-γ production following IL12/IL18 stimulation

Liver biopsies from 18 out of 37 HCV-infected patients were mechanically disrupted and cultured in RPMI medium in a 5% CO_2 incubator at 37°C with or without IL12 (20 ng/mL; R&D Systems) and IL18 (80 ng/mL; MBL Clinisciences) as described [31]. Brefeldin A (GolgiPlug, Becton Dickinson) was then added to detect intracellular IFN-γ 6 h after initiation of stimulation and culture was maintained for another 6 h before harvesting. Finally, cells were washed and stained prior to flow cytometric analysis. IFN-γ released by liver-infiltrating immune cells was performed on 3 HCV-infected patients with or without incubation with IL12+IL18 over 24 h. Supernatant samples were recovered at 0, 2, 4, 6, 8, 10, 12 and 24 h post stimulation and IFN-γ secretion was measured by Cytometric Bead Array (CBA) assay according manufacturer's instruction and analyzed by flow cytometry.

Degranulation activity following K562 target cells activation

IH or PBMC immune cells were incubated for 3 h at 37°C with or without K562 target cells (Cell:Target = 1:1). Cells were then harvested, washed and stained for flow cytometric analysis. Degranulation activity was monitored by detection of membranous presence of CD107a marker [12,14,15,32].

Immunohistochemical study

Double perforin/CD56 and perforin/CD3 immunostainings were performed on consecutive 4 µm thick liver sections (n = 4) from formalin-fixed, paraffin-embedded tissue, as described in [33]. Slides were first immunostained with the anti-perforin Ab2 antibody (Clone 5B10, Neomarkers) and revealed with the N-Histofine kit (Nichirei Biosciences Inc). Fast red was used as the chromogen for perforin immunodetection. Then, antigen retrieval was performed in Tris-citrate buffer for CD56 or citrate buffer for CD3. Slides were incubated with the primary anti-CD56 (clone 1B6, Novocastra) or anti-CD3 (polyclonal rabbit CD3, Dako) antibodies and then incubated with the secondary antibody using the Envision kit. DAB was used as the chromogen for CD56 or CD3 immunodetection. All sections were counterstained with Harris hematoxylin, washed in tap water and mounted in aquamount (Merck). Sur-fixation in glutaraldehyde (0.05% in PBS pH 8.6) followed each incubation with the primary or secondary antibody.

Statistical methods

Statistical analysis was performed using SPSS 19.0 software (*SPSS Inc., Chicago, IL, USA*) as previously described [33] and included the following statistical tests: Mann-Whitney U test, Pearson and Wilcoxon matched-t test. Two-sided P values < 0.05 were considered to be significant.

Supporting Information

Figure S1 Flow cytometry strategy to investigate intracellular production of IFN-γ and degranulation activity of NK cells. IH lymphocytes were first identified according their FSC and SSC parameters (gate 1) and further gated on their $CD45^+$ expression (gate 2). Among the $CD45^+$ population, NK cells ($CD56^+CD3^-$) were then analyzed for their intracellular contents of IFN-γ cytokine or perforin and CD107a expression.

Figure S2 Detection of IFN-γ IH-NK cells production from chronic HCV-infected patients after stimulation with IL12/IL18. Monitoring of IFN-γ production was performed on 3 liver biopsies from HCV-infected patients incubated or not with IL12/IL18 over 24 h. Supernatant was recovered at 0, 2, 4, 6, 8, 10, 12 and 24 hours and IFN-γ release was measured by CBA assays, and analyzed by flow cytometry.

Figure S3 Relationship between IH-NK cells functions and HCV viral genotypes. **A**) The number of $IFN\text{-}\gamma^+$IH-NK cells and (**B**) degradulation activity in patients stratified according to HCV viral genotype. Each patient is represented by a symbol and median values are indicated by dark lines.

Figure S4 The frequencies of IH-NK cells in studies. NK cells from fresh liver biopsies and from blood samples of HCV-infected patients were analyzed during IFN gamma and CD107 study. The frequencies of IH-NK cells (mean ± SD) were determined.

Table S1 Main characteristics of the patients. Demographic, biochemical and clinical parameters of chronic HCV-infected patients and of NASH individuals studied for production of IFN-γ and CD107a expression. Necroinflammatory activity and fibrosis stage of NASH patients were expressed according Metavir classification, allowing the comparison between HCV and NASH patients.

Acknowledgments

We would like to thank the patients enrolled in this study for their participation. We are grateful to Alice Marlu for providing clinical characteristics on patient cohorts and Aurélie Dariz-Soldini for the technical assistance. We deeply thank Thomas Decaens for scientific discussions and Stanislas Tomavo for the language editing.

Author Contributions

Conceived and designed the experiments: EJM PNM. Performed the experiments: EF MAT HM ZMJ NVC TDD. Analyzed the data: EF MAT NS JPZ EJM. Contributed reagents/materials/analysis tools: VL JPZ NS. Wrote the paper: EF MAT ZMJ PNM EJM. Clinical data analysis and advices: JPZ NS.

References

1. Bowen DG, Walker CM (2005) Adaptive immune responses in acute and chronic hepatitis C virus infection. Nature 436: 946–952.
2. Hoofnagle JH (2002) Course and outcome of hepatitis C. Hepatology 36: S21–29.
3. Lunemann S, Schlaphoff V, Cornberg M, Wedemeyer H (2012) NK cells in hepatitis C: role in disease susceptibility and therapy. Dig Dis 30 Suppl 1: 48–54.
4. Vivier E, Raulet DH, Moretta A, Caligiuri MA, Zitvogel L, et al. (2011) Innate or adaptive immunity? The example of natural killer cells. Science 331: 44–49.
5. Saez-Borderias A, Romo N, Magri G, Guma M, Angulo A, et al. (2009) IL-12-dependent inducible expression of the CD94/NKG2A inhibitory receptor regulates CD94/NKG2C+ NK cell function. J Immunol 182: 829–836.
6. Mondelli MU, Varchetta S, Oliviero B (2010) Natural killer cells in viral hepatitis: facts and controversies. Eur J Clin Invest 40: 851–863.
7. Sene D, Levasseur F, Abel M, Lambert M, Camous X, et al. (2010) Hepatitis C virus (HCV) evades NKG2D-dependent NK cell responses through NS5A-mediated imbalance of inflammatory cytokines. PLoS Pathog 6: e1001184.
8. Kawarabayashi N, Seki S, Hatsuse K, Ohkawa T, Koike Y, et al. (2000) Decrease of CD56(+)T cells and natural killer cells in cirrhotic livers with hepatitis C may be involved in their susceptibility to hepatocellular carcinoma. Hepatology 32: 962–969.
9. Morishima C, Paschal DM, Wang CC, Yoshihara CS, Wood BL, et al. (2006) Decreased NK cell frequency in chronic hepatitis C does not affect ex vivo cytolytic killing. Hepatology 43: 573–580.
10. Notas G, Kisseleva T, Brenner D (2009) NK and NKT cells in liver injury and fibrosis. Clin Immunol 130: 16–26.
11. Bonorino P, Ramzan M, Camous X, Dufeu-Duchesne T, Thelu MA, et al. (2009) Fine characterization of intrahepatic NK cells expressing natural killer receptors in chronic hepatitis B and C. J Hepatol 51: 458–467.
12. Kramer B, Korner C, Kebschull M, Glassner A, Eisenhardt M, et al. (2012) Natural killer p46High expression defines a natural killer cell subset that is potentially involved in control of hepatitis C virus replication and modulation of liver fibrosis. Hepatology 56: 1201–1213.
13. Gur C, Doron S, Kfir-Erenfeld S, Horwitz E, Abu-Tair L, et al. (2012) NKp46-mediated killing of human and mouse hepatic stellate cells attenuates liver fibrosis. Gut 61: 885–893.
14. Varchetta S, Mele D, Mantovani S, Oliviero B, Cremonesi E, et al. (2012) Impaired intrahepatic natural killer cell cytotoxic function in chronic hepatitis C virus infection. Hepatology 56: 841–849.
15. Ahlenstiel G, Edlich B, Hogdal LJ, Rotman Y, Noureddin M, et al. (2011) Early changes in natural killer cell function indicate virologic response to interferon therapy for hepatitis C. Gastroenterology 141: 1231-1239, 1239 e1231–1232.
16. Brunt EM, Kleiner DE, Wilson LA, Belt P, Neuschwander-Tetri BA (2011) Nonalcoholic fatty liver disease (NAFLD) activity score and the histopathologic diagnosis in NAFLD: distinct clinicopathologic meanings. Hepatology 53: 810–820.
17. Kleiner DE, Brunt EM, Van Natta M, Behling C, Contos MJ, et al. (2005) Design and validation of a histological scoring system for nonalcoholic fatty liver disease. Hepatology 41: 1313–1321.
18. Narni-Mancinelli E, Jaeger BN, Bernat C, Fenis A, Kung S, et al. (2012) Tuning of natural killer cell reactivity by NKp46 and Helios calibrates T cell responses. Science 335: 344–348.
19. Pelletier S, Drouin C, Bedard N, Khakoo SI, Bruneau J, et al. (2010) Increased degranulation of natural killer cells during acute HCV correlates with the magnitude of virus-specific T cell responses. J Hepatol 53: 805–816.
20. Howell J, Visvanathan K (2013) The role of natural killer cells in hepatitis C infection. Antivir Ther 18: 853–865.

21. Tian Z, Chen Y, Gao B (2013) Natural killer cells in liver disease. Hepatology 57: 1654–1662.
22. Ahlenstiel G, Titerence RH, Koh C, Edlich B, Feld JJ, et al. (2010) Natural killer cells are polarized toward cytotoxicity in chronic hepatitis C in an interferon-alfa-dependent manner. Gastroenterology 138: 325–335 e321–322.
23. Ryan EJ, Stevenson NJ, Hegarty JE, O'Farrelly C (2011) Chronic hepatitis C infection blocks the ability of dendritic cells to secrete IFN-alpha and stimulate T-cell proliferation. J Viral Hepat 18: 840–851.
24. Wang FS, Zhang Z (2013) Liver: How can acute-on-chronic liver failure be accurately identified? Nat Rev Gastroenterol Hepatol 10: 390–391.
25. Bozzano F, Marras F, Biassoni R, De Maria A (2012) Natural killer cells in hepatitis C virus infection. Expert Rev Clin Immunol 8: 775–788.
26. Yoon JC, Lim JB, Park JH, Lee JM (2011) Cell-to-cell contact with hepatitis C virus-infected cells reduces functional capacity of natural killer cells. J Virol 85: 12557–12569.
27. Andrews DM, Estcourt MJ, Andoniou CE, Wikstrom ME, Khong A, et al. (2010) Innate immunity defines the capacity of antiviral T cells to limit persistent infection. J Exp Med 207: 1333–1343.
28. Jaeger BN, Donadieu J, Cognet C, Bernat C, Ordonez-Rueda D, et al. (2012) Neutrophil depletion impairs natural killer cell maturation, function, and homeostasis. J Exp Med 209: 565–580.
29. Mondelli MU, Oliviero B, Mele D, Mantovani S, Gazzabin C, et al. (2012) Natural killer cell functional dichotomy: a feature of chronic viral hepatitis? Front Immunol 3: 351.
30. Pernollet M, Jouvin-Marche E, Leroy V, Vigan I, Zarski JP, et al. (2002) Simultaneous evaluation of lymphocyte subpopulations in the liver and in peripheral blood mononuclear cells of HCV-infected patients: relationship with histological lesions. Clin Exp Immunol 130: 518–525.
31. Fehniger TA, Shah MH, Turner MJ, VanDeusen JB, Whitman SP, et al. (1999) Differential cytokine and chemokine gene expression by human NK cells following activation with IL-18 or IL-15 in combination with IL-12: implications for the innate immune response. J Immunol 162: 4511–4520.
32. Betts MR, Brenchley JM, Price DA, De Rosa SC, Douek DC, et al. (2003) Sensitive and viable identification of antigen-specific CD8+ T cells by a flow cytometric assay for degranulation. J Immunol Methods 281: 65–78.
33. Sturm N, Thelu MA, Camous X, Dimitrov G, Ramzan M, et al. (2010) Characterization and role of intra-hepatic regulatory T cells in chronic hepatitis C pathogenesis. J Hepatol 53: 25–35.

12

Liver Stiffness by Transient Elastography Predicts Liver-Related Complications and Mortality in Patients with Chronic Liver Disease

Jack X. Q. Pang[1,2], Scott Zimmer[3], Sophia Niu[3], Pam Crotty[1], Jenna Tracey[1], Faruq Pradhan[1], Abdel Aziz M. Shaheen[1], Carla S. Coffin[1], Steven J. Heitman[1,2], Gilaad G. Kaplan[1,2], Mark G. Swain[1], Robert P. Myers[1,2]*

1 Liver Unit, Division of Gastroenterology and Hepatology, Department of Medicine, University of Calgary, Calgary, Alberta, Canada, **2** Department of Community Health Sciences, University of Calgary, Calgary, Alberta, Canada, **3** Medical Services, Alberta Health Services, Calgary, Alberta, Canada

Abstract

Background: Liver stiffness measurement (LSM) by transient elastography (TE, FibroScan) is a validated method for noninvasively staging liver fibrosis. Most hepatic complications occur in patients with advanced fibrosis. Our objective was to determine the ability of LSM by TE to predict hepatic complications and mortality in a large cohort of patients with chronic liver disease.

Methods: In consecutive adults who underwent LSM by TE between July 2008 and June 2011, we used Cox regression to determine the independent association between liver stiffness and death or hepatic complications (decompensation, hepatocellular carcinoma, and liver transplantation). The performance of LSM to predict complications was determined using the c-statistic.

Results: Among 2,052 patients (median age 51 years, 65% with hepatitis B or C), 87 patients (4.2%) died or developed a hepatic complication during a median follow-up period of 15.6 months (interquartile range, 11.0–23.5 months). Patients with complications had higher median liver stiffness than those without complications (13.5 vs. 6.0 kPa; $P<0.00005$). The 2-year incidence rates of death or hepatic complications were 2.6%, 9%, 19%, and 34% in patients with liver stiffness <10, 10–19.9, 20–39.9, and ≥40 kPa, respectively ($P<0.00005$). After adjustment for potential confounders, liver stiffness by TE was an independent predictor of complications (hazard ratio [HR] 1.05 per kPa; 95% confidence interval [CI] 1.03–1.06). The c-statistic of liver-stiffness for predicting complications was 0.80 (95% CI 0.75–0.85). A liver stiffness below 20 kPa effectively excluded complications (specificity 93%, negative predictive value 97%); however, the positive predictive value of higher results was sub-optimal (20%).

Conclusions: Liver stiffness by TE accurately predicts the risk of death or hepatic complications in patients with chronic liver disease. TE may facilitate the estimation of prognosis and guide management of these patients.

Editor: Seung Up Kim, Yonsei University College of Medicine, Republic of Korea

Funding: Drs. Myers, Coffin, and Kaplan are supported by awards from the Canadian Institutes for Health Research (CIHR). Dr. Kaplan is also supported by Alberta Innovates-Health Solutions (AIHS). Dr. Swain is supported by the Cal Wenzel Family Foundation Chair in Hepatology. This study was supported in part by grants from CIHR, AIHS, and the Canadian Liver Foundation, and is based in part on data provided by Alberta Health. The interpretation and conclusions are those of the researchers and do not necessarily represent the views of the Government of Alberta. Neither the Government nor Alberta Health expresses any opinion in relation to this study. The funders had no role in study design, data collection and analysis, decision to publish, or preparation of the manuscript.

* E-mail: rpmyers@ucalgary.ca

Introduction

Liver fibrosis assessment is a vital aspect of the management of patients with chronic liver disease, both for guiding therapy and estimating prognosis. Most hepatic complications occur in patients with advanced fibrosis. Although liver biopsy had traditionally been used to stage fibrosis, it is limited by invasiveness, potential complications, cost, and difficulty of repetition for monitoring changes over time [1,2]. Moreover, the accuracy of biopsy is influenced by subjectivity in histological interpretation and sampling error, which may lead to discordance in staging in up to 40% of patients [3]. In light of these limitations, noninvasive means for staging fibrosis have been developed including serum biomarkers (e.g. FibroTest [4], ELF Panel [5], FibroMeter [6]) and elastography (e.g. transient elastography [TE] [7–9] and magnetic resonance elastography) [10]. A wealth of literature has confirmed the accuracy of these tools for staging fibrosis [11] leading to their widespread use. More recently, attention has turned to the prognostic significance of these tools. Traditionally, the Child-Pugh score and Model for End-Stage Liver Disease (MELD) have been used to estimate prognosis in cirrhotic patients [12]; however, their utility in milder disease is unclear. On the contrary, emerging data suggest that in addition to the surrogate endpoint of fibrosis, the aforementioned noninvasive methods can predict mortality and liver-related complications. For example, the FibroTest is correlated with survival and has similar 5-year prognostic value to that of biopsy in patients with hepatitis B (HBV) [13], hepatitis C (HCV) [14,15], and alcoholic liver disease [16]. Similar data has been reported for the ELF panel [17], AST-platelet ratio index (APRI) [18], FIB-4 [18], and TE (FibroScan; Echosens, Paris, France) [15,19–24].

TE is an ultrasound-based tool for measuring liver stiffness as a surrogate of fibrosis that is widely used due to its high accuracy for the diagnosis of advanced fibrosis [25,26]. Liver stiffness correlates with cirrhosis complications including variceal hemorrhage, ascites, and hepatocellular carcinoma (HCC) [27]. Many of these complications are portal hypertension-related; indeed, liver stiffness correlates with the hepatic venous pressure gradient [28,29]. Furthermore, recent studies have shown an association between liver stiffness and survival. Among 1,457 patients with chronic HCV, Vergniol *et al.* reported that LSM by TE had superior diagnostic performance for predicting 5-year survival compared with biopsy [15]. In another study of patients with various conditions, Klibansky reported excellent diagnostic performance of TE for predicting a composite outcome including death, decompensation, and HCC (area under the receiver operating characteristic curve [AUROC], 0.87) [19].

The objective of our study was to examine the association between liver stiffness and the risk of death or liver-related complications in a large cohort of patients with diverse hepatic disorders and severities to reflect routine clinical practice. We report risk estimates at clinically relevant liver stiffness thresholds that that may help physicians estimate the prognosis of their patients and guide their management.

Methods

Study Population

This retrospective-prospective study included consecutive adults (≥18 years) with chronic liver disease (i.e. chronically elevated liver biochemistry and/or abnormal liver imaging) who underwent LSM by TE at the University of Calgary Liver Unit (UCLU) between July 2008 and June 2011. The UCLU is the major referral center for patients with liver disease in southern Alberta serving a catchment population of ~1.5 million individuals. LSM by TE is performed routinely in all UCLU patients without overt evidence of hepatic decompensation. Patients with any of the following criteria were excluded: 1) non-residents of Alberta; 2) invalid provincial health numbers and/or the inability to link clinical information with administrative data (see below); 3) liver-related complications prior to or at the time of their FibroScan (see below); and 4) FibroScan failure, defined as no valid LSMs after ≥ 10 attempts. The Research Ethics Board at the University of Calgary approved the study protocol. The requirement for individual informed consent was waived for the study; however, patient records were anonymized and de-identified prior to analysis.

Liver Stiffness Measurement

Two experienced operators performed all FibroScan examinations as per the manufacturer's recommendations. Between July 2008 and July 2009, the M probe was used in all patients; thereafter, the XL probe was used in obese patients (body mass index [BMI]≥30 kg/m^2). Briefly, with the patient lying in the dorsal decubitus position and the right arm in maximal abduction, the tip of the FibroScan transducer probe was placed on the skin between the ribs over the right lobe of the liver. Assisted by a sonographic image, a portion of the liver ≥6 cm thick and free of large vascular structures was identified and an attempt was made to collect ≥10 valid LSMs. The median liver stiffness value was considered representative of the elastic modulus of the liver. Fasting prior to the examination was not routinely required. As an indicator of variability, the ratio of the interquartile range (IQR) of liver stiffness to the median (IQR/M) was calculated. As recommended by Boursier and colleagues [30], examinations with median stiffness ≥7.1 kPa and an IQR/M >30% were considered poorly reliable [31]. Analysis of the results according to a prior definition of reliability (≥10 valid measurements, success rate ≥60%, and IQR/M ≤30%) [32] revealed similar results (data not shown).

Administrative Data Sources

This study utilized three administrative databases with linkage using a unique identifier to identify the underlying liver disease etiologies, comorbidities, hepatic complications, and mortality of study participants. These databases have been used to examine the epidemiology [33,34], outcomes [2,35,36], and coding accuracy [33,37] of various medical conditions.

1. *Physician Claims Database.* This database includes claims submitted for payment by Alberta physicians for services provided to registrants of the Alberta Health Care Insurance Plan, a universal plan that covers over 99% of Alberta residents [38]. Each record includes the service provided, date, and up to three diagnosis fields. The database was queried from April 2001 to March 2011.
2. *Inpatient Discharge Abstract Database.* This database contains diagnosis, procedure, and mortality information on all discharges from Alberta hospitals. Chart validation studies have shown rates of agreement >95% for demographics and 75–96% for most responsible diagnosis codes [39]. The database was queried from January 1991 to January 2012.
3. *National Ambulatory Care Reporting System/Ambulatory Care Classification System Database.* This database contains information on facility-based ambulatory care including clinic and emergency department visits, same-day surgery, and day procedures [38]. The database was queried from July 1996 to December 2011.

Outcomes and Predictor Variables

Patients were managed as per consensus recommendations and followed according to the discretion of their hepatologist. Our primary outcome measure was a composite that included overall mortality and hepatic complications, including features of decompensation (ascites, spontaneous bacterial peritonitis, jaundice, hepatic encephalopathy, variceal hemorrhage, hepatorenal syndrome), HCC, and liver transplantation. Complications were identified by querying the administrative databases for relevant diagnosis and procedure codes according to the *International Classification of Disease, Ninth Revision, Clinical Modification* (ICD-9-CM) [40], the *Tenth Revision of the ICD* (ICD-10) [41], the *Canadian Classification of Diagnostic, Therapeutic, and Surgical Procedures (CCP)* [42], and the *Canadian Classification of Health Interventions* [43] after the FibroScan examination (see Appendix S1). Since the administrative databases do not include data regarding the underlying cause of death, we could not examine liver-related mortality specifically.

The primary predictor variable was median liver stiffness examined as a continuous variable; according to established cut-offs (F0–1: stiffness <7.1 kPa; F2:7.1–9.4 kPa; F3 (bridging fibrosis): 9.5–12.4 kPa; and F4 (cirrhosis): ≥12.5 kPa) [44]; and according to the following clinically-relevant thresholds: <10, 10–19.9, 20–39.9, and ≥40 kPa. Previous studies have used similar thresholds [15,20,45,46]. Additional covariates included age, gender, the underlying liver disease, comorbidities, and FibroScan reliability [32]. Hepatic diagnoses were categorized according to a hierarchy as follows: HBV, HCV, autoimmune (including primary biliary cirrhosis, primary sclerosing cholangitis, and autoimmune hepatitis), hemochromatosis, alcoholic liver disease, nonalcoholic fatty liver disease (NAFLD), and other (see Appendix S1). For example, a patient with any diagnosis code for HBV with or without other hepatic diagnoses would be categorized as having HBV. Comorbidities occurring before the FibroScan were defined using the Elixhauser algorithm (liver diseases excluded), which has been validated in patients with hepatic and non-hepatic disorders [47,48]. Based on literature describing an adverse relationship between several comorbidities and outcomes in this population (i.e. diabetes, renal failure, fluid and electrolyte disorders, coagulopathy, HIV/AIDS, alcohol and drug abuse, and malignancy) [48], we *a priori* examined these comorbidities individually and the remainder were categorized (as 0, 1, or ≥2). We also examined the type of FibroScan probe because the XL probe gives lower readings than the M probe [9]. Moreover, use of the XL probe was considered a surrogate marker for obesity since BMI is not available in the administrative data.

Statistical Analyses

All analyses were performed using Stata v11.0 (StataCorp; College Station, TX). Between groups comparisons were made using Fisher's exact, chi-square, and Mann-Whitney tests, as appropriate. Two-sided *P*-values <0.05 were considered statistically significant. The association between liver stiffness and hepatic complications or mortality was assessed using the Kaplan-Meier method and Cox proportional hazards regression [49]. The proportional hazards assumption was confirmed. Patients were followed from the date of their FibroScan until a complication or the end of follow-up of the administrative data (31 January 2012). Multivariate Cox models adjusted for age, gender, liver stiffness, FibroScan probe, and variables that were statistically significant in univariate analyses. Due to differences in liver stiffness measured using the XL and M probes [9], an interaction term between liver stiffness and probe was examined, but it was not statistically significant (data not shown).

To assess the performance of LSM by TE in predicting death or hepatic complications during follow-up, we calculated the sensitivity, specificity, accuracy, and positive (PPV) and negative predictive values (NPV) of a threshold of ≥20 kPa. Previous studies have shown that this threshold reliably excludes hepatic complications during medium-term follow-up [19,21,22]. Finally, to determine the ability of LSM to discriminate between patients who will and will not develop complications, the c-statistic with a modification for survival data was calculated. The c-statistic from the Cox model is conceptually analogous to the AUROC estimated for logistic models (1.0 indicates perfect discrimination and 0.5 is equivalent to chance) [50].

Results

Patient Characteristics and Liver Stiffness Results

In total, 2,437 patients had a LSM by TE during the study period. After excluding 385 ineligible patients, 2,052 were included in the study cohort (Figure 1 and Table 1). The median age was 51 years (IQR 40–58) and 55% were male. The majority had HCV (36%) or HBV (29%), while 7% had NAFLD, 5% had autoimmune liver disease, 3% had hemochromatosis, and 2% had alcoholic liver disease. FibroScans were performed using the M probe in the majority (87%) of patients; 4.5% (n = 93) were poorly reliable. The median liver stiffness value was 6.1 kPa (range, 2.3–75 kPa; IQR 4.6–9.0 kPa). According to cut-offs recommended by Castera *et al.* [44], an estimated 61% of patients had F0–1 fibrosis, 15% had F2, 8% had F3, and 15% had F4 (cirrhosis).

Predictors of Hepatic Complications and Mortality

During a median follow-up period of 15.6 months (IQR 11.0–23.5), 87 patients (4.2%) died or developed a hepatic complication, corresponding to an overall incidence of 2.8 cases per 100 person-years (95% confidence interval [CI] 2.3–3.5). In the subpopulation of 315 patients with presumed cirrhosis, 46 cases (14.6%) developed a complication, corresponding to an overall incidence of 10.1 (95% CI 7.5–13.4) per 100 person-years (vs. 1.6 [95% CI 1.1–2.1] per 100 person-years in 1,737 non-cirrhotic patients; *P*< 0.00005). Of the 124 total complications, specific events are outlined in Table 2. The median intervals between LSM and a complication, including transplantation (n = 5) specifically, were 5.7 months (IQR 1.5–10.6) and 4.1 months (IQR 0.7–8.4), respectively.

Patients who died or developed a hepatic complication during follow-up had higher median liver stiffness than patients without complications (13.5 kPa vs. 6.0 kPa; *P*<0.00005; Table 1). Survival free of complications was reduced in patients with an estimated fibrosis stage of F2, F3, or F4 compared with F0–1 (*P*< 0.00005; Figure 2). Similarly, the risk of complications increased with liver stiffness within the advanced range (*P*<0.00005; Figure 3). Specifically, the overall incidence rates of death or hepatic complications in patients with liver stiffness <10 (n = 1,597), 10–19.9 (n = 274), 20–39.9 (n = 135), and ≥40 kPa (n = 46) were 1.23 (95% CI 0.9–1.8), 4.9 (3.2–7.5), 11.3 (7.4–17.1), and 29.0 (17.2–49.0) cases per 100 person-years, respectively (*P*< 0.00005). In patients with liver stiffness <10, 10–19.9, 20–39.9, and ≥40 kPa, actuarial rates of death or hepatic complications at 1, 2 and 3 years were 1.3% (95% CI 0.8–2.0%), 2.6% (1.7–4.0%) and 3.9% (2.2–6.7%); 6.6% (4.1–10.4%), 8.8% (5.6–13.6%) and 10% (6.4–15.6%); 14% (9.4–22%), 19% (12–28%) and 19% (12–28%); and 29% (18–44%), 34% (21–52%) and 34% (21–52%), respectively (*P*<0.00005).

After adjustment for age, gender, hepatic diagnosis, comorbidities, and FibroScan probe and reliability, liver stiffness was an independent predictor of hepatic complications or mortality (Table 3). Specifically, the adjusted risk of complications increased 5% per 1-kPa increase in liver stiffness (hazard ratio [HR] 1.05; 95% CI 1.03–1.06). In subgroup analyses according to liver disease etiology, liver stiffness was predictive of complications in patients with HBV (HR 1.04; 95% CI 1.00–1.08), HCV (HR 1.06; 1.04–1.07), and other conditions (HR 1.05; 1.03–1.06). Additional predictors included diabetes (HR 1.79; 95% CI 1.02–3.14) and coagulopathy (HR 2.20; 1.27–3.81). In supplemental analyses in which liver stiffness was categorized rather than examined as a continuous variable, similar results were obtained (Table 3). For example, compared with patients with liver stiffness below 10 kPa, the risk of complications increased 3-fold in those with liver stiffness from 10 to 19.9 kPa (HR 3.22; 95% CI 1.81–5.75), 7-fold between 20 and 39.9 kPa (HR 7.02; 3.88–12.7), and 12-fold with liver stiffness ≥40 kPa (HR 12.5; 6.21–25.0).

Performance of Liver Stiffness for Predicting Complications

The c-statistic of liver-stiffness for the prediction of hepatic complications and mortality was 0.80 (95% CI 0.75–0.85). The

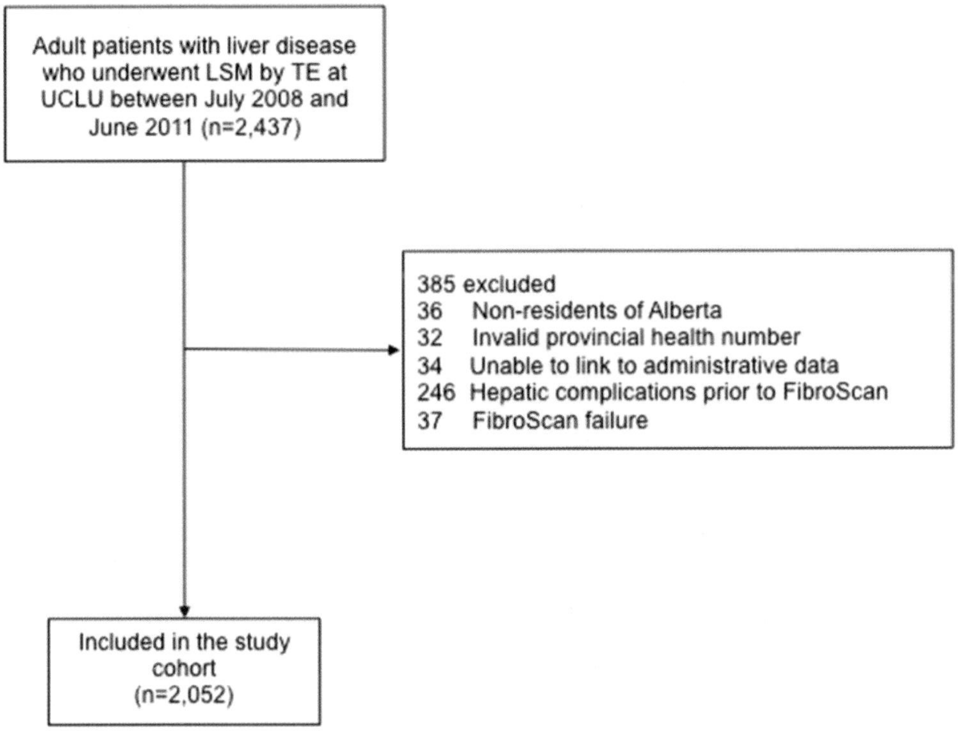

Figure 1. Flow diagram of study participants.

sensitivity, specificity, PPV, NPV, and accuracy of a liver stiffness value ≥20 kPa for predicting complications were 41% (95% CI 31–52%), 93% (91–94%), 20% (14–26%), 97% (96–98%), and 90% (89–92%), respectively. The actuarial rates of death or hepatic complications at 3 years in patients with liver stiffness ≥ 20 kPa and <20 kPa were 23% (95% CI 16–30%) and 4.7% (3.2–7.0%), respectively (Figure 4; *P*<0.0005). For the secondary outcomes of hepatic decompensation or HCC (n = 76) and overall mortality (n = 17), the c-statistics of liver stiffness were 0.82 (95% CI 0.77–0.87) and 0.67 (0.55–0.80), respectively.

Discussion

This is the largest study to examine the prognostic significance of liver stiffness by TE. In over 2,000 patients with various liver disease etiologies, we demonstrate that liver stiffness is an independent predictor of hepatic complications and mortality after adjustment for age, gender, underlying disease, comorbidities, and other potential confounders. Specifically, for every 1-kPa increase in liver stiffness, the adjusted risk of complications increased 5%. Importantly, we have generated risk estimates stratified according to clinically relevant stiffness categories that may help physicians to estimate the prognosis of their patients and guide their management. Specifically, the 3-year actuarial rates of death or hepatic complications in patients with liver stiffness <10, 10 to <20, 20 to <40, and ≥40 kPa were 3.9%, 10%, 19%, and 34%, respectively (Figure 3). Corresponding incidence rates of complications were 1.2, 4.9, 11.3, and 29.0 cases per 100 person-years, respectively.

These data are consistent with other reports. For example, in patients with HCV, Vergniol and colleagues reported that the 5-year risk of death increased from 4% in patients with liver stiffness ≤9.5 kPa, to 34% with stiffness >20 kPa and 53% with stiffness > 40 kPa [15]. In another study of HIV/HCV-coinfected, cirrhotic subjects, the risk of death or HCC at 3 years was 19% in patients with liver stiffness <40 kPa compared with 37% among those with higher values [20]. The event rates of complications that we report according to liver stiffness are clinically relevant, particularly since the proportion of patients undergoing biopsy is declining as use of TE increases. Our data suggest that in patients with stiffness > 10 kPa, and particularly those with stiffness >20 kPa, enhanced follow-up to monitor for complications is advisable. On the contrary, patients with liver stiffness <10 kPa can be safely reassured that their risk during several years of follow-up is low (< 5%). As the burden of liver disease increases (e.g. due to NAFLD), the ability to defer close surveillance in patients with low liver stiffness values will be important for providing reassurance and minimizing healthcare expenditures.

The stepwise increase in risk of complications that we observed according to liver stiffness categories within the cirrhotic range (Figure 3) suggests that TE offers prognostic information above and beyond that provided by liver biopsy. Whereas the stage of cirrhosis is traditionally defined by histological evidence of regenerative nodules with one or two qualitative categories (e.g. METAVIR stage 4 or Ishak stages 5 and 6), the dynamic range of LSM is much greater. Since the quantity of fibrous tissue deposition varies widely in cirrhosis, it is clear that the risk of complications is not uniform among cirrhotic patients. In this regard, the ability to express liver stiffness as a continuous variable (from ~12.5 to 75 kPa in cirrhosis) or in an arbitrary number of categories represents an advantage for prognostication compared with biopsy. Indeed, several studies have shown better performance of FibroScan (and other non-invasive tools) compared with biopsy for predicting hepatic complications [15,19]. For example, in the study of Vergniol *et al.* [15], the AUROCs for 5-year survival of FibroScan, FibroTest, and biopsy were 0.82, 0.80, and 0.76, respectively. The AUROC observed for TE (0.80) in our study is consistent with these reports, and supports its excellent

Table 1. Characteristics of the Study Cohort According to the Occurrence of Hepatic Complications or Mortality During Follow-Up.

Variable	Total Cohort* (n = 2,052)	Without Complications (n = 1,965)	With Complications* (n = 87)	Unadjusted Hazard Ratio (95% CI)
Male	55% (1,134)	55% (1,081)	61% (53)	1.23 (0.80–1.89)
Age, *years*	50 (40–58)	50 (40–57)	55 (46–60)	**1.03 (1.01–10.5)**
Hepatic diagnosis				
Hepatitis B	29% (588)	29% (569)	22% (19)	0.85 (0.42–1.73)
Hepatitis C	36% (736)	36% (699)	43% (37)	1.30 (0.69–2.46)
Autoimmune	5.0% (102)	4.9% (96)	6.9% (6)	1.75 (0.66–4.60)
Hemochromatosis	3.0% (61)	3.0% (60)	1.2% (1)	0.44 (0.06–3.40)
Alcohol	2.2% (45)	2.2% (40)	5.8% (5)	**3.41 (1.22–9.57)**
NAFLD	6.8% (140)	6.8% (134)	6.9% (6)	1.16 (0.44–3.04)
Other/unknown	19% (380)	19% (367)	15% (13)	Ref
Comorbidities				
Diabetes mellitus	10% (205)	9.4% (184)	24% (21)	**3.04 (1.87–4.99)**
Renal failure	3.9% (80)	3.7% (72)	9.2% (8)	**2.69 (1.30–5.56)**
Fluid/electrolyte disorders	12% (238)	11% (221)	20% (17)	**1.94 (1.14–3.30)**
Coagulopathy	6.0% (123)	5.3% (105)	21% (18)	**4.21 (2.51–7.08)**
Malignancy †	26% (542)	26% (516)	30% (26)	1.11 (0.70–1.76)
Alcohol abuse	10% (208)	10% (198)	11% (10)	1.22 (0.63–2.35)
Drug abuse	9.4% (192)	9.0% (177)	17% (15)	**2.15 (1.23–3.75)**
HIV	1.0% (21)	1.0% (20)	1.2% (1)	0.95 (0.13–6.81)
Other comorbidities				
0	28% (580)	28% (559)	24% (21)	Ref
1	29% (590)	29% (567)	26% (23)	1.07 (0.59–1.93)
≥2	43% (882)	43% (839)	49% (43)	1.38 (0.82–2.32)
Liver stiffness, *kPa*				
Median (IQR)	6.1 (4.6–9.0)	6.0 (4.6–8.8)	13.5 (7.8–29.9)	**1.05 (1.04–1.06)**
F0–1 (<7.1 kPa)	61% (1,253)	63% (1,235)	21% (18)	Ref
F2 (7.1–9.4 kPa)	15% (316)	15% (305)	13% (11)	**2.46 (1.16–5.22)**
F3 (9.5–12.4 kPa)	8.2% (168)	8.0% (156)	14% (12)	**4.98 (2.40–10.3)**
F4 (≥12.5 kPa)	15% (315)	14% (269)	53% (46)	**10.71 (6.21–18.48)**
M probe (vs. XL probe)	87% (1,788)	88% (1,720)	78% (68)	**0.47 (0.28–0.79)**
Poorly reliable liver stiffness measurement	4.5% (93)	4.1% (81)	14% (12)	**3.21 (1.74–5.91)**

Data are median (IQR) or proportions (% [n]). Hazard ratios in bold are statistically significant ($P<0.05$).
*Complications include hepatic decompensation, HCC, liver transplantation, or death.
†Malignancy includes lymphoma, solid tumors without metastases, and metastatic cancer.

discriminatory ability. At a threshold liver stiffness value ≥20 kPa, TE had a sensitivity, specificity, and accuracy of 41%, 93%, and 90%, respectively. Liver stiffness values <20 kPa effectively exclude complications (NPV 97%; Figure 4); however, the PPV of higher results (20%) does not allow one to adequately identify which patients will go on to develop a complication. The latter patients should perhaps undergo enhanced follow-up.

Our study includes several additional findings worthy of discussion. First, we identified an increased risk of complications among patients with liver stiffness corresponding to each of F2, F3, and F4 fibrosis compared with F0–1 fibrosis (Figure 2). For example, patients with liver stiffness between 7.1 and 9.4 kPa (~F2) at baseline had a two-fold risk of complications compared with those with lower liver stiffness (F0–1; Table 3). Since progression to cirrhosis over this time frame in a patient with F2 fibrosis is unexpected, we hypothesize that this relates to underestimation of fibrosis by TE in some cases. This is not unexpected since the sensitivity of a liver stiffness ≥9.5 kPa for advanced fibrosis (F3–F4) is only 73% [44]. Second, our data suggest that the influence of liver stiffness on complications is independent of which FibroScan probe is used. A unique aspect of our study is the inclusion of patients scanned using the XL probe, not available in most prior studies. Confirmation of this association is important because liver stiffness measured using the XL probe is typically 1–2 kPa lower than with the M probe [9]. Also, we considered the XL probe a surrogate marker for obesity, which we could not reliably identify using our databases. Surprisingly, this was not a significant predictor of complications, although the study may have been underpowered to detect this association. On the contrary, diabetes and coagulopathy were independently associated with complications. Diabetes is an important risk factor for all-cause mortality in general, plus the progression of chronic liver

Table 2. Specific Hepatic Complications and Mortality (n = 87)*.

Complication	% (n)
Hepatic decompensation	3.3% (67)
Variceal hemorrhage	2.0% (40)
Ascites	1.3% (26)
Hepatic encephalopathy	0.5% (11)
Jaundice	0.3% (6)
Hepatorenal syndrome	0.2% (3)
Spontaneous bacterial peritonitis	0.05% (1)
HCC	0.7% (15)
Liver transplantation	0.2% (5)
Death	0.8% (17)

*Individual patients could have multiple complications; hence the total (n = 124) exceeds 87 patients.

diseases including HBV, HCV, and NAFLD [51]. The association between coagulopathy and liver-related complications is largely due to recorded diagnoses of thrombocytopenia in the administrative data, although some patients had hereditary and acquired coagulation defects (data not shown). Although we attempted to exclude patients with hepatic decompensation prior to their FibroScan, it is possible that some patients were coagulopathic, yet clinically compensated. Nevertheless, exclusion of the 123 patients with coagulopathy did not influence the association between liver stiffness and complications (data not shown).

Our study has several limitations. First, our findings rely on the validity of the administrative databases that we used. Although chart abstraction studies have confirmed their accuracy for many hepatic [33,36,37] and non-hepatic [52] conditions, additional validation is necessary. Likewise, it is possible that patients developed a complication (e.g. mild ascites), yet did not seek medical attention or had a medical visit without capture of the diagnosis in the administrative data. Second, the databases lack laboratory data to confirm the diagnosis and assess disease severity (e.g. with the Child-Pugh or MELD scores). Prior studies have suggested that the discrimination of liver stiffness can be improved by considering additional laboratory variables. For example, Klibansky *et al.* reported that a composite score including TE, AST/ALT ratio, and MELD outperformed TE for predicting clinical outcomes (AUROCs 0.93 vs. 0.86) [19]. In addition, since liver biochemistry is not available in the administrative databases, we cannot exclude an impact of non-fibrotic histologic features impacting liver stiffness (e.g. marked ALT elevation due to severe hepatic inflammation). Similarly, information regarding alcohol consumption, obesity, dyslipidemia, and specific treatments (e.g. antiviral therapy) that can have disease-modifying effects are not available or poorly coded in the administrative databases. Nevertheless, it is unlikely that over the restricted follow-up in our study that these factors would have had a significant impact on

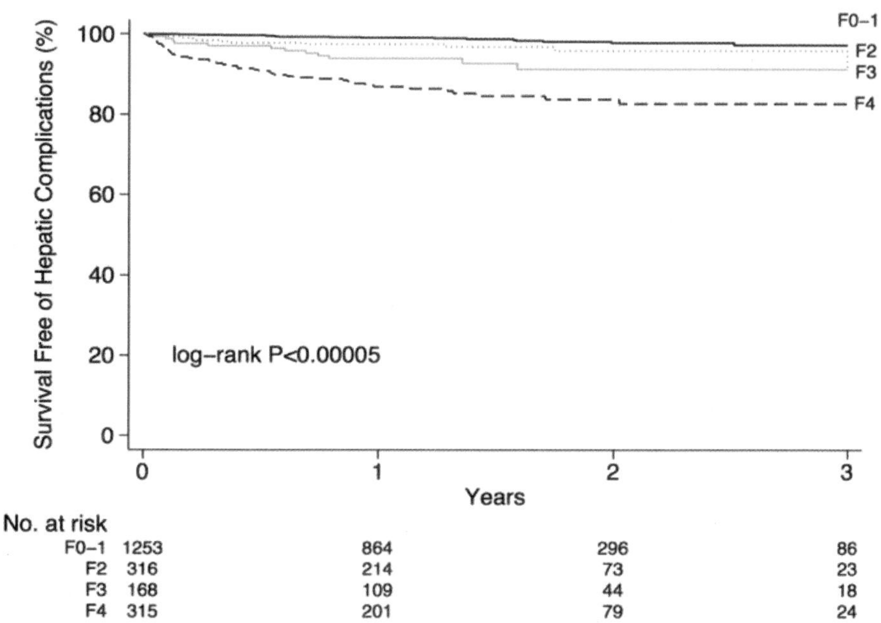

Figure 2. Unadjusted survival free of hepatic complications according to LSM by TE categorized as F0–1 (liver stiffness <7.1 kPa), F2 (7.1–9.4 kPa), F3 (9.5–12.4 kPa), and F4 (cirrhosis; ≥12.5 kPa).

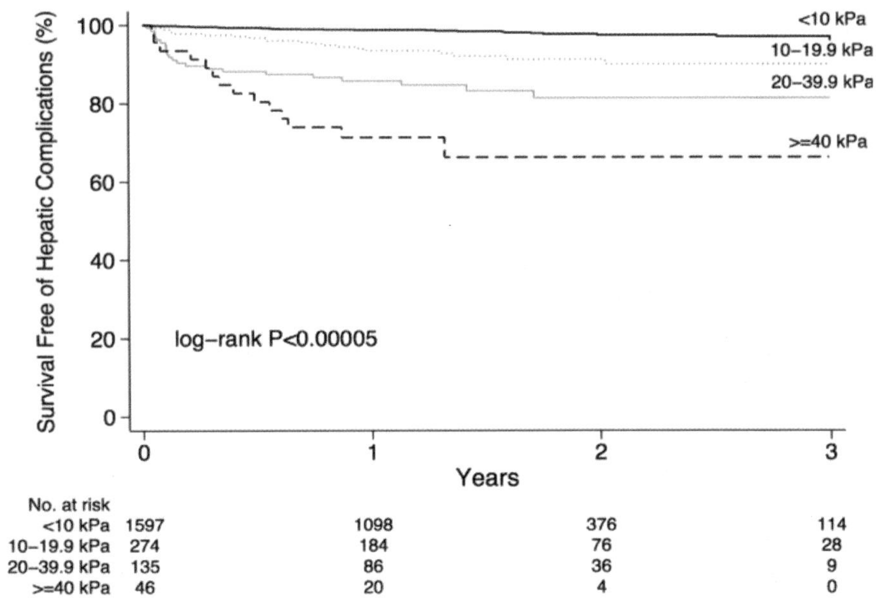

Figure 3. Unadjusted survival free of hepatic complications according to LSM by TE categorized as <10 kPa, 10–19.9 kPa, 20–39.9 kPa, and ≥40 kPa.

the clinical course of most patients. Moreover, a prior study in patients with HCV showed that the prognostic significance of liver stiffness persists after adjustment for antiviral treatment [15]. Third, we considered liver stiffness cut-offs validated for HCV despite the diverse etiologies of liver disease in our cohort. We chose this approach for simplicity despite literature showing that these thresholds may be disease-dependent. Finally, our study is limited by a relatively small number of events that precluded an

Table 3. Multivariate Analysis of Predictors of Hepatic Complications and Mortality (n = 2,052)*.

Variable	Hazard Ratio (95% CI)	*P*-value
Age, *per year*	1.01 (0.99–1.03)	0.16
Male gender	1.10 (0.71–1.70)	0.68
Alcoholic liver disease	1.03 (0.39–2.69)	0.95
Diabetes mellitus	**1.79 (1.02–3.14)**	**0.04**
Renal failure	1.66 (0.74–3.71)	0.22
Fluid and electolyte disorders	1.16 (0.65–2.07)	0.63
Coagulopathy	**2.20 (1.27–3.81)**	**0.005**
Drug abuse	1.71 (0.96–3.06)	0.07
FibroScan probe (M vs. XL)	0.81 (0.47–1.40)	0.45
Poorly reliable liver stiffness measurement	1.58 (0.84–2.99)	0.16
Liver stiffness		
Per 1-kPa increase	**1.05 (1.03–1.06)**	**<0.0005**
F0–1 (<7.1 kPa)	Ref	Ref
F2 (7.1–9.4 kPa)	**2.16 (1.01–4.64)**	**0.05**
F3 (9.5–12.4 kPa)	**4.23 (2.01–8.90)**	**<0.0005**
F4 (≥12.5 kPa)	**7.64 (4.22–13.8)**	**<0.0005**
<10 kPa	Ref	Ref
10–19.9 kPa	**3.22 (1.81–5.75)**	**<0.0005**
20–39.9 kPa	**7.02 (3.88–12.7)**	**<0.0005**
≥40 kPa	**12.5 (6.21–25.0)**	**<0.0005**

*Hazard ratios for all variables (except those listed for specific liver stiffness categories) were obtained from a model including liver stiffness examined as a continuous variable.

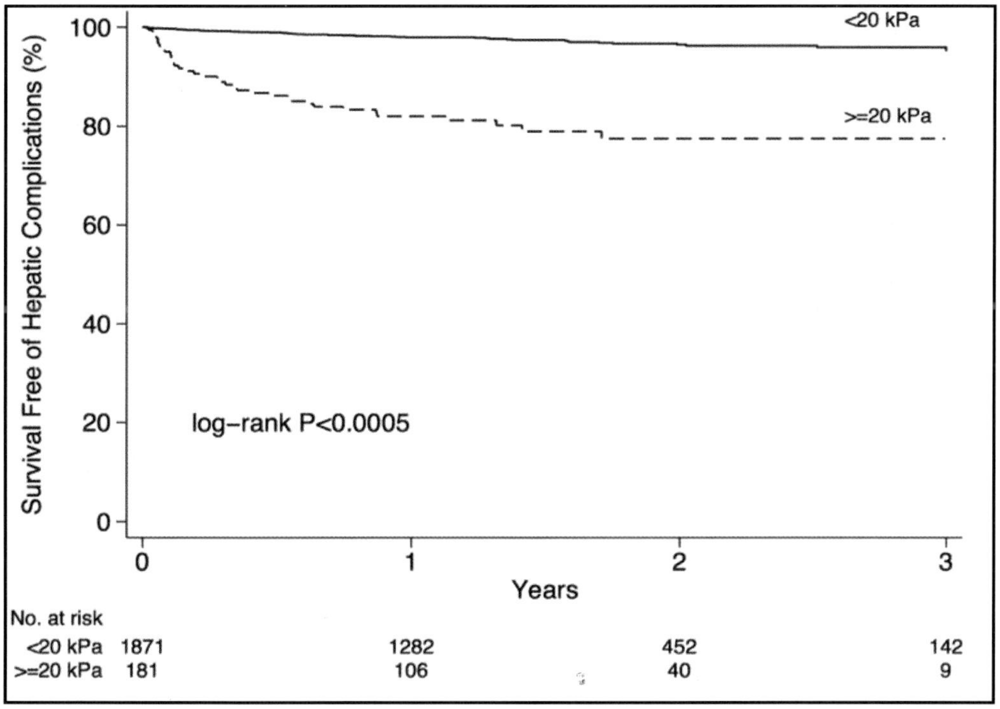

Figure 4. Unadjusted survival free of hepatic complications according to the 20 kPa-threshold for liver stiffness.

analysis of the associations between liver stiffness and individual complications. Nevertheless, other studies have shown a correlation between liver stiffness and sequelae including death, HCC, variceal hemorrhage, and hepatic insufficiency following surgical resection [15,19–24,53].

In conclusion, liver stiffness measured by TE is an independent predictor of hepatic complications and mortality in patients with chronic liver disease. The risk estimates that we report at clinically relevant liver stiffness cut-offs will provide valuable information to physicians and assist them in counseling their patients regarding their prognosis and may help guide their follow-up.

Author Contributions

Conceived and designed the experiments: RPM. Performed the experiments: JXQP SZ SN PC JT FP AAS RPM. Analyzed the data: JXQP RPM. Contributed reagents/materials/analysis tools: JXQP SZ SN PC JT FP AAS CSC SH GGK MGS RPM. Wrote the paper: JXQP RPM. Revised the manuscript for important intellectual content: JXQP SZ SN PC JT FP AAS CSC SH GGK MGS RPM.

References

1. Rockey DC, Caldwell SH, Goodman ZD, Nelson RC, Smith AD (2009) Liver biopsy. Hepatology 49: 1017–1044.
2. Myers RP, Fong A, Shaheen AA (2008) Utilization rates, complications and costs of percutaneous liver biopsy: a population-based study including 4275 biopsies. Liver Int 28: 705–712.
3. Bedossa P, Dargere D, Paradis V (2003) Sampling variability of liver fibrosis in chronic hepatitis C. Hepatology 38: 1449–1457.
4. Poynard T, Imbert-Bismut F, Munteanu M, Messous D, Myers RP, et al. (2004) Overview of the diagnostic value of biochemical markers of liver fibrosis (FibroTest, HCV FibroSure) and necrosis (ActiTest) in patients with chronic hepatitis C. Comp Hepatol 3: 8.
5. Rosenberg WM, Voelker M, Thiel R, Becka M, Burt A, et al. (2004) Serum markers detect the presence of liver fibrosis: a cohort study. Gastroenterology 127: 1704–1713.
6. Cales P, Oberti F, Michalak S, Hubert-Fouchard I, Rousselet MC, et al. (2005) A novel panel of blood markers to assess the degree of liver fibrosis. Hepatology 42: 1373–1381.
7. Sandrin L, Fourquet B, Hasquenoph JM, Yon S, Fournier C, et al. (2003) Transient elastography: a new noninvasive method for assessment of hepatic fibrosis. Ultrasound Med Biol 29: 1705–1713.
8. Myers RP, Elkashab M, Ma M, Crotty P, Pomier-Layrargues G (2010) Transient elastography for the noninvasive assessment of liver fibrosis: a multicentre Canadian study. Can J Gastroenterol 24: 661–670.
9. Myers RP, Pomier-Layrargues G, Kirsch R, Pollett A, Duarte-Rojo A, et al. (2012) Feasibility and diagnostic performance of the FibroScan XL probe for liver stiffness measurement in overweight and obese patients. Hepatology 55: 199–208.
10. Yin M, Chen J, Glaser KJ, Talwalkar JA, Ehman RL (2009) Abdominal magnetic resonance elastography. Top Magn Reson Imaging 20: 79–87.
11. Guha IN, Myers RP, Patel K, Talwalkar JA (2011) Biomarkers of liver fibrosis: What lies beneath the receiver operating characteristic curve? Hepatology 54: 1454–1462.
12. Kamath PS, Kim WR (2007) The model for end-stage liver disease (MELD). Hepatology 45: 797–805.
13. Ngo Y, Benhamou Y, Thibault V, Ingiliz P, Munteanu M, et al. (2008) An accurate definition of the status of inactive hepatitis B virus carrier by a combination of biomarkers (FibroTest-ActiTest) and viral load. PLoS One 3: e2573.
14. Ngo Y, Munteanu M, Messous D, Charlotte F, Imbert-Bismut F, et al. (2006) A prospective analysis of the prognostic value of biomarkers (FibroTest) in patients with chronic hepatitis C. Clin Chem 52: 1887–1896.
15. Vergniol J, Foucher J, Terrebonne E, Bernard PH, le Bail B, et al. (2011) Noninvasive tests for fibrosis and liver stiffness predict 5-year outcomes of patients with chronic hepatitis C. Gastroenterology 140: 1970–1979, 1979 e1971–1973.
16. Naveau S, Gaude G, Asnacios A, Agostini H, Abella A, et al. (2009) Diagnostic and prognostic values of noninvasive biomarkers of fibrosis in patients with alcoholic liver disease. Hepatology 49: 97–105.
17. Parkes J, Roderick P, Harris S, Day CP, Mutimer D, et al. (2010) Enhanced liver fibrosis test can predict clinical outcomes in patients with chronic liver disease. Gut 59: 1245–1251.
18. Nunes D, Fleming C, Offner G, Craven D, Fix O, et al. (2010) Noninvasive markers of liver fibrosis are highly predictive of liver-related death in a cohort of HCV-infected individuals with and without HIV infection. Am J Gastroenterol 105: 1346–1353.
19. Klibansky DA, Mehta SH, Curry M, Nasser I, Challies T, et al. (2012) Transient elastography for predicting clinical outcomes in patients with chronic liver disease. J Viral Hepat 19: e184–193.

20. Merchante N, Rivero-Juarez A, Tellez F, Merino D, Jose Rios-Villegas M, et al. (2012) Liver stiffness predicts clinical outcome in human immunodeficiency virus/hepatitis C virus-coinfected patients with compensated liver cirrhosis. Hepatology 56: 228–238.
21. Robic MA, Procopet B, Metivier S, Peron JM, Selves J, et al. (2011) Liver stiffness accurately predicts portal hypertension related complications in patients with chronic liver disease: a prospective study. J Hepatol 55: 1017–1024.
22. Kim SU, Lee JH, Kim do Y, Ahn SH, Jung KS, et al. (2012) Prediction of liver-related events using fibroscan in chronic hepatitis B patients showing advanced liver fibrosis. PLoS One 7: e36676.
23. Masuzaki R, Tateishi R, Yoshida H, Goto E, Sato T, et al. (2009) Prospective risk assessment for hepatocellular carcinoma development in patients with chronic hepatitis C by transient elastography. Hepatology 49: 1954–1961.
24. Jung KS, Kim SU, Ahn SH, Park YN, Kim do Y, et al. (2011) Risk assessment of hepatitis B virus-related hepatocellular carcinoma development using liver stiffness measurement (FibroScan). Hepatology 53: 885–894.
25. Friedrich-Rust M, Ong MF, Martens S, Sarrazin C, Bojunga J, et al. (2008) Performance of transient elastography for the staging of liver fibrosis: a meta-analysis. Gastroenterology 134: 960–974.
26. Steadman R, Myers RP, Leggett L, Lorenzetti D, Noseworthy T, et al. (2013) A health technology assessment of transient elastography in adult liver disease. Can J Gastroenterol 27: 149–158.
27. Foucher J, Chanteloup E, Vergniol J, Castera L, Le Bail B, et al. (2006) Diagnosis of cirrhosis by transient elastography (FibroScan): a prospective study. Gut 55: 403–408.
28. Bureau C, Metivier S, Peron JM, Selves J, Robic MA, et al. (2008) Transient elastography accurately predicts presence of significant portal hypertension in patients with chronic liver disease. Aliment Pharmacol Ther 27: 1261–1268.
29. Vizzutti F, Arena U, Romanelli RG, Rega L, Foschi M, et al. (2007) Liver stiffness measurement predicts severe portal hypertension in patients with HCV-related cirrhosis. Hepatology 45: 1290–1297.
30. Boursier J, Zarski JP, de Ledinghen V, Rousselet MC, Sturm N, et al. (2013) Determination of reliability criteria for liver stiffness evaluation by transient elastography. Hepatology 57: 1182–1191.
31. Pang JX, Pradhan F, Zimmer S, Niu S, Crotty P, et al. (2014) The feasibility and reliability of transient elastography using Fibroscan(R): A practice audit of 2335 examinations. Can J Gastroenterol Hepatol 28: 143–149.
32. Castera L, Foucher J, Bernard PH, Carvalho F, Allaix D, et al. (2010) Pitfalls of liver stiffness measurement: a 5-year prospective study of 13,369 examinations. Hepatology 51: 828–835.
33. Myers RP, Liu M, Shaheen AA (2008) The burden of hepatitis C virus infection is growing: a Canadian population-based study of hospitalizations from 1994 to 2004. Can J Gastroenterol 22: 381–387.
34. Kaplan GG, Gregson DB, Laupland KB (2004) Population-based study of the epidemiology of and the risk factors for pyogenic liver abscess. Clin Gastroenterol Hepatol 2: 1032–1038.
35. Myers RP, Shaheen AA, Li B, Dean S, Quan H (2008) Impact of liver disease, alcohol abuse, and unintentional ingestions on the outcomes of acetaminophen overdose. Clin Gastroenterol Hepatol 6: 918–925; quiz 837.
36. Myers RP, Shaheen AA, Fong A, Burak KW, Wan A, et al. (2009) Epidemiology and natural history of primary biliary cirrhosis in a Canadian health region: a population-based study. Hepatology 50: 1884–1892.
37. Myers RP, Leung Y, Shaheen AA, Li B (2007) Validation of ICD-9-CM/ICD-10 coding algorithms for the identification of patients with acetaminophen overdose and hepatotoxicity using administrative data. BMC Health Serv Res 7: 159.
38. (2003) Data Disclosure Handbook. Alberta Health and Wellness. 1–15.
39. Williams JI, Young W (1996) A summary of studies on the quality of health care administrative databases in Canada. In: Goel V, Williams JI, Anderson GM, Blackstein-Hirsch P, Fooks C et al., editors. Patterns of Health Care in Ontario: The ICES Practice Atlas. 2nd ed. Ottawa, ON: The Canadian Medical Association. 339–345.
40. (2001) International Classificiation of Diseases, 9th Revision, Clinical Modification (ICD-9-CM). Los Angeles: Practice Management Information Corporation.
41. WHO (1992) International Statistical Classification of Diseases and Related Health Problems, Tenth Revision (ICD-10) Geneva: World Health Organization.
42. (1993. Cat no 82–562.) Canadian Classification of Diagnostic, Therapeutic, and Surgical Procedures. Ottawa: Statistics Canada.
43. (2001) Canadian Classification of Health Interventions (CCI) 2001. Ottawa: Canadian Institute for Health Information (CIHI).
44. Castera L, Vergniol J, Foucher J, Le Bail B, Chanteloup E, et al. (2005) Prospective comparison of transient elastography, Fibrotest, APRI, and liver biopsy for the assessment of fibrosis in chronic hepatitis C. Gastroenterology 128: 343–350.
45. Kazemi F, Kettaneh A, N'Kontchou G, Pinto E, Ganne-Carrie N, et al. (2006) Liver stiffness measurement selects patients with cirrhosis at risk of bearing large oesophageal varices. J Hepatol 45: 230–235.
46. Robic MA, Procopet B, Metivier S, Peron JM, Selves J, et al. (2011) Liver stiffness accurately predicts portal hypertension related complications in patients with chronic liver disease: a prospective study. J Hepatol.
47. Elixhauser A, Steiner C, Harris DR, Coffey RM (1998) Comorbidity measures for use with administrative data. Med Care 36: 8–27.
48. Myers RP, Quan H, Hubbard JN, Shaheen AA, Kaplan GG (2009) Predicting in-hospital mortality in patients with cirrhosis: results differ across risk adjustment methods. Hepatology 49: 568–577.
49. Therneau TM, Grambsch PM (2000) Modeling survival data: extending the Cox model. New York, NY: Springer-Verlag. 107–111 p.
50. D'Agostino RB, Nam BH (2004) Evaluation of the performance of survival analysis models: discrimination and calibration measures. In: Balakrishnan N, Rao CR, editors. Advances in survival analysis. Amsterdam: Elsevier. 1–25.
51. Powell EE, Jonsson JR, Clouston AD (2005) Steatosis: co-factor in other liver diseases. Hepatology 42: 5–13.
52. Quan H, Li B, Saunders LD, Parsons GA, Nilsson CI, et al. (2008) Assessing validity of ICD-9-CM and ICD-10 administrative data in recording clinical conditions in a unique dually coded database. Health Serv Res 43: 1424–1441.
53. Cescon M, Colecchia A, Cucchetti A, Peri E, Montrone L, et al. (2012) Value of transient elastography measured with FibroScan in predicting the outcome of hepatic resection for hepatocellular carcinoma. Ann Surg 256: 706–712; discussion 712–703.

13

Angiopoietin-2 and Biliary Diseases: Elevated Serum, but Not Bile Levels Are Associated with Cholangiocarcinoma

Torsten Voigtländer[1,2]¶, Sascha David[3]¶, Kristina Thamm[3], Jerome Schlué[4], Jochen Metzger[5], Michael P. Manns[1,2], Tim O. Lankisch[1,2]*

1 Department of Gastroenterology, Hepatology and Endocrinology, Hannover Medical School, Hannover, Germany, **2** Integrated Research and Treatment Center – Transplantation (IFB-Tx), Hannover Medical School, Hannover, Germany, **3** Department of Nephrology & Hypertension, Hannover Medical School, Hannover, Germany, **4** Institute of Pathology, Hannover Medical School, Hannover, Germany, **5** Mosaiques diagnostics GmbH, Hannover, Germany

Abstract

Background: The diagnosis of cholangiocarcinoma (CC) is challenging especially in patients with primary sclerosing cholangitis (PSC) and often delayed due to the lack of reliable markers. Angiopoietin-2 (Angpt-2) has been employed as a biomarker of angiogenesis and might be involved in tumor neoangiogenesis.

Aim: To evaluate the diagnostic potential of Angpt-2 as a biomarker to detect patients with CC.

Methods: Bile and serum Angpt-2 levels were measured in patients with CC (n = 45), PSC (n = 74), CC complicating PSC (CC/PSC) (n = 11) and patients with bile duct stones (n = 37) in a cross sectional study. Diagnostic accuracy of Angpt-2 was compared to carbohydrate antigen 19-9 (CA19-9). Fluorescent immunohistochemistry from human CC liver tissue samples was performed to localize the origin of Angpt-2.

Results: Serum Angpt-2 concentration was significantly elevated in patients with CC compared to control patients ($p<0.05$). Diagnostic accuracy of Angpt-2 as determined by receiver operating characteristic (ROC) analysis resulted in a higher area under the curve (AUC) value compared to CA19-9 (AUC: 0.85 versus 0.77; 95% confidence interval (CI): 0.74–0.93 versus 0.65–0.87, respectively). Angpt-2 was also detectable in bile, but was not associated with the presence of CC. Immunohistochemistry revealed a strong induction of Angpt-2 expression in the tumor vasculature.

Conclusions: Circulating Angpt-2 in serum might be a promising protein candidate locally derived from the tumor vasculature in patients with CC. Measurement of Angpt-2 in serum may be useful for diagnosis and further clinical management of patients with CC.

Editor: Niklas K. Björkström, Karolinska Institutet, Sweden

Funding: The authors have no support or funding to report.

* E-mail: lankisch.tim@mh-hannover.de

¶ These authors contributed equally to this work.

Introduction

Cholangiocarcinoma (CC) is the second most common primary liver cancer world-wide after hepatocellular carcinoma [1]. CC originates from the biliary epithelium and is classified by its localization in intrahepatic (ICC) and extrahepatic CC (ECC) [2], [3]. Growing evidence indicates that ICC and ECC differ regarding incidence and risk factors [1], [2]. In western countries, primary sclerosing cholangitis (PSC) is the main risk factor for later CC development [4–6]. PSC is complicated by CC in up to 13% of cases underlining the impact of this precancerous condition [6]. CC is regularly diagnosed at advanced stages due to the lack of early symptoms or reliable tumor biomarkers. Carbohydrate antigen (CA) 19-9 is often used as a biomarker for CC. However, CA 19-9 remains unspecific as it is also increased in benign biliary disorders such as cholestasis or cholangitis [7], [8]. In addition, the diagnostic accuracy of CA 19-9 in patients with PSC remains limited [9].

Consequently, there is a need for new diagnostic approaches (e.g. potent surrogate parameters for a reliable risk stratification) to improve the ability of an early detection and subsequently the clinical management of patients with CC.

The angiopoietin (Angpt)/Tie2 system consists of the transmembrane endothelial tyrosine kinase Tie2 and its antagonistic circulating ligands Angpt-1, and Angpt-2 [10]. The balance between the canonical agonist Angpt-1 and its competitive inhibitor, Angpt-2, regulates basal endothelial quiescence [11], [12]. Angpt-2 is strongly expressed in the vasculature of many tumors and it has been suggested that Angpt-2 may act synergistically with other cytokines to promote tumor-associated angiogenesis and tumor progression. It has been proposed that Angpt-2 might play a proangiogenic role in CC [13].

We therefore hypothesized that circulating levels of Angpt-2 might serve as a biomarker for the detection of CC. As the action of CC takes place at the biliary epithelium, we performed Angpt-2 analysis not only in serum, but also in bile in patients with CC, PSC, CC complicating PSC or bile duct stones and investigated Angpt-2 expression in human biopsies by immunohistochemistry.

Patients and Methods

We included 167 patients (74 patients with PSC, 11 patients with CC/PSC, 45 patients with CC and 37 patients with bile duct stones) from the endoscopic unit of Hannover Medical School in a cross-sectional study during 2010 and 2012. The diagnosis of PSC was based on typical cholangiographic findings such as strictures or irregularity of intrahepatic and/or extrahepatic bile ducts after exclusion of secondary causes for sclerosing cholangitis. CC was confirmed histologically in 41 out of 45 patients. In four patients histology was not available, but clinical, laboratory, radiological and endoscopic retrograde cholangiography (ERC) findings were consistent with diagnosis of CC. The diagnosis of bile duct stones was based on ultrasound and/or endoscopic ultrasound and confirmed by ERC. Demographic data and laboratory values at day of ERC were recorded.

Angpt-2 Measurement in Bile and Serum

Bile samples from patients were obtained during ERC as described before [14]. Serum samples were drawn whenever possible at day of ERC before endoscopic examination. Serum and bile Angpt-2 concentrations were measured by enzyme-linked immunosorbent assay (ELISA) according to the manufacturer's instructions (R&D Systems, Minneapolis, MN, United States). The average value intra-assay coefficient of variation for Angpt-2 was 4.2%, and the average value inter-assay coefficient of variation was 7.4%. The sensitivity threshold was 8.29 pg/mL. All assays were performed in duplicate by investigators blinded to patients' characteristics and outcome.

The study protocol was approved by the ethics commission of Hannover Medical School and is in accordance with the Declaration of Helsinki. Written informed consent was obtained from all patients.

Fluorescent Immunohistochemistry from Human CC Samples

Slides from formalin-fixed, paraffin-embedded human CC samples were blocked for 60 min in 10% donkey serum, incubated with the primary antibody (polyclonal anti-human Angpt-2 AF 623, R&D Systems) in a dilution of 1:50 overnight at 4°C, followed by fluorescence-conjugated affinity-purified secondary antibody labeling (60 min, 1:500; Jackson ImmunoResearch, West Grove, PA), and mounted with ProLong Gold/4,6-diamidino-2-phenylindole (Life Technologies, Grand Island, NY). All images were taken by a Leica DMI 6000B (Leica Microscopy, Mannheim, Germany) immunofluorescence system at ×63 magnification. Of note, all images were obtained with the same laser power, gain, and offset conditions.

Statistical Analysis

Group data are presented as number/percentages or median with interquartile range (IQR). All data were tested for normality (Shapiro-Wilk test, Kolmogorov-Smirnov test). Continuous data of the study groups were compared using Kruskal Wallis test. In case of statistical differences, Mann–Whitney or Wilcoxon test was used to compare groups. Receiver operating characteristics (ROC) curves were applied to determine diagnostic accuracy of the serological markers. Angpt-2 and CA 19-9 were included in a logistic regression model to detect an improvement in diagnostic accuracy of patients with CC. Correlation analysis was performed using Pearson or Spearman correlation as appropriate. P values < 0.05 were considered statistically significant. The software used was the SPSS Statistical Package (version 19.0, SPSS Inc, USA), GraphPad Prism (version 6.01, GraphPad Inc, USA) and MedCalc Software (version 12.7.5.0, Belgium).

Results

Characteristics of the Study Cohort

Bile samples from 130 patients (68 PSC, 8 CC/PSC, 20 CC and 34 patients with bile duct stones) were obtained during ERC and corresponding serum samples at the same day were drawn from a total of 60 patients (27 PSC, 5 CC/PSC, 17 CC and 11 patients with bile duct stones). Additional 37 serum samples were analyzed (7 PSC, 2 CC/PSC, 25 CC and 3 patients with bile duct stones). Demographic characteristics and laboratory findings of the patient groups on day of ERC/day of blood collection are given in **Table 1**.

Serum Angpt-2 Levels are Significantly Elevated in Patients with CC

Serum Angpt-2 concentrations among different groups are illustrated in **Figure 1A**. CC patients had the highest median serum concentration with 6497 (3789–9314) pg/ml ($p = 0.01$). PSC patients showed lower concentrations with 2771 (2013–4559) pg/ml. Patients with CC complicating PSC (2746 [2618–4595] pg/ml) and patients with bile duct stones (2807 [1956–4723] pg/ml) displayed lower concentrations, respectively. Regarding ECC and ICC, metastatic disease and pre-treatment with chemotherapy no significant differences in Angpt-2 serum concentration among CC patients were detected ($p > 0.05$).

Angpt-2 is Detectable in Bile but is not Associated with CC

Angpt-2 levels in bile were measured in 130 patients. Results are shown in **Figure 1B**. CC patients had the highest median Angpt-2 concentration in bile (470 [238–1267] pg/ml). In contrast, PSC patients (331 [163–516] pg/ml), CC/PSC patients (304 [161–511] pg/ml) and patients with bile duct stones (358 [259–613] pg/ml) showed lower concentrations. However, these differences did not reach statistical significance ($p = 0.23$). Correlation analysis between serum and bile Angpt-2 concentration showed no significant correlation ($p > 0.05$).

Diagnostic Accuracy of Serum Angpt-2 and CA 19–9

In order to compare the diagnostic potential of serum Angpt-2 and CA 19-9 in patients with CC a receiver operating characteristic (ROC) curve analysis was performed. The area under the curve (AUC) for Angpt-2 was 0.85 (95% confidence interval 0.74–0.93, $p = 0.01$) (**Figure 2**). The sensitivity and specificity for Angpt-2 to diagnose CC was 74% and 94%, respectively (cut off value 5333 pg/ml). In contrast, the AUC for CA 19-9 in this patient cohort was 0.77 (95% confidence interval 0.65–0.87, $p = 0.01$). The sensitivity and specificity for CA 19-9 to diagnose CC was 53% and 82%, respectively (cut off value 130 U/ml). A combination of Angpt-2 and CA 19-9 in a logistic regression model did not improve the detection of CC patients (AUC 0.85, 95% confidence interval 0.74–0.93, $p = 0.01$).

Table 1. Demographic characteristics, clinical features and laboratory findings of the patient groups on day of ERC/day of blood collection.

	All patients (n = 167)	Cholangiocarcinoma (CC) (n = 45)	Primary sclerosing cholangitis (PSC) (n = 74)	CC complicating PSC (n = 11)	Bile duct stones (n = 37)	Reference value	p-value
Gender	M104, F63	M29, F16	M52, F22	M7, F4	M16, F21	–	0.05
Age (years)	51 (41–64)	64 (53–71)	42 (36–50)	52 (33–59)	60 (55–68)	–	0.001
ECC/ICC	–	37/8	–	7/4	–	–	–
Metastatic disease (y/n)	–	30/15	–	6/5	–	–	–
Chemotherapy (y/n)	–	21/24	–	4/7	–	–	–
Laboratory values							
ALT	52 (27–102)	54 (30–106)	54 (30–92)	51 (27–255)	40 (16–95)	<45 U/L	0.15
AST	51 (30–91)	58 (36–136)	52 (38–86)	71 (28–197)	31 (25–67)	<35 U/L	0.007
AP	253 (128–380)	336 (210–408)	244 (127–345)	263 (163–670)	134 (72–380)	40–129 U/L	0.006
GGT	198 (73–444)	364 (127–776)	166 (72–336)	114 (83–229)	159 (35–552)	<55 U/L	0.011
Bilirubin	18 (10–61)	48 (10–208)	16 (10–32)	41 (9–385)	13 (8–29)	<2–21 μmol/L	0.016
CRP	12 (4–41)	31 (5–80)	8 (3–28)	29 (6–36)	7 (3–31)	<8 mg/L	0.019
WBC	6.8 (5.5–9.8)	8.5 (6–11.8)	6.6 (5.2–9.7)	6.7 (5.8–7.2)	6.3 (5.4–8.4)	4.4 - 11.3/nL	0.058
LDH	191 (166–220)	191 (164–239)	181 (163–210)	180 (135–207)	206 (193–228)	<248 U/L	0.095
Tumor markers							
CA 19–9	41 (14–160)	142 (35–592)	29 (11–56)	43 (14–1820)	40 (13–91)	–	0.001
CEA	2 (2–4)	4 (2–6)	2 (1–3)	2 (2–3)	2 (2–4)	–	0.002
Angiopoietin-2							
Angpt-2 serum	4076 (2535–6881)	6497 (3789–9314)	2771 (2013–4559)	2746 (2618–4595)	2807 (1956–4723)	–	0.001
Angpt-2 bile	348 (190–604)	470 (238–1267)	331 (163–516)	304 (161–511)	358 (259–613)	–	0.227

Abbreviations: ECC, extrahepatic cholangiocarcinoma; ICC, intrahepatic cholangiocarcinoma; y, yes; n, no; M, male; F, female; ALT, alanine aminotransferase; AST, aspartate aminotransferase; AP, alkaline phosphatase; GGT, gamma-glutamyl transferase; CRP, C-reactive protein; WBC, white blood cells; LDH, lactate dehydrogenase; CA 19-9, carbohydrate antigen 19-9; CEA, carcinoembryonic antigen; angpt-2, angiopoietin-2.

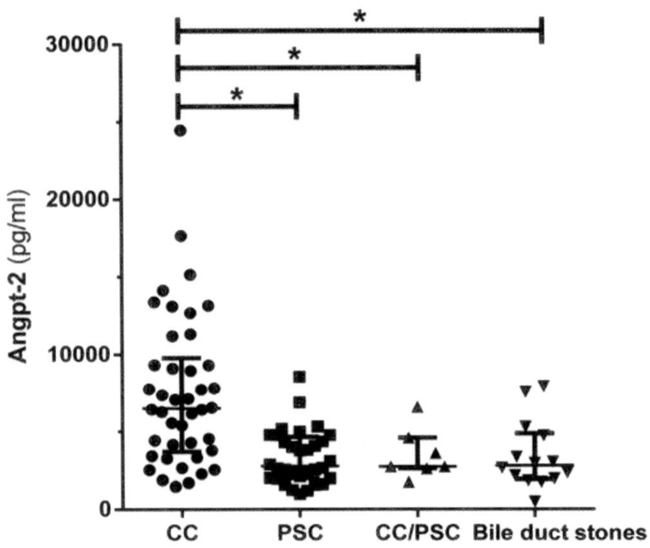

Figure 1. Serum Angpt-2 is elevated in patients with CC, (A). Angpt-2 was measured in patients with CC (n = 42), PSC (n = 34), CC/PSC (n = 7) and patients with bile duct stones (n = 14). Serum Angpt-2 was significantly elevated in patients with CC compared to control patients ($p<0.01$). Angpt-2 in bile is not associated with CC, (B). Bile concentration of Angpt-2 was measured in patients with CC (n = 20), PSC (n = 68), CC/PSC (n = 8) and patients with bile duct stones (n = 34). Four values (CC) are outside the scale of the Y-axis. No significant differences were detected among the groups.

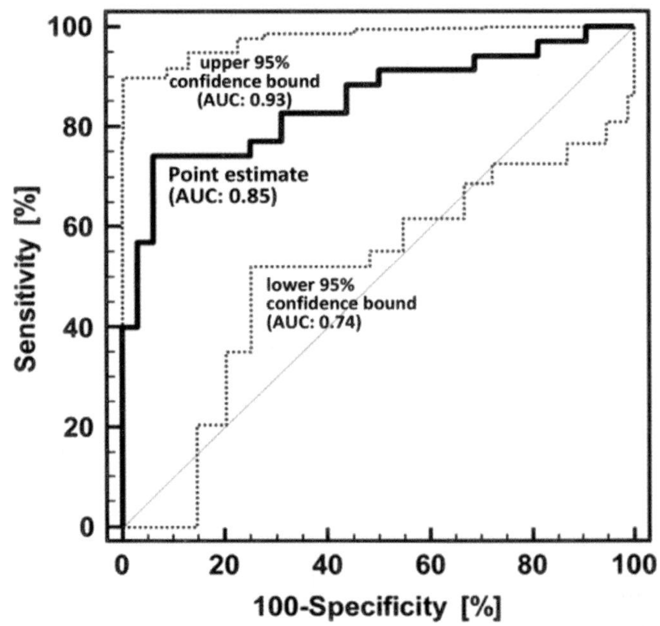

Figure 2. Receiver operating characteristic (ROC) curve analysis of serum Angpt-2 to diagnose CC. ROC analysis allows the evaluation of the binary classification variable (presence of CC = 1, absence of CC = 0) at different thresholds of Angpt-2 levels. The area under the curve (AUC) value for the point estimate (thick solid line) was calculated to be 0.85. The 95% confidence interval (CI) as the probability range in which the estimate is expected in 100 different cohorts of patients with equally distributed Angpt-2 levels ranges from an AUC of 0.74 in the worst case to 0.93 in the best case (thin dotted lines). The 95% CI is therefore a measure for the reliability of Angpt-2-based CC diagnosis. For testing the performance of Angpt-2 the departure of its AUC from 0.5 (a random classifier) was assessed by using a standard t test, which resulted in a p-value of <0.0001 for the point estimate.

Angpt-2 Expression is Induced in the Tumor Vasculature

To investigate the origin of Angpt- 2 levels we performed an immunohistochemical analysis for Angpt-2 from liver tissue from patients with PSC or CC. Indeed, we observed a strong expression of Angpt-2 protein on the tissue level mostly limited to the tumor vasculature. **Figure 3** shows an exemplary comparison highlighting extensive Angpt-2 biosynthesis within the CC vasculature.

Discussion

The detection of CC and differentiation from benign biliary strictures is challenging in clinical practice [15], [16]. Consequently, new diagnostic approaches are needed in order to improve the clinical management of patients with CC and tumor-predisposing conditions such as PSC. Proteomic analysis of bile and urine is a new promising technique as it analyzes a complete protein pattern in contrast to classical biochemical methods [17], [18]. However, these studies are complex, time-consuming and expensive and therefore supporting diagnostic tests are of special interest.

As the malignant transformation in CC takes place at the biliary epithelium analysis of bile might detect tumor-derived proteins in higher concentrations compared to serum specimens. To date, none of the single markers studied in bile has been implemented in clinical routine so far [19], [20].

Carcinogenesis in patients with CC includes a complex interaction between cancer-associated fibroblasts, remodeling of the extracellular matrix, immune cell migration and stimulation of proangiogenic factors [1], [16], [21]. Particularly, formation of new blood vessels is crucial for tumor maintenance, growth and metastasis as it supplies the neoplasia with essential nutrients and oxygen [22], [23]. Vascular endothelial growth factor (VEGF), VEGF receptors and nerve growth factor-β (NGF-β) are crucial mediators of pathological neoangiogenesis in the tumor environment and are also overexpressed in human CC samples favoring neoangiogenesis [24], [25]. Tang *et. al* analyzed surgically resected human CC samples and reported an association between tissue expression of VEGF, Angpt-2 and tumor microvessel density [13]. The role of the Angpt/Tie2 system, a second class of tyrosine kinase receptors, has not been fully evaluated in CC, but may play a role in tumor angiogenesis of other malignancies. Therefore, we hypothesized that Angpt-2 might also be involved in CC and may serve as a putative novel biomarker. This hypothesis is of high translational relevance as recently function-blocking antibodies against the Tie2 antagonist Angpt-2 have been developed and are currently investigated in ongoing clinical trials.

Initially, our study was designed to analyze circulating levels of Angpt-2 in patients' sera, potential effects of the tumor on the local environment in terms of bile concentration of Angpt-2, and local Angpt-2 expression directly within the tumor by fluorescent immunohistochemistry from human tissue samples.

We found increased circulating levels of Angpt-2 in patients with CC compared to those with non-malignant pathologies. Our data indicate that Angpt-2 is useful as an additional novel marker. More importantly the data indicate a putative mechanistic involvement of Angpt-2 in tumor angiogenesis and might therefore represent a promising candidate for future therapeutic intervention. However, this aspect is clearly beyond the scope of the current project but warrants further investigation. We assume that elevated Angpt-2 in the serum reflects its potent - but most likely unspecific – mediator function in tumor neoangiogenesis as it has been demonstrated for other entities [26–29].

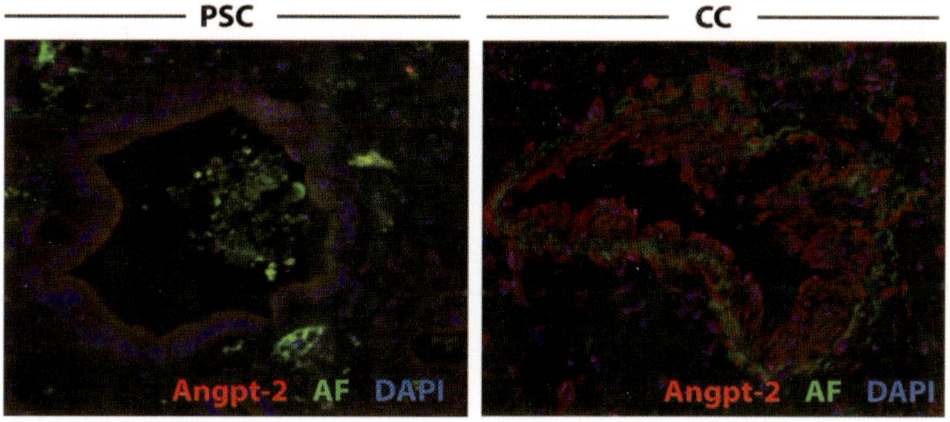

Figure 3. Angpt-2 expression in human CC samples. In human biopsies Angpt-2 expression is induced within CC vasculature. Fluorescent immunohistochemistry for Angiopoietin-2 (Angpt-2) showing an exemplary biopsy sample from individuals with primary sclerosis cholangitis (PSC, left panel) and cholangiocarcinoma (CC, right panel). Nuclear staining (DAPI) is shown in blue, tissue autofluorescence (AF) in green.

For the first time, we demonstrate that Angpt-2 is detectable in bile of CC patients. However, its pathophysiological role in bile is completely unknown. We hypothesize that in the sense of a "demand and supply" strategy the tumor cells might be able to produce Angpt-2 to maintain neoangiogensis at a high level. The detection of Angpt-2 in bile might be the result of tumor involvement of the large bile ducts and secretion of Angpt-2 from tumor vessels. A passive diffusion of Angpt-2 from blood vessels into the bile seems unlikely as no correlation was found for serum and bile Angpt-2 levels.

Taking the current Angpt/Tie2 knowledge in healthy conditions into account, one would assume that the tumor vasculature is the primary source of Angpt-2 biosynthesis as Angpt-2 is synthesized in the endothelium. With respect to this theoretical assumption and our earlier observation that Angpt-2 is also detectable in the bile we performed immunohistochemical stainings for Angpt-2. Of note, our histological data did show that it is indeed the vasculature where Angpt-2 is expressed in biopsies from human CC samples.

PSC patients are at special risk to develop CC and need accurate monitoring. In many patients, PSC is complicated by CC development despite regular surveillance [4–6]. Consequently, new diagnostic approaches are required. However, Angpt-2 measurement did not help to detect CC/PSC in our cohort.

Unfortunately, serum samples were not available for all patients which is a limitation of our study. Therefore we measured Angpt-2 in additional serum samples without concomitant bile specimens to provide sufficient data for statistical analysis.

In summary, we show that Angpt-2 is significantly elevated in patients with CC and has a higher AUC value in ROC analysis than CA 19-9 in our cohort. More importantly, Angpt-2 is expressed in the tumor vasculature and thus is of interest for the diagnosis and therapy in patients with CC.

Author Contributions

Conceived and designed the experiments: TV SD TOL. Performed the experiments: TV SD KT. Analyzed the data: TV SD MPM TOL JM. Contributed reagents/materials/analysis tools: TV SD JS JM. Wrote the paper: TV SD TOL MPM.

References

1. Tyson GL, El-Serag HB (2011) Risk factors for cholangiocarcinoma. Hepatology 54: 173–184. doi: 10.1002/hep.24351.
2. Khan SA, Toledano MB, Taylor-Robinson SD (2008) Epidemiology, risk factors, and pathogenesis of cholangiocarcinoma. HPB 10: 77–82. doi: 10.1080/13651820801992641.
3. Razumilava N, Gores GJ (2013) Classification, diagnosis, and management of cholangiocarcinoma. Clin Gastroenterol Hepatol 11: 13–21. doi: 10.1016/j.cgh.2012.09.009.
4. Karlsen TH, Boberg KM (2013) Update on primary sclerosing cholangitis. J Hepatol 59: 571–582. doi: 10.1016/j.jhep.2013.03.015.
5. Chapman MH, Webster GJM, Bannoo S, Johnson GJ, Wittmann J, et al. (2012) Cholangiocarcinoma and dominant strictures in patients with primary sclerosing cholangitis: a 25-year single-centre experience. Eur J Gastroenterol Hepatol 24: 1051–1058. doi: 10.1097/MEG.0b013e3283554bbf.
6. Boberg KM, Lind GE (2011) Primary sclerosing cholangitis and malignancy. Best Pract Res Clin Gastroenterol 25: 753–764. doi: 10.1016/j.bpg.2011.10.002.
7. Alvaro D (2009) Serum and bile biomarkers for cholangiocarcinoma. Curr Opin Gastroenterol 25: 279–284. doi: 10.1097/MOG.0b013e328325a894.
8. Nehls O, Gregor M, Klump B (2004) Serum and bile markers for cholangiocarcinoma. Semin Liver Dis 24: 139–154. doi: 10.1055/s-2004-828891.
9. Sinakos E, Saenger AK, Keach J, Kim WR, Lindor KD (2011) Many patients with primary sclerosing cholangitis and increased serum levels of carbohydrate antigen 19–9 do not have cholangiocarcinoma. Clin Gastroenterol Hepatol 9: 434–9.e1. doi: 10.1016/j.cgh.2011.02.007.
10. Augustin HG, Koh GY, Thurston G, Alitalo K (2009) Control of vascular morphogenesis and homeostasis through the angiopoietin-Tie system. Nat Rev Mol Cell Biol 10: 165–177. doi: 10.1038/nrm2639.
11. Suri C, Jones PF, Patan S, Bartunkova S, Maisonpierre PC et al. (1996) Requisite role of angiopoietin-1, a ligand for the TIE2 receptor, during embryonic angiogenesis. Cell 87: 1171–1180. doi: 10.1016/S0092-8674(00)81813-9.
12. Maisonpierre PC, Suri C, Jones PF, Bartunkova S, Wiegand SJ, et al. (1997) Angiopoietin-2, a natural antagonist for Tie2 that disrupts in vivo angiogenesis. Science 277: 55–60. doi: 10.1126/science.277.5322.55.
13. Tang D, Nagano H, Yamamoto H, Wada H, Nakamura M, et al. (2006) Angiogenesis in cholangiocellular carcinoma: expression of vascular endothelial growth factor, angiopoietin-1/2, thrombospondin-1 and clinicopathological significance. Oncol Rep15: 525–532. doi: 10.3892/or.15.3.525.
14. Negm AA, Schott A, Vonberg R-P, Weismueller TJ, Schneider AS, et al. (2010) Routine bile collection for microbiological analysis during cholangiography and its impact on the management of cholangitis. Gastrointest Endosc 72: 284–291. doi: 10.1016/j.gie.2010.02.043.
15. Malhi H, Gores GJ (2006) Review article: the modern diagnosis and therapy of cholangiocarcinoma. Aliment Pharmacol Ther 23: 1287–1296. doi: 10.1111/j.1365-2036.2006.02900.x.
16. Rizvi S, Gores GJ (2013) Pathogenesis, diagnosis, and management of cholangiocarcinoma. Gastroenterology 145: 1215–1229. doi: 10.1053/j.gastro.2013.10.013.

17. Lankisch TO, Metzger J, Negm AA, Vosskuhl K, Schiffer E, et al. (2011) Bile proteomic profiles differentiate cholangiocarcinoma from primary sclerosing cholangitis and choledocholithiasis. Hepatology 53: 875–884. doi: 10.1002/hep.24103.
18. Metzger J, Negm AA, Plentz RR, Weismüller TJ, Wedemeyer J, et al. (2013) Urine proteomic analysis differentiates cholangiocarcinoma from primary sclerosing cholangitis and other benign biliary disorders. Gut 62: 122–130. doi: 10.1136/gutjnl-2012-302047.
19. Koopmann J, Thuluvath PJ, Zahurak ML, Kristiansen TZ, Pandey A, et al. (2004) Mac-2-binding protein is a diagnostic marker for biliary tract carcinoma. Cancer 101: 1609–1615. doi: 10.1002/cncr.20469.
20. Alvaro D, Macarri G, Mancino MG, Marzioni M, Bragazzi M, et al. (2007) Serum and biliary insulin-like growth factor I and vascular endothelial growth factor in determining the cause of obstructive cholestasis. Ann Intern Med 147: 451–459. doi:10.7326/0003-4819-147-7-200710020-00003.
21. Everhart JE, Ruhl CE (2009) Burden of digestive diseases in the United States Part III: Liver, biliary tract, and pancreas. Gastroenterology 136: 1134–1144. doi: 10.1053/j.gastro.2009.02.038.
22. Leyva-Illades D, McMillin M, Quinn M, Demorrow S (2012) Cholangiocarcinoma pathogenesis: Role of the tumor microenvironment. Transl Gastrointest Cancer 1: 71–80. doi: 10.3978/j.issn.2224-4778. 2011.11.05.
23. McDougall SR, Anderson AR, Chaplain MA (2006) Mathematical modelling of dynamic adaptive tumour-induced angiogenesis: clinical implications and therapeutic targeting strategies. J Theor Biol 241: 564–589. doi: 10.1016/j.jtbi.2005.12.022.
24. Möbius C, Demuth C, Aigner T, Wiedmann M, Wittekind C, et al. (2007) Evaluation of VEGF A expression and microvascular density as prognostic factors in extrahepatic cholangiocarcinoma. Eur J Surg Oncol 33: 1025–1029. doi: 10.1016/j.ejso.2007.02.020.
25. Xu LB, Liu C, Gao GQ, Yu XH, Zhang R, et al. (2010) Nerve growth factor-beta expression is associated with lymph node metastasis and nerve infiltration in human hilar cholangiocarcinoma. World J Surg 34: 1039–45. doi: 10.1007/s00268-010-0417-4.
26. Naumnik W, Naumnik B, Niewiarowska K, Ossolinska M, Chyczewska E (2013) Angiogenic axis angiopoietin-1 and angiopoietin-2/Tie-2 in non-small cell lung cancer: a bronchoalveolar lavage and serum study. Adv Exp Med Biol 788: 341–348. doi: 10.1007/978-94-007-6627-3_46.
27. Li C, Sun CJ, Fan JC, Geng N, Li CH, et al. (2013) Angiopoietin-2 expression is correlated with angiogenesis and overall survival in oral squamous cell carcinoma. Med Oncol 30: 571. doi: 10.1007/s12032-013-0571-2.
28. Scholz A, Rehm VA, Rieke S, Derkow K, Schulz P, et al. (2007) Angiopoietin-2 serum levels are elevated in patients with liver cirrhosis and hepatocellular carcinoma. Am J Gastroenterol 102: 2471–2481. doi:10.1111/j.1572-0241.2007.01377.x.
29. Diaz-Sanchez A, Matilla A, Nuñez O, Lorente R, Fernandez A, et al. (2013) Serum angiopoietin-2 level as a predictor of tumor invasiveness in patients with hepatocellular carcinoma. Scand J Gastroenterol 48: 334–343. doi: 10.3109/00365521.2012.746391.

14

An Interferon Response Gene Signature Is Associated with the Therapeutic Response of Hepatitis C Patients

Lawrence M. Pfeffer[1]*, Kui Li[2], Jaquelyn F. Fleckenstein[3], Tony N. Marion[2], Joel Diament[1], Chuan He Yang[1], Susan R. Pfeffer[1], Meiyun Fan[1], Elizabeth Handorf[4], Charles R. Handorf[1]

1 Department of Pathology and Laboratory Medicine, and the Center for Cancer Research, University of Tennessee Health Science Center, Memphis, Tennessee, United States of America, **2** Department of Microbiology, Immunology and Biochemistry, University of Tennessee Health Science Center, Memphis, Tennessee, United States of America, **3** The Department of Medicine, Division of Gastroenterology, Washington University School of Medicine, St. Louis, Missouri, United States of America, **4** Biostatistics and Bioinformatics Facility, Fox Chase Cancer Center, Philadelphia, Pennsylvania, United States of America

Abstract

Infection with the hepatitis C virus (HCV) is a major cause of chronic liver diseases and hepatocellular carcinoma worldwide, and thus represents a significant public health problem. The type I interferon (IFN), IFNα, has been successful in treating HCV-infected patients, but current IFN-based treatment regimens for HCV have suboptimal efficacy, and relatively little is known about why IFN therapy eliminates the virus in some patients but not in others. Therefore, it is critical to understand the basic mechanisms that underlie the therapeutic resistance to IFN action in HCV-infected individuals, and there is an urgent need to identify those patients most likely to respond to IFN therapy for HCV. To characterize the response of HCV-infected patients to treatment with IFNα, the expression of an IFN-response gene signature comprised of IFN-stimulated genes and genes that play an important role in the innate immune response was examined in liver biopsies from HCV-infected patients enrolled in a clinical trial. In the present study we found that the expression of a subset of IFN-response genes was dysregulated in liver biopsy samples from nonresponsive hepatitis C patients as compared with virologic responders. Based on these findings, a statistical model was developed to help predict the response of patients to IFN therapy, and compared to results obtained to the IL28 mutation model, which is highly predictive of the response to IFN-based therapy in HCV-infected patients. We found that a model incorporating gene expression data can improve predictions of IFN responsiveness compared to IL28 mutation status alone.

Editor: Naglaa H. Shoukry, University of Montreal Hospital Research Center (CRCHUM), Canada

Funding: 1. National Institute of Health grants U19 AI066316, R01-AI069285, General Clinical Research Center Grant M01-RR00211, a maturation grant from the University of Tennessee Research Foundation, and by funds from the Muirhead Chair Endowment and the Gerwin Endowment at the University of Tennessee Health Science Center. 2. The funders had no role in study design, data collection and analysis, decision to publish, or preparation of the manuscript.

* Email: LPFEFFER@UTHSC.EDU

Introduction

Hepatitis C virus (HCV) is estimated to infect ~170 million people worldwide, causing a wide spectrum of liver diseases that varies from the asymptomatic carrier state to end-stage liver diseases [1]. These include chronic hepatitis, cirrhosis, liver failure, and hepatocellular carcinoma. Classified within the Flaviviridae family of enveloped, single-stranded, positive-sense RNA viruses, HCV has a tightly restricted host range confined to humans and chimpanzees, and replicates predominantly in hepatocytes. For reasons that have remained elusive, only a fraction of HCV-infected individuals spontaneously clear the virus, while the majority of HCV-infected individuals (70–80%) develop a chronic infection. Several structural and nonstructural proteins of HCV have been shown to antagonize the host innate immune response that is normally triggered by viral infection [2]. Viral RNA is a potent inducer of the host immune response and is recognized by specific Toll-like receptors in endosomal compartments or by the RNA helicases RIG-I and MDA5 in cytoplasm [3]. Rapid induction of the interferon (IFN) system, type I IFNs (IFNα, IFNβ and IFNω, type II IFN (IFNγ) and type III IFN (IL29, IL28A and IL28B), is a central event in establishing the host innate antiviral response that is downstream of TLR (Toll-like receptor)-dependent and TLR–independent pathways [4]. IFN acts in a paracrine and autocrine fashion to regulate gene expression that results in the induction of an antiviral state [5]. HCV control of the innate antiviral responses, especially at the level of IFN production, may provide a cellular foundation for viral persistence [6].

The pegylated derivative of IFNα (peg-IFN) and the antiviral drug ribavirin combined with a protease inhibitor is the current standard-of-care for HCV-infected patients [7]. IFNα has antiviral activity against a diverse variety of RNA and DNA viruses. When IFNα has been utilized as a monotherapy in chronically infected HCV patients, the success rate is ~20%. Peg-IFNα, which has an improved half-life over standard IFNα, appears to have a somewhat higher success rate. However, it is unknown why IFNα therapy causes a sustained virological response in only a fraction of the patient population, as determined by the clearance of HCV. Moreover, several studies have identified specific cohorts of patients that have a relatively low response to these therapeutic regimens. For example, several studies established that the response rate of African-Americans is significantly lower than non-Hispanic whites [8–10]. This finding is of major health concern in the United States, since African-Americans account for ~22% of the HCV-infected patients. Recently, single nucleotide polymorphisms within the IL28B locus, which encodes members of the IFNλ family, have been found to be highly predictive of the response to IFN/ribavirin therapy in HCV-infected patients [11–15]. While this represents a major advance in the field, the underlying mechanism for differential response in HCV-infected patients remains elusive.

To characterize the response of HCV-infected patients to treatment with type I IFN, the expression of an IFN-response gene signature was examined in liver biopsies. Based on microarray analysis we previously performed on IFN-treated human and mouse cells as well as a public database of IFN-stimulated genes (ISGs) [16–19], ISGs were stratified into genes that are most commonly induced by IFN and had putative binding sites with strong DNA binding scores for STAT2 (ISRE), STAT3/STAT1 (SIE), and NF-κB. The IFN-induced expression of these ISGs in Huh7 hepatoma cells was verified by quantitative real time PCR as being strongly IFN-induced (>10-fold) and the ISGs were placed into the following categories: 1) ISGs whose expression is predominantly driven by an ISRE; 2) ISGs whose expression is predominantly driven by an ISRE and potentially regulated by NF-κB; 3) ISGs whose expression is predominantly driven by an SIE; and 4) ISGs whose expression is predominantly driven by an SIE, and potentially regulated by NF-κB. An IFN signature gene list of 39 genes was then established based on a bioinformatic search of these genes as potentially playing important roles in the biological actions of IFN. The expression of this gene signature was examined in samples of formalin-fixed paraffin embedded (FFPE) tissue from liver biopsies obtained prior to the onset of any therapy in patients whose clinical course and response to IFN/ribavirin therapy was subsequently characterized in a clinical trial at UTHSC. Our results suggest that only a subset of the IFN-response gene signature was dysregulated in liver biopsies from chronically infected HCV patients. Moreover, we determined the predictive value of this gene signature and that of polymorphisms of IL-28 locus. Our results indicate that, besides nucleotide polymorphisms of IL-28 locus, this IFN response gene signature has important predictive value in determining which patients will most likely fail to respond to standard IFN-based hepatitis C therapy.

Materials and Methods

Patient Selection

Adult African American (AA) and Caucasian (C) patients with compensated chronic HCV were enrolled and treated at the UTHSC General Clinical Research Center as part of our clinical trial entitled "Racial Differences in HCV-Host Interaction". Patients were required to be adult, AA or C with genotype 1A or 1B chronic hepatitis C with positive HCV RNA and no prior attempt at treatment. A liver biopsy was required with the histological diagnosis of chronic hepatitis. Patients with histological diagnosis of cirrhosis were enrolled if they did not have symptomatic portal hypertension and if they had a neutrophil count greater than $1500/mm^3$, platelet count of $85{,}000/mm^3$, albumin level greater than 3.0 g/dL and serum creatinine less than 1.4 mg/dL. All clinical investigation was conducted according to the principles expressed in the Declaration of Helsinki. All patients signed written informed consent specific for this protocol that was approved by the UTHSC IRB before entry into the study. Exclusion criteria included any cause of chronic liver disease other than HCV, HIV infection, active hemolytic anemia, evidence of decompensated cirrhosis with ascites, bleeding varices or portosystemic encephalopathy. In addition, patients with any known preexisting medical conditions that could interfere with participation such as uncontrolled seizure disorders, poorly controlled diabetes, serious pulmonary disease, immunologically-mediated disease, gout or any medical condition likely to require steroids during the course of the study were excluded from this study. Patients with cardiac ischemia, significant arrhythmia, cardiac failure, active substance abuse, retinal abnormalities, organ transplantation, HIV infection or serious psychiatric disease were also excluded. General clinical patient information is shown in Table 1.

Treatment Regimen

All patients were treated with standard weight-based therapy with 1.5 mg/kg of pegylated IFNα2b subcutaneously once per week and 13 mg/kg of ribavirin PO daily for up to 48 weeks. Therapy was discontinued after 24 weeks if patients did not have a negative HCV RNA level. Use of erythropoietin was allowed.

Patients who completed at least 12 weeks of therapy were classified as Sustained Viral Responders (SVR) if they cleared virus on treatment and remained virus-free for 6 months after completion of therapy. Non–responders (NR) were defined as patients who never cleared virus. Patients who initially had a negative HCV RNA level upon treatment but subsequently became positive again for HCV RNA (either during continued treatment or within 6 months after completing therapy) were defined as Relapsers (R).

Gene expression analysis of RNA obtained from FFPE liver biopsies

Formalin-fixed paraffin embedded (FFPE) pre-treatment liver biopsy specimens from ~130 patients were retrieved, 3–5 (5 μm) curls were cut from each liver biopsy and RNA isolated using the RecoverAll Total Nucleic Acid Isolation Kit (Ambion Inc.) according to the manufacturer's directions. Gene expression analysis was conducted on the nCounter Analysis System (NanoString Technologies) using a codeset designed to target 43 genes (39 genes in an IFN gene signature and 4 potential house-keeping genes: ACTB, GAPDH, GUSB, PGK1) and 15 controls (58-plex codeset). The 39 genes in the IFN gene signature targeted in the gene array are listed in Table 2. In brief, 100 ng of total RNA was mixed with pairs of capture and reporter probes and hybridized on the nCounter Prep Station. Upon removal of unbound probes, the purified ternary complexes were bound to the imaging surface, elongated, immobilized, and quantified on the nCounter digital analyzer. To account for differences in hybridization and purification, data were normalized to the average counts for all control spikes in each sample and analyzed with nSolver software. The expression data was normalized by using a geometric mean of the four housekeeping genes (ACTB, GAPDH, GUSB, PGK1) in our codeset as previously described [20]. Only two RNA samples out of the 132 samples prepared from FFPE liver biopsies were not used in further analysis due to low retrieved RNA levels or marked degradation of RNA extracted from the FFPE tissue. Thus, gene expression in 130 samples was subjected to analysis and represented 43 hepatitis C-infected patients who responded to IFNα-ribavirin therapy (responders), 56 hepatitis C-infected patients who did not respond to therapy (nonresponders), and 31 patients who had an initial virological response but then relapsed and exhibited high viral HCV titers (relapsers). FFPE

Table 1. Enrolled patient information.

	AA	C
Patients enrolled	145	82
Male	54	38
Average age (s.d.)	48.5 (7.97)	44.3 (9.51)
Average weight[1] (s.d.)	198.6 (32.91)	205.0 (39.76)
Female	91	44
Average age (s.d.)	48.9 (42.1)	46.0 (7.99)
Average weight[1] (s.d.)	185.2 (41.92)	170.9 (56.18)
Il28B rs12979860 Genotype[2]	CC 9 (8.4%)	20 (33%)
	TT 39 (36%)	6 (10%)
	C/T 59 (55%)	34 (57%)
Infected with genotype 1a[3]	99	69
1b	45	10
Average years infected (max/min)	22 (43/1)	21 (47/3)
Average pre-therapy serum HCV IU/ml[4] (s.d.)	1,064,878 (1,377,098)	1,599,894 (2,451,571)
Average ALT (s.d.)	88 (62)	103 (65)
Average fibrosis score (s.d.)[5]	2.0 (1.1)	1.9 (0.9)
Mild fibrosis (0–2)	104	56
Advanced fibrosis (3–4)	39	26

[1]Weight is in US pounds.
[2]Likelihood ratio = 24.72, $p = 4.3\times10^{-6}$. *Il28B* rs12979860 SNP genotypes were determined for 107 AA and 60 C.

tissue from 80 African-American and 50 Caucasian hepatitis C-infected patients were studied in this dataset.

IL28B SNP sequence analysis

The 184 bp genomic DNA fragment that included the *19q13* rs12979860 SNP at nucleotide 92 was amplified by PCR using the following primers: forward 5′-CTGCACAGTCTGGGATTCC-3′ and reverse 5′-TCACAGAAGGGAGCCCTGC-3′. Nucleotide sequences were generated with an ABI Model 3130XL Gene Analyzer (Applied Biosystems, Life Technologies, Carlsbad, CA) in the UTHSC Molecular Resource Center, and the sequence at position 92 of the PCR fragment was determined using Sequence Scanner v.1.0 (Applied Biosystems).

Statistical analysis and modeling

The data on expression of the IFN gene signature in the different patient subgroups were subjected to nonparametric Mann-Whitney analysis using Graphpad InStat 3 software, with p-values <0.05 considered statistically significant. We then built a predictive model for response using logistic regression. Only full responders were considered successfully treated, with relapsers and non-responders considered unsuccessful. In our initial model, self-reported race and continuous expression of each statistically significant genes identified in univariable analysis were included as predictors of response to interferon. We then refined our model using a backwards selection procedure, where the model was fit repeatedly, removing the least informative genes at each step. Patients with a model-based probability of >0.5 were categorized as predicted responders. We used 10-fold cross validation to test the predictive ability of each model [21], so that our final model demonstrated the highest agreement with true response across the validation sets. We also considered models in the subset of patients whose IL28B SNP data was available. Under a per-allele model, we added IL28B status to the logistic regression models and compared the results to expression-based models. The regression procedures were performed using R software (version 2.13).

Results

The expression of an IFN-response gene signature in liver biopsies

Total RNA was extracted from curls cut from FFPE liver biopsies collected from patients prior to the initiation of therapy, and assayed on a Nanostring nCounter for expression of an IFN gene signature that we designed based on our own microarray results, databases of IFN-stimulated genes (ISGs), and regulatory elements in gene promoter regions. The expression of these genes was then normalized to the expression of four housekeeping genes (Actin B, GAPDH, GUSB and PGK1) that was included in the Nanostring analysis. As shown in Table 1 there was a large sample-to-sample variation in the expression of the genes in the IFN signature. Some genes were expressed at low but detectable levels such as cytokine and growth factors, including ANGPT2, IFNB1, IL6 and VEGFC, as well as classical IFN-stimulated genes such as Mx1, SOCS1 and TLR3. In addition a number of genes critical in the IFN response pathway, which included GBP1, MAVS, TNFSF10 (TRAIL), and XAF1, were expressed at relatively high levels in liver biopsies. These results are consistent with our previous finding that low levels of type I IFNs could be detected in the sera of patients chronically infected with HCV [22], as well as the findings that ISG expression could be detected in the livers of HCV-infected patients and in experimentally-infected chimpanzees [23–26].

Table 2. Expression of the IFN Gene Signature.

Gene	Minimum	Maximum	Mean	Std Error	Median
ANGPT2 [b]	1	132.8	7. 7	1.4	2.3
CASP4 [c]	54.4	214.6	102.9	2.8	95.4
CCL5 [b]	49.1	469.2	160.5	6.6	143.6
DDX58 [b]	60.7	450.9	200.8	7.3	189.7
DHX58 [a]	84.9	507.1	223.7	8.1	215.4
EIF2AK2 [a]	117.6	554.1	311.7	9.6	309.3
GADD45B [d]	56.6	584.2	158.5	6.9	144.6
GADD45G [d]	1	112.6	16.9	1.7	12.3
GBP1 [b]	94.8	482.9	266.2	7.38	260.4
HIF3A [d]	1	202.2	8.6	2.5	1
IFI16 [a]	43.3	280.1	132.5	4.5	125.6
IFI6 [a]	258.6	11402.8	5904.4	289.9	6385.7
IFIH1 [b]	51.6	316.4	158.4	5.9	157
IFNB1 [b]	1	274	5.8	2.5	1
IL6 [b]	1	79.2	6.9	1.4	1
IRF1 [d]	27.9	208.7	78.8	3.1	69.5
IRF2 [a]	95.2	422.7	188.8	4.4	184
IRF5 [b]	10.8	253.8	45.9	2.9	39
IRF7 [b]	107.5	1121	323.8	15.08	302.5
IRF9 [b]	293.3	1524.4	635.5	17.0	631
ISG20 [b]	23.8	395	111.8	6.0	97. 7
MAVS [c]	108	939.5	282.6	10.8	261.6
MX1 [a]	1	96.8	24.7	2.0	20.1
MYD88 [d]	107	378.6	217.2	4.8	219.3
OAS1 [a]	198.5	1660.4	905.5	35.7	932.2
PLSCR1 [a]	96.5	560	248.2	8.5	244.8
PML [a]	49.1	798.3	207.5	10.7	184.1
RARRES3 [a]	200	797.6	405.0	11.0	393.7
RSAD2 [a]	1.6	346.5	118.3	7.4	108.6
SOCS1 [a]	1	99.6	10.4	1.4	5.1
STAT1 [b]	347.8	3343.8	1492.0	53.2	1456.6
STAT2 [a]	413	1532.1	818.0	21.0	816.3
TAP1 [a]	28.1	253.8	86.8	3.2	84.6
TLR2 [a]	21.3	213.5	59.5	3.2	51.3
TLR3 [a]	4.2	193.3	45.9	2.3	43.1
TNFRSF10B [c]	33.7	194.8	77.5	2.7	72.8
TNFSF10 [a]	303.1	1929.8	898.1	29.7	857
VEGFC [c]	1	92.4	17.9	1.6	12.4
XAF1 [d]	101.9	988	403.9	15.6	421.5

Key: [a] ISRE-driven ISGs, [b] ISRE-driven ISGs potentially regulated by NF-κB, [c] SIE-driven ISGs, and [d] SIE-driven ISGs potentially regulated by NF-κB.

The expression of a subset of the IFN gene signature correlates with the patient response to therapy

In the 130 liver samples subjected to Nanostring analysis, 43 were obtained from HCV-infected patients who responded to IFN-ribavirin therapy (responders), 56 from HCV-infected patients who did not respond to therapy (nonresponders), and 31 from patients who had an initial virological response to therapy, but then relapsed during therapy and had high viral HCV titers (relapsers). Of these 130 patient samples, 112 had their IL28B genotype determined (Table 3). The liver tissue was obtained from 80 African-American (AA) and 50 Caucasian hepatitis C-infected patients (Table 4). Consistent with the previous findings that African Americans demonstrate a lower response rate to IFN than Caucasians, in the African American group of patients 27.5% were classified as responders, 57.5% as non-responders and 15% as relapsers. In contrast, in the Caucasian group of patients 50% were classified as responders, 22.1% as non-responders and 27.9% as relapsers. Initial analysis of differences in gene expression

Table 3. IL28 Genotype analysis (112/130 patients).

Genotype	R	NR	Relapser	AA	CA
CT	21 (35%)	22 (37%)	17 (28%)	35 (58%)	25 (52%)
TT	4 (11%)	21 (60%)	10 (29%)	29 (83%)	6 (17%)
CC	10 (59%)	3 (18%)	4 (23%)	5 (29%)	12 (71%)

between responders and non-responders (excluding relapsers) revealed statistically significant differences ($p<0.05$) in the expression of 16 out of the 39 genes examined, which included CCL5, DDX58/RIG-I, DHX58/LGP2, EIF2AK2, IFI6, IFI16, IFIH1/MDA5, IRF7, ISG20, MX1, OAS1, PLSCR1, RSAD2, STAT1, TLR3 and XAF1 (Figure 1). Most interestingly, these genes were expressed at higher levels in liver biopsies from patients that did not respond to IFN-ribavirin therapy as compared to the responders to therapy. The higher expression levels of ISGs prior to therapy in nonresponders compared with responders was consistent with several previous reports [27–30]. It is important to note that there was no relationship found between the expression of the IFNβ gene in liver biopsies, and responsiveness to exogenous IFN therapy. This finding is consistent with our previous report that serum levels of type I IFNs in patients chronically infected with HCV did not correlate with the response to exogenous IFN therapy [22].

In addition we subjected the data collected on gene expression from relapsers and compared it to the data from responders and nonresponders. Although there was no statistical difference between the various genes in nonresponders and relapsers, the expression of CASP4, GADD45G and IFI16 was found to be statistically different between the relapsers and the responders to IFN-ribavirin therapy. As shown in Figure 2, while CASP4 and IFI16 expression was higher in the group of relapsers, GADD45G expression was found to be somewhat lower. In addition, we compared the expression of the IFN gene signature according to race and found no statistical differences according to race, i.e. AA responders did not differ from Caucasian responders, etc.

Cellular functions of genes associated with IFN responsiveness

To gain insights into the cellular functions of the genes that were found associated with IFN responsiveness, we performed signaling pathway analysis using the Ingenuity Pathway analysis (IPA) software. As shown in Figure 3, 4 and 5, several critical antiviral signaling pathways were overrepresented in the genes that are associated with IFN responsiveness, For example TLR3, RIG-I/DDX58, MDA5/IFIH1, PKR/EIF2AK2, OAS1, IRF7 and RANTES/CCL5 are expressed at higher levels in nonresponders and are components in the pattern recognition receptor (PRR) pathway that is involved in the recognition of bacteria and viruses (Figure 4). Of these, TLR3 is known to recognize dsRNA intermediates produced during HCV RNA replication [31,32], while RIG-I senses 5′-triphosphate-bearing, genomic or antigenomic HCV RNAs [33]. Activation of either pathway in hepatocytes leads to an IFN response that restricts HCV replication. PKR has also been shown to recognize HCV RNA [34], although it is uncertain whether PKR has an antiviral and/or proviral effect [2]. OAS1 is a component of the OAS-RNase L system that had been shown to detect and degrade HCV RNA in HeLa cytoplasmic extracts [35]. In addition, RIG-I, LGP2, MDA5, IRF7 and STAT1 are also expressed at higher levels in nonresponders (Figure 5) and are components of the pathways leading to IRF activation by cytosolic PRRs or signaling to ISG induction downstream of the IFN receptors, which result in an innate immune response against viruses and bacteria. Furthermore, genes with significantly higher expression in nonresponders included two ISGs that possess anti-HCV activity in cell culture, i.e. RSAD2/viperin and ISG20 [24,36].

Table 4. Patient Demographics.

Patient Response	AA	Caucasians
Responders	22 (17%)	25 (19%)
Nonresponders	46 (35%)	11 (9%)
Relapsers	12 (9%)	14 (11%)

Nucleotide polymorphism in the IL28B gene is highly predictive of the response to IFN/ribavirin in HCV-infected patients

AA in the present study had ~three-fold higher inheritance of the homozygous *TT* genotype at the *Il28B*-associated rs12979860 SNP compared to homozygous *CC* (Table 3). In contrast, C had ~four-fold higher inheritance of *CC* compared to *TT*. These results are consistent with the well-established racially associated difference in inheritance at rs12979860 in chronic HCV infection [11–14]. The inheritance of the CC versus TT or CT genotypes at rs12979860 was highly correlated with (OR = 3.17, 95% CI 1.004 – 9.989, $p = 0.049$) a sustained response of HCV-infected patients to IFN-ribavirin therapy (responders). In addition, failure to respond to therapy (nonresponders), or an initial virological response to therapy but then relapsed with high viral HCV titers (relapsers) was highly dependent upon rs12979860 genotype ($p = 0.000972$) and race ($p = 0.00861$). Although rs12979860 genotype and other *il28B*-associated SNPs in linkage disequilibrium may be the most important correlates for racially associated differences in response to IFN-ribavirin therapy for hepatitis C, factors not associated with the *il28B* locus also contribute to racially associated response differences.

The development of a predictive model for the patient response to therapy based on the expression of IFN signature genes, and nucleotide polymorphism in the IL28B gene

Using logistic regression with cross validation, we found that the best model contained RSAD2, IFI6, IFI16, STAT1, CCL5, and XAF1. We show the results of the logistic regression models in Table 5. We note that not all variables were statistically significant in the final models. Although we used statistical significance to help develop candidate models, we selected the final model based

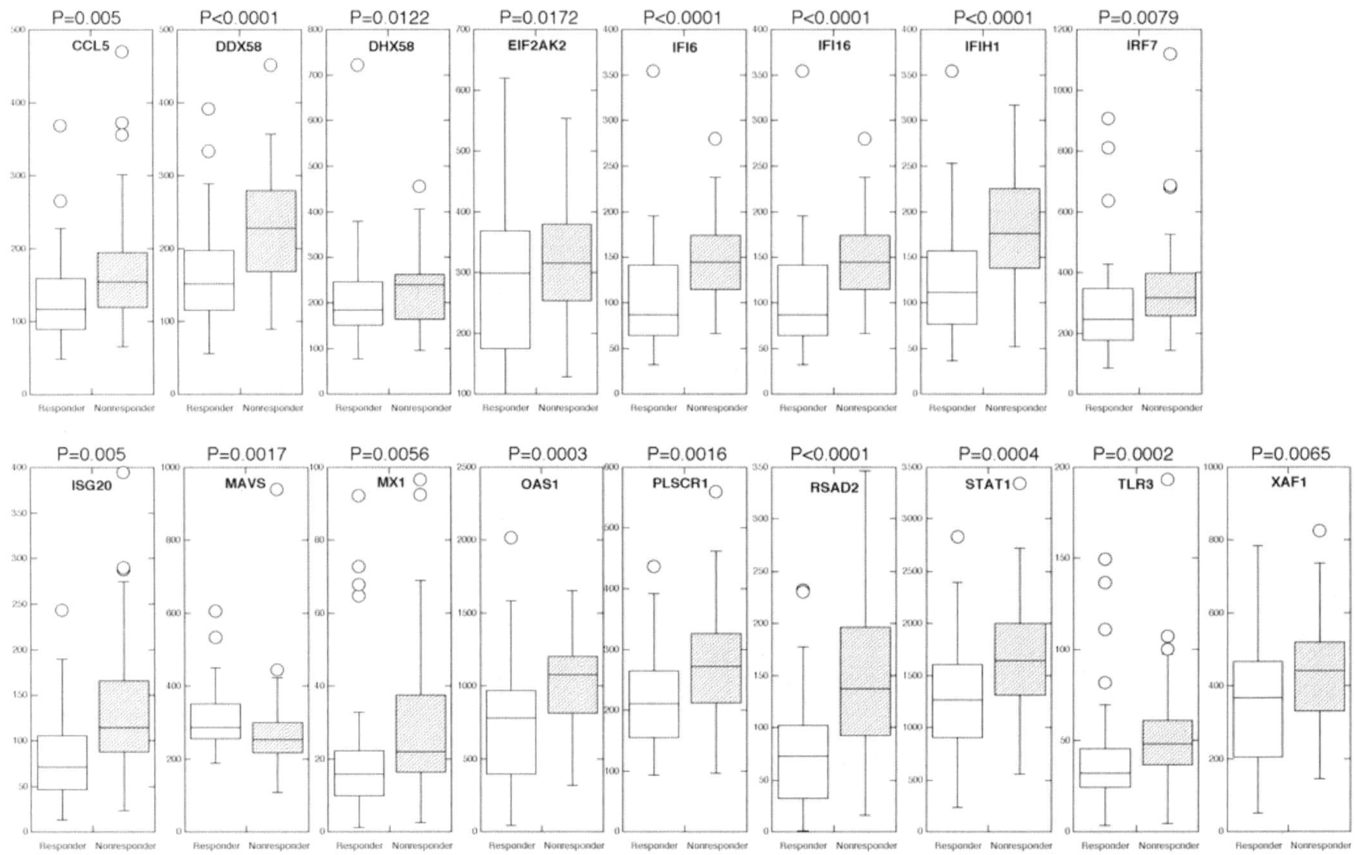

Figure 1. Differential expression of an IFN-regulated signature geneset in responders versus nonresponders to therapy. Expression of an IFN-regulated signature geneset was determined in RNA extracted from FFPE liver biopsies by nCounter analysis. Boxplots of genes found to be statistically differentially expressed by nonparametric Mann-Whitney analysis ($p<0.05$).

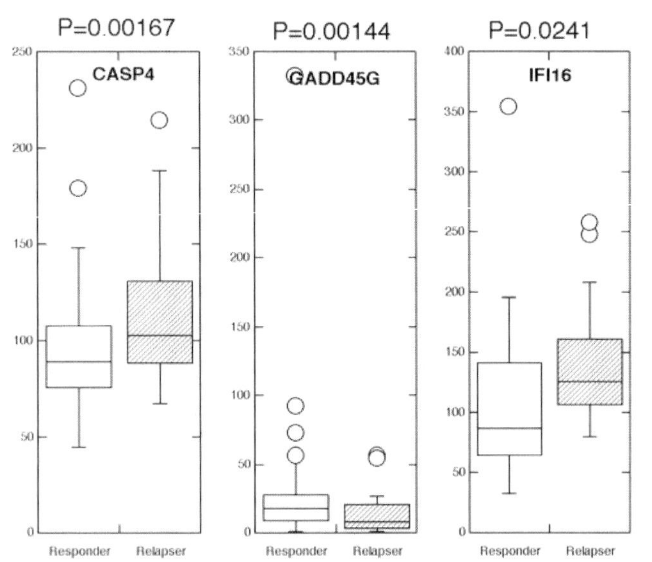

Figure 2. Differential expression of an IFN-regulated signature geneset in relapsers versus responders to IFN-ribavirin therapy to therapy. Expression of an IFN signature geneset was determined in RNA extracted from FFPE liver biopsies by nCounter analysis. Boxplots of genes found to be statistically differentially expressed by nonparametric Mann-Whitney analysis ($p<0.05$).

on its predictive potential in the 10-fold cross validation procedure. Higher expression levels of RSAD2, IFI6, IFI16, and CCL5 were associated with a reduced probability of patient response to IFN. Lower expression of STAT1 and XAF1 were associated with increased probability of response. Interestingly, race was not strongly predictive of response when controlling for the effects of these genes, indicating that we may have identified some of the genetic factors that reduce response rates among African Americans. Our model accurately predicted response for 79.2% of individuals, with a specificity of 90% and sensitivity of 58% (See Figure 6). Therefore, although the model rarely predicted response when the true outcome was nonresponse/relapse (false positives), it lacked sensitivity with several false negatives. Model-based predictions were superior to race alone, which was not very predictive of response with only 60% overall accuracy.

IL28B status was available in 112 out of the 130 patients whose IFN-response gene signature was examined. In this subset of patients, our expression-based model using RSAD2, IFI6, IFI16, CCL5, XAF1, and STAT1 was 73.0% accurate. Although this was lower than accuracy for the cohort as a whole, it still performed better than other expression-based models. We found that we could improve performance by including IL28B status. Combining this with RSAD2, IFI6, IFI16, and CCL5 had 74.9% accuracy. Importantly, this model had improved accuracy over a model with IL28B and race alone (without expression data), which had an accuracy of 67.8%.

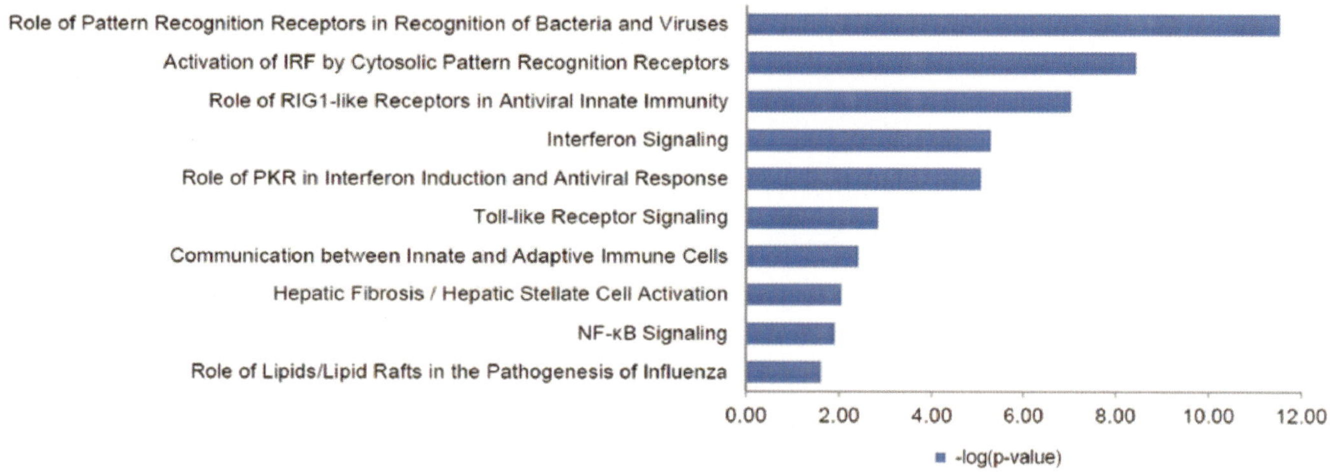

Figure 3. Signaling networks of genes that are associated with IFN responsiveness. The gene network was generated using Ingenuity Pathway Analysis software.

Discussion

Approximately 3% of the world's population is infected with HCV, and ~80% of HCV-infected individuals eventually become chronically infected. While long-term persistence results predominantly from evasion of the adaptive immune response to viral infection, evasion of host innate immune response is believed to contribute to establishing persistent HCV infection [6]. The IFN system is a key player in the innate immune response against viral infections, by inducing an antiviral state in the host against a variety of viral pathogens. Moreover, HCV is highly sensitive to treatment with type I and type III IFNs in vitro, and IFN remains

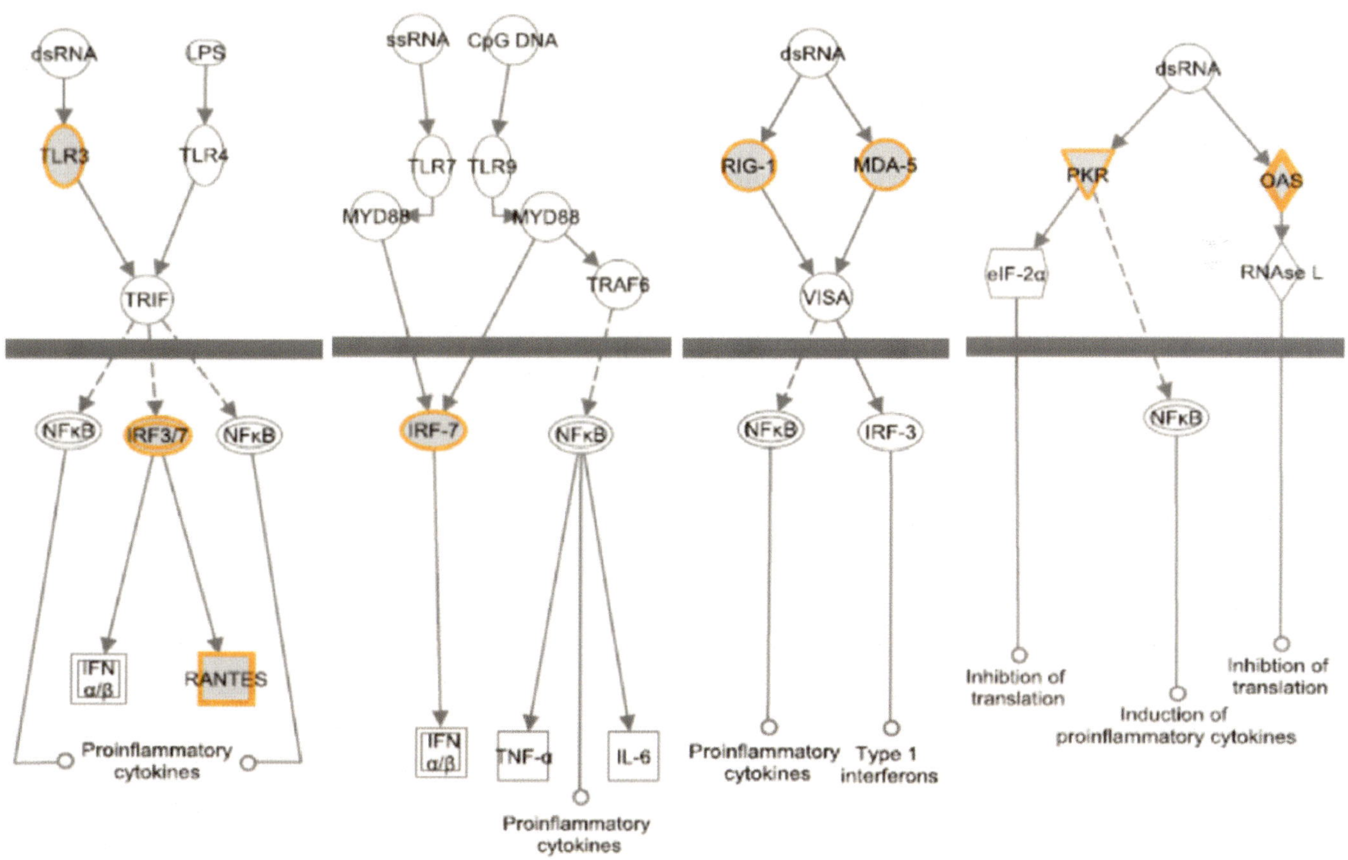

Figure 4. Genes in the pattern recognition receptor pathway are associated with IFN responsiveness. The gene network was generated using Ingenuity Pathway Analysis software. Genes upregulated in nonresponders (shown in Figure 1) were highlighted. As expected, several antiviral signaling pathways were overrepresented in these genes.

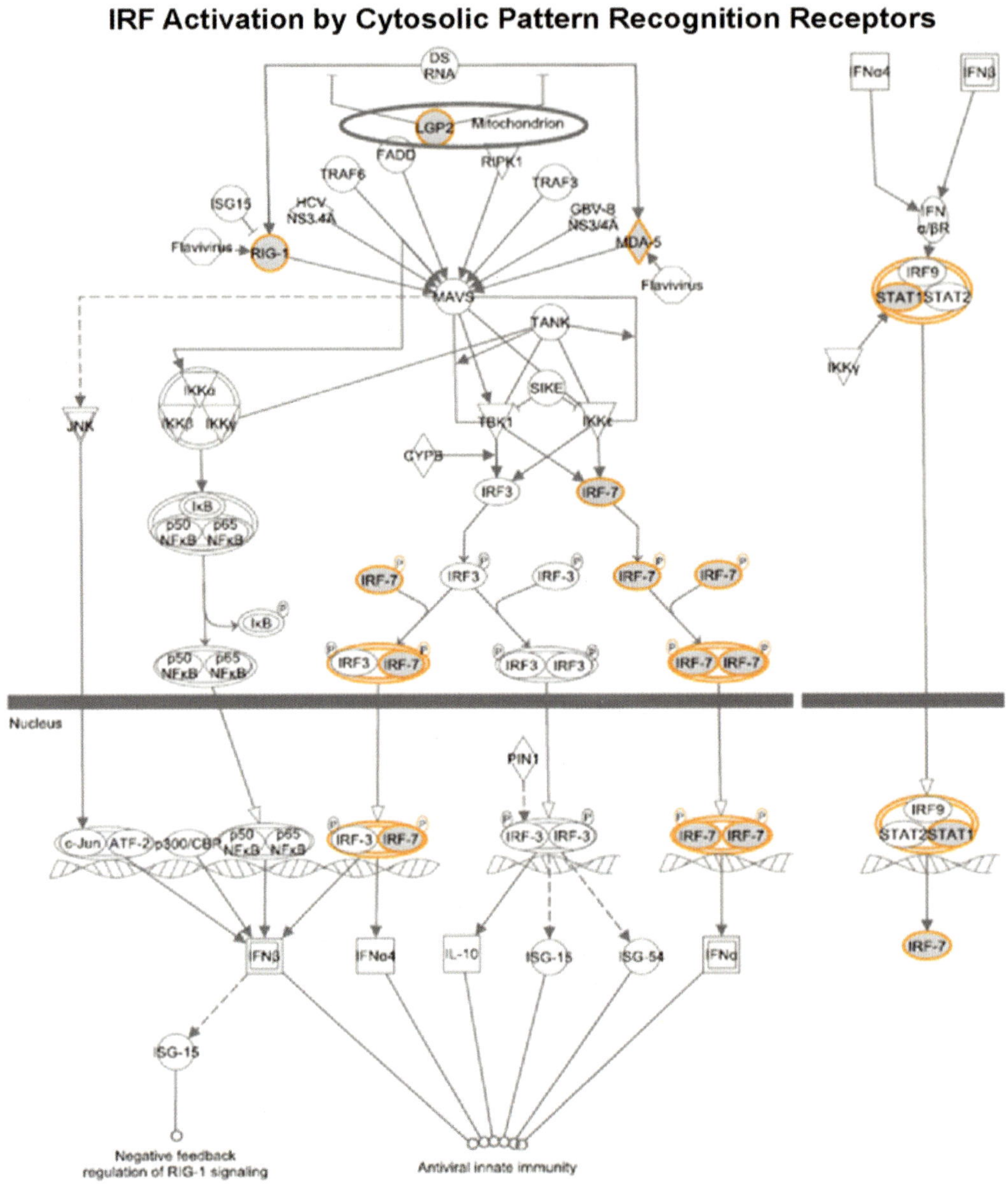

Figure 5. Genes in IRF activation by cytosolic pattern recognition receptors are associated with IFN responsiveness. The gene network was generated using Ingenuity Pathway Analysis software. Genes upregulated in nonresponders (shown in Figure 1 and 2) were highlighted.

a mainstay of treatment of HCV infected patients [37]. However, precisely why the current IFNα-based therapy is only effective in a proportion of treated patients remains largely a mystery, and this has been an area of intensive investigation. In the present study we compared expression of an IFN-response geneset in FFPE derived from liver biopsies from patients enrolled in an IFN-ribavirin trial conduced at UTHSC, which were taken before therapy was initiated. Our goal was to establish an IFN-response gene signature that can be used to predict IFN-responsiveness in hepatitis C patients.

The IFN-response signature geneset was based on our own microarray studies on IFN-induced genes in human and mouse cell lines, a database of IFN-stimulated genes from a variety of cells, and regulatory elements of gene promoter regions. Our strategy was to focus on genes that may play an important role in the antiviral innate immune response, and that were induced by various IFN activated signaling pathways. Thus genes such as Mx1 and PKR/EIF2AK2 contain an ISRE (IFN-stimulated response element), and are induced by the classical IFN-activated signaling that involved JAK1 and TYK2 activation and STAT1 and STAT2 transcription factors [38]. However ISGs such as RIG-I/DDX58 and MDA5/IFIH1 may be induced through an NF-κB-dependent pathway as well [16]. In addition, a number of ISGs such as VISA/MAVS and Casp4 do not contain an ISRE but rather an SIE (c-sis-inducible element) and appear to be regulated by STAT1 and STAT3 homodimers and heterodimers [39]. In addition, some SIE-containing ISGs such as IRF1 and MYD88 may also be regulated through an NF-κB-dependent pathway [18]. All 39 members of the IFN-regulated signature gene set were induced upon IFNα treatment of Huh7 hepatoma cells (data not shown).

Table 5. Logistic regression modeling of patient data.

Gene	OR*	95% CI	
Expression-based model (N = 130)			
RSAD2	0.863	0.755	0.986
IFI6	0.997	0.994	0.999
IFI16	0.867	0.758	0.992
STAT1	1.014	1.000	1.029
CCL5	0.927	0.857	1.002
XAF1	1.053	1.008	1.100
Expression and IL28 model (N = 115)			
Gene	OR*	95% CI	
RSAD2	0.947	0.850	1.056
IFI6	1.000	0.997	1.002
IFI16	0.978	0.869	1.101
CCL5	0.910	0.833	0.993
IL28B	2.988	1.271	7.024

*OR for gene expression is for a change of 10 units.

We found that nearly all 39 of the IFN-response signature genes were expressed in liver biopsies from chronically HCV-infected patients enrolled in the clinical trial of IFN-ribavirin at UTHSC. Previous studies using microarrays to determine global gene expression of liver biopsies from chronically HCV-infected patients and from experimentally HCV-infected chimpanzees show elevated ISG expression [23–26]. In addition, there was a great deal of heterogeneity in the expression level of the signature genes in the different patients. For example, genes that were expressed at relatively low levels such as IFNβ, IL6, TNFRSF10B, VEGFC and ANGPT2 were expressed only in a subset of patient samples. In contrast, genes that were expressed at relatively high levels such as TNFSF10 (TRAIL), OAS1, RANTES (CCL5) and IRF9 were detected in all liver biopsies. It is of particular interest that only a small fraction of liver biopsies (~10%) from patients chronically infected with HCV expressed the IFNβ gene. While this seems to conflict with our previous finding that ~50% of the serum samples from a smaller patient population in the clinical

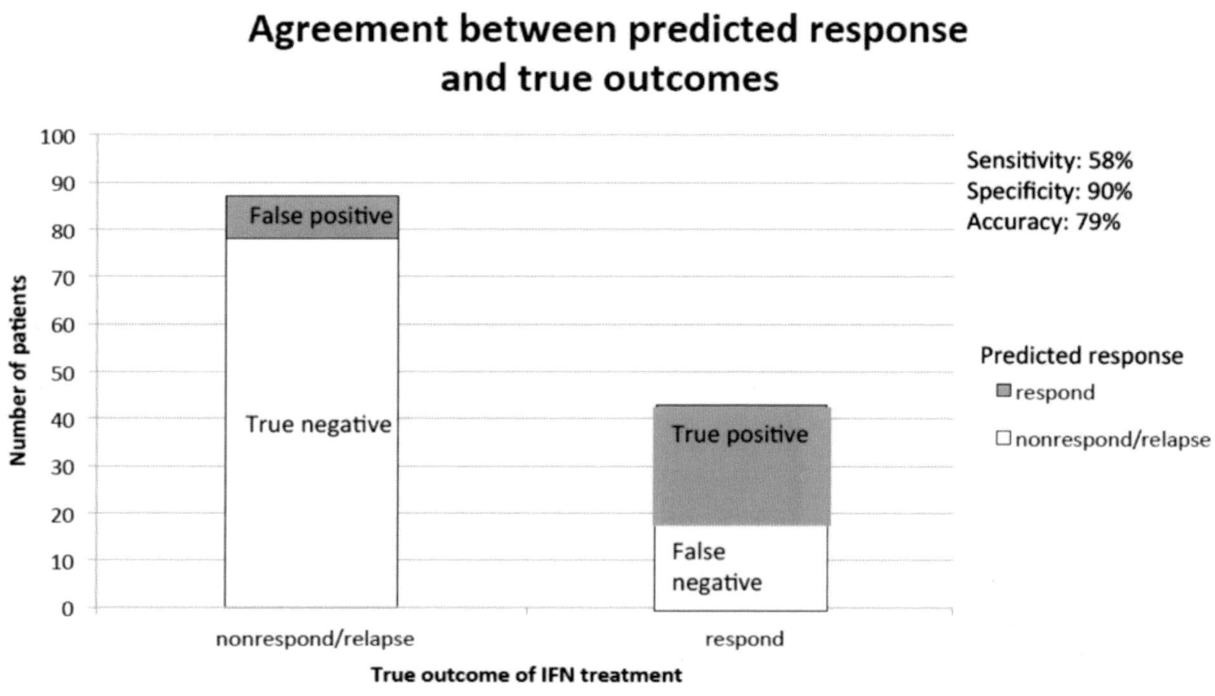

Figure 6. The distribution of predicted probability of therapeutic response (with relapsers included). We found that those who actually responded to IFN-ribavirin treatment had higher predicted probabilities of response in the model.

trial of IFN-ribavirin had detectable levels of type I IFN [22], it is conceivable that most of the circulating levels of type I IFN derive from extrahepatic sources such as the plasmacytoid dendritic cells. Consistent with our data, two recent studies have shown that type III IFNs rather than type I IFNs are induced in the liver of experimentally HCV-infected chimpanzees and that the intrahepatic level of type III IFNs correlates with that of ISG expression [40,41]. Our IFN-response geneset did not contain type III IFN genes, since when this study was initiated and the geneset was constructed a role for IL29/IL28B in hepatic innate immunity to HCV infection was not recognized. Nevertheless, it is worth noting that intrahepatic type III IFN level was not found to associate with the outcome of acute HCV infection [40], nor was it related to response to IFN therapy in patients with chronic hepatitis C [42].

Another important finding from these studies is that expression of a subset of these genes in liver biopsies inversely correlated with the responsiveness to IFN-ribavirin therapy, i.e. higher expression was observed in nonresponders as compared to responders. Although this finding is counterintuitive, as one would expect an active IFN system would help eliminate the virus during therapy, it is supported by a number of studies, which have shown that patients with a high ISG expression prior to the initiation of IFN therapy seem to respond poorly to IFN therapy [27–30]. Additional support is lent from a study showing that the expression of intrahepatic ISGs was already maximally induced in chimpanzees chronically infected with HCV. Consequently, when exogenous IFN was administered, there was no further ISG upregulation [43]. Although the underlying mechanism remains elusive, nonresponder hepatitis C patients tend to have pre-activated Jak-STAT pathway prior to therapy, which may connect to IFN refractoriness [27].

However, it is important to note that in our study only a subset of the IFN-regulated genes examined were expressed at a statistically significant higher level in patients that were nonresponsive to IFN therapy. Of particular interest, some of these overexpressed genes were either involved in viral sensing (TLR3, RIG-I/DDX58, DHX58/LGP2, MDA5) or effector functions of IFNs (ISG20, RSAD2, PKR, etc.). Both TLR3 and RIG-I can sense HCV RNA (although they recognize different viral ligand forms) early after infection and initiate signaling pathways culminating in the induction of an IFN response that curtails HCV replication [32,33]. However, HCV has evolved to disarm both mechanisms by NS3/4A-mediated cleavage of the essential adaptor proteins, TRIF (Toll/interleukin receptor domain-containing adapter-inducing interferon), and MAVS, once the infection is established in hepatocytes [44–46]. Among the ISG effectors, ISG20 and RSAD2 have been shown to inhibit HCV replication, while controversial results have been reported for PKR [2]. There are several possibilities that may explain why induction of the endogenous anti-viral ISGs prior to IFN therapy fails to contain HCV infection [47]. The anti-HCV ISGs may only be transcriptionally upregulated in uninfected surrounding cells but not in HCV-infected hepatocytes. Alternatively, ISG transcripts may be made in both infected and uninfected cells but ISG proteins are only made in uninfected cells because of PKR activation in infected cells [48]. Third, some HCV proteins may inhibit the effector functions of the antiviral ISGs. Regardless of the infection/treatment outcome, the induction of a subset of IFN-regulated signature genes we identified in treatment-naïve patient liver underscores the important roles these genes/pathways may play in host attempts to control HCV infection in the liver.

In addition, we found CCL5/RANTES to be over-expressed in both nonresponders and relapsers to IFN therapy. CCL5 is a chemokine produced by monocyte/macrophage subsets in the liver, which contributes to recruiting T cells and other leukocytes to the infection site and also to the progression and resolution of liver fibrosis [49]. A recent study from our group suggests that infected hepatocytes represent a cellular source for CCL5 production at early phase of HCV infection, through TLR3-mediated sensing of HCV dsRNA intermediates and subsequent activation of NF-κB, a transcription factor pivotal for RANTES synthesis [31]. CCL5 is associated with a Th1 lymphocyte-related cytokine/chemokine profile and HCV clearance [50]. However, CCL5 may also shape the IFN response in the liver by altering the infiltration and activation of hepatic stellate cells, which maintains chronic HCV infection in the liver in part by inhibiting liver fibrosis [51]. Exactly how pre-activated intrahepatic RANTES expression affects IFN responsiveness will require further study.

Our study also presents a predictive model for IFN responsiveness based on a small number of signature genes. Although variants of the IL28B/IFNλ3 gene have recently been found to be highly predictive of the response to IFN/ribavirin in HCV-infected patients [11–15], there has been a paucity of mechanistic insights. Clearly, intrahepatic type III IFN levels of hepatitis C patients are not affected by IL28B polymorphism [42,52], nor is it the case in primary hepatocyte cultures infected by HCV in vitro [40,53]. Thus, the underlying mechanism for differential response in HCV-infected patients remains largely unknown. In our study we show that the expression of RSAD2, IFI6, IFI16, STAT1, CCL5, and XAF1 was highly predictive of the eventual IFN responsiveness to IFN/ribavirin therapy. Future studies will elucidate why lower expression of STAT1 and XAF1 were predictive of IFN responsiveness while expression of RSAD2, IFI6, IFI16, and CCL5 were associated with a poorer response to therapy. The model must also be validated with external data, and though our model had high specificity, further refinement is needed to improve model sensitivity.

Author Contributions

Conceived and designed the experiments: LMP KL JFF TNM JD CHY SRP MF EH CRH. Performed the experiments: TNM JD. Analyzed the data: LMP KL JFF TNM EH CRH. Contributed reagents/materials/analysis tools: MF TNM EH. Contributed to the writing of the manuscript: LMP KL JFF TNM SRP MF EH CRH.

References

1. Lemon SM (2010) Induction and evasion of innate antiviral responses by hepatitis C virus. J Biol Chem 285: 22741–22747.
2. Li K, Lemon SM (2013) Innate immune responses in hepatitis C virus infection. Semin Immunopathol 35: 53–72.
3. Meylan E, Tschopp J, Karin M (2006) Intracellular pattern recognition receptors in the host response. Nature 442: 39–44.
4. Lester SN, Li K (2014) Toll-Like Receptors in Antiviral Innate Immunity. J Mol Biol 426: 1246–1264.
5. Pfeffer LM, Dinarello CA, Herberman RB, Williams BR, Borden EC, et al. (1998) Biological properties of recombinant alpha-interferons: 40th anniversary of the discovery of interferons. Cancer Res 58: 2489–2499.
6. Gale M, Jr., Foy EM (2005) Evasion of intracellular host defence by hepatitis C virus. Nature 436: 939–945.
7. Ghany MG, Nelson DR, Strader DB, Thomas DL, Seeff LB (2011) An update on treatment of genotype 1 chronic hepatitis C virus infection: 2011 practice guideline by the American Association for the Study of Liver Diseases. Hepatology 54: 1433–1444.
8. Fleckenstein J (2004) Chronic hepatitis C in African Americans and other minority groups. Curr Gastroenterol Rep 6: 66–70.
9. Castellino S, Lensing S, Riely C, Rai SN, Davila R, et al. (2004) The epidemiology of chronic hepatitis C infection in survivors of childhood cancer: an update of the St Jude Children's Research Hospital hepatitis C seropositive cohort. Blood 103: 2460–2466.

10. Muir AJ, Bornstein JD, Killenberg PG (2004) Peginterferon alfa-2b and ribavirin for the treatment of chronic hepatitis C in blacks and non-Hispanic whites. N Engl J Med 350: 2265–2271.
11. Ge D, Fellay J, Thompson AJ, Simon JS, Shianna KV, et al. (2009) Genetic variation in IL28B predicts hepatitis C treatment-induced viral clearance. Nature 461: 399–401.
12. Suppiah V, Moldovan M, Ahlenstiel G, Berg T, Weltman M, et al. (2009) IL28B is associated with response to chronic hepatitis C interferon-alpha and ribavirin therapy. Nat Genet 41: 1100–1104.
13. Tanaka Y, Nishida N, Sugiyama M, Kurosaki M, Matsuura K, et al. (2009) Genome-wide association of IL28B with response to pegylated interferon-alpha and ribavirin therapy for chronic hepatitis C. Nat Genet 41: 1105–1109.
14. Thomas DL, Thio CL, Martin MP, Qi Y, Ge D, et al. (2009) Genetic variation in IL28B and spontaneous clearance of hepatitis C virus. Nature 461: 798–801.
15. Rauch A, Kutalik Z, Descombes P, Cai T, Di Iulio J, et al. (2010) Genetic variation in IL28B is associated with chronic hepatitis C and treatment failure: a genome-wide association study. Gastroenterology 138: 1338–1345, 1345 e1331–1337.
16. Pfeffer LM, Kim JG, Pfeffer SR, Carrigan DJ, Baker DP, et al. (2004) The role of NF-κB in the antiviral action of interferon and interferon-regulated gene expression. J Biol Chem 279: 31304–31311.
17. Wei L, Fan M, Xu L, Heinrich K, Berry MW, et al. (2008) Bioinformatic analysis reveals cRel as a regulator of a subset of interferon-stimulated genes. J Interferon Cytokine Res 28: 541–551.
18. Wei L, Sandbulte MR, Thomas PG, Webby RJ, Homayouni R, et al. (2006) NFκB negatively regulates interferon-induced gene expression and anti-influenza activity. J Biol Chem 281: 11678–11684.
19. Rusinova I, Forster S, Yu S, Kannan A, Masse M, et al. (2013) Interferome v2.0: an updated database of annotated interferon-regulated genes. Nucleic Acids Res 41: D1040–1046.
20. Vandesompele J, De Preter K, Pattyn F, Poppe B, Van Roy N, et al. (2002) Accurate normalization of real-time quantitative RT-PCR data by geometric averaging of multiple internal control genes. Genome Biol 3: RESEARCH0034.
21. Hastie T, Tibishirani R, Friedman J (2009) Elements of Statistical Learning: Data Mining, Inference and Prediction (Second Edition). New York: Springer-Verlag.
22. Pfeffer LM, Madey MA, Riely CA, Fleckenstein JF (2009) The Induction of Type I Interferon Production in Hepatitis C-Infected Patients. J Interferon Cytokine Res 29: 299–306.
23. Bigger CB, Brasky KM, Lanford RE (2001) DNA microarray analysis of chimpanzee liver during acute resolving hepatitis C virus infection. J Virol 75: 7059–7066.
24. Helbig KJ, Lau DT, Semendric L, Harley HA, Beard MR (2005) Analysis of ISG expression in chronic hepatitis C identifies viperin as a potential antiviral effector. Hepatology 42: 702–710.
25. Lau DT, Fish PM, Sinha M, Owen DM, Lemon SM, et al. (2008) Interferon regulatory factor-3 activation, hepatic interferon-stimulated gene expression, and immune cell infiltration in hepatitis C virus patients. Hepatology 47: 799–809.
26. Su AI, Pezacki JP, Wodicka L, Brideau AD, Supekova L, et al. (2002) Genomic analysis of the host response to hepatitis C virus infection. Proc Natl Acad Sci U S A 99: 15669–15674.
27. Sarasin-Filipowicz M, Oakeley EJ, Duong FH, Christen V, Terracciano L, et al. (2008) Interferon signaling and treatment outcome in chronic hepatitis C. Proc Natl Acad Sci U S A 105: 7034–7039.
28. Chen J, Young NL, Subbarao S, Warachit P, Saguanwongse S, et al. (1999) HIV type 1 subtypes in Guangxi Province, China, 1996. AIDS Res Hum Retroviruses 15: 81–84.
29. Feld JJ, Nanda S, Huang Y, Chen W, Cam M, et al. (2007) Hepatic gene expression during treatment with peginterferon and ribavirin: Identifying molecular pathways for treatment response. Hepatology 46: 1548–1563.
30. Asselah T, Bieche I, Sabbagh A, Bedossa P, Moreau R, et al. (2009) Gene expression and hepatitis C virus infection. Gut 58: 846–858.
31. Li K, Li NL, Wei D, Pfeffer SR, Fan M, et al. (2012) Activation of chemokine and inflammatory cytokine response in hepatitis C virus-infected hepatocytes depends on Toll-like receptor 3 sensing of hepatitis C virus double-stranded RNA intermediates. Hepatology 55: 666–675.
32. Wang N, Liang Y, Devaraj S, Wang J, Lemon SM, et al. (2009) Toll-like receptor 3 mediates establishment of an antiviral state against hepatitis C virus in hepatoma cells. J Virol 83: 9824–9834.
33. Saito T, Owen DM, Jiang F, Marcotrigiano J, Gale M, Jr. (2008) Innate immunity induced by composition-dependent RIG-I recognition of hepatitis C virus RNA. Nature 454: 523–527.
34. Arnaud N, Dabo S, Akazawa D, Fukasawa M, Shinkai-Ouchi F, et al. (2011) Hepatitis C virus reveals a novel early control in acute immune response. PLoS Pathog 7: e1002289.
35. Han JQ, Barton DJ (2002) Activation and evasion of the antiviral 2'-5' oligoadenylate synthetase/ribonuclease L pathway by hepatitis C virus mRNA. RNA 8: 512–525.
36. Zhou Z, Wang N, Woodson SE, Dong Q, Wang J, et al. (2011) Antiviral activities of ISG20 in positive-strand RNA virus infections. Virology 409: 175–188.
37. Strader DB, Wright T, Thomas DL, Seeff LB (2004) Diagnosis, management, and treatment of hepatitis C. Hepatology 39: 1147–1171.
38. Levy DE, Darnell JEJ (1990) Interferon-dependent transcriptional activation: Signal transduction without second messenger involvement. New Biol 2: 923–928.
39. Pine R, Canova A, Schindler C (1994) Tyrosine phosphorylated p91 binds to a single element in the ISGF2/IRF-1 promoter to mediate induction by IFNa and IFNg, and is likely to autoregulate the p91 gene. EMBO J 13: 158–167.
40. Park H, Serti E, Eke O, Muchmore B, Prokunina-Olsson L, et al. (2012) IL-29 is the dominant type III interferon produced by hepatocytes during acute hepatitis C virus infection. Hepatology 56: 2060–2070.
41. Thomas E, Gonzalez VD, Li Q, Modi AA, Chen W, et al. (2012) HCV infection induces a unique hepatic innate immune response associated with robust production of type III interferons. Gastroenterology 142: 978–988.
42. Honda M, Sakai A, Yamashita T, Nakamoto Y, Mizukoshi E, et al. (2010) Hepatic ISG expression is associated with genetic variation in interleukin 28B and the outcome of IFN therapy for chronic hepatitis C. Gastroenterology 139: 499–509.
43. Lanford RE, Guerra B, Bigger CB, Lee H, Chavez D, et al. (2007) Lack of response to exogenous interferon-alpha in the liver of chimpanzees chronically infected with hepatitis C virus. Hepatology 46: 999–1008.
44. Li K, Foy E, Ferreon JC, Nakamura M, Ferreon AC, et al. (2005) Immune evasion by hepatitis C virus NS3/4A protease-mediated cleavage of the Toll-like receptor 3 adaptor protein TRIF. Proc Natl Acad Sci U S A 102: 2992–2997.
45. Meylan E, Curran J, Hofmann K, Moradpour D, Binder M, et al. (2005) Cardif is an adaptor protein in the RIG-I antiviral pathway and is targeted by hepatitis C virus. Nature 437: 1167–1172.
46. Li XD, Sun L, Seth RB, Pineda G, Chen ZJ (2005) Hepatitis C virus protease NS3/4A cleaves mitochondrial antiviral signaling protein off the mitochondria to evade innate immunity. Proc Natl Acad Sci U S A 102: 17717–17722.
47. Heim MH (2013) Innate immunity and HCV. J Hepatol 58: 564–574.
48. Garaigorta U, Chisari FV (2009) Hepatitis C virus blocks interferon effector function by inducing protein kinase R phosphorylation. Cell Host Microbe 6: 513–522.
49. Berres ML, Koenen RR, Rueland A, Zaldivar MM, Heinrichs D, et al. (2010) Antagonism of the chemokine Ccl5 ameliorates experimental liver fibrosis in mice. The Journal of clinical investigation 120: 4129–4140.
50. Katsounas A, Trippler M, Kottilil S, Lempicki RA, Gerken G, et al. (2012) Cytokine/chemokine patterns connect host and viral characteristics with clinics during chronic hepatitis C. Eur J Med Res 17: 9.
51. Schulze-Krebs A, Preimel D, Popov Y, Bartenschlager R, Lohmann V, et al. (2005) Hepatitis C virus-replicating hepatocytes induce fibrogenic activation of hepatic stellate cells. Gastroenterology 129: 246–258.
52. Urban TJ, Thompson AJ, Bradrick SS, Fellay J, Schuppan D, et al. (2010) IL28B genotype is associated with differential expression of intrahepatic interferon-stimulated genes in patients with chronic hepatitis C. Hepatology 52: 1888–1896.
53. Marukian S, Andrus L, Sheahan TP, Jones CT, Charles ED, et al. (2011) Hepatitis C virus induces interferon-lambda and interferon-stimulated genes in primary liver cultures. Hepatology 54: 1913–1923.

15

The Development of the Pediatric NAFLD Fibrosis Score (PNFS) to Predict the Presence of Advanced Fibrosis in Children with Nonalcoholic Fatty Liver Disease

Naim Alkhouri[1,2]*, Sana Mansoor[1], Paola Giammaria[4], Daniela Liccardo[4], Rocio Lopez[3], Valerio Nobili[4]

1 Department of Pediatric Gastroenterology and Hepatology, Cleveland Clinic, Cleveland, Ohio, United States of America, 2 Digestive Disease Institute, Cleveland Clinic, Cleveland, Ohio, United States of America, 3 Department of Quantitative Health Sciences, Cleveland Clinic, Cleveland, Ohio, United States of America, 4 The Liver Unit, Bambino Gesu Children's Hospital, Rome, Italy

Abstract

Background: Noninvasive hepatic fibrosis scores that predict the presence of advanced fibrosis have been developed and validated in adult patients with NAFLD. The aims of our study were to assess the utility of commonly used adult fibrosis scores in pediatric NAFLD and to develop a pediatric specific fibrosis score that can predict advanced fibrosis.

Methods: Consecutive children with biopsy-proven NAFLD were included. Fibrosis was determined by an experienced pathologist (F0–4). Advanced fibrosis was defined as fibrosis stage ≥3. The following adult fibrosis scores were calculated for each child: AST/ALT ratio, AST/platelet ratio index (APRI), NAFLD fibrosis score (NFS), and FIB-4 Index. Multivariable logistic regression analysis was performed to build a new pediatric model for predicting advanced fibrosis.

Results: Our cohort consisted of 242 children with a mean age of 12.4±3.1 years and 63% were female. 36 (15%) subjects had advanced fibrosis. APRI and FIB-4 were higher in patients with advanced fibrosis compared to those with fibrosis stage 0–2; however, AST/ALT ratio and NFS were not different between the two groups. We used our data to develop a new model to predict advanced fibrosis which included: ALT, alkaline phosphatase, platelet counts and GGT. The multivariable logistic regression model (z) was defined as follows: z = 1.1+(0.34*sqrt(ALT))+(0.002*alkaline phosphatase) – (1.1*log(platelets) – (0.02*GGT). This value was then converted into a probability distribution (p) with a value between 0 to 100 by the following formula: p = 100×exp(z)/[1+exp(z)]. The AUCROC for this model was 0.74 (95% CI: 0.66, 0.82). This was found to be significantly better than APRI, NAFLD Fibrosis Score and FIB-4 Index.

Conclusion: Noninvasive hepatic fibrosis scores developed in adults had poor performance in diagnosing advanced fibrosis in children with NAFLD. We developed a new pediatric NAFLD fibrosis score with improved performance characteristics.

Editor: Maria Tsokos, BIDMC, United States of America

Funding: The authors have no support or funding to report.

* Email: alkhoun@ccf.org

Introduction

Due to the epidemic of childhood obesity, nonalcoholic fatty liver disease (NAFLD) has become the most common chronic liver disease in children [1,2]. Pediatric NAFLD is relatively benign but some children can develop major hepatic complications including cirrhosis and the need for liver transplantation [3]. The presence of advanced fibrosis, which includes bridging fibrosis and cirrhosis, may be the most important factor in determining the prognosis of NAFLD and its risk of progression to end-stage liver disease. Liver biopsy remains the gold standard for assessing NAFLD severity and staging of fibrosis [4]; however, with a disease that affects approximately 10% of American children, performing a liver biopsy is neither practical nor ethical. Moreover, children with bridging fibrosis are very likely to progress to developing cirrhosis in the absence of effective treatment for NAFLD which requires close monitoring for signs of portal hypertension and hepatic decompensation. Therefore, there is an urgent need to develop simple noninvasive tests to identify children with advanced fibrosis. Several noninvasive fibrosis scoring systems comprised of routinely measured clinical and laboratory variables have been developed in adult patients with NAFLD to identify those with advanced fibrosis including the AST/ALT ratio, NAFLD fibrosis score (NFS), the AST/platelet ratio index (APR), and the FIB4-score [5]. However, recent data from our group and others have suggested that these adult scores may not be accurate to predict advanced fibrosis in children [6,7].

The aims of the current study were to assess the utility of commonly used adult fibrosis scores in a large cohort of pediatric patients with biopsy-proven NAFLD and to develop a pediatric specific fibrosis score that can predict advanced fibrosis.

Materials and Methods

Patients

A written informed consent was obtained from the parents, caretakers, or guardians on behalf of the minors/children enrolled in the study. Consecutive patients diagnosed with NAFLD seen at the Bambino Gesù Children's Hospital were included in the study. Study was approved by Ethics committee of the Bambino Gesù Children's Hospital and Research Institute in Rome, Italy. Inclusion criteria were persistently elevated serum aminotransferase levels, diffusely hyperechogenic liver on ultrasonography suggestive of fatty liver, and biopsy consistent with the diagnosis of NAFLD [8,9]. Exclusion criteria were hepatic virus infections (hepatitis A, B, C, and D, cytomegalovirus and Epstein-Barr virus), alcohol consumption, history of parenteral nutrition, and use of drugs known to induce steatosis (e.g. valproate, amiodarone or prednisone) or to affect body weight and carbohydrate metabolism. Autoimmune liver disease, metabolic liver disease, Wilson disease, celiac disease and α-1-antitrypsin deficiency were ruled out using standard clinical, laboratory and histological criteria. A blood sample for laboratory tests was taken within one week of the liver biopsy.

The body mass index (BMI) and its standard deviation score (Z-score) were calculated [10,11]. The metabolic syndrome (MetS) was defined as the presence of ≥3 of the following 5 criteria [12]: abdominal obesity as defined by a waist circumference $\geq 90^{th}$ percentile for age [13]; hypertriglyceridemia as defined by TG > 95th percentile for age and sex [14]; low HDL cholesterol as defined by $<5^{th}$ percentile for age and sex [14]; elevated blood pressure (BP) as defined by systolic or diastolic BP>95th percentile for age and sex [15]; and impaired fasting glucose, impaired glucose tolerance (IGT) or known type 2 diabetes mellitus as described in detail elsewhere [16]. The homeostasis model assessment index of insulin resistance (HOMA-IR) was calculated as surrogate markers of insulin sensitivity [17].

Liver Histology and Noninvasive Fibrosis Scores

The clinical indication for biopsy was either to assess the presence of NASH and degree of fibrosis or other likely independent or competing liver diseases. Liver biopsy was performed in all children, after an overnight fast, using an automatic core biopsy 18 Gauge needle (Biopince, Amedic, Sweden) under general anaesthesia and ultrasound guidance. A Sonoline Omnia Ultrasound machine (Siemens, Germany) equipped with a 5-MHz probe (5.0 C 50, Siemens) and a biopsy adaptor was employed. Two biopsy passes within different liver segments were performed for each subject. The length of liver specimen (in millimetres) was recorded. Only samples with a length ≥15 mm and including at least 6 complete portal tracts [18] were considered adequate for the purpose of the study. Biopsies were evaluated by a single pathologist who was blinded to clinical and laboratory data. Biopsies were routinely processed (*i.e.*, formalin-fixed and paraffin-embedded) and sections of liver tissue, 5 μm thick, were stained with Hematoxylin-Eosin, Van Gieson, PAS-D, and Prussian blue stain. Liver biopsy features were graded according to the NAFLD activity scoring (NAS) system proposed by Kleiner et al [19]. Fibrosis was scored as 0 = none; 1 = periportal or perisinusoidal fibrosis; 2 = perisinusoidal and portal/periportal fibrosis; 3 = bridging fibrosis; and 4 = cirrhosis. Advanced fibrosis was defined as fibrosis stage ≥3.

APRI was calculated as AST/ULN (upper limit of normal)/Platelets×100 [20]. The AST/ALT ratio was calculated as ratio of AST to ALT values. The FIB –4 index was calculated using the following formula: FIB - 4 = (Age×AST)/[Platelet count (10.9/L)×$\sqrt{ALT}$] [21] [18]. NAFLD Fibrosis Score (NFS) was obtained using the formula: −1.675+0.037×age (years)+0.094×BMI (kg/m2)+1.13×IFG/diabetes (yes = 1, no = 0)+0.99×AST/ALT ratio −0.013×platelet (×109/l) −0.66×albumin (g/dl) [22].

Statistical analysis

Descriptive statistics were computed for all variables. These include means, standard deviations and percentiles for continuous variables and frequencies and percentages for categorical factors. A univariable analysis was done to assess differences between subjects with and without advanced fibrosis; ANOVA or the non-parametric Kruskal-Wallis tests were used to compare continuous and ordinal factors and Pearson's chi-square tests were used to compare categorical variables. Multivariable logistic regression analysis was performed to build a model for prediction of advanced fibrosis. An automated stepwise variable selection method performed on 1000 bootstrap samples was used to choose the final model. All non-invasive factors were assessed and the 4 variables with highest inclusion rates were included in the final model.

Discrimination was used for internal model validation; this measures the ability to rank patients by risk of advanced fibrosis such that patients with a higher predicted risk are more likely to have advanced fibrosis. Discrimination was measured by the area under the Receiver Operating Characteristics curve (AUROC). The method described by Harrell [23] was used to compute the validation metric with over-fitting bias correction through bootstrap resampling. A thousand bootstrap samples (B = 1000) were drawn from the original data set and a new model with the same model settings was built on each bootstrap resample. Prediction on patients that were not chosen in the resample was calculated. An optimism factor was calculated over the 1000 new models and the bias-corrected validation metric was obtained by subtracting this optimism value from the AUROC directly measured from the original model. A $P<0.05$ was considered statistically significant. All analyses were performed using SAS (version 9.2, The SAS Institute, Cary, NC) and R (version 3.0.1, The R Foundation for Statistical Computing, Vienna, Austria; packages used: Hmisc and ROCR).

Results

Patient Characteristics

A total of 242 pediatric patients with biopsy-proven NAFLD were included in the analysis. 63% were female and the mean age was 12.4±3.1 years. The majority were obese (85%) with a mean BMI percentile of 93.4±7.6. MetS and its individual components were commonly present in our cohort (MetS in 53%). Thirty six patients (15%) had advanced fibrosis F ≥3 (only two patients with cirrhosis). None of the patient had complications from cirrhosis or portal hypertension. Table 1 presents a summary of patient clinical and laboratory characteristics. Hypertension, higher triglycerides, ALT, and AST were significantly associated with presence of advanced fibrosis (p value <0.005 for all).

Histological Features of NAFLD

Table 2 presents a summary of the histological features of the biopsy specimens. Approximately 90% of patients had some degree of lobular inflammation while two-thirds revealed at least mild portal inflammation. Ballooning was present in only 50% of patients. Subjects with advanced fibrosis were more likely to have higher grades of steatosis, lobular inflammation, portal inflammation, and ballooning, p value <0.05 for all. The mean NAS was 3.9+1.8 (significantly higher in patients with advanced fibrosis

Table 1. Demographic and Clinical Characteristics.

Factor	Overall (N = 242)	Fibrosis stage 0–2 (N = 206)	Fibrosis stage 3–4 (N = 36)	p-value
Male (%)	90(37.2)	79(38.3)	11(30.6)	0.37
Age at first visit (years)	12.4±3.1	12.3±3.1	13.1±2.6	0.12
BMI Percentile	93.4±7.6	93.4±7.5	93.3±8.4	0.91
Obese (%)	205(84.7)	174(84.5)	31(86.1)	0.80
Low HDL (%)	127(52.5)	108(52.4)	19(52.8)	0.97
Hypertriglyceridemia (%)	154(63.6)	130(63.1)	24(66.7)	0.68
Hypertension (%)	77(31.8)	57(27.7)	20(55.6)	**<0.001**
IGT/Diabetes (%)	95(39.3)	76(36.9)	19(52.8)	0.072
Metabolic syndrome (%)	120(53.1)	107(51.9)	13(65.0)	0.26
Cholesterol (mg/dL)	156.7±29.9	156.0±29.8	160.7±30.6	0.39
HDL (mg/dL)	54[40,73]	55.5[40,73]	52.5[43,72]	0.86
Triglycerides (mg/dL)	90[66,122]	88.5[63,118]	118.0[77,136.5]	**0.006**
ALT (IU/L)	75[55,99]	72[52,89]	100.5[72.5,122.5]	**<0.001**
AST (IU/L)	49[40,66]	48[39,65]	57.5[48,87.5]	**0.002**
GGT (IU/L)	25[19,38]	25[19.0,37]	27[20.5,45.5]	0.19
Total bilirubin (mg/dL)	0.66±0.24	0.67±0.24	0.64±0.22	0.58
Albumin (g/dL)	4.6±0.54	4.6±0.57	4.6±0.36	0.79
Alkaline phosphatase (IU/L)	629.5[481,790]	626[481,771]	714[471.5,857.5]	0.28
Platelet count (10^9/L)	295.5[261,343]	296.5[263,348]	289.5[241,332]	0.16
HOMA-IR	2.2[1.4,3.2]	2.1[1.4,3.1]	2.6[1.7,3.5]	0.051

Values presented as Mean ± SD, Median [P25, P75], or N (column %).
P-values: a = ANOVA, b = Kruskal-Wallis test, c = Pearson's chi-square test. P-values in bold are statistically significant.

compared to fibrosis stage 0–2, 6±1.5 and 3.5±1.5, respectively; p value <0.001).

Adult Noninvasive Fibrosis Scores in Children with NAFLD

Of the commonly used fibrosis scores shown in Table 3, APRI and FIB-4 index were found to be significantly higher in patients with advanced fibrosis (APRI values were 0.51 [0.39, 0.80] in children with advanced fibrosis and 0.40 [0.30, 0.55] in those without, p value = 0.001. FIB-4 index values were 0.26±0.15 and 0.32±0.14, respectively, p value = 0.037). Of note, these values for both APRI and FIB-4 index in children with advanced fibrosis were much lower than the proposed cutoff values to identify advanced fibrosis in adult patients with NAFLD (1.5 for APRI and 2.67 for FIB-4 index). More importantly, there was no difference in the AST/ALT ratio or the NFS between those with and without advanced fibrosis.

The Development of the Pediatric NAFLD Fibrosis Score (PNFS)

We performed a multivariable logistic regression analysis to build a model for prediction of advanced fibrosis using available clinical variables. The final proposed model consists of ALT, alkaline phosphatase, platelet count and GGT. The multivariable logistic regression model (z) for prediction of advanced fibrosis was defined as follows:

$$z = 1.1 + (0.34 \times \sqrt{ALT}) + (0.002 \times Alkaline Phosphatase) - (1.1 \times \log(Platelets)) - (0.02 \times GGT)$$

This value was then converted into a probability distribution (p) with a value between 0 to 100 by the following formula:

$$p = \left[\frac{e^z}{1+e^z}\right] \times 100$$

The mean PNFS for patients with stage 0–2 fibrosis was 13.2±10.1 compared to 24.7±18.7 for those with advanced fibrosis, p value <0.001, as shown in Figure 1.

The AUROC for the new PNFS model was 0.74 (95% CI: 0.66, 0.82) which was higher than the AUROC for APRI, NAFLD Fibrosis Score and FIB-4 Index (Figure 2). A cutoff of 26% would provide specificity, sensitivity, positive and negative predictive values of 92%, 31%, 41% and 88%, respectively, for predicting advanced fibrosis. The proportion of false positives would be 8% for the 26% cut off value (high specificity). On the other hand, a cutoff of 8% would provide specificity, sensitivity, positive and negative predictive values of 33%, 97%, 20% and 99%, respectively. The proportion of false negatives would be 3% for the 8% cutoff value (high sensitivity).

Internal validation of the model using bootstrapping showed an AUROC of 0.71 (Figure 3).

Table 2. Histological Features and NAFLD Activity Score.

Factor	Overall (N = 242)	Fibrosis stage 0–2 (N = 206)	Fibrosis stage 3–4 (N = 36)	p-value
Steatosis				*<0.001*
. <5%	2(0.83)	0(0.0)	2(5.6)	
. 5–33%	85(35.1)	85(41.3)	0(0.0)	
. 34–65%	80(33.1)	69(33.5)	11(30.6)	
. >=66%	75(31.0)	52(25.2)	23(63.9)	
Lobular inflammation				*<0.001*
. None	20(8.3)	20(9.7)	0(0.0)	
. <2 under 20x	166(68.6)	159(77.2)	7(19.4)	
. 2–4 under 20x	54(22.3)	25(12.1)	29(80.6)	
. >4 under 20x	2(0.83)	2(0.97)	0(0.0)	
Portal inflammation				***0.030***
. None	90(37.2)	81(39.3)	9(25.0)	
. Mild	134(55.4)	113(54.9)	21(58.3)	
. More than mild	18(7.4)	12(5.8)	6(16.7)	
Ballooning				*<0.001*
. None	121(50.4)	118(57.8)	3(8.3)	
. Few	46(19.2)	39(19.1)	7(19.4)	
. Many	73(30.4)	47(23.0)	26(72.2)	
NAS	3.9±1.8	3.5±1.5	6.0±1.5	*<0.001*

Values presented as Mean ± SD, or N (column %).
P-values in bold are statistically significant.

An online calculator was developed to allow for increased ease of utilizing PNFS in pediatric patients with NAFLD. This calculator can be found at:

http://www.r-calc.com/calculator.aspx?calculator_id=JYAVKOWT.

In Table 4, two study patient examples (with and without biopsy proven advanced fibrosis) are provided to reflect the implementation of PNFS to assess for the probability of having advanced fibrosis.

Discussion

As the prevalence of pediatric NAFLD continues to remain high especially among obese children, the development of reliable and simple scoring systems that can predict the presence of advanced disease is crucial. The main findings of this large study in children with biopsy-proven NAFLD are that: (1) simple noninvasive scores that have been validated to predict advanced fibrosis in adult patients with NAFLD are not accurate in children, (2) the newly developed PNFS is more accurate than APRI, FIB-4 index or NFS for predicting the presence of advanced fibrosis in children with fatty liver disease and may become a useful tool to determine patients that need more intensive evaluation and management.

NAFLD represents a disease spectrum that ranges from simple steatosis to non-alcoholic steatohepatitis (NASH), to advanced fibrosis and ultimately cirrhosis [24]. The presence and stage of fibrosis is considered an important factor in the prognosis of NAFLD and the prediction of the risk of developing cirrhosis [25]. Studies on natural history of pediatric NAFLD showed that fibrosis can progress to cirrhosis and its feared complications during childhood [3]. Therefore this brings the necessity of early diagnosis of advanced fibrosis in NAFLD to light as that can play an important role in preventing development of further compli-

Table 3. Adult Noninvasive Fibrosis Scores in Children with NAFLD.

Score	Overall (N = 242)	Fibrosis stage 0–2 (N = 206)	Fibrosis stage 3–4 (N = 36)	p-value
AST/ALT ratio	0.65[0.52,0.87]	0.66[0.54,0.88]	0.55[0.47,0.79]	0.059
APRI	0.41[0.30,0.56]	0.40[0.30,0.55]	0.51[0.39,0.80]	**0.001**
NAFLD Fibrosis Score	−4.6±1.3	−4.7±1.4	−4.3±1.2	0.14
FIB-4 Index	0.27±0.15	0.26±0.15	0.32±0.14	**0.037**
PNFS	14.9±12.5	13.2±10.1	24.7±18.7	**<0.001**

Values presented as Mean ± SD or Median [P25, P75].
P-values in bold are statistically significant.

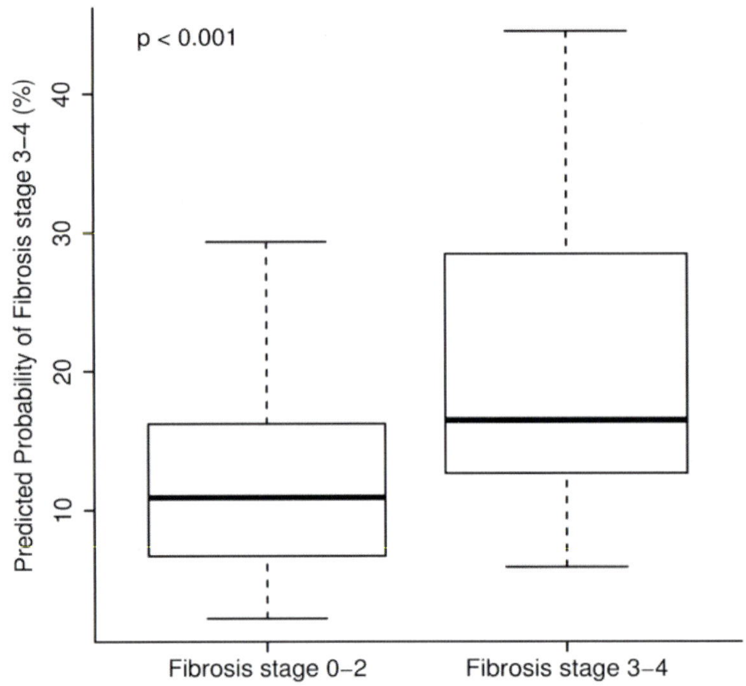

Figure 1. Pediatric NAFLD Fibrosis Score Values are significantly higher in children with advanced fibrosis. The lower boundary of the box-and-whisker plot corresponds to the 25th percentile, the line within the box to the median, and the upper boundary of the box to the 75th percentile. The whiskers extend to the most extreme data point which is no more than 1.5 times the interquartile range from the box.

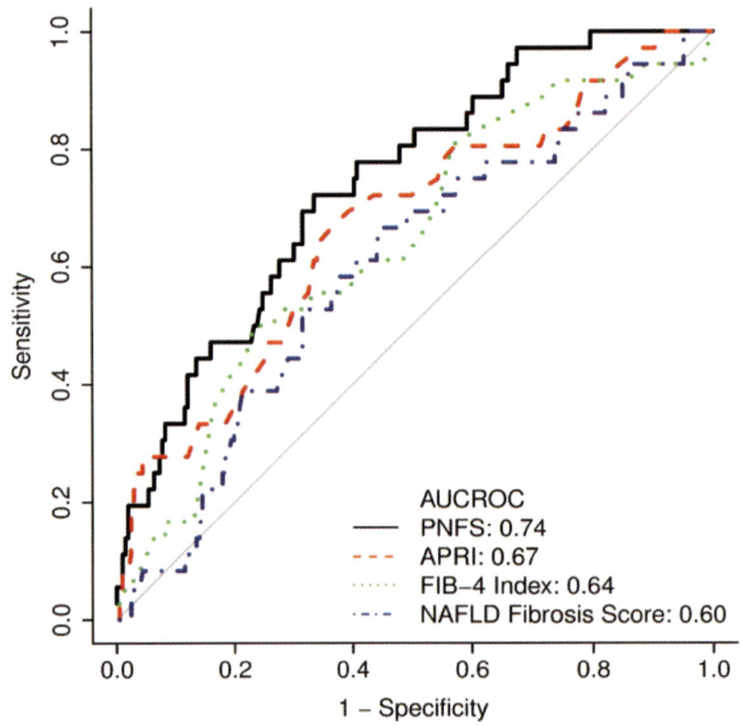

Figure 2. Performance characteristics of the Pediatric NAFLD Fibrosis Score (PNFS) in comparison to APRI, FIB-4, and NFS. The new model (PNFS) was more accurate for predicting advanced fibrosis than APRI, FIB-4 index and NAFLD fibrosis score as assessed by the area under the ROC curve (AUROC).

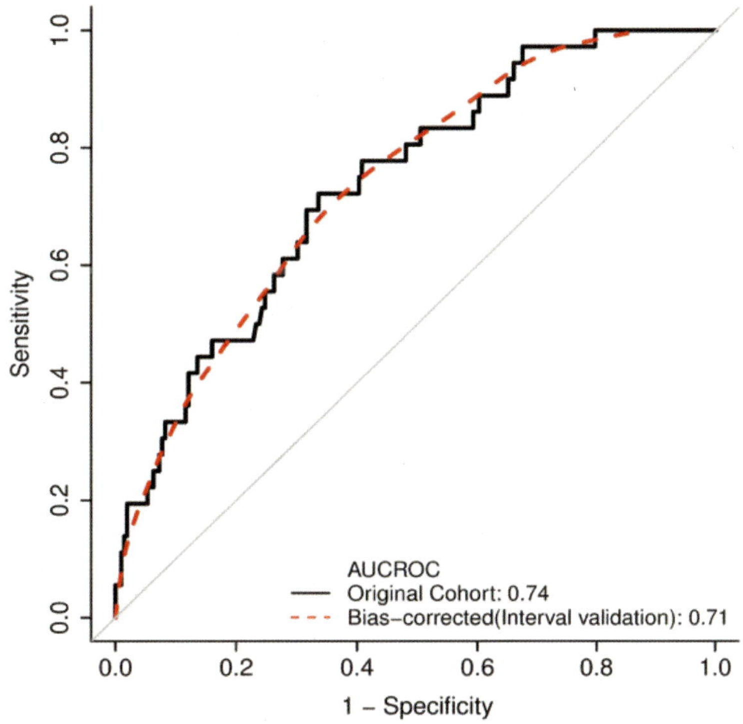

Figure 3. Bootstrap Validation of the Proposed PNFS Model. Internal validation of the model using bootstrapping showed an area under the ROC curve (AUROC) of 0.71.

cations [26]. The gold standard of diagnosis remains percutaneous liver biopsy which is not only a costly procedure but is invasive with high risk of complications and sampling error [27]. Several fibrosis scores have been developed and validated to predict advanced fibrosis in large studies on adults with NAFLD. In fact, the NFS was recommended as a clinically useful tool for identifying NAFLD patients with higher likelihood of having bridging fibrosis and/or cirrhosis by the recent practice guidelines endorsed by all the major gastroenterology and hepatology societies in the United States [4]. Furthermore, recent data demonstrated that these simple scoring systems can predict long-term outcomes of adult patients with NAFLD including liver-related complications and death with the best indicator being the NFS followed by APRI and FIB-4 scores [28]. However, none of these scores has been developed or validated in children with NAFLD. To date, only one fibrosis score has been developed by our group for children with NAFLD, namely the Pediatric NAFLD Fibrosis Index (PNFI) [29]. Due to the fact that the majority of children in the original PNFI cohort had only mild fibrosis (stage 1) and none had cirrhosis, we could not develop a predictor of advanced fibrosis. A recent study from South Korea that included 77 children with biopsy-proven NAFLD showed that the PNFI did not perform well for predicting significant fibrosis [6].

The ability of the new PNFS to separate children with advanced fibrosis may be explained by some of the variables included in the score. Low platelet count indicates more advanced liver disease and portal hypertension. ALT level is a surrogate for necroinflammatory activity and may server as a proxy for disease activity. Interestingly, alkaline phosphatase and GGT levels correlated with the presence of advanced fibrosis and further investigations are warranted to explain this phenomenon. If validated externally, PNFS may become a useful tool to rule in the presence of advanced fibrosis in children referred to large centers for management of fatty liver disease. By using a cutoff value that maximizes specificity, we propose that children with PNFS values above that cutoff should undergo a liver biopsy to confirm the presence of advanced fibrosis. This will minimize the number of children with no advanced fibrosis that will undergo liver biopsy. These children with mild disease do not need more aggressive monitoring for liver related morbidities during childhood and they should be encouraged to maintain a healthy lifestyle and lose weight if indicated. On the other hand, if the biopsy confirms the presence of advanced fibrosis in children with high PNFS, they should be monitored closely for the development of cirrhosis, complications of portal hypertension and potentially hepatocellular carcinoma.

Table 4. Utilization of the PNFS in Two Patients with and without Advanced Fibrosis.

	ALT	Alkaline Phosphatase	Platelet Count	GGT	Probability	Fibrosis
Patient One	280	845	180	50	77.1	Fibrosis 3–4
Patient Two	28	652	343	15	5.0	Fibrosis 0–2

We recognize that our study has several limitations, mainly related to selection bias and the fact that our study consisted of children followed at a tertiary hospital specialized in pediatric hepatology which may provide a skewed representation of the true prevalence of advanced fibrosis. Most of our children were white, making it difficult to determine the utility of PNFS among other ethnic groups. External cross-validation is needed before PNFS can be used to predict advanced fibrosis in children with NAFLD.

This study has several strengths including the large number of children with biopsy-proven NAFLD with adequate samples for interpretation by pathologist. Sampling issues associated with the quality of liver biopsies were excluded by not including any biopsy that was fragmented, <15 mm in length or had <6 portal tracts. The inclusion of a large number of children with advanced fibrosis (including two patients with cirrhosis) represents another unique strength of this study.

In conclusion, we have demonstrated clearly that noninvasive hepatic fibrosis scores developed in adults had poor performance in diagnosing advanced fibrosis in children with NAFLD. We have developed a new pediatric specific score called the PNFS, with improved performance characteristics. PNFS may help clinicians select children with NAFLD who are at high risk for advanced disease to undergo liver biopsy and more aggressive monitoring. The score must be validated in other populations before it can be recommended for this purpose.

Author Contributions

Conceived and designed the experiments: NA SM PG DL RL VN. Performed the experiments: NA SM PG DL RL VN. Analyzed the data: NA SM PG DL RL VN. Contributed to the writing of the manuscript: NA SM PG DL RL VN.

References

1. Chan DF, Li AM, Chu WC, Chan MH, Wong EM, et al. (2004) Hepatic steatosis in obese Chinese children. Int J Obes Relat Metab Disord 28: 1257–1263.
2. Schwimmer JB, Deutsch R, Kahen T, Lavine JE, Stanley C, et al. (2006) Prevalence of fatty liver in children and adolescents. Pediatrics 118: 1388–1393.
3. Feldstein AE, Charatcharoenwitthaya P, Treeprasertsuk S, Benson JT, Enders FB, et al. (2009) The natural history of non-alcoholic fatty liver disease in children: a follow-up study for up to 20 years. Gut 58: 1538–1544.
4. Chalasani N, Younossi Z, Lavine JE, Diehl AM, Brunt EM, et al. (2012) The diagnosis and management of non-alcoholic fatty liver disease: Practice Guideline by the American Association for the Study of Liver Diseases, American College of Gastroenterology, and the American Gastroenterological Association. Hepatology 55: 2005–2023.
5. Alkhouri N, McCullough A (2012) Noninvasive Diagnosis of NASH and Liver Fibrosis Within the Spectrum of NAFLD. Gastroenterology and Hepatology 8: 661–668.
6. Yang HR, Kim HR, Kim MJ, Ko JS, Seo JK (2012) Noninvasive parameters and hepatic fibrosis scores in children with nonalcoholic fatty liver disease. World J Gastroenterol 18: 1525–1530.
7. Mansoor S, Yerian L, Lopez R, Kohli R, Xanthakos S, et al. (2013) The Evaluation of Hepatic Fibrosis Scores in Children with Nonalcoholic Fatty Liver Disease. Am J Gastroenterol 108: Abstrac 2055.
8. Nobili V, Manco M, Devito R, Ciampalini P, Piemonte F, et al. (2006) Effect of vitamin E on aminotransferase levels and insulin resistance in children with non-alcoholic fatty liver disease. Aliment Pharmacol Ther 24: 1553–1561.
9. Manco M, Nobili V (2008) Intensive treatment and dietary fats in adolescents with nonalcoholic fatty liver disease. J Pediatr Gastroenterol Nutr 46: 224.
10. Kuczmarski RJ, Ogden CL, Grummer-Strawn LM, Flegal KM, Guo SS, et al. (2000) CDC growth charts: United States. Adv Data 314: 1–27.
11. Cole TJ, Bellizzi MC, Flegal KM, Dietz WH (2000) Establishing a standard definition for child overweight and obesity worldwide: international survey. Bmj 320: 1240–1243.
12. Boney CM, Verma A, Tucker R, Vohr BR (2005) Metabolic syndrome in childhood: association with birth weight, maternal obesity, and gestational diabetes mellitus. Pediatrics 115: e290–296.
13. Fernandez JR, Redden DT, Pietrobelli A, Allison DB (2004) Waist circumference percentiles in nationally representative samples of African-American, European-American, and Mexican-American children and adolescents. J Pediatr 145: 439–444.
14. (1992) American Academy of Pediatrics. National Cholesterol Education Program: Report of the Expert Panel on Blood Cholesterol Levels in Children and Adolescents. Pediatrics 89: 525–584.
15. (1987) Report of the Second Task Force on Blood Pressure Control in Children–1987. Task Force on Blood Pressure Control in Children. National Heart, Lung, and Blood Institute, Bethesda, Maryland. Pediatrics 79: 1–25.
16. Genuth S, Alberti KG, Bennett P, Buse J, Defronzo R, et al. (2003) Follow-up report on the diagnosis of diabetes mellitus. Diabetes Care 26: 3160–3167.
17. Matthews DR, Hosker JP, Rudenski AS, Naylor BA, Treacher DF, et al. (1985) Homeostasis model assessment: insulin resistance and beta-cell function from fasting plasma glucose and insulin concentrations in man. Diabetologia 28: 412–419.
18. Poynard T, Halfon P, Castera L, Charlotte F, Le Bail B, et al. (2007) Variability of the area under the receiver operating characteristic curves in the diagnostic evaluation of liver fibrosis markers: impact of biopsy length and fragmentation. Aliment Pharmacol Ther 25: 733–739.
19. Kleiner DE, Brunt EM, Van Natta M, Behling C, Contos MJ, et al. (2005) Design and validation of a histological scoring system for nonalcoholic fatty liver disease. Hepatology 41: 1313–1321.
20. Wai CT, Greenson JK, Fontana RJ, Kalbfleisch JD, Marrero JA, et al. (2003) A simple noninvasive index can predict both significant fibrosis and cirrhosis in patients with chronic hepatitis C. Hepatology 38: 518–526.
21. Sterling RK, Lissen E, Clumeck N, Sola R, Correa MC, et al. (2006) Development of a simple noninvasive index to predict significant fibrosis in patients with HIV/HCV coinfection. Hepatology 43: 1317–1325.
22. Angulo P, Hui JM, Marchesini G, Bugianesi E, George J, et al. (2007) The NAFLD fibrosis score: a noninvasive system that identifies liver fibrosis in patients with NAFLD. Hepatology 45: 846–854.
23. Harrell FE, Jr., Califf RM, Pryor DB, Lee KL, Rosati RA (1982) Evaluating the yield of medical tests. Jama 247: 2543–2546.
24. Aggarwal A, Puri K, Thangada S, Zein N, Alkhouri N (2013) Nonalcoholic Fatty Liver Disease In Children: Recent Practice Guidelines, Where Do They Take Us?. Current Pediatric Reviews Volume 9, 4 Issues: E-Pub Ahead of Print.
25. Angulo P (2010) Long-term mortality in nonalcoholic fatty liver disease: is liver histology of any prognostic significance? Hepatology 51: 373–375.
26. Nobili V, Marcellini M, Devito R, Ciampalini P, Piemonte F, et al. (2006) NAFLD in children: a prospective clinical-pathological study and effect of lifestyle advice. Hepatology 44: 458–465.
27. Bravo AA, Sheth SG, Chopra S (2001) Liver biopsy. N Engl J Med 344: 495–500.
28. Angulo P, Bugianesi E, Bjornsson ES, Charatcharoenwitthaya P, Mills PR, et al. (2013) Simple noninvasive systems predict long-term outcomes of patients with nonalcoholic fatty liver disease. Gastroenterology 145: 782–789 e784.
29. Nobili V, Alisi A, Vania A, Tiribelli C, Pietrobattista A, et al. (2009) The pediatric NAFLD fibrosis index: a predictor of liver fibrosis in children with non-alcoholic fatty liver disease. BMC Med 7: 21.

16

The Diagnostic Value of the FIB-4 Index for Staging Hepatitis B-Related Fibrosis: A Meta-Analysis

Yuanyuan Li, Yu Chen*, Ying Zhao

Department of Laboratory Medicine, The First Affiliated Hospital of the Medical College, Zhejiang University, Hangzhou, China

Abstract

Background: Liver fibrosis stage is an important factor in determining prognosis and need for treatment in patients infected with hepatitis B virus (HBV). Liver biopsies are typically used to assess liver fibrosis; however, noninvasive alternatives such as the FIB-4 index have also been developed.

Aims: To quantify the accuracy of the FIB-4 index in the diagnosis of HBV related fibrosis and cirrhosis.

Methods: A meta-analysis of studies comparing the diagnostic accuracy of the FIB-4 index vs. liver biopsy in HBV-infected patients was performed using studies retrieved from the following databases: PubMed, Ovid, EMBASE, the Cochrane Library, the Chinese National Knowledge Infrastructure and the Chinese Biology Medicine disc. A hierarchical summary receiver operating curves model and bivariate model were used to produce summary receiver operating characteristic curves and pooled estimates of sensitivity and specificity. The heterogeneity was explored with meta-regression analysis. Publication bias was detected using Egger's test and the trim and fill method.

Results: 12 studies ($N = 1,908$) and 10 studies ($N = 2,105$) were included in the meta-analysis for significant fibrosis and cirrhosis, respectively. For significant fibrosis, the area under the hierarchical summary receiver operating curve (AUHSROC) was 0.78 (95% CI = 0.74–0.81). The recommended cutoff value was between 1.45 and 1.62, and the AUHSROC, summary sensitivity and specificity were 0.78 (95% CI = 0.74–0.81), 0.65 (95% CI = 0.56–0.73) and 0.77 (95% CI = 0.7–0.83), respectively. For cirrhosis, the AUHSROC was 0.89 (95% CI = 0.85–0.91). The recommended cutoff value was between 2.9 and 3.6, and the AUHSROC, summary sensitivity and specificity were 0.96 (95% CI = 0.92–1.00), 0.42 (95% CI = 0.36–0.48) and 0.96 (95% CI = 0.95–0.97), respectively. No publication bias was detected.

Conclusions: The FIB-4 index is valuable for detecting significant fibrosis and cirrhosis in HBV-infected patients, but has suboptimal accuracy in excluding fibrosis and cirrhosis.

Editor: Robert Lane Schmidt, University of Utah School of Medicine, United States of America

Funding: The authors have no support or funding to report.

* Email: yuchenyuchen666@126.com

Introduction

An accurate assessment of liver fibrosis in patients with hepatitis virus B (HBV) infection is essential not only in determining whether and when to initiate antiviral therapy, but also in predicting long-term clinical prognosis [1–3]. For example, with regard to antiviral therapy, it is known that maintenance of viral suppression can reduce liver-related complications in chronic hepatitis B (CHB) patients [1–3]. Furthermore, assessing prognosis in patients with cirrhosis is required to closely follow the potential development of hepatocellular carcinoma and other complications [2,4].

To date, liver biopsy remains the gold standard for assessing liver fibrosis; however, it does have some limitations. The invasive nature of the biopsy is associated with patient discomfort, and can cause rare but important complications [5]. Furthermore, its accuracy is affected by sampling error and variability in pathological interpretation [6,7], and the dynamic process of liver fibrosis related to disease progression and regression cannot be easily quantified. An ideal diagnostic index should be accurate, noninvasive, inexpensive, convenient and readily available. The limitations of the liver biopsy have lead many clinicians to develop noninvasive indexes, and most attention has been focused on whether noninvasive indexes can detect the presence or absence of significant fibrosis (i.e., ≥F2), severe fibrosis (i.e., ≥F3) and cirrhosis (i.e., ≥F4) according to the METAVIR histological score [8].

Currently, there are several categories of non-invasive indexes. Measures of hyaluronic acid, collagen, laminin and YKL-40 are direct laboratory indexes, but these are usually not routinely available. Indirect laboratory indexes are calculated from routine laboratory data, and include the aspartate aminotransferase (AST) to alanine aminotransferase (ALT) ratio (AAR), the AST to platelet (PLT) ratio index (APRI), the cirrhosis discriminant score

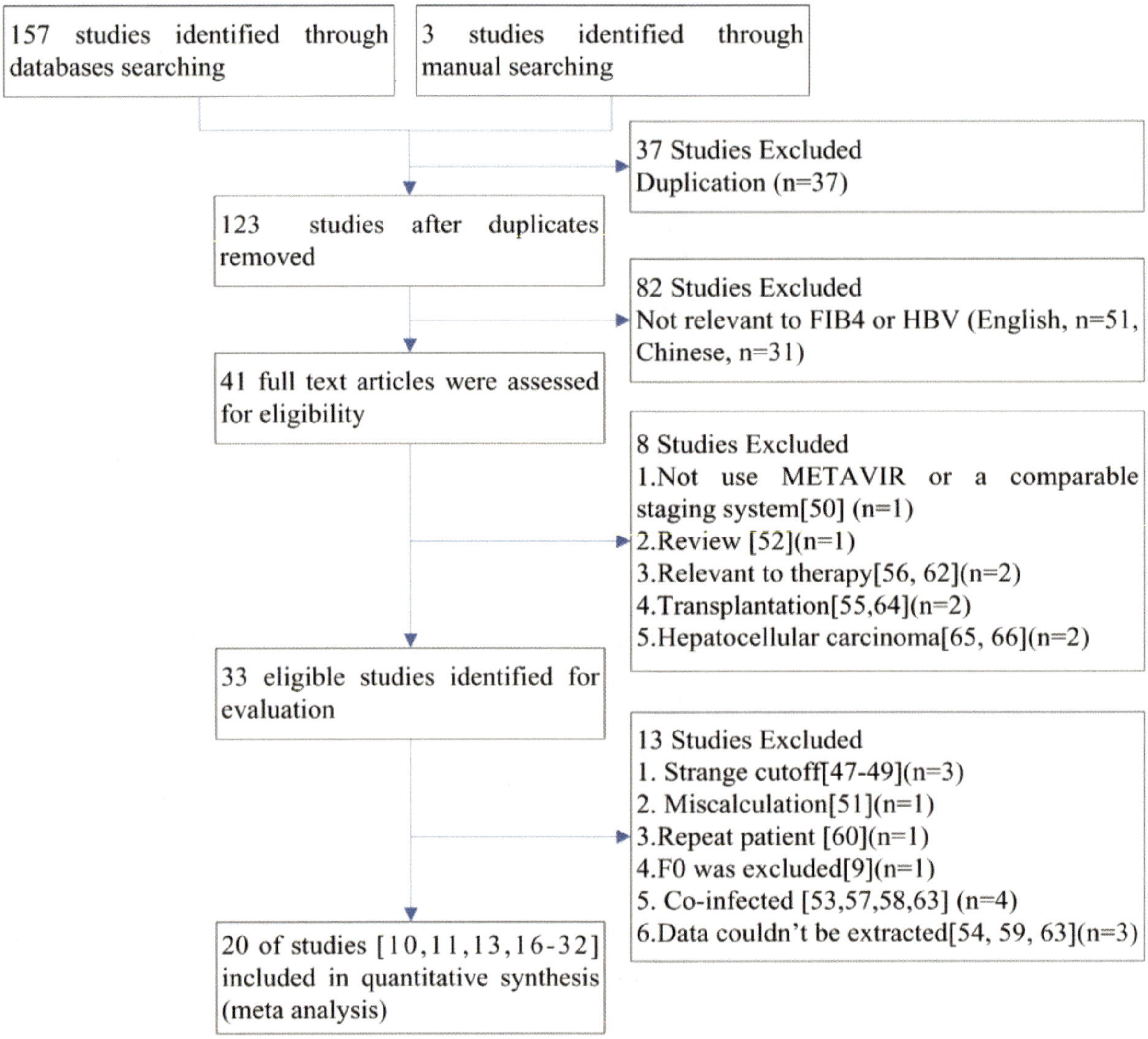

Figure 1. Flow chart of article selection.

(CDS), the age-PLT index (API), the FIB-4 index (see below), Lok's model and the red cell distribution width (RDW) to platelet ratio [9–11]. While some of the calculations for these indexes are simple and accessible, some are more complex [11]. Assessment of these indexes has been reviewed and found to vary from bad to excellent [9,11]; however, relevant systematic reviews in the context of HBV are rare. Thus, no current index has satisfied all the standards of the ideal diagnostic index [12].

The FIB-4 index is calculated using the formula: FIB-4 = Age (years) × AST (U/L)/[PLT(10^9/L) × ALT$^{1/2}$ (U/L)]. The theoretical basis for this index has been previously described [13], and adheres to the following logic: (1) age is considered to be relevant to disease duration and is associated with more severe fibrosis; (2) elevations in AST more than ALT has been related to both delayed clearance of AST relative to ALT, and to the mitochondrial injury associated with more advanced fibrosis; (3) thrombocytopenia has been associated with the progression of fibrosis and worsening portal hypertension that not only destroys platelets by sequestration in the enlarged spleen, but also decreases the production of thrombopoietin by hepatocytes. Based on these foundations, the FIB-4 index was first applied to assess hepatic fibrosis in the context of human immunodeficiency virus (HIV) and hepatitis C virus (HCV) infection [14,15].

The diagnostic value of the FIB-4 index is attractive because measures of AST, ALT and PLT are routine and inexpensive tests in the clinical laboratory, and the calculation is simple. Numerous studies have assessed the diagnostic performance of the FIB-4 index in HBV-related fibrosis and cirrhosis [10,11,13,16–32], with several showing that the FIB-4 index was superior in comparison to other non-invasive indexes [9,13,16]. Despite the benefit shown by these studies, the utility of the FIB-4 index remains controversial. Thus, the aim of the current study was to perform a meta-analysis of diagnostic tests for predicting the accuracy of the FIB-4 index in predicting significant fibrosis (F2–F4 vs. F0–F1), severe fibrosis (F3–F4 vs. F0–F2) and cirrhosis (F4 vs. F0–F3) in patients with HBV infection.

Materials and Methods

Ethics statement

The data of this meta-analysis was extracted from published studies. So the data were analyzed anonymously.

Table 1. Characteristics of studies eligible for meta-analysis.

Author, Year, Region	Number (male%)	Age (years)	Interval Between Biopsy and FIB-4	Liver Biopsy Scoring system	Liver Biopsy Length	Blinded
Chen[10], 2013, China	148 (66%)	40.36±11.2	≤7d	Metavir	>15 mm	Yes
Kim[13], 2010, Korea	668 (66%)	39.1±14.8	≤2d	Batts and Ludwig	>15 mm	Yes
Zhu[29], 2012, China	159 (71%)	42 (18~62)	unclear	METAVIR	≥15 mm	unclear
Ucar[18], 2013, Turkey	73 (64%)	42.81±12.86	unclear	METAVIR	unclear	Yes
Gong[21], 2013, China	41 (73%)	50.8±10.3	unclear	METAVIR	unclear	unclear
Wang[20], 2013, China	231 (68%)	34.1±9.8	<1d	Scheuer	>15 mm	Yes
Ji[17], 2011, China	313 (69%)	35.6±11.2	1d	METAVIR	20 mm	unclear
Başar[25], 2013, Turkey	76 (55%)	unclear	<1d	METAVIR	>10 mm	Yes
Bonnard[19], 2010, France	59 (68%)	35±9	0.5–10 m	METAVIR	21±6 mm	Yes
Erdogan[11], 2013, Turkey	221 (63%)	43.68±12.56	≤1d	Ishak	unclear	Yes
Wu[30], 2010, China	78 (85%)	32.6±12.3	unclear	METAVIR	>15 mm	unclear
Mallet[16], 2009, France	138 (71%)	42±15	<1d	METAVIR	17.6±6.8	unclear
Seto[24], 2011, China	237 (68%)	38.2 (18~63)	same time	Ishak	≥15 mm	Yes
Zhu[27], 2011, China	175 (78%)	36.5±9.4	≤7d	METAVIR	>15 mm	Yes
Liu[23], 2012, China	114 (80%)	38.32±11.36	same time	METAVIR	15~20 mm	unclear
Wang[26], 2013, China	149 (93%)	37 (30~42)	≤2d	Scheuer	>10 mm	Yes
Xun[28], 2013, China	197 (76%)	31 (21–45)	same time	Scheuer	>15 mm	unclear
Zhang[32], 2009, China	86 (60%)	39 (16-64)	<1d	METAVIR	15~20 mm	unclear
Zhang[22], 2012, China	361 (62%)	36±11	≤7d	Scheuer	unclear	unclear
Zhang[31], 2010, China	212 (88%)	31±7	1day	Scheuer	20 mm	Yes

Literature and search strategy

The following databases were searched without the use of time limitations: PubMed, Ovid, EMBASE, the Cochrane Library, the Chinese National Knowledge Infrastructure (CNKI) and the Chinese Biology Medicine disc (CBMdisc). The search strategy to identify all relevant articles involved the use of the following key words: FIB-4, aspartate aminotransferase, AST, alanine aminotransferase, ALT, platelet, PLT, hepatitis B, fibrosis and cirrhosis. For example, File S1 and S2 displayed the search strategy of Ovid and PubMed respectively. Additional studies were identified via a manual review of the reference lists of identified studies and review articles. This literature search was performed in November 2013.

Inclusion criteria

Studies were deemed eligible if they met the following inclusion criteria: 1) the study evaluated the performance of the FIB-4 index for the diagnosis of fibrosis in mono-HBV-infected patients before antiviral therapy. Studies including patients with other causes of liver disease were included if data of HBV-infected patients could be extracted. 2) Liver biopsy was used as the reference standard for assessing fibrosis. METAVIR [8] or comparable staging systems

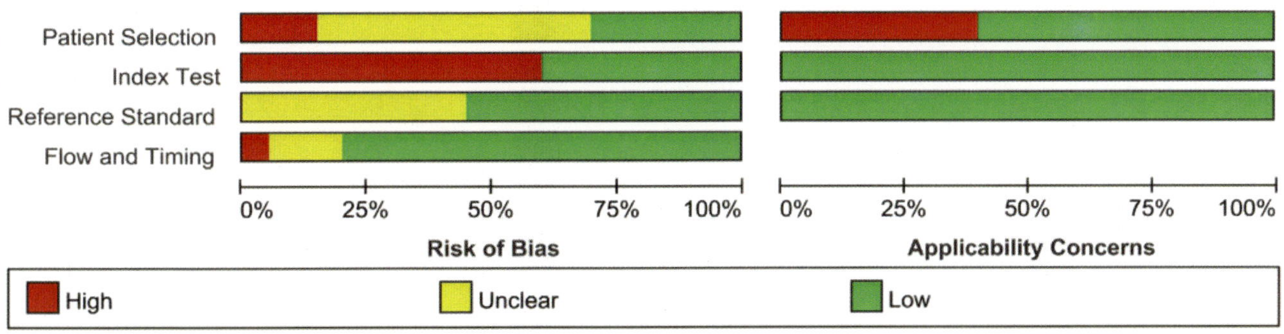

Figure 2. Methodological quality graph. Summary of methodological quality of studies according to Quality Assessment of Diagnostic Accuracy Studies-2 (QUADAS-2) tool concerning risk of bias and applicability in review authors' judgments about each domain for each included study and review authors' judgments about each domain, presented as percentages across included studies.

Table 2. The diagnostic performance of the FIB-4 index for detecting significant fibrosis, severe fibrosis and cirrhosis.

Study characteristics	Number of studies	Summary estimates (95% CI)			Likelihood ratio (95% CI)		AUHSROC (95% CI)
		Sensitivity	Specificity	DOR	PLR	NLR	
Significant fibrosis							
All	12	0.71 (0.64–0.77)	0.73 (0.67–0.78)	6.52 (4.53–9.39)	2.61 (2.12–3.21)	0.4 (0.32 to 0.49)	0.78 (0.74–0.81)
Exclude improper spectrum^Δ^	7	0.73 (0.63–0.81)	0.79 (0.73–0.84)	10.31 (6.52–16.30)	3.52 (2.75–4.51)	0.341 (0.25–0.47)	0.83 (0.80–0.86)
Blindness*	7	0.68 (0.61–0.74)	0.68 (0.61–0.73)	4.39 (3.3–5.82)	2.09 (1.78–2.45)	0.48 (0.40–0.57)	0.73 (0.69–0.77)
Non blindness	5	0.75 (0.62–0.84)	0.78 (0.69–0.85)	10.74 (5.60–20.59)	3.45 (2.39–4.98)	0.32 (0.21–0.49)	0.83 (0.80–0.86)
Proper interval※	8	0.69 (0.62–0.75)	0.71 (0.64–0.78)	5.39 (4.02–7.22)	2.38 (1.95–2.90)	0.44 (0.37–0.52)	0.76 (0.72–0.79)
Improper interval	4	0.76 (0.64–0.84)	0.75 (0.63–0.84)	9.45 (4.02–22.2)	3.04 (1.92–4.83)	0.32 (0.20–0.51)	0.82 (0.78–0.85)
Exclude repeat patient#	11	0.69 (0.63–0.75)	0.73 (0.66–0.79)	6.09 (4.23–8.76)	2.56 (2.06–3.19)	0.42 (0.35–0.51)	0.77 (0.73–0.81)
Severe fibrosis							
All	6	0.76 (0.64–0.85)	0.74 (0.70–0.79)	9.14 (5.35–15.60)	2.96 (2.48–3.53)	0.32 (0.21–0.49)	0.79 (0.75–82)
Exclude improper spectrum^Δ^	5	0.79 (0.67–0.87)	0.72 (0.68–0.75)	9.17 (4.91–17.1)	2.76 (2.28–3.33)	0.3 (0.19–0.48)	0.73 (0.69–0.77)
Blindness*	5	0.76 (0.62–0.86)	0.75 (0.70–0.79)	9.54 (5.18–17.58)	3.03 (2.50–3.68)	0.32 (0.19–0.52)	0.79 (0.76–0.83)
Cirrhosis							
All	10	0.83 (0.78–0.88)	0.80 (0.73–0.86)	20.64 (11.54–36.93)	4.26 (3.04–5.96)	0.21 (0.15–0.28)	0.89 (0.85–0.91)
Exclude improper spectrum^Δ^	6	0.85 (0.80–0.89)	0.77 (0.7–0.83)	19.10 (10.41–35.03)	3.75 (2.72–5.16)	0.2 (0.14–0.27)	0.88 (0.85–0.91)
Blindness*	5	0.80 (0.7–0.87)	0.77 (0.72–0.82)	13.25 (6.5–27.05)	3.48 (2.59–4.69)	0.26 (0.17–0.41)	0.85 (0.81–0.88)
Non blindness	5	0.85 (0.80–0.90)	0.85 (0.72–0.92)	32.53 (14.48–73.08)	5.6 (3–10.57)	0.17 (0.12–0.25)	0.87 (0.84–0.90)
Proper interval※	8	0.83 (0.77–0.88)	0.80 (0.72–0.86)	20.04 (10.32–38.92)	4.18 (2.9–6.04)	0.21 (0.15–0.30)	0.88 (0.85–0.91)
Exclude repeat patient#	9	0.83 (0.77–0.88)	0.82 (0.75–0.87)	21.93 (11.75–40.95)	4.52 (3.15–6.47)	0.21 (0.15–0.29)	0.89 (0.86–0.91)

ΔThe disease spectrum of some studies [11,17,19–21,24,26–28] were not in good accordance with our study, thus they were excluded for sensitivity analysis.
*The studies in which the reference standard results were interpreted without knowledge of the results of the index tests, were grouped into "Blindness".
※The "proper interval" was defined as the time interval between the determination of the FIB-4 index and liver biopsy was no longer than 7 days.
#As two studies [22,32] were written by the same author, the study [32] with the smaller sample size was excluded for sensitivity analysis. 95% CI: 95% confidence interval. DOR: diagnostic odds ratio. PLR: positive likelihood ratio; NLR: negative likelihood ratio. AUHSROC: area under the hierarchical summary receiver operating characteristic curve.

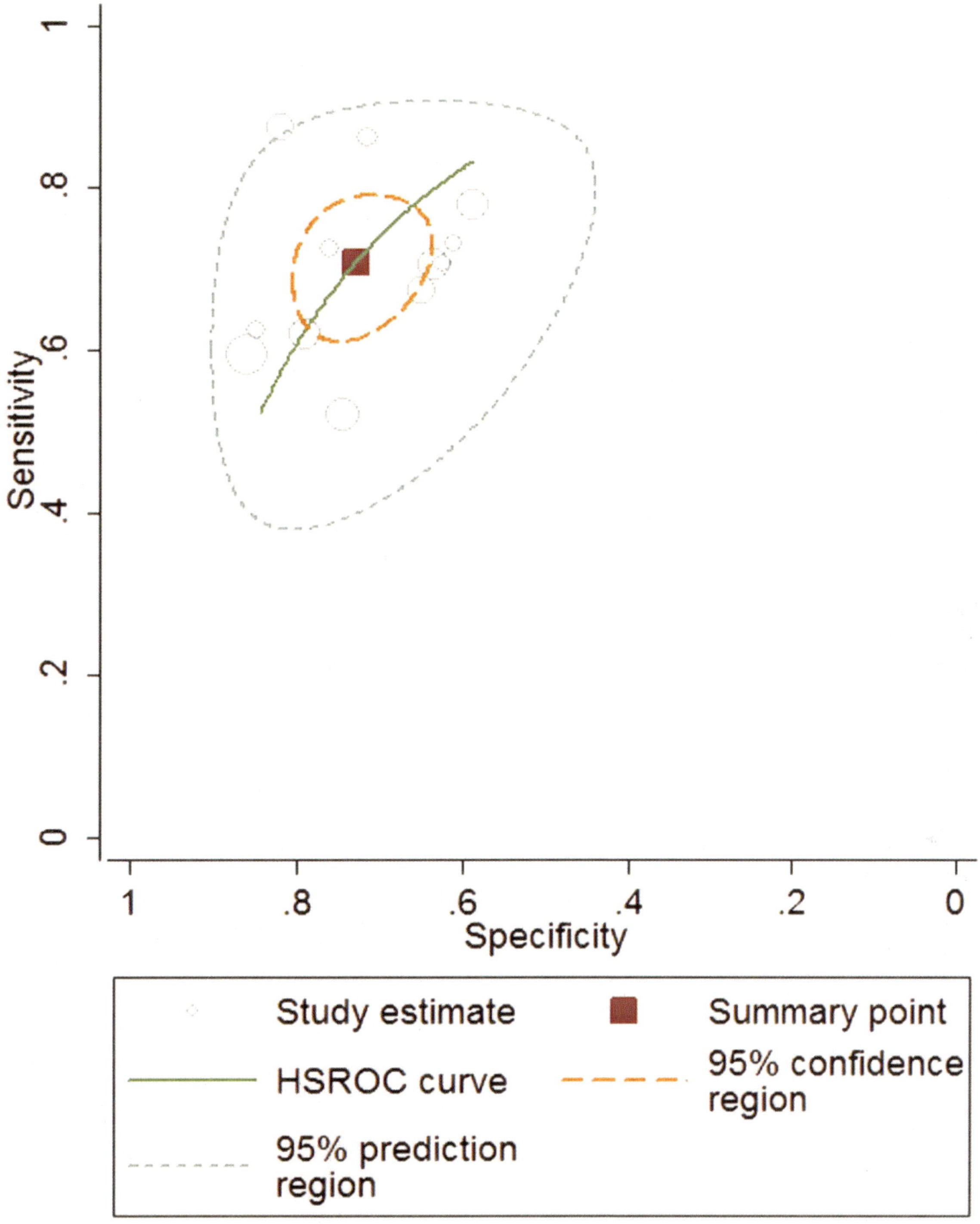

Figure 3. The hierarchical summary receiver operating characteristic (HSROC) curve of FIB-4 index for predicting significant fibrosis. The size of circles indicates the weight of the individual studies. The marked point on the curve represents the summary sensitivity and specificity. The area delimited by dashed line represents 95% confidence interval of the summary estimate. The area delimited by the dots represents the 95% prediction region, within which there is a 95%confidence that the true sensitivity and specificity of a future study should lie.

(i.e., Batts and Ludwig [33], Scheuer [34] or Ishak [35]) were applied to stage fibrosis. Significant fibrosis was defined as F≥2 for METAVIR, Batts and Ludwig, and Scheuer staging systems; or F≥3 for the Ishak system. Severe fibrosis was defined as F≥3 for METAVIR, Batts and Ludwig, and Scheuer staging systems. Cirrhosis was defined as F≥4 for METAVIR, Batts and Ludwig, and Scheuer staging systems; or F≥5 for the Ishak system. 3) Data could be extracted to allow the construction of at least one 2×2 table of test performance. 4) The study included more than 40

Study	TP	FP	FN	TN	Sensitivity (95% CI)	Specificity (95% CI)
Basar2013	37	6	14	19	0.73 [0.58, 0.84]	0.76 [0.55, 0.91]
Bonnard2010	30	7	11	11	0.73 [0.57, 0.86]	0.61 [0.36, 0.83]
Erdogan2013	53	63	15	90	0.78 [0.66, 0.87]	0.59 [0.51, 0.67]
Seto2011	40	41	37	119	0.52 [0.40, 0.63]	0.74 [0.67, 0.81]
Ucar2013	29	12	12	20	0.71 [0.54, 0.84]	0.63 [0.44, 0.79]
Wang Y2013	60	21	29	39	0.67 [0.57, 0.77]	0.65 [0.52, 0.77]
Wu2010	20	7	12	39	0.63 [0.44, 0.79]	0.85 [0.71, 0.94]
Xun2013	79	31	33	54	0.71 [0.61, 0.79]	0.64 [0.52, 0.74]
Zhang2009	50	8	8	20	0.86 [0.75, 0.94]	0.71 [0.51, 0.87]
Zhang2010	99	11	61	41	0.62 [0.54, 0.69]	0.79 [0.65, 0.89]
Zhang2012	143	17	98	103	0.59 [0.53, 0.66]	0.86 [0.78, 0.92]
Zhu2012	91	10	13	45	0.88 [0.80, 0.93]	0.82 [0.69, 0.91]

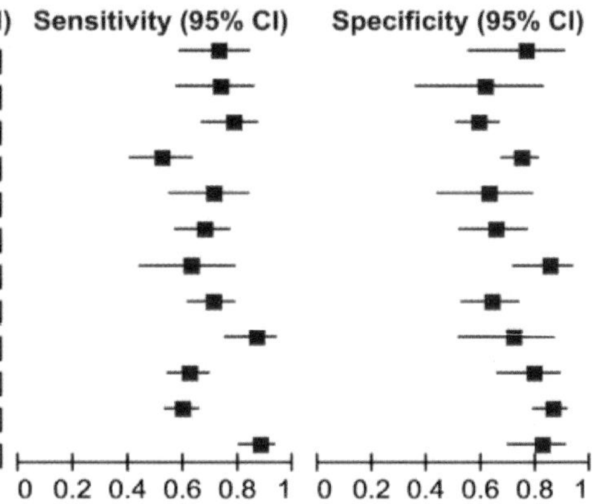

Figure 4. The forest plot of the FIB-4 index for predicting significant fibrosis.

patients; otherwise it was excluded because of low statistical power and poor reliability.

Quality assessment and data extraction

Two reviewers (Drs. Li and Zhao) independently evaluated the eligibility of each study according to the inclusion criteria described above, and assessed methodological quality according to the Quality Assessment of Diagnostic Accuracy Studies-2 (QUADAS-2) tool [36]. Discrepancies were resolved by consensus agreement. Note – some specific issues were defined before assessment, e.g. CHB was defined as hepatitis B surface antigen positive for more than 6 months. With regard to disease progression bias, the time interval between the determination of the FIB-4 index and liver biopsy was no longer than 7 days. As the FIB-4 index was calculated from four objective measures (ALT, AST, PLT and age), the item relating to blinding of the test interpreter to results of the reference standard was omitted. In addition to 2×2 tables of test performance, two kinds of data (patient related data and study related data) were also extracted. The patient related data included mean age, gender distribution, region and prevalence of the fibrosis stages. The study related data included sample size, interval time between determination of the FIB-4 index and liver biopsy, the size of liver biopsy, histological scoring system, blinded interpretation of the biopsy, and the cutoff value of the FIB-4. To avoid double counting of data, when multiple pairs of sensitivity or specificity were reported in one study, we consistently used the data with the highest Youden index (sensitivity + specificity-1) for meta-analysis [37], except for subgroup analysis based on different cutoff values.

Statistical analyses

For meta-analyses, a bivariate random effects model [38] was used to calculate summary estimates of sensitivity, specificity, positive likelihood ratio (PLR) and negative likelihood ratio (NLR), and to fit a hierarchical summary receiver-operating characteristic (HSROC) curve [39]. These models take into account potential threshold effects and the correlation between sensitivity and specificity. They also allow addition of covariates for investigation of potential sources of heterogeneity, thus are standard methods recommended for meta-analyses of diagnostic tests [40,41]. Additionally, the following guidelines have been suggested for interpretation of the area under the hierarchical summary receiver-operating characteristic curve (AUHSROC): an area of 1.0 indicates perfect discrimination, and 0.90 to 1.0 has been classified as excellent, 0.80 to less than 0.90 as good, 0.70 to less than 0.80 as fair, and less than 0.70 as poor [42,43].

Multiple sources of heterogeneity frequently exist in diagnostic studies. In addition to visual assessment with the use of the forest plots, we formally quantified the extent of heterogeneity by calculating the inconsistency index (I^2 statistics) [44]. Statistically significant heterogeneity was considered present at I^2>50%. To explore the source of heterogeneity, meta-regression and subgroup analysis were performed. The potential factors evaluated by meta-regression analysis were mean age of subjects, prevalence of fibrosis stages, disease spectrum, a consecutive or random sample enrollment, interval between FIB-4 index determination and liver biopsy, the liver blinded biopsy interpretation and a predefined cutoff value.

With respect to publication bias, the funnel plot is a basic and routine method for detecting biases, but it is subjective and qualitative. To counter these limitations, several quantitative methods such as Egger's test [45] and the trim and fill method [46] have been developed. Egger's test quantifies the degree of funnel plot asymmetry as measured by the intercept from regression of standard normal deviates against precision, but its capacity to detect bias is limited when meta-analyses are based on a limited number of small trials [45]. The trim and fill method is a nonparametric method for estimating the number of missing studies that might exist in a meta-analysis and the effect that these studies might have had on its outcome. This method also provides effective and relatively powerful tests for evaluating the existence of such publication bias [46]. To be cautious, the publication bias was assessed with two distinct methods. Statistical analyses were conducted using Review Manager 5.2 (The Cochrane Collaboration) and STATA 11.0 (Stata Corp., College Station, TX, USA), notably with the user-written 'midas' and 'metandi' programs for STATA.

Results

Search results

One hundred and sixty studies were retrieved based on the described search strategies. One hundred and forty studies [9,47–66] were excluded in accord with our exclusion criteria (Figure 1). Xu et al. defined cutoff values for the FIB-4 index as 223.70 for predicting significant fibrosis and 808.77 for cirrhosis [47], and Gumusay et al. reported that the average FIB-4 index for healthy controls was 11.7±5.8 [48]. These cutoff values were much larger

Table 3. Subgroup analysis based on different FIB-4 index cutoff values.

Thresholds	Number of studies	Summary estimates(95% CI)			Likelihood ratio (95%CI)		AUHSROC (95% CI)
		Sensitivity	Specificity	DOR	PLR	NLR	
Significant fibrosis							
0.8–1.085	5	0.73 (0.68–0.77)	0.62 (0.56–0.67)	4 (3–6)	1.9 (1.6–2.2)	0.44 (0.36–0.54)	0.73 (0.69–0.77)
1.45–1.62	6	0.65 (0.56–0.73)	0.77 (0.7–0.83)	6.24 (4.06–9.61)	2.83 (2.16–3.71)	0.45 (0.36–0.57)	0.78 (0.74–0.81)
3.25	3	0.18 (0.13–0.24)	0.98 (0.95–0.99)	7.53 (3.06–18.54)	6.04 (2.61–13.96)	0.85 (0.76–0.95)	0.61 (0.57–0.65)
Severe fibrosis							
1.45–1.65	4	0.68 (0.6–0.75)	0.75 (0.69–0.81)	6.44 (4.44–9.35)	2.75 (2.21–3.43)	0.42 (0.34–0.53)	0.77 (0.73–0.80)
Cirrhosis							
1.6–2.29	7	0.82 (0.75–0.88)	0.77 (0.71–0.82)	15.55 (8.69–27.80)	3.59 (2.73–4.74)	0.23 (0.16–0.33)	0.87 (0.84–0.90)
2.9–3.6	3	0.42 (0.36–0.48)	0.96 (0.95–0.97)	46.28 (18.3–117.04)	13.38 (9.24–19.37)	0.3 (0.06–0.45)	0.96 (0.92–1.00)

95% CI: 95% confidence interval. DOR: diagnostic odds ratio. PLR: positive likelihood ratio; NLR: negative likelihood ratio. AUHSROC: area under the hierarchical summary receiver operating characteristic curve.

than that of other studies, which ranged from 0.8 to 4.9, and we could not calculate similar cutoff values from the data included in these articles, thus they were excluded [47,48]. Wong et al. calculated cutoff values based on a >90% sensitivity to exclude and >90% specificity to confirm advanced liver fibrosis [49]. This method was different from other studies, so it was also excluded. Two studies [13,60] included the same patient populations, thus the study with the smaller sample size and data that could not be extracted was excluded [60]. As the true negative and false positive patients of the study by Jing et al. were underestimated because they excluded non-fibrotic samples (i.e.,F0), we excluded it [9]. Ultimately, 20 studies [10,11,13,16–32] were eligible for evaluation, and their characteristics are listed in Table 1. Although two studies [22,32] were written by the same author, the patients were collected at different times and the study with the smaller sample size [32] was excluded for further sensitivity analysis.

A cumulative bar plot of risk of bias and applicability concerns across all studies derived from QUADAS-2 was constructed (Figure 2). Unfortunately, a few studies stated that a consecutive or random sample of patients were enrolled, so there were not enough studies to do further subgroup analysis or sensitivity analysis. Despite this limitation, these factors were assessed in meta-regression for exploring sources of heterogeneity. The disease spectrum of 9 studies [11,17,19–21,24,26–28] were not in good accordance with our study and were excluded for further sensitivity analysis. Specifically, three of these studies [20,24,27] focused on patients with limited ALT (normal or less than 2× upper limit of normal), one focused on Hepatitis B virus e antigen (HBeAg)-positive patients [28], one focused on HBeAg-negative patients [26], one defined the urea nitrogen limitation when collecting samples [11], one included patients after therapy [19], one only included inpatients [17], and one did not describe the objective of the study clearly [21]. The bias of index test was mainly because many studies didn't predefine the cutoff value. Five studies were found to have a disease progression bias [18,19,21,29,30], and nine studies did not describe whether interpretation of liver biopsy specimens was blinded to other test results [16,17,21–23,28–30,32].

Diagnostic accuracy of the FIB-4 index for predicting significant fibrosis

Twelve studies, including 1,908 patients (male: 71%; average age: 37.1 years; average prevalence 57.4%) were used in our meta-analysis for testing the diagnostic accuracy of the FIB-4 index for predicting significant fibrosis (i.e. METAVIR F2–F4 vs. F0–F1; Table 2). The area under the HSROC was 0.78 (95% CI = 0.74–0.81; Figure 3). The summary sensitivity and specificity were 0.71 (95% CI = 0.64–0.77) and 0.73 (95% CI = 0.67–0.78), respectively (Figure 4). The heterogeneity was significant ($I^2 = 94\%$), and the meta-regression showed that disease spectrum ($P = 0.00$) and blindness ($P = 0.05$) lead to the heterogeneity. The diagnostic performance of the FIB-4 index was improved after excluding studies with improper disease spectrum (Table 2). Although the data derived from blinded tests was more reliable, it was understandable that the diagnostic performance of the non-blinded subgroup (AUHSROC = 0.83) was better than that of the blinded subgroup (AUHSROC = 0.73). We also performed a subgroup analysis based on different cutoff values (Table 3). Based on the highest AUHSROC, the most appropriate cutoff value for detecting significant fibrosis was between 1.45 and 1.62, with a PLR of 2.83, and a NLR of 0.45. This means that patients with significant fibrosis have about 3-fold higher chance of being FIB-4 positive (above 1.62) compared with patients without significant fibrosis. If the FIB-4 was below the cutoff value, the probability

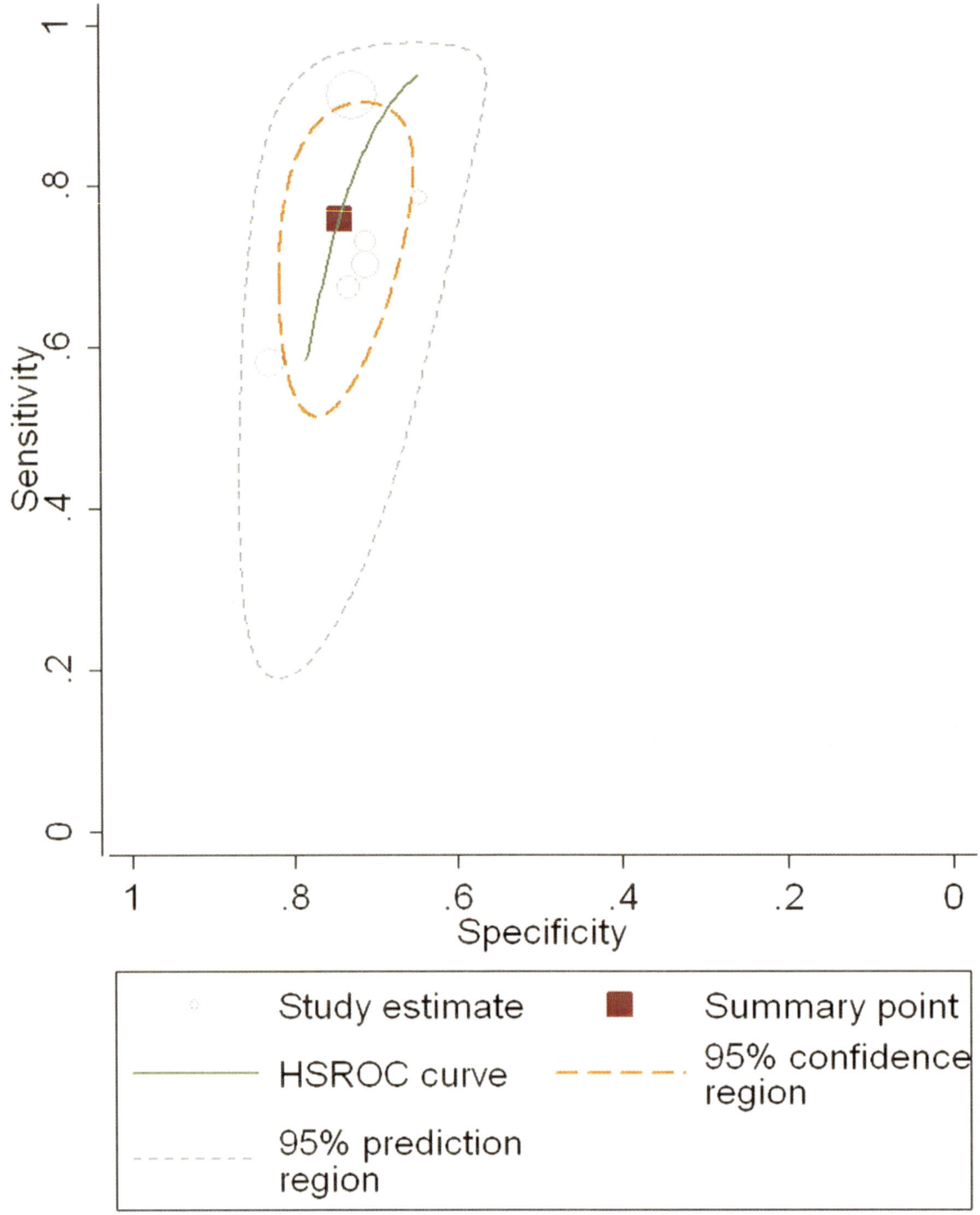

Figure 5. The hierarchical summary receiver operating characteristic (HSROC) curve of FIB-4 index for predicting severe fibrosis. The size of circles indicates the weight of the individual studies. The marked point on the curve represents the summary sensitivity and specificity. The area delimited by dashed line represents 95% confidence interval of the summary estimate. The area delimited by the dots represents the 95% prediction region, within which there is a 95% confidence that the true sensitivity and specificity of a future study should lie.

that the patient has significant fibrosis was 45%. Thus, the FIB-4 index with a cutoff value between 1.45 and 1.62 was not suitable as a test for excluding the presence of significant fibrosis. Additionally, when a cutoff value of 3.25 is used, the PLR (6.04, 95% CI = 2.61–13.96) of the FIB-4 index is high enough to be used as a test to identify significant fibrosis. As none of subgroups (Table 3) has a sufficiently low NLR to be used to exclude significant fibrosis, FIB-4 index has suboptimal accuracy in excluding significant fibrosis.

Study	TP	FP	FN	TN	Sensitivity (95% CI)	Specificity (95% CI)
Basar2013	22	17	6	31	0.79 [0.59, 0.92]	0.65 [0.49, 0.78]
Chen2013	27	29	13	79	0.68 [0.51, 0.81]	0.73 [0.64, 0.81]
Kim2010	301	92	29	246	0.91 [0.88, 0.94]	0.73 [0.68, 0.77]
Mallet2009	30	28	11	69	0.73 [0.57, 0.86]	0.71 [0.61, 0.80]
Wang H2013	18	34	13	166	0.58 [0.39, 0.75]	0.83 [0.77, 0.88]
Zhang2010	66	34	28	84	0.70 [0.60, 0.79]	0.71 [0.62, 0.79]

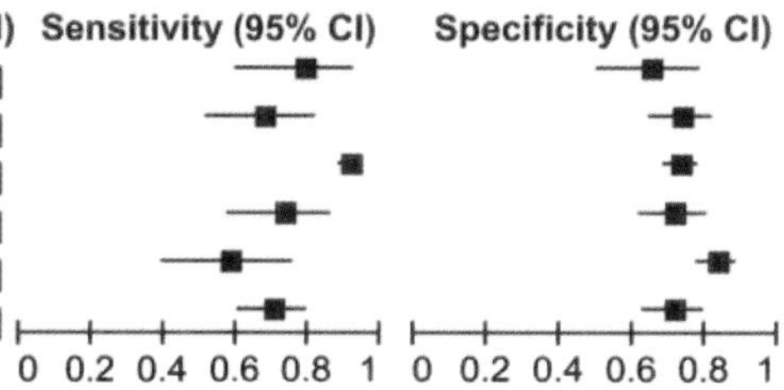

Figure 6. The forest plot of the FIB-4 index for predicting severe fibrosis.

Diagnostic accuracy of the FIB-4 index for predicting severe fibrosis

Six studies of 1,473 patients (male: 68.9%; average age: 37.3 years, average prevalence: 33.5%) were involved in the meta-analysis for testing the diagnostic accuracy of the FIB-4 index for predicting severe fibrosis (i.e., METAVIR F3–F4 vs. F0–F2). The cutoff values ranged from 1 to 3.25. The area under the HSROC was 0.79 (95% CI = 0.75-82; Figure 5). The summary sensitivity and specificity were 0.76 (95% CI = 0.64–0.85) and 0.74 (95% CI = 0.70–0.79), respectively (Figure 6). The heterogeneity was significant (I^2 = 93%), and the meta-regression showed that disease spectrum (P = 0.01) and prevalence (P = 0.01) lead to the heterogeneity. There was only one study with improper disease spectrum [26]. At the same time, disease prevalence of this study (prevalence = 0.13) was also much lower than that of the others. After excluding this study, the area under HSROC dropped from 0.79 to 0.73. Subgroup analysis (Table 3) showed that in four studies with cutoff values ranging from 1.45 to 1.65, the area under the summary receiver-operating characteristic curve (AUROC) was 0.77 (95% CI = 0.73–0.80). The corresponding PLR (2.75, 95% CI = 2.21–3.43) and NLR (0.42, 95% CI = 0.34–0.53) indicated that using the FIB-4 index with a cutoff value between 1.45 and 1.65 has a suboptimal accuracy in identifying and excluding severe fibrosis.

Diagnostic accuracy of the FIB-4 index for predicting cirrhosis

Ten studies of 2,105 patients (male: 69.9%, average age: 37.9 years, average prevalence of cirrhosis 20.8%) were involved in the meta-analysis for testing the diagnostic accuracy of the FIB-4 index for predicting cirrhosis (i.e., METAVIR F4 vs. F0–F3). The cutoff values ranged from 1.05 to 3.6, and the area under the HSROC was 0.89 (95% CI = 0.85–0.91; Figure 7), so the diagnostic performance was nearly excellent [42,43]. The summary sensitivity and specificity were 0.83 (95% CI = 0.78–0.88) and 0.80 (95% CI = 0.73–0.86), respectively (Figure 8). The heterogeneity was significant (I^2 = 67%), and the meta-regression showed that the potential factors described above didn't lead to the heterogeneity (P>0.05). The most appropriate cutoff value for detecting significant fibrosis was between 2.9 and 3.6. At this range, the AUROC was 0.96 (95% CI = 0.92–1.00), so it was classified as excellent. The PLR (13.38, 95% CI = 9.24–19.37) for the FIB-4 index was high enough to be used to identify cirrhosis, although the NLR (0.3, 95% CI = 0.06–0.45) was not low enough to exclude cirrhosis.

Publication bias

A publication bias was not detected when tested using Egger's test or the trim and fill method (Table 4). For Egger's test, the publication bias 95% CI of every group included zero and the P-value was >0.05, so there was no statistical difference between publication bias and zero. This means that no publication bias was present. For the trim and fill method, the summary diagnostic odds ratio (SDOR) was always >1 both before and after trim and fill, meaning that trimming and filling studies didn't influence the outcome of the meta-analysis (SDOR always >1). Taken together this means that publication bias was nonexistent in our meta-analysis.

Discussion

Accurate diagnosis of liver fibrosis is clinically advantageous. Liver biopsy is the gold standard for diagnosing fibrosis; however, its clinical application is hampered by various limitations. Despite these limitations, an ideal alternative to liver biopsies has not been found [67,68]. In this meta-analysis we assessed the diagnostic accuracy of the FIB-4 index as a non-invasive alternative to liver biopsy.

The FIB-4 index is a simple and inexpensive noninvasive marker of liver fibrosis. Recently, the diagnostic value of the FIB-4 index in predicting the extent of fibrosis has been substantiated, and is even considered by some to be the best noninvasive index [11,13]; however, others have highlighted its weaknesses [10,26]. The current study comprehensively analyzed the predictive power of the FIB-4 index using a meta-analysis of previously published studies. The area under the HSROC for the FIB-4 index was 0.78, and 0.79 and 0.89 for predicting significant and severe fibrosis, and cirrhosis, respectively. Thus, the summary diagnostic performance of FIB-4 for significant and severe fibrosis was nearly good, and for cirrhosis was nearly excellent.

As the summary estimates of all cutoff values was deemed difficult to interpret and use in clinical practice, a subgroup analysis based on different cutoff values was performed. The recommended cutoff value for predicting significant fibrosis was between 1.45 and 1.62 based on the highest AUHSROC, but it still had suboptimal accuracy in excluding significant fibrosis. Fortunately, we found that the FIB-4 index with a cutoff value of 3.25 was suitable for identifying significant fibrosis. For severe fibrosis, the recommended cutoff value was between 1.45 and 1.65, and it has a suboptimal accuracy in identifying and excluding severe fibrosis. For cirrhosis, the recommended cutoff value was between 2.9 and 3.6, and the diagnostic performance was excellent (AUROC = 0.96). Thus, patient's with a FIB-4 index above 3.6 can almost be diagnosed with cirrhosis, with a PLR = 13.38.

In terms of other noninvasive indexes, the APRI has the advantage of including only two inexpensive laboratory tests, which are performed routinely, and the FibroTest/Fibrosure is one of the most investigated and most frequently used tools for assessing liver fibrosis. The diagnostic performance of these two non-invasive indexes has been evaluated by meta-analysis [67,69]. If we compare our meta-analysis of the FIB-4 index with these

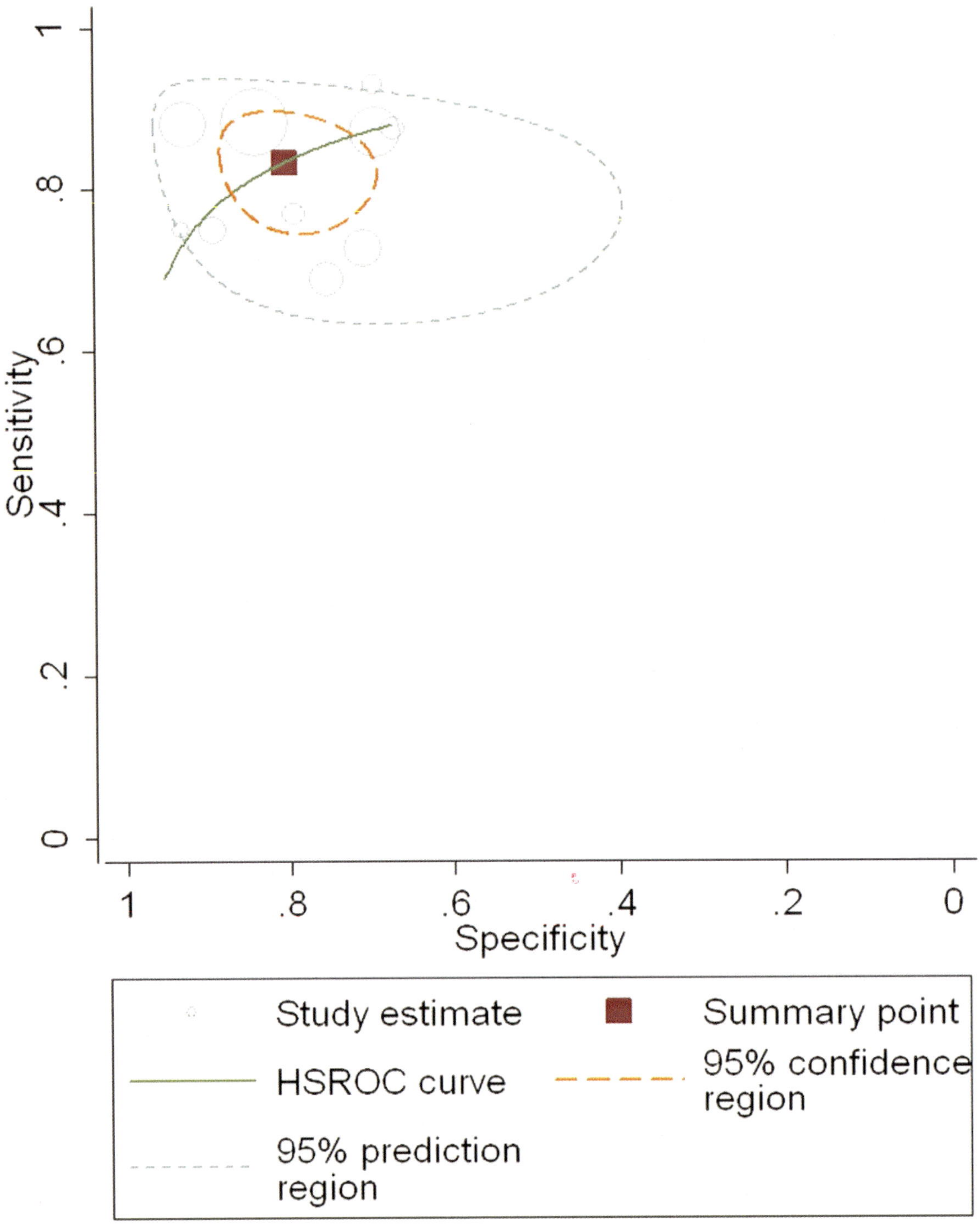

Figure 7. The hierarchical summary receiver operating characteristic (HSROC) curve of FIB-4 index for predicting cirrhosis. The size of circles indicates the weight of the individual studies. The marked point on the curve represents the summary sensitivity and specificity. The area delimited by dashed line represents 95% confidence interval of the summary estimate. The area delimited by the dots represents the 95% prediction region, within which there is a 95% confidence that the true sensitivity and specificity of a future study should lie.

studies we can see that for significant fibrosis, AUROC of the APRI and FibroTest/Fibrosure was 0.79 (SE = 0.0243) and 0.84 (95% CI = 0.78–0.88), respectively. Thus, the diagnostic accuracy of the FIB-4 was similar to that of the APRI, and worse than the FibroTest/Fibrosure. For cirrhosis, the AUROC of the APRI and FibroTest/Fibrosure was 0.75 (SE = 0.0237) and 0.87 (95% CI = 0.85–0.90), respectively. Thus, based on our meta-analysis, the FIB-4 index was superior to that of the APRI, and similar to that of the FibroTest/Fibrosure for diagnosing cirrhosis. Additionally, another meta-analysis revealed that the AUROC of the FIB-4 index for significant fibrosis and cirrhosis with HCV infection was 0.74 and 0.87, respectively [70]. Thus, the diagnostic

Study	TP	FP	FN	TN	Sensitivity (95% CI)	Specificity (95% CI)
Basar2013	10	13	3	50	0.77 [0.46, 0.95]	0.79 [0.67, 0.89]
Bonnard2010	13	14	1	32	0.93 [0.66, 1.00]	0.70 [0.54, 0.82]
Gong2013	9	2	3	27	0.75 [0.43, 0.95]	0.93 [0.77, 0.99]
Ji2011	44	19	6	244	0.88 [0.76, 0.95]	0.93 [0.89, 0.96]
Kim2010	203	70	27	368	0.88 [0.83, 0.92]	0.84 [0.80, 0.87]
Liu2012	9	11	3	91	0.75 [0.43, 0.95]	0.89 [0.82, 0.94]
Zhang2009	14	23	2	47	0.88 [0.62, 0.98]	0.67 [0.55, 0.78]
Zhang2010	32	49	12	119	0.73 [0.57, 0.85]	0.71 [0.63, 0.78]
Zhang2012	67	87	10	197	0.87 [0.77, 0.94]	0.69 [0.64, 0.75]
Zhu2011	20	36	9	110	0.69 [0.49, 0.85]	0.75 [0.68, 0.82]

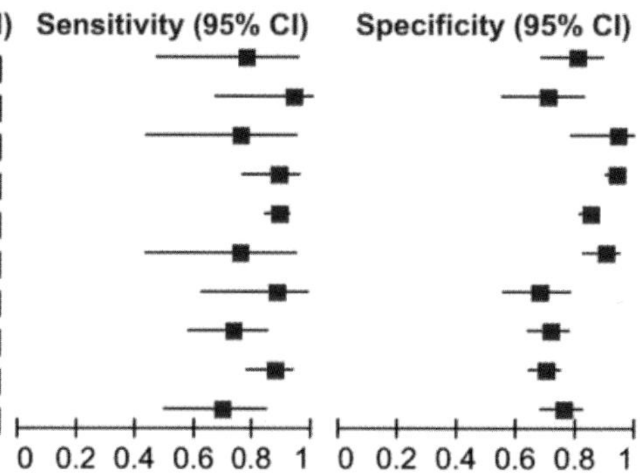

Figure 8. The forest plot of the FIB-4 index for predicting cirrhosis.

value of the FIB-4 index for predicting HBV-related fibrosis was also slightly better than that for HCV, although it was originally applied to HCV and HIV co-infection [14,15]. Unfortunately, meta-analyses of other non-invasive tests for predicting HBV related fibrosis was not found, so comparison with the FIB-4 index was not possible.

There are two strengths to the current meta-analysis. First, although the diagnostic performance of the FIB-4 index for HBV-related fibrosis has previously been assessed by several studies [10,11,13,16–32], our evaluation combined the data from previously published work in a meta-analysis, thereby strengthening its accuracy. Second, we searched the CNKI and CBMdisc databases that provided authoritative and comprehensive data from Chinese populations. This is important because the prevalence of HBV infection is much higher than that of HCV infection in Chinese populations [71]. Additionally, we found that of the 15 eligible studies written in English for this meta-analysis [10,11,13,16,18–20,23–30], nine were written by Chinese groups [10,20,23,24,26–30]. Thus, authors not searching Chinese databases may have overlooked some valuable studies.

There are three limitations to the current meta-analysis. First, there were 20 eligible studies included in the meta-analysis, but this number was too small for further subgroup analysis. This limitation was compounded by the fact that there were few studies with a large sample size and multiple centers. The second limitation was the significant heterogeneity of included studies. A considerable variation between the results of diagnostic studies is a common occurrence, possibly to a greater extent than is seen for therapeutic interventions [72]. One of the potential sources of heterogeneity and a direct consequence of the fact that the importance of rigorous design has been less well appreciated for diagnostic studies than for therapeutic interventions, is poor adherence to methodological constraints [69,73]. This is noticeable in many studies that we included, and can be considered as a general problem in many studies dealing with the diagnostic accuracy of liver fibrosis markers, as already noted by others [73]. In our study, although disease spectrum, blindness and prevalence were found to be the factors causing heterogeneity, and further sensitivity analysis and/or subgroup analysis were performed in our study, more detailed subgroup analysis, such as grouping by both proper disease spectrum and blindness, is needed. Unfortunately, the eligible studies were too few to perform this. Finally, we only included published manuscripts, so bias in the selection of search channels may have influenced our results.

Our meta-analysis has several implications for future research. For example, we believe that more studies on the diagnostic accuracy for liver fibrosis are needed in patient populations with CHB. In the future, authors of studies exploring the performance of the FIB-4 index in CHB patients should be encouraged to insist on a rigorous design and methodology. In this regard, QUADAS-2 [36] describes what is required for a rigorous study design and methodology, and is a good tool for guiding diagnostic study design. As common flaws in design and methodology found in our eligible studies, we emphasize two points: first, a study should ideally enroll all consecutive, or a random sample of, eligible patients with suspected disease – otherwise there is potential for bias. Second, selecting the test threshold to optimize sensitivity and/or specificity may lead to overoptimistic estimates of test performance, which is likely to be poorer in an independent sample of patients in whom the same threshold is used [74]. As a result, if a threshold was used, it should be pre-specified.

Implications for practice deriving from our results suggest that the FIB-4 index is of excellent utility for detecting cirrhosis in patients with CHB, and has moderate accuracy in detecting significant fibrosis. On the other hand, it has suboptimal performance in the exclusion of significant and severe fibrosis, and cirrhosis. Thus, it is necessary to further improve the test or

Table 4. Analysis of publication bias for studies.

Staging	P value of bias	95%CI of bias	SDOR after trim and fill
Significant fibrosis	0.18	(−1.34~6.26)	6.394 (4.44~9.21)
Severe fibrosis	0.08	(−12.56~1.07)	8.38 (4.27~16.43)
Cirrhosis	0.75	(−3.93~2.94)	19.67 (10.53~36.74)

95% CI: 95% confidence interval. SDOR: summary diagnostic odds ratio.

combine it with other noninvasive modalities in order to improve its accuracy.

Supporting Information

File S1 Search strategy of Ovid database. This literature search was performed in November 2013.

File S2 Search strategy of Pubmed database. This literature search was performed in November 2013.

Checklist S1 PRISMA 2009 checklist.

Acknowledgments

The authors thank Guocai Lv, PhD and Renyong Guo, PhD (Department of Laboratory Medicine, the First Affiliated Hospital, College of Medicine, Zhejiang University, Hangzhou 310003, China) for critical comments on research design and statistics. We thank Elixigen Corporation (Huntington Beach, California, USA) for helping in proofreading and editing the English of final manuscript.

Author Contributions

Conceived and designed the experiments: YC YL. Performed the experiments: YL YZ. Analyzed the data: YL YZ. Contributed reagents/materials/analysis tools: YC. Contributed to the writing of the manuscript: YL YZ.

References

1. Liaw YF, Sung JJ, Chow WC, Farrell G, Lee CZ, et al. (2004) Lamivudine for patients with chronic hepatitis B and advanced liver disease. N Engl J Med 351: 1521–1531.
2. Lok AS, McMahon BJ (2007) Chronic hepatitis B. Hepatology 45: 507–539.
3. (2012) EASL clinical practice guidelines: Management of chronic hepatitis B virus infection. J Hepatol 57: 167–185.
4. de Franchis R (2008) Non-invasive (and minimally invasive) diagnosis of oesophageal varices. J Hepatol 49: 520–527.
5. Bravo AA, Sheth SG, Chopra S (2001) Liver biopsy. N Engl J Med 344: 495–500.
6. Bedossa P, Dargere D, Paradis V (2003) Sampling variability of liver fibrosis in chronic hepatitis C. Hepatology 38: 1449–1457.
7. Friedman LS (2004) Controversies in liver biopsy: who, where, when, how, why? Curr Gastroenterol Rep 6: 30–36.
8. Bedossa P, Poynard T (1996) An algorithm for the grading of activity in chronic hepatitis C. The METAVIR Cooperative Study Group. Hepatology 24: 289–293.
9. Ma J, Jiang Y, Gong G (2013) Evaluation of seven noninvasive models in staging liver fibrosis in patients with chronic hepatitis B virus infection. Eur J Gastroenterol Hepatol 25: 428–434.
10. Chen B, Ye B, Zhang J, Ying L, Chen Y (2013) RDW to Platelet Ratio: A Novel Noninvasive Index for Predicting Hepatic Fibrosis and Cirrhosis in Chronic Hepatitis B. PLOS ONE 8: e68780.
11. Erdogan S, Dogan HO, Sezer S, Uysal S, Ozhamam E, et al. (2013) The diagnostic value of non-invasive tests for the evaluation of liver fi brosis in chronic hepatitis B patients. Scandinavian Journal of Clinical & Laboratory Investigation, 73: 300–308.
12. Lin ZH, Xin YN, Dong QJ, Wang Q, Jiang XJ, et al. (2011) Performance of the aspartate aminotransferase-to-platelet ratio index for the staging of hepatitis C-related fibrosis: an updated meta-analysis. Hepatology 53: 726–736.
13. Kim BK, Kim DY, Park JY, Ahn SH, Chon CY, et al. (2010) Validation of FIB-4 and comparison with other simple noninvasive indices for predicting liver fibrosis and cirrhosis in hepatitis B virus-infected patients. Liver International 30: 546–553.
14. Sterling RK, Lissen E, Clumeck N, Sola R, Correa MC, et al. (2006) Development of a simple noninvasive index to predict significant fibrosis in patients with HIV/HCV coinfection. Hepatology 43: 1317–1325.
15. Torriani FJ, Rodriguez-Torres M, Rockstroh JK, Lissen E, Gonzalez-Garcia J, et al. (2004) Peginterferon Alfa-2a plus ribavirin for chronic hepatitis C virus infection in HIV-infected patients. N Engl J Med 351: 438–450.
16. Mallet V, Dhalluin-Venier V, Roussin C, Bourliere M, Pettinelli ME, et al. (2009) The accuracy of the FIB-4 index for the diagnosis of mild fibrosis in chronic hepatitis B. Alimentary Pharmacology & Therapeutics 29: 409–415.
17. Ji D, Shao Q; Han P, Zhang J, Niu X, et al. (2011) Analysis of the efficiency of Fibroscan combined with serologic markers for diagnosing liver fibrosis. Med J Clin PLA 36.
18. Ucar F, Sezer S, Ginis Z, Ozturk G, Albayrak A, et al. (2013) APRI, the FIB-4 score, and Forn's index have noninvasive diagnostic value for liver fibrosis in patients with chronic hepatitis B. European Journal of Gastroenterology & Hepatology 25: 1076–1081.
19. Bonnard P, Sombie R, Lescure F-X, Bougouma A, Guiard-Schmid JB, et al. (2010) Comparison of Elastography, Serum Marker Scores, and Histology for the Assessment of Liver Fibrosis in Hepatitis B Virus (HBV)-Infected Patients in Burkina Faso. American Journal of Tropical Medicine & Hygiene 82: 454–458.
20. Wang H, Xue L, Yan R, Zhou Y, Wang MS, et al. (2013) Comparison of FIB-4 and APRI in Chinese HBV-infected patients with persistently normal ALT and mildly elevated ALT. Journal of Viral Hepatitis 20: e3–e10.
21. Gong H, Hu Y, Ye X, Lin H (2013) Diagnostic efficiency of real-time tissue elastography in evaluating liver fibrosis. ACTA UNIVERSITATIS MEDICINALIS NANJING (Natural Science) 33: 131–134.
22. Zhang Y, Zeng J, Fan Q, Zheng J, Li Q (2012) Four noninvasive score systems for diagnosis of liver fibrosis in patients with chronic hepatitis B. Chin J Clin Infect Dis 5: 338–341.
23. Liu XD, Wu JL, Liang J, Zhang T, Sheng QS (2012) Globulin-platelet model predicts minimal fibrosis and cirrhosis in chronic hepatitis B virus infected patients. World J Gastroenterol 18: 2784–2792.
24. Seto W-K, Lee C-F, Lai C-L, Ip PPC, Fong DY-T, et al. (2011) A New Model Using Routinely Available Clinical Parameters to Predict Significant Liver Fibrosis in Chronic Hepatitis B. PLoS One 6: Article No. e23077.
25. Başar Ö, Yımaz B, Ekiz F, Giniş Z, Altınbaş A, et al. (2013) Non-invasive tests in prediction of liver fibrosis in chronic hepatitis B and comparison with post-antiviral treatment results. Clinics and Research in Hepatology and Gastroenterology 37: 152–158.
26. Wang Y, Xu M-Y, Zheng R-D, Xian J-C, Xu H-T, et al. (2013) Prediction of significant fibrosis and cirrhosis in hepatitis B e-antigen negative patients with chronic hepatitis B using routine parameters. Hepatology Research 43: 441–451.
27. Zhu X, Wang L-C, Chen E-Q, Chen X-B, Chen L-Y, et al. (2011) Prospective Evaluation of FibroScan for the Diagnosis of Hepatic Fibrosis Compared with Liver Biopsy/AST Platelet Ratio Index and FIB-4 in Patients with Chronic HBV Infection. Digestive Diseases & Sciences 56: 2742–2749.
28. Xun Y-h, Zang G-q, Guo J-c, Yu X-l, Liu H, et al. (2013) Serum hepatitis B surface antigen quantification as a useful assessment for significant fibrosis in hepatitis B e antigen-positive hepatitis B virus carriers. Journal of Gastroenterology & Hepatology 28: 1746–1755.
29. Zhu CL, Li WT, Li Y, Gao RT (2012) Serum levels of tissue inhibitor of metalloproteinase-1 are correlated with liver fibrosis in patients with chronic hepatitis B. Journal of Digestive Diseases 13: 558–563.
30. Wu SD, Wang JY, Li L (2010) Staging of liver fibrosis in chronic hepatitis B patients with a composite predictive model: a comparative study. World J Gastroenterol 16: 501–507.
31. Zhang YF, Shi H, Chen LB, Xu QH (2010) Value of FIB-4 for the diagnosis of liver fibrosis in chronic hepatitis B. Zhonghua Shi Yan He Lin Chuang Bing Du Xue Za Zhi 24: 215–217.
32. Zhang Y, Hong D, Bian W, Shen Y, Yan N (2009) Value of FIB-4 for the diagnosis of liver fibrosis in patients with chronic hepatitis B. Ch in J Gastroentero lH epato, l: 213–214.
33. Batts KP, Ludwig J (1995) Chronic hepatitis. An update on terminology and reporting. Am J Surg Pathol 19: 1409–1417.
34. Scheuer PJ (1991) Classification of chronic viral hepatitis: a need for reassessment. J Hepatol 13: 372–374.
35. Ishak K, Baptista A, Bianchi L, Callea F, De Groote J, et al. (1995) Histological grading and staging of chronic hepatitis. J Hepatol 22: 696–699.
36. Whiting PF, Rutjes AW, Westwood ME, Mallett S, Deeks JJ, et al. (2011) QUADAS-2: a revised tool for the quality assessment of diagnostic accuracy studies. Ann Intern Med 155: 529–536.
37. Lu XL, Xiao ZH, Yang MY, Zhu YM (2013) Diagnostic value of serum procalcitonin in patients with chronic renal insufficiency: a systematic review and meta-analysis. Nephrol Dial Transplant 28: 122–129.
38. Chu H, Cole SR (2006) Bivariate meta-analysis of sensitivity and specificity with sparse data: a generalized linear mixed model approach. J Clin Epidemiol 59: 1331–1332; author reply 1332–1333.
39. Wang F, Gatsonis CA (2008) Hierarchical models for ROC curve summary measures: design and analysis of multi-reader, multi-modality studies of medical tests. Stat Med 27: 243–256.
40. Leeflang MM (2014) Systematic reviews and meta-analyses of diagnostic test accuracy. Clin Microbiol Infect 20: 105–113.
41. Leeflang MM, Deeks JJ, Gatsonis C, Bossuyt PM (2008) Systematic reviews of diagnostic test accuracy. Ann Intern Med 149: 889–897.
42. Zweig MH, Campbell G (1993) Receiver-operating characteristic (ROC) plots: a fundamental evaluation tool in clinical medicine. Clinical Chemistry 39: 561–577.
43. Altman DG, Bland JM (1994) Diagnostic tests 3: receiver operating characteristic plots. BMJ 309: 188.
44. Lijmer JG, Bossuyt PM, Heisterkamp SH (2002) Exploring sources of heterogeneity in systematic reviews of diagnostic tests. Stat Med 21: 1525–1537.

45. Egger M, Davey Smith G, Schneider M, Minder C (1997) Bias in meta-analysis detected by a simple, graphical test. BMJ 315: 629–634.
46. Duval S, Tweedie R (2000) Trim and fill: A simple funnel-plot-based method of testing and adjusting for publication bias in meta-analysis. Biometrics 56: 455–463.
47. Xu M-Y, Qu Y, Jia X-F, Wang M-L, Liu H, et al. (2013) Serum proteomic MRM identify peptide ions of transferrin as new fibrosis markers in chronic hepatitis B. Biomedicine & Pharmacotherapy 67: 561–567.
48. Gumusay O, Ozenirler S, Atak A, Sonmez C, Ozkan S, et al. (2013) Diagnostic potential of serum direct markers and non-invasive fibrosis models in patients with chronic hepatitis B. Hepatology Research 43: 228–237.
49. Wong GLH, Wong VWS, Choi PCL, Chan AWH, Chan HLY (2010) Development of a non-invasive algorithm with transient elastography (Fibroscan) and serum test formula for advanced liver fibrosis in chronic hepatitis B. Alimentary Pharmacology & Therapeutics 31: 1095–1103.
50. Ding D, Meng Z, Ke C, Li D, Chen Y (2013) The Correlation of FIB-4 Index with Child-Pugh Classification in Patients with HBV-related Cirrhosis. J HBUM: 245–247.
51. Zhou J (2013) Application of FibroScan combined with other serologic markers on the diagnosis of liver fibrosis. Int J Lab Med: 409–411.
52. Li X (2012) Developments in hepatic fibrosis diagnosis with the combination of serological indexes and Fibroscan. J Clin Hepatol 15: 472–474.
53. Stibbe KJ, Verveer C, Francke J, Hansen BE, Zondervan PE, et al. (2011) Comparison of non-invasive assessment to diagnose liver fibrosis in chronic hepatitis B and C patients. Scand J Gastroenterol 46: 962–972.
54. Sebastiani G, Castera L, Halfon P, Pol S, Mangia A, et al. (2011) The impact of liver disease aetiology and the stages of hepatic fibrosis on the performance of non-invasive fibrosis biomarkers: an international study of 2411 cases. Aliment Pharmacol Ther 34: 1202–1216.
55. Pissaia A Jr, Borderie D, Bernard D, Scatton O, Calmus Y, et al. (2009) APRI and FIB-4 Scores Are Useful After Liver Transplantation Independently of Etiology. Transplantation Proceedings 41: 679–681.
56. Nalpas B, Mallet V, Vallet-Pichard A, Fontaine H, Pol S (2009) 374 THE FIB-4 INDEX IS ACCURATE TO ASSESS LIVER FIBROSIS BEFORE AND DURING TREATMENT IN CHRONIC HEPATITIS B. Journal of Hepatology 50, Supplement 1: S142–S143.
57. Molto J, Llibre JM, Ribera E, Minguez C, del Rio JS, et al. (2009) Saquinavir exposure in HIV-infected patients with chronic viral hepatitis. Journal of Antimicrobial Chemotherapy 63: 992–997.
58. Lee MH, Cheong JY, Um SH, Seo YS, Kim DJ, et al. (2010) Comparison of Surrogate Serum Markers and Transient Elastography (Fibroscan) for Assessing Cirrhosis in Patients with Chronic Viral Hepatitis. Digestive Diseases & Sciences 55: 3552–3560.
59. Lee JH, Yoon JH, Lee CH, Myung SJ, Keam B, et al. (2009) Complete blood count reflects the degree of oesophageal varices and liver fibrosis in virus-related chronic liver disease patients. Journal of Viral Hepatitis 16: 444–452.
60. Kim BK, Han KH, Park JY, Ahn SH, Chon CY, et al. (2010) External Validation of P2/MS and Comparison with Other Simple Non-invasive Indices for Predicting Liver Fibrosis in HBV-Infected Patients. Digestive Diseases & Sciences 55: 2636–2643.
61. Jain MK, Seremba E, Bhore R, Dao D, Joshi R, et al. (2012) Change in fibrosis score as a predictor of mortality among HIV-infected patients with viral hepatitis. AIDS Patient Care STDS 26: 73–80.
62. de Ledinghen V, Vergniol J, Barthe C, Foucher J, Chermak F, et al. (2013) Non-invasive tests for fibrosis and liver stiffness predict 5-year survival of patients chronically infected with hepatitis B virus. Alimentary Pharmacology & Therapeutics 37: 979–988.
63. Cheong JY, Um SH, Seo YS, Kim DJ, Hwang SG, et al. (2011) Non-invasive index for predicting significant liver fibrosis: comparison of diagnostic performances in patients with chronic hepatitis B and C. Dig Dis Sci 56: 555–563.
64. Beckebaum S, Iacob S, Klein CG, Dechene A, Varghese J, et al. (2010) Assessment of Allograft Fibrosis by Transient Elastography and Noninvasive Biomarker Scoring Systems in Liver Transplant Patients. Transplantation 89: 983–993.
65. Huang YC, Huang CF, Chang KC, Hung SF, Wang JH, et al. (2011) Community-based screening for hepatocellular carcinoma in elderly residents in a hepatitis B- and C-endemic area. J Gastroenterol Hepatol 26: 129–134.
66. Chon YE, Jung ES, Park JY, Kim do Y, Ahn SH, et al. (2012) The accuracy of noninvasive methods in predicting the development of hepatocellular carcinoma and hepatic decompensation in patients with chronic hepatitis B. J Clin Gastroenterol 46: 518–525.
67. Jin W, Lin Z, Xin Y, Jiang X, Dong Q, et al. (2012) Diagnostic accuracy of the aspartate aminotransferase-to-platelet ratio index for the prediction of hepatitis B-related fibrosis: a leading meta-analysis. BMC Gastroenterol 12: 14.
68. Castera L, Vergniol J, Foucher J, Le Bail B, Chanteloup E, et al. (2005) Prospective comparison of transient elastography, Fibrotest, APRI, and liver biopsy for the assessment of fibrosis in chronic hepatitis C. Gastroenterology 128: 343–350.
69. Salkic NN, Jovanovic P, Hauser G, Brcic M (2014) FibroTest/Fibrosure for Significant Liver Fibrosis and Cirrhosis in Chronic Hepatitis B: A Meta-Analysis. Am J Gastroenterol 109: 796–809.
70. Chou R, Wasson N (2013) Blood tests to diagnose fibrosis or cirrhosis in patients with chronic hepatitis C virus infection: a systematic review. Ann Intern Med 158: 807–820.
71. Lan X (2012) Study on the area distribution of viral hepatitis in China. Chinese Journal of Health Laboratory Technology: 2467–2469.
72. Dinnes J, Deeks J, Kirby J, Roderick P (2005) A methodological review of how heterogeneity has been examined in systematic reviews of diagnostic test accuracy. Health Technol Assess 9: 1–113, iii.
73. Regev A, Berho M, Jeffers LJ, Milikowski C, Molina EG, et al. (2002) Sampling error and intraobserver variation in liver biopsy in patients with chronic HCV infection. Am J Gastroenterol 97: 2614–2618.
74. Leeflang MM, Moons KG, Reitsma JB, Zwinderman AH (2008) Bias in sensitivity and specificity caused by data-driven selection of optimal cutoff values: mechanisms, magnitude, and solutions. Clin Chem 54: 729–737.

17

Limited Utility of Plasma M30 in Discriminating Non-Alcoholic Steatohepatitis from Steatosis – A Comparison with Routine Biochemical Markers

Wah-Kheong Chan[1]*, Pavai Sthaneshwar[2], Nik Raihan Nik Mustapha[3], Sanjiv Mahadeva[1]

1 Gastroenterology and Hepatology Unit, Gastrointestinal Endoscopy Unit, Department of Medicine, Faculty of Medicine, University of Malaya, Kuala Lumpur, Malaysia, **2** Division of Laboratory Medicine, Department of Pathology, Faculty of Medicine, University of Malaya, Kuala Lumpur, Malaysia, **3** Department of Pathology, Hospital Alor Setar, Alor Setar, Kedah, Malaysia

Abstract

Introduction: The utility of Cytokeratin-18 fragment, namely CK18Asp396 (M30), for the diagnosis of non-alcoholic steatohepatitis (NASH) is currently uncertain. We aimed to provide further data in this area among multi-ethnic Asian subjects with NAFLD.

Materials and Methods: The accuracy of M30 for detecting NASH was compared with serum alanine aminotransferase (ALT), aspartate aminotransferase (AST) and gamma glutamyl transpeptidase (GGT) levels in consecutive adult subjects with biopsy-proven non-alcoholic fatty liver disease (NAFLD).

Results: Data for 93 NAFLD subjects (mean age 51.0±11.1 years old and 51.6% males) and 20 healthy controls (mean age 50.2±16.4 years old and 33.3% males) were analyzed. There were 39 NASH subjects (41.9%) and 54 non-NASH subjects (58.1%) among the NAFLD subjects. Plasma M30 (349 U/L vs. 162 U/L), and serum ALT (70 IU/L vs. 26 IU/L), AST (41 IU/L vs. 20 IU/L) and GGT (75 IU/L vs. 33 IU/L) were significantly higher in NAFLD subjects than in healthy controls. Serum ALT (86 IU/L vs. 61 IU/L), AST (58 IU/L vs. 34 IU/L) and GGT (97 IU/L vs. 56 IU/L) were significantly higher in NASH subjects compared to non-NASH subjects, but no significant difference was observed with plasma M30 (435 U/L vs. 331 U/L). The accuracy of plasma M30, and serum ALT, AST and GGT was good for predicting NAFLD (AUROC 0.91, 0.95, 0.87 and 0.85, respectively) but less so for NASH (AUROC 0.59, 0.64, 0.75 and 0.68, respectively). Serum ALT and AST, but not plasma M30 showed a significant trend with increasing grades of ballooning and lobular inflammation.

Conclusion: The utility of M30 in the detection of NASH in clinical practice appears limited, in comparison to routine biochemical markers.

Editor: Anna Alisi, Bambino Gesu' Children Hospital, Italy

Funding: This study was funded by the University of Malaya Research Grant. Project No.: RG536-13HTM. URL: http://umresearch.um.edu.my/mainpage.php?module=Maklumat&kategori=86&id=62&papar=1. The funders had no role in study design, data collection and analysis, decision to publish, or preparation of the manuscript.

Competing Interests: The authors have declared that no competing interests exist.

* Email: wahkheong2003@hotmail.com

Introduction

The prevalence of non-alcoholic fatty liver disease (NAFLD) has increased rapidly over the years, parallel to the increase in metabolic syndrome, and it is recognized as one of the most common causes of chronic liver disease worldwide [1]. NAFLD encompasses a spectrum of liver conditions, ranging from simple steatosis to non-alcoholic steatohepatitis (NASH) to fibrosis and cirrhosis. While simple steatosis is generally considered benign, NASH may lead to fibrosis and eventually cirrhosis, with an increased risk of morbidity and mortality [2,3].

The diagnosis of NASH is made by histopathological examination of a liver biopsy specimen. However, liver biopsy is invasive and it is associated with a small risk of serious complications [4]. It is not practical to subject all subjects with NAFLD to a liver biopsy to diagnose NASH. Furthermore, repeated liver biopsies to monitor disease progression in clinical practice is not acceptable either. A simple and reliable non-invasive test is needed for the diagnosis and follow-up of NASH.

Cytokeratin 18 (CK-18) is the major intermediate filament protein in liver cells and it is cleaved by caspases that are activated during apoptosis of liver cells, a process which plays an important role in NASH [5]. CK-18 fragment, namely CK18Asp396 (M30), has been studied for the diagnosis of NASH with varying results [6–13]. Whilst some studies have suggested that specific cut-off levels of CK-18 can reliably detect NASH in a cohort of NAFLD subjects [6–10], others have not shown such promising results [11–13]. These contrasting data may have been due to studies with a small sample size or from inadequate samples of cases with a range of NAFLD histology.

In an effort to provide more balanced data on the role of M30 in NAFLD, we have conducted a study in multi-ethnic Asian subjects with NAFLD. In this study, we aimed to evaluate the accuracy of plasma M30 in detecting NASH, and to compare it with some routine biochemical markers, namely serum alanine aminotransferase (ALT), aspartate aminotransferase (AST) and gamma glutamyl transpeptidase (GGT).

Materials and Methods

Consecutive adult subjects (aged ≥18 years) with NAFLD who were scheduled for a liver biopsy were prospectively recruited between November 2012 and October 2013 for this study. The diagnosis of NAFLD was based on ultrasonography finding of fatty liver and exclusion of significant alcohol intake, use of medications that can cause fatty liver, viral hepatitis B and C infection, and other causes of chronic liver disease where indicated [14].

Demographic, anthropometric, relevant clinical and laboratory data were obtained using a standard protocol on the day of the liver biopsy procedure. Weight and height were measured using standard equipment. Body mass index (BMI) was calculated by dividing weight in kilogram by the square of height in meters. Waist circumference (WC) was measured at the mid-point between the lowest margin of the least palpable rib and the top of the iliac crest in the standing position. Blood pressure was measured in the sitting position using standardized equipment. A patient was considered hypertensive if there was a self-reported history of hypertension, if the patient was on anti-hypertensive medication(s), if the systolic blood pressure was ≥130 mmHg, or if the diastolic blood pressure was ≥85 mmHg.

All subjects had venous blood drawn after an overnight fast on the day of the liver biopsy procedure for complete blood count, blood glucose, glycated haemoglobin (HbA1c), lipid profile, liver profile, tests for viral hepatitis B and C infection, and for measurement of plasma M30 level. Biochemical measurements were performed using standard laboratory procedures. A patient was considered to have diabetes mellitus if there was a self-reported history of diabetes mellitus, if the patient was on anti-diabetic medication(s), or if fasting blood sugar was ≥7.0 mmol/L. A patient was considered to have dyslipidemia if there was a self-reported history of dyslipidemia, if the patient was on lipid-lowering medication(s), if the serum total cholesterol (TC) was ≥ 5.2 mmol/L, if the serum triglyceride (TG) was ≥1.7 mmol/L, if the serum high-density lipoprotein (HDL) was <1.0 mmol/L for men or <1.3 mmol/L for women, or if the serum low-density lipoprotein (LDL) was ≥3.4 mmol/L. Our laboratory's upper limit of normal for liver enzymes were as follow: alkaline phosphatase (ALP) 136 IU/L, aspartate aminotransferase (AST) 37 IU/L, alanine aminotransferase (ALT) 65 IU/L and gamma-glutamyl transpeptidase (GGT) 55 IU/L. The Elecsys HBsAg II assay and the Elecsys Anti-HCV II assay (Roche, Mannheim, Germany) were used to test for viral hepatitis B and C infection, respectively.

Controls were recruited from persons attending the Endoscopy Unit, University of Malaya Medical Centre for investigation of dyspepsia or screening colonoscopy. All controls had no history of chronic liver disease and had an ultrasound examination to exclude fatty liver. The presence of hypertension, diabetes mellitus and dyslipidemia was based on self-report. BMI and WC was determined as described above. Venous blood was drawn after an overnight fast for liver profile and for measurement of plasma M30 level.

Measurement of plasma M30 level

The blood sample for measurement of plasma M30 level was collected in a plain tube on the same day of the liver biopsy procedure. The blood sample was processed to plasma and stored at −80°C until further analysis. The plasma was subsequently used for quantitative measurement of M30 using the M30-Apoptosense ELISA kit (PEVIVA, Bromma, Sweden). The test was performed for all samples in a single session by a single investigator (PS).

Liver biopsy and histological assessment

Ultrasonography-guided percutaneous liver biopsy was performed by either one of two experienced operators (WKC, SM) using 18 G Temno ® II semi-automatic biopsy needle (Cardinal Health, Dublin, Ohio, USA). Liver biopsy specimens were processed using standard laboratory procedures. Liver biopsy slides were stained with hematoxylin and eosin stain and masson trichrome stain. Liver biopsy slides were examined by an experienced histopathologist (NRNM) who was blinded to clinical data. Histopathological findings were reported according to the Non-Alcoholic Steatohepatitis Clinical Research Network Scoring System [15]. The NAFLD activity score (NAS) is the sum of scores for hepatic steatosis (0–3), lobular inflammation (0–3) and hepatocyte ballooning (0–2). NAS 0–2 is not diagnostic of NASH, 3–4 is probable NASH and 5–8 is definite NASH. Subjects with NAS<5 was considered as non-NASH while subjects with NAS≥ 5 were considered to have NASH. Fibrosis was staged 0–4 (0 = no fibrosis, 1 = mild fibrosis, 2 = moderate fibrosis, 3 = severe fibrosis, 4 = cirrhosis).

Ethics statement

This study was approved by the University of Malaya Medical Centre's Medical Ethics Committee and conformed to the Declaration of Helsinki. All subjects who participated provided written informed consent.

Statistical analysis

Data were analysed using a standard statistical software program (SPSS 15.0). Continuous variables were expressed as mean ± standard deviation or median (interquartile range) and analyzed using t-test, ANOVA, Mann-Whitney test or Kruskal-Wallis test, as appropriate. Categorical variables were expressed as percentages and analyzed using chi-square test or Fisher's exact test, as appropriate. Significance was assumed when $p<0.05$. The performance of plasma M30 and serum ALT, AST and GGT levels for prediction of NAFLD and NASH was determined using area under receiver-operating characteristics curve (AUROC). AUROC was interpreted as follows: 0.90–1.00 = excellent, 0.80–0.90 = good, 0.70–0.80 = fair, <0.70 = poor. The sensitivity, specificity, positive predictive value and negative predictive value using cut-off values for high sensitivity, highest overall accuracy and high specificity were determined. Boxplots were used to compare the distribution of plasma M30 and serum ALT, AST and GGT levels across the different grades of steatosis, lobular inflammation and ballooning, and across the different stages of fibrosis.

Results

Patient characteristics

Ninety-three NAFLD subjects and 20 controls were recruited during the period of study. The characteristics of subjects are shown in Table 1. Controls and NAFLD subjects were well-matched in age and gender. NAFLD subjects had a greater BMI and WC and had higher prevalence of diabetes mellitus, hypertension and dyslipidemia compared to controls. There was a lower proportion of males among NASH subjects compared to non-NASH subjects. NASH and non-NASH subjects were similar in age, BMI, WC and prevalence of diabetes mellitus, hypertension and dyslipidemia. The quality of liver biopsy specimen as reflected by its length and the number of portal tracts, were also similar between NASH and non-NASH subjects. NASH subjects showed greater steatosis, lobular inflammation, ballooning and fibrosis.

Plasma M30 and serum ALT, AST and GGT levels in controls and NAFLD subjects

Plasma M30 levels were significantly higher in subjects with NAFLD (median 349 U/L, IQR 257 U/L–612 U/L) than in controls (median 162 U/L, IQR 103 U/L–215 U/L, $p<0.001$). Although plasma M30 levels were higher in subjects with NASH (median 435 U/L, IQR 279 U/L–758 U/L) compared to non-NASH subjects (median 332 U/L, IQR 249 U/L–534 U/L), the difference was not significant statistically ($p=0.145$).

Serum ALT levels were significantly higher in subjects with NAFLD (median 70 IU/L, IQR 44 IU/L–109 IU/L) than in

Table 1. Patient characteristics.

	Controls, n = 20	NAFLD patients, n = 93	Non-NASH patients, n = 54	NASH patients, n = 39
Age, years	50.6±16.8	51.0±11.1	50.2±11.3	52.2±10.8
Male, %†	30.0	51.6	63.0	35.9
BMI, kg per m^2*	22.5±2.8	29.4±3.8	29.1±3.7	29.8±4.0
WC, cm*	81.8±7.6	97.7±9.7	96.8±9.7	98.8±9.7
Diabetes mellitus, %*	0	59.1	51.9	69.2
Hypertension, %*	20.0	88.2	85.2	92.3
Dyslipidemia, %*	40.0	96.8	94.4	100
Serum ALT, IU/L*†	26 (22–32)	70 (44–109)	61 (44–93)	86 (55–121)
Serum AST, IU/L*‡	20 (18–27)	41 (28–64)	34 (25–46)	58 (38–78)
Serum GGT, IU/L*†	33 (22–45)	75 (47–125)	56 (40–101)	97 (53–151)
Plasma M30, U/L*	162 (103–215)	349 (257–612)	332 (249–534)	435 (279–758)
Liver biopsy length, mm	–	15.0±3.9	14.5±4.2	15.7±3.5
Number of portal tracts	–	8 (7–10)	8 (6–10)	9 (7–11)
Steatosis†				
0	–	3.2	5.6	0
1	–	34.4	42.6	23.1
2	–	47.3	48.1	46.2
3	–	15.1	3.7	30.8
Lobular inflammation‡				
0	–	4.3	7.4	0
1	–	53.8	81.5	15.4
2	–	38.7	11.1	76.9
3	–	3.2	0	7.7
Ballooning‡				
0	–	14.0	24.1	0
1	–	60.2	70.4	46.2
2	–	25.8	5.6	53.8
Fibrosis‡				
0	–	30.1	44.4	10.3
1	–	43.0	42.6	43.6
2	–	6.5	1.9	12.8
3	–	18.3	7.4	33.3
4	–	2.2	3.7	0

NAFLD, non-alcoholic fatty liver disease; NASH, non-alcoholic steatohepatitis; BMI, body mass index; WC, waist circumference; ALT, alanine aminotransferase; AST, aspartate aminotransferase; GGT, gamma glutamyl transpeptidase.
* Significant at $p<0.001$ between healthy controls and NAFLD patients.
†Significant at $p<0.05$.
‡Significant at $p<0.001$, between non-NASH and NASH patients.

controls (median 26 IU/L, IQR 22 IU/L–32 IU/L, $p<0.001$). More importantly, serum ALT levels were significantly higher in NASH subjects (median 86 IU/L, IQR 55 IU/L–121 IU/L) compared to non-NASH subjects (median 61 IU/L, IQR 44 IU/L–93 IU/L, $p<0.05$).

Serum AST levels were significantly higher in subjects with NAFLD (median 41 IU/L, IQR 28 IU/L–64 IU/L) than in controls (median 20 IU/L, IQR 18 IU/L–27 IU/L, $p<0.001$). Serum AST levels were also significantly higher in NASH subjects (median 58 IU/L, IQR 38 IU/L–78 IU/L) compared to non-NASH subjects (median 34 IU/L, IQR 25 IU/L–46 IU/L, $p<0.001$).

Serum GGT levels were significantly higher in subjects with NAFLD (median 75 IU/L, IQR 47 IU/L–125 IU/L) than in controls (median 33 IU/L, IQR 22 IU/L–45 IU/L, $p<0.001$). Serum GGT levels were also significantly higher in NASH subjects (median 97 IU/L, IQR 53 IU/L–151 IU/L) compared to non-NASH subjects (median 56 IU/L, IQR 40 IU/L–101 IU/L, $p<0.05$).

Prediction of NAFLD and NASH

The receiver operating characteristic curves of plasma M30 and serum ALT, AST and GGT for prediction of NAFLD and NASH are shown in Figure 1a–b. Plasma M30 and serum ALT levels were excellent for predicting NAFLD with an AUROC of 0.91 and 0.95, respectively. Serum AST and GGT levels were good for predicting NAFLD with an AUROC of 0.87 and 0.85, respectively. Serum AST level was fair for predicting NASH among NAFLD subjects with AUROC of 0.75. Plasma M30 and serum ALT and GGT levels were poor for predicting NASH among NAFLD subjects with an AUROC of 0.59, 0.64 and 0.68, respectively. The sensitivity, specificity, positive predictive value and negative predictive value when using the different cut-offs of plasma M30 and serum ALT, AST and GGT levels for prediction of NAFLD and NASH are shown in Tables 2 and 3.

When global histological assessment was used for the diagnosis of NASH, 44 patients who were considered as non-NASH using the NAS had NASH. The characteristics of patients with and without NASH and the receiver operating characteristic curves of plasma M30 and serum ALT, AST and GGT for prediction of NASH when global histological assessment was used can be found as supplementary material (Table S1 and Figure S1, respectively). The findings were similar regardless of whether NAS or global histological assessment was used for the diagnosis of NASH.

Plasma M30 and serum ALT, AST and GGT according to steatosis, ballooning, lobular inflammation and fibrosis

Plasma M30 and serum ALT and AST levels did not show any significant trend when analyzed according to steatosis grades. Although serum GGT level showed a significant trend when analyzed according to steatosis grades, the difference in serum GGT level was only significant between subjects with grade 2 and 3 steatosis (Figure S2).

Serum ALT and AST levels showed a significant trend with increasing grades of ballooning. However, this was not seen with plasma M30 and serum GGT levels. Serum ALT levels were significantly higher in subjects with grade 1 compared to subjects without ballooning. However, serum ALT levels were not significantly different between subjects with grade 1 and grade 2 ballooning. Serum AST levels were significantly higher in subjects with grade 2 compared to grade 1 ballooning and in subjects with grade 1 compared to subjects without ballooning (Figure S3).

Serum ALT and AST levels also showed a significant trend with increasing grades of lobular inflammation. Once again, this was not seen with plasma M30 and serum GGT levels. Serum ALT and AST levels were significantly higher in subjects with grade 2 compared to grade 1 lobular inflammation. However, serum ALT and AST levels were not significantly different between subjects with grade 2 and grade 3 lobular inflammation, and between subjects with grade 1 and subjects without lobular inflammation (Figure S4).

Plasma M30 level did not show any significant trend when analyzed according to fibrosis stages. There was a significant difference in serum ALT, AST and GGT levels across fibrosis stages. However, only differences in serum ALT and AST for stage 1 and stage 2 fibrosis was significant (Figure 2).

Prediction of ballooning and lobular inflammation

In view of the above findings, analysis was carried out to determine the accuracy of plasma M30 and serum ALT, AST and GGT levels for prediction of presence of ballooning and presence of more severe lobular inflammation. Lobular inflammation grade 0 and grade 1 were considered less severe while grade 2 and grade 3 were considered more severe. The results are shown in Figure 3a–b. Serum ALT and AST levels were fair for prediction of presence of ballooning with AUROC of 0.72 and 0.77, respectively. Serum AST level was fair for prediction of presence of more severe lobular inflammation with AUROC of 0.78. Plasma M30 and serum GGT levels were poor for prediction of presence of ballooning and presence of more severe lobular inflammation. The sensitivity, specificity, positive predictive value

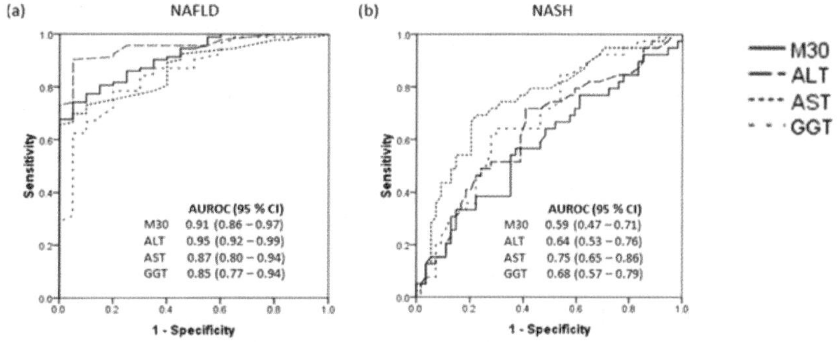

Figure 1. The receiver operating characteristic curves of plasma M30 and serum ALT, AST and GGT for prediction of (a) NAFLD, and (b) NASH. AUROC was interpreted as follows: 0.90–1.00 = excellent, 0.80–0.90 = good, 0.70–0.80 = fair, <0.70 = poor. ALT, alanine aminotransferase; AST, aspartate aminotransferase; GGT; gamma glutamyl transpeptidase; NAFLD, non-alcoholic fatty liver disease; NASH, non-alcoholic steatohepatitis.

Table 2. Accuracy of plasma M30 and serum ALT, AST and GGT for prediction of NAFLD.

	Cut-off, U/L or IU/L*	Sensitivity, %	Specificity, %	PPV, %	NPV, %
Plasma M30	162	95.7	45.0	89.0	69.2
	263	74.2	95.0	98.6	44.2
	278	67.7	100	100	40.0
Serum ALT	27	95.7	55.0	90.8	73.3
	35	90.3	95.0	98.8	67.9
	47	73.1	100	100	44.4
Serum AST	21	92.5	55.0	90.5	61.1
	33†	65.6	100	100	38.5
Serum GGT	32	90.3	50.0	89.4	52.6
	46	78.5	80.0	94.8	44.4
	55	62.4	95.0	98.3	35.2

ALT, alanine aminotransferase; AST, aspartate aminotransferase; GGT, gamma glutamyl transpeptidase; NAFLD, non-alcoholic fatty liver disease; PPV, positive predictive value; NPV, negative predictive value.
* Cut-off with high sensitivity, highest overall accuracy and high specificity were presented.
†Cut-off for highest overall accuracy and high specificity were the same.

and negative predictive value when using the different cut-offs of plasma M30 and serum ALT, AST and GGT levels for prediction of presence of ballooning and more severe lobular inflammation can be found as supplementary material (Table S2 and S3).

Characteristics of patients according to plasma M30 tertiles and factors associated with plasma M30 level

The characteristics of patients according to plasma M30 tertiles can be found as supplementary material (Table S4). The only variables that showed significant difference across tertiles were serum ALT and GGT. On bivariate correlation, plasma M30 level was significantly correlated with BMI ($r = 0.23$, $p < 0.05$), and serum ALT ($r = 0.32$, $p < 0.01$) and AST ($r = 0.35$, $p < 0.01$). Age, BMI, and serum ALT, AST and GGT were entered into multiple linear regression analysis but none of the variables were found to be significant (data not shown).

Discussion

The potential use of plasma M30 level as a non-invasive biomarker to determine histological disease severity in NAFLD subjects was first reported by Wieckowska et al. In their study of 44 consecutive subjects with suspected NAFLD at the time of liver biopsy, plasma CK-18 levels were markedly increased in adults with NASH compared to those with simple steatosis or normal liver biopsies. Plasma M30 level had a high accuracy in distinguishing subjects with NASH from those with simple steatosis or normal liver biopsies with an AUROC of 0.93. Two subjects with borderline NASH were not included in the analysis [6]. In a subsequent multi-centre validation study consisting of 139 subjects, Feldstein et al demonstrated that plasma M30 level had an AUROC of 0.83 in detecting NASH. However, it is important to note that this population consisted of a relatively small percentage

Table 3. Accuracy of plasma M30 and serum ALT, AST and GGT for prediction of NASH.

	Cut-off, U/L or IU/L*	Sensitivity, %	Specificity, %	PPV, %	NPV, %
Plasma M30	293	71.8	40.7	46.7	66.7
	432	56.4	63.0	52.4	66.7
	474	43.6	64.8	47.2	61.4
Serum ALT	53	79.5	40.7	49.2	73.3
	67	71.8	59.3	56.0	74.4
	100	41.0	79.6	59.3	65.2
Serum AST	30	84.6	40.7	50.8	78.6
	48	69.2	77.8	69.2	77.8
	65	43.6	90.7	77.3	69.0
Serum GGT	49	84.6	42.6	51.6	79.3
	84	64.1	70.4	61.0	73.1
	109	46.2	77.8	60.0	66.7

ALT, alanine aminotransferase; AST, aspartate aminotransferase; GGT, gamma glutamyl transpeptidase; NASH, non-alcoholic steatohepatitis; PPV, positive predictive value; NPV, negative predictive value.
* Cut-off with high sensitivity, highest overall accuracy and high specificity were presented.

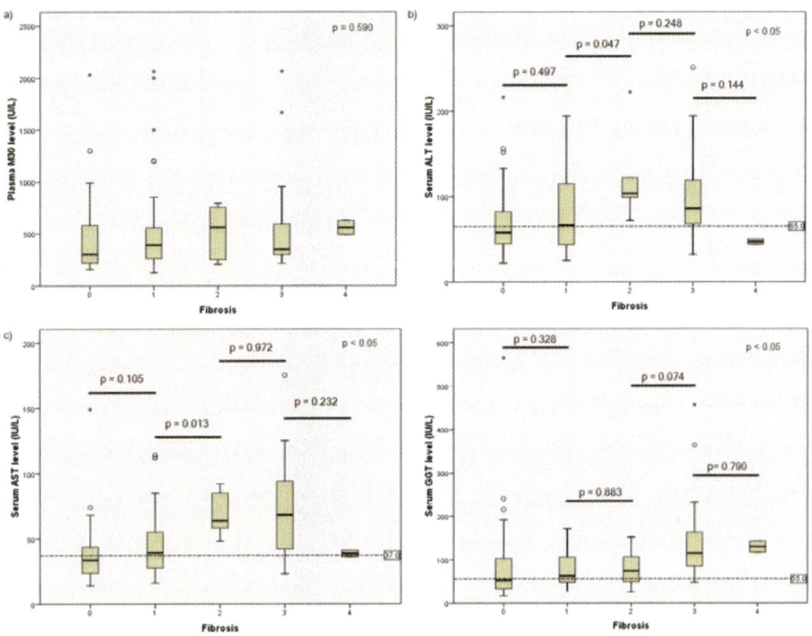

Figure 2. Plasma M30 and serum ALT, AST and GGT levels according to fibrosis stages. The data between and across groups were analyzed using Mann-Whitney test and Kruskal-Wallis test, respectively. The p value between groups were only shown when there was a significant difference across groups. Fibrosis was staged 0–4 (0 = no fibrosis, 1 = mild fibrosis, 2 = moderate fibrosis, 3 = severe fibrosis, 4 = cirrhosis). F, fibrosis stage; ALT, alanine aminotransferase; AST, aspartate aminotransferase; GGT; gamma glutamyl transpeptidase.

of subjects with borderline NASH (19%) [7]. Subsequently, Shen et al reported that M30 had an AUROC of 0.66 for detecting NASH in a study population which consisted of a larger percentage of subjects with borderline NASH (49.7%) [12]. In our study population which consisted of a similar proportion of subjects with borderline NASH (52.7%), we similarly demonstrated that plasma M30 was less useful for distinguishing NAFLD subjects with NASH from those without NASH with an AUROC of 0.59. In a recently published study consisting of 318 subjects, Cusi et al similarly reported that plasma M30 level was less useful for NASH diagnosis with an AUROC of 0.65 [13].

Although M30 appeared to have a limited value for detecting NASH in this study, we found that serum AST level had a reasonable accuracy in distinguishing NASH from non-NASH subjects with an AUROC of 0.75. Furthermore, serum AST level had a greater accuracy in predicting the presence of ballooning and the presence of more severe lobular inflammation in contrast to serum ALT and GGT levels. Other tests for the diagnosis of NASH such as measurement of total cell death markers M65 and M65ED, adipocyte fatty acid binding protein (AFABP) and fibroblast growth factors 21 (FGF21) have been studied but were not better with AUROC of 0.71, 0.70, 0.59 and 0.62, respectively [11,12].

It appears that an accurate non-invasive test for NASH remains elusive. However, we should not forget that NASH is a continuous spectrum and markers may be variably expressed in each individual so that finding a test that confirms the presence or absence of NASH using a pre-determined cut-off may be difficult if not impossible. It may be more realistic to aim for a test that would reflect changes in severity of NASH when followed over time. For example, Suzuki et al reported that the combination of a baseline and rate of change of serum ALT and AST levels had an AUROC of 0.72 and 0.73, respectively, in predicting improvement, and an AUROC of 0.75 and 0.77, respectively, in

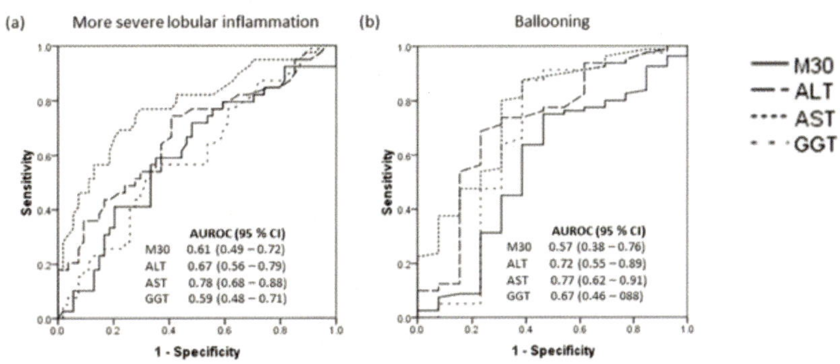

Figure 3. The receiver operating characteristic curves of plasma M30 and serum ALT, AST and GGT for prediction of (a) more severe lobular inflammation, and (b) ballooning. AUROC was interpreted as follows: 0.90–1.00 = excellent, 0.80–0.90 = good, 0.70–0.80 = fair, < 0.70 = poor. ALT, alanine aminotransferase; AST, aspartate aminotransferase; GGT; gamma glutamyl transpeptidase.

predicting worsening of histological inflammation in NASH subjects. The AUROC improved to 0.88 and 0.89, respectively, when baseline histology was taken into consideration [16]. In another study of 36 subjects without NASH at baseline, Shen et al showed that changes in M30 was quite accurate in predicting the development of NASH with an AUROC of 0.82. Using 35 U/L as the cut-off for increment in M30, development of NASH could be predicted with a sensitivity and specificity of 80.0% and 81.5%, respectively [12]. The use of changes in plasma M30 and serum ALT and AST levels to predict changes in histology, particularly inflammation and ballooning, should be compared and deserves further studies in a larger group of subjects. A combination of various parameters, including diabetes mellitus, gender, BMI, triglycerides, M30 and M65–M30 has been proposed for non-invasive diagnosis of NASH [17]. Separately, a support vector machine-based panel using osteoprotegerin, fibroblast growth factor 21 and M30 also appeared promising for this purpose [18]. However, these requires further study and validation.

Our study was carried out prospectively and collection of blood samples were done on the same day as the liver biopsy procedure to minimize differences due to changes over time. Despite our best effort, the study had several limitations. Firstly, as in any study using histopathological examination of liver biopsy specimen as a reference, there may have been sampling and observer variability. Secondly, the absence of NAFLD in controls was based on ultrasonography, which may lack sensitivity in detection of mild hepatic steatosis. However, performing a liver biopsy to exclude NAFLD in these subjects was not deemed to be ethical in this study.

In conclusion, plasma M30 appears to have a limited utility in detecting NASH in clinical practice, particularly when compared to serum ALT, AST or GGT levels subjects. While other more accurate yet non-invasive tests are needed for the diagnosis of NASH, the use of changes in plasma M30 and serum ALT and AST levels to predict changes in histology, particularly inflammation and ballooning, should be compared and deserves further study in a larger group of subjects.

Supporting Information

Figure S1 The receiver operating characteristic curves of plasma M30 and serum ALT, AST and GGT for prediction of NASH when global histological assessment was used for the diagnosis of NASH. AUROC was interpreted as follows: 0.90–1.00 = excellent, 0.80–0.90 = good, 0.70–0.80 = fair, <0.70 = poor. ALT, alanine aminotransferase; AST, aspartate aminotransferase; GGT; gamma glutamyl transpeptidase; NASH, non-alcoholic steatohepatitis.

Figure S2 Plasma M30 and serum ALT, AST and GGT levels according to steatosis grades. The data between and across groups were analyzed using Mann-Whitney test and Kruskal-Wallis test, respectively. The p value between groups were only shown when there was a significant difference across groups. Steatosis was graded 0–3 (0 = less than 5%, 1 = 5–33%, 2 = 34–66%, 3 = more than 66%). ALT, alanine aminotransferase; AST, aspartate aminotransferase; GGT; gamma glutamyl transpeptidase.

Figure S3 Plasma M30 and serum ALT, AST and GGT levels according to ballooning grades. The data between and across groups were analyzed using Mann-Whitney test and Kruskal-Wallis test, respectively. The p value between groups were only shown when there was a significant difference across groups. Ballooning was graded 0–2 (0 = none, 1 = few/mild, 2 = many/prominent). ALT, alanine aminotransferase; AST, aspartate aminotransferase; GGT; gamma glutamyl transpeptidase.

Figure S4 Plasma M30 and serum ALT, AST and GGT levels according to lobular inflammation grades. The data between and across groups were analyzed using Mann-Whitney test and Kruskal-Wallis test, respectively. The p value between groups were only shown when there was a significant difference across groups. Lobular inflammation was graded 0–3 (0 = none, 1 = less than 2 foci, 2 = 2–4 foci, 3 = more than 4 foci) ALT, alanine aminotransferase; AST, aspartate aminotransferase; GGT; gamma glutamyl transpeptidase.

Table S1 Patient characteristics (diagnosis of NASH based on global histological assessment).

Table S2 The sensitivity, specificity, positive predictive value and negative predictive value when using the different cut-offs of plasma M30 and serum ALT, AST and GGT levels for prediction of presence of more severe lobular inflammation.

Table S3 The sensitivity, specificity, positive predictive value and negative predictive value when using the different cut-offs of plasma M30 and serum ALT, AST and GGT levels for prediction of presence of ballooning.

Table S4 Characteristics of patients according to plasma M30 tertiles.

Data S1 This file contains data underlying the findings described in this manuscript.

Acknowledgments

The authors would like to acknowledge the help from Madam Talvant Kaur and Ms. Nurliyana Adzhar.

Author Contributions

Conceived and designed the experiments: WKC. Performed the experiments: WKC NRNM PS SM. Analyzed the data: WKC. Contributed reagents/materials/analysis tools: NRNM PS. Contributed to the writing of the manuscript: WKC SM.

References

1. Chan WK, Goh KL (2013) Epidemiology of a fast-emerging disease in the Asia-Pacific region: non-alcoholic fatty liver disease. Hepatol Int 7: 65–71.
2. Ekstedt M, Franzen LE, Mathiesen UL, Thorelius L, Holmqvist M, et al. (2006) Long-term follow-up of patients with NAFLD and elevated liver enzymes. Hepatology 44: 865–73.
3. Sanyal AJ, Banas C, Sargeant C, Luketic VA, Sterling RK, et al. (2006) Similarities and differences in outcomes of cirrhosis due to nonalcoholic steatohepatitis and hepatitis C. Hepatology 43: 682–9.
4. Piccinino F, Sagnelli E, Pasquale G, Giusti G (1986) Complications following percutaneous liver biopsy. A multicentre retrospective study on 68,276 biopsies. Journal of hepatology 2: 165–73.

5. Feldstein AE, Canbay A, Angulo P, Taniai M, Burgart LJ, et al. (2003) Hepatocyte apoptosis and fas expression are prominent features of human nonalcoholic steatohepatitis. Gastroenterology 125: 437–43.
6. Wieckowska A, Zein NN, Yerian LM, Lopez AR, McCullough AJ, et al. (2006) In vivo assessment of liver cell apoptosis as a novel biomarker of disease severity in nonalcoholic fatty liver disease. Hepatology 44: 27–33.
7. Feldstein AE, Wieckowska A, Lopez AR, Liu YC, Zein NN, et al. (2009) Cytokeratin-18 fragment levels as noninvasive biomarkers for nonalcoholic steatohepatitis: a multicenter validation study. Hepatology 50: 1072–8.
8. Diab DL, Yerian L, Schauer P, Kashyap SR, Lopez R, et al. (2008) Cytokeratin 18 fragment levels as a noninvasive biomarker for nonalcoholic steatohepatitis in bariatric surgery patients. Clinical gastroenterology and hepatology : the official clinical practice journal of the American Gastroenterological Association 6: 1249–54.
9. Tamimi TI, Elgouhari HM, Alkhouri N, Yerian LM, Berk MP, et al. (2011) An apoptosis panel for nonalcoholic steatohepatitis diagnosis. Journal of hepatology 54: 1224–9.
10. Yilmaz Y, Dolar E, Ulukaya E, Akgoz S, Keskin M, et al. (2007) Soluble forms of extracellular cytokeratin 18 may differentiate simple steatosis from nonalcoholic steatohepatitis. World journal of gastroenterology : WJG 13: 837–44.
11. Shen J, Chan HL, Wong GL, Choi PC, Chan AW, et al. (2012) Non-invasive diagnosis of non-alcoholic steatohepatitis by combined serum biomarkers. Journal of hepatology 56: 1363–70.
12. Shen J, Chan HL, Wong GL, Chan AW, Choi PC, et al. (2012) Assessment of non-alcoholic fatty liver disease using serum total cell death and apoptosis markers. Alimentary pharmacology & therapeutics 36: 1057–66.
13. Cusi K, Chang Z, Harrison S, Lomonaco R, Bril F, et al. (2014) Limited value of plasma cytokeratin-18 as a biomarker for NASH and fibrosis in patients with non-alcoholic fatty liver disease. Journal of hepatology 60: 167–74.
14. Chalasani N, Younossi Z, Lavine JE, Diehl AM, Brunt EM, et al. (2012) The diagnosis and management of non-alcoholic fatty liver disease: practice Guideline by the American Association for the Study of Liver Diseases, American College of Gastroenterology, and the American Gastroenterological Association. Hepatology 55: 2005–23.
15. Kleiner DE, Brunt EM, Van Natta M, Behling C, Contos MJ, et al. (2005) Design and validation of a histological scoring system for nonalcoholic fatty liver disease. Hepatology 41: 1313–21.
16. Suzuki A, Lymp J, Sauver JS, Angulo P, Lindor K (2006) Values and limitations of serum aminotransferases in clinical trials of nonalcoholic steatohepatitis. Liver international : official journal of the International Association for the Study of the Liver 26: 1209–16.
17. Younossi ZM, Page S, Rafiq N, Birerdinc A, Stepanova M, et al. (2011) A biomarker panel for non-alcoholic steatohepatitis (NASH) and NASH-related fibrosis. Obes Surg 21: 431–9.
18. Yilmaz Y, Eren F (2012) Identification of a support vector machine-based biomarker panel with high sensitivity and specificity for nonalcoholic steatohepatitis. Clin Chim Acta 24: 154–7.

18

Interaction between *PNPLA3* I148M Variant and Age at Infection in Determining Fibrosis Progression in Chronic Hepatitis C

Stella De Nicola[1], Paola Dongiovanni[2], Alessio Aghemo[1], Cristina Cheroni[3], Roberta D'Ambrosio[1,4], Michele Pedrazzini[4], Francesco Marabita[3¤], Lorena Donnici[3], Marco Maggioni[5], Silvia Fargion[2,4], Massimo Colombo[1,4], Raffaele De Francesco[3*], Luca Valenti[2,4*]

1 Department of Gastroenterology, Fondazione IRCCS Ca' Granda Ospedale Policlinico Milano, Milano, Italy, **2** Department of Internal Medicine, Fondazione IRCCS Ca' Granda Ospedale Policlinico Milano, Milano, Italy, **3** Virology Program, INGM - Istituto Nazionale di Genetica Molecolare "Romeo ed Enrica Invernizzi," Milano, Italy, **4** Department of Pathophysiology and Transplantation, Università degli Studi di Milano, Milano, Italy, **5** Department of Pathology, Fondazione IRCCS Ca' Granda Ospedale Policlinico Milano, Milano, Italy

Abstract

Background and Aims: The *PNPLA3* I148M sequence variant favors hepatic lipid accumulation and confers susceptibility to hepatic fibrosis and hepatocellular carcinoma. The aim of this study was to estimate the effect size of homozygosity for the *PNPLA3* I148M variant (148M/M) on the fibrosis progression rate (FPR) and the interaction with age at infection in chronic hepatitis C (CHC).

Methods: FPR was estimated in a prospective cohort of 247 CHC patients without alcohol intake and diabetes, with careful estimation of age at infection and determination of fibrosis stage by Ishak score.

Results: Older age at infection was the strongest determinant of FPR ($p<0.0001$). *PNPLA3* 148M/M was associated with faster FPR in individuals infected at older age (above the median, 21 years; -0.64 ± 0.2, $n=8$ vs. -0.95 ± 0.3, $n=166$ $\log_{10}$ FPR respectively; $p=0.001$; confirmed for lower age thresholds, $p<0.05$), but not in those infected at younger age (p = ns). The negative impact of *PNPLA3* 148M/M on fibrosis progression was more marked in subjects at risk of altered hepatic lipid metabolism (those with grade 2–3 steatosis, genotype 3, and overweight; $p<0.05$). At multivariate analysis, *PNPLA3* 148M/M was associated with FPR (incremental effect 0.08 ± 0.03 $\log_{10}$ fibrosis unit per year; $p=0.022$), independently of several confounders, and there was a significant interaction between 148M/M and older age at infection ($p=0.025$). The association between 148M/M and FPR remained significant even after adjustment for steatosis severity ($p=0.032$).

Conclusions: We observed an interaction between homozygosity for the *PNPLA3* I148M variant and age at infection in determining fibrosis progression in CHC patients.

Editor: Matias A. Avila, University of Navarra School of Medicine and Center for Applied Medical Research (CIMA), Spain

Funding: This manuscript was supported by Ricerca Corrente Fondazione IRCCS Ca' Granda (Institutional core funds; no grant number is available), and Associazione Malattie Metaboliche del Fegato ONLUS (non-profit organization for the study and the cure of metabolic liver diseases). The funders had no role in study design, data collection and analysis, decision to publish, or preparation of the manuscript.

* Email: luca.valenti@unimi.it (LV); defrancesco@ingm.it (RDF)

Competing Interests: The authors have declared that no competing interests exist.

These authors contributed equally to this work.

¤ Current address: Unit of Computational Medicine, Center for Molecular Medicine, Department of Medicine, Karolinska Institutet, Stockholm, Sweden

Introduction

Hepatitis C virus (HCV) infection affects roughly 130–170 million people worldwide. Individuals with chronic HCV-related hepatitis (CHC) are at high risk of liver fibrosis, an in about 20% of cases CHC progresses to cirrhosis. Therefore, HCV is a leading cause of end-stage liver disease and hepatocellular carcinoma [1]. Older age at infection, genotype 3, coexistent liver diseases, male gender, alcohol abuse, obesity and diabetes, and steatosis are risk factors for disease evolution [2–5].

However, even after taking into account all known viral, host related, and environmental factors, the rate of progression to advanced fibrosis is highly variable among individuals, thereby suggesting a role for inherited variants. Indeed, single-nucleotide polymorphisms at different genetic loci have been associated with fibrosis progression in candidate gene studies [6,7].

The rs738409 C>G polymorphism of *Patatin-like phospholipase domain-containing 3* (*PNPLA3*), encoding for the I148M protein sequence variant, is the major common genetic determinant of hepatic fat content. The I148M variant influences the metabolism of triglycerides, lipid droplets remodeling, and lipoprotein secretion in hepatocytes [8–13]. *PNPLA3* I148M is the major risk factor for both alcoholic and nonalcoholic steatohepatitis, showing an age-modulated effect on liver damage susceptibility and fibrogenesis [14–19]. Recently, it has been reported that homozygosity for the 148M risk allele (henceforth *PNPLA3* 148M/M) also influences the risk of advanced fibrosis and hepatocellular carcinoma in CHC [20–25]. However, scant data are derived from prospective studies [23,25], and the interaction with age at infection has not been evaluated so far.

Therefore, the aim of this study was to estimate the effect size of *PNPLA3* 148M/M on fibrosis progression rate (FPR) and the interaction with age at infection in a unique validated cohort of 247 CHC subjects without significant alcohol intake and diabetes, characterized by a careful estimation of age at infection and with histological determination of liver damage [3].

Materials and Methods

Patients

We analyzed a previous published cohort of 247 CHC patients followed-up at the Migliavacca Liver Disease Center at the Fondazione IRCCS Ca' Granda Policlinico of Milan [3]. Briefly, inclusion criteria comprised a precise estimate of the date of infection based on the date of the first reported risk factor, a diagnostic liver biopsy before any antiviral therapy performed at least 4 years after the date of infection, and no history of past or current alcohol abuse. Patients with viral co-infections or other liver diseases were excluded, as well as patients with either type 1 or type 2 diabetes. Disease duration was calculated considering the time elapsed from the date of infection to the time of liver biopsy. The study protocol conformed to the Declaration of Helsinki and was approved by the Institutional Review Board of the Fondazione IRCCS Ca' Granda. Each patient signed a written informed consent.

The baseline features of the study cohort stratified by *PNPLA3* 148M/M status are presented in table 1. The study database has been uploaded as supplementary material (Data S1).

Histological evaluation

Liver histology was evaluated by a single expert pathologist. Mean biopsy length was 26.3 mm. The severity of hepatic inflammation was evaluated by the Ishak score [26], entailing a maximum of 18 points for grading (G) and 6 points for liver staging (S). All specimens were also evaluated for steatosis severity (grade 0: absent or <5%; grade 1: 5–33%; grade 2: 34–66%; grade 3: >66% of hepatocytes affected) [27]. Steatosis assessment is missing for 14 patients due to the inability to recollect the original histological slides re-evaluated for fibrosis stage. To analyze the effect of steatosis severity in the whole study cohort, additional analyses were conducted estimating the severity of steatosis in these 14 subjects by ultrasonography [28].

Genetic analysis

Genomic DNA was obtained from peripheral whole blood as previously described [3]. The *PNPLA3* rs738409 C>G single nucleotide polymorphism, encoding for the I148M protein sequence variant, was genotyped by a 5′ nuclease Taqman assay (LifeTechnologies, Carlsbad, CA, USA) at the Metabolic Liver Diseases lab at the Fondazione Ca' Granda IRCCS. Success rate was 100% and perfect concordance between duplicates and internal controls was observed.

Statistical analysis

For descriptive statistics, variables were shown as mean ± SD and frequencies, and compared by Student's t-test or chi-square test according to data distribution. P values were considered significant when <0.05 (two-tailed). FPR was calculated by taking the ratio between the staging value of Ishak score and the disease duration (years), and it was treated as a continuous variable. Mean disease duration was 25±10 years. Log_{10} transformation of FPR was employed to obtain linearity. FPR estimation assumes that no significant liver fibrosis was present at the time of infection, and that liver fibrosis progression is constant during time [2]. A first generalized linear model was formulated and fitted to the data, specifying the presence of *PNPLA3* 148M/M at risk genotype [21–23], and the covariates as explanatory variables. We considered as covariated the independent predictors of FPR in a previously reported analysis of the same cohort [3]: age at infection (encoded as > or ≤ the median value, 21 years), gender, and HCV genotype. The product term age at infection x *PNPLA3* 148M/M was fitted into the model to test the interaction between *PNPLA3* genotype and age at infection on FPR. To account for other potential confounders, a second model was tested, with further adjustement for the route of HCV transmission (intra-venous drug use: IVDU or other), body-mass (BMI < or ≥25 Kg/m^2), and age at liver biopsy. Finally, to check whether the relationship between *PNPLA3* genotype and FPR was independent of steatosis, a final model further adjusted for the histological severity of steatosis (grade 2–3 vs. 0–1) was evaluated. Models were checked through the regression diagnostic plots to verify normality, linearity of the data, and constant variance. The effect of the explanatory variables was considered significant if $p < 0.05$ (two-tailed). Analyses were performed by the SPSS 21.0 (IBM, Burbank, NY, USA) statistical analysis software.

Results

Study cohort

Detailed characterization of the study cohort has previously been reported [3]. Briefly, 52% of patients were males, the majority infected by genotype 1 (52%), during blood transfusion (75%). Median age at infection was 21 years and disease duration 25 years. At the time of histological evaluation, 16% of patients had cirrhosis, whereas severe steatosis (grade 2–3) was observed in 20% of cases. The frequency distribution of the *PNPLA3* I148M variant did not violate Hardy-Weinberg equilibrium (p>0.8), and was in line with that expected unselected subjects: 120 patients were *PNPLA3* 148I/I (48%), 106 148I/M (43%), and 21 had the unfavorable 148M/M genotype (9%).

Clinical features of patients stratified by *PNPLA3* 148M/M status are presented in table 1. Demographic and anthropometric features, viral genotype distribution, age and route of infection, and duration of follow-up did not differ according to *PNPLA3* 148M/M status (p = ns). There was no statistically significant difference in the prevalence of grade 2–3 steatosis according to *PNPLA3* 148M/M status (p = ns), although a nonsignificant trend was observed in the whole cohort including subjects with ultrasonographic estimation of steatosis severity (7/21, 33% vs. 44/226, 19% in 148M/M vs. individuals carrying other *PNPLA3* genotypes, p = 0.15).

Table 1. Clinical features of 247 CHC patients subdivided according to the presence of homozygosity for *PNPLA3* I148M variant (148M/M).

	PNPLA3 **I148M genotype**		**p value**
	148I/I or I/M	**148M/M**	
	n = 226 (91)	**n = 21 (9)**	
Age at infection years	21.5±13	21.7±16	0.96
Sex F	109 (48)	9 (43)	0.66
BMI Kg/m²	26.1±13	24.9±6	0.69
Age at biopsy years	46.8±12	48.4±13	0.70
HCV genotype			0.64
G1	116 (51)	13 (62)	
G2	68 (30)	6 (28)	
G3	32 (14)	2 (10)	
G4	10 (5)	0	
Route of infection			0.83
Transfusion	169 (75)	16 (76)	
IVDU	53 (23)	5 (24)	
Other	4 (2)	0	
Steatosis grade 2–3	42 (19)	5 (26)	0.48
Disease activity (grade)	6 {5–7}	6 {5–7}	0.78
Fibrosis stage	2 {1–3}	3 {2–5}	0.22

Continous variables are shown as mean ± SD (normally distributed) or median {interquartile range} (skewed variables); (): % values; F: female; BMI: body mass index; G: genotype; IVDU: intra-venous drug user; Other: needlestick, mother-to-child, sexual transmission.

Effect of age at infection and *PNPLA3* 148M/M on fibrosis progression

Older age at infection was strongly associated with FPR ($\log_{10}$ FPR -1.1 ± 0.3 vs. -0.9 ± 0.3 in subjects younger or older than 21 years, median value, respectively; $p<0.0001$). The FPR stratified by age at infection ($>$ or $\leq$ median value, 21 years) and *PNPLA3* 148M/M and is presented in figure 1 and in table 2. *PNPLA3* 148M/M was associated with faster FPR in older ($p = 0.001$), but not in younger patients ($p = ns$). The positive association between *PNPLA3* 148M/M and FPR in older patients was confirmed in sensitivity analyses using different age cut-offs (table 2): 15 years, the 25th centile ($p = 0.038$), 18 years ($p = 0.045$), and 27 years, the 75th centile ($p = 0.01$).

Steatogenic factors, *PNPLA3* 148M/M, and fibrosis progression

Moderate-severe steatosis was associated with faster FPR ($\log_{10}$ FPR -1.1 ± 0.3 vs. -0.9 ± 0.3 in subjects with steatosis grade 0–1, n = 186 vs. grade 2–3, n = 47, respectively; $p = 0.016$). The association between steatosis grade 2–3 and FPR was confirmed in the whole cohort including subjects with ultrasonographic estimation of steatosis severity ($\log_{10}$ FPR -1.1 ± 0.3 vs. -0.9 ± 0.3 in subjects with steatosis grade 0–1, n = 196 vs. grade 2–3, n = 51, respectively; $p = 0.012$). Since PNPLA3 I148M interferes with hepatocellular lipid metabolism, we next evaluated whether the effect of *PNPLA3* 148M/M on FPR was influenced by steatosis severity and risk factors for derangement of hepatic lipid metabolism. Results are shown in table 3. The association of *PNPLA3* 148M/M with FPR was more consistent in the presence of grade 2–3 steatosis ($p = 0.024$), or in the presence of other steatogenic factors: namely infection with genotype 3 ($p = 0.005$), or overweight ($p = 0.05$). The association between *PNPLA3* 148M/M and FPR was nearly significant in patients with steatosis grade 2–3 including subjects with ultrasonographic estimation of steatosis severity ($p = 0.056$).

Independent predictors of fibrosis progression

At the multivariate generalized linear model considering known determinants of FPR (age at infection, gender, and viral genotype: shown in model 1, table 4) *PNPLA3* 148M/M was an independent predictor of FPR ($p = 0.022$). The model estimated an incremental progression of 0.08 ± 0.03 $\log_{10}$ unit of fibrosis per year conferred by 148M/M status. Furthermore, there was a significant interaction between *PNPLA3* 148M/M and older age at infection in determining FPR ($p = 0.025$; estimate $+0.07\pm0.03$). In exploratory analyses, there was no significant interaction between *PNPLA3* 148M/M and other determinants of FPR.

To test the robustness of the association between *PNPLA3* genotype and FPR, we extended the model with further adjustment for additional potential confounders: age at biopsy, presence of overweight, and route of infection (model 2; table 4). In this extended model, the association of *PNPLA3* 148M/M with FPR (estimate $+0.08\pm0.03$, $p = 0.018$), as well as the interaction with older age at infection (estimate $+0.07\pm0.03$, $p = 0.021$) remained unaffected.

Finally, to test whether the effect of 148M/M status on fibrosis progression was independent of the histological severity of steatosis, we further adjusted the extended model for the presence of grade 2–3 steatosis (model 3; table 4). Again, *PNPLA3* 148M/M (estimate $+0.07\pm0.03$, $p = 0.032$) and the interaction with older age at infection (estimate $+0.07\pm0.03$, $p = 0.045$) remained significantly associated with FPR independently of the steatosis severity (grade 2–3 vs. 0–1; estimate $+0.04\pm0.02$, $p = 0.03$). In the overall series of patients including those with ultrasonographic

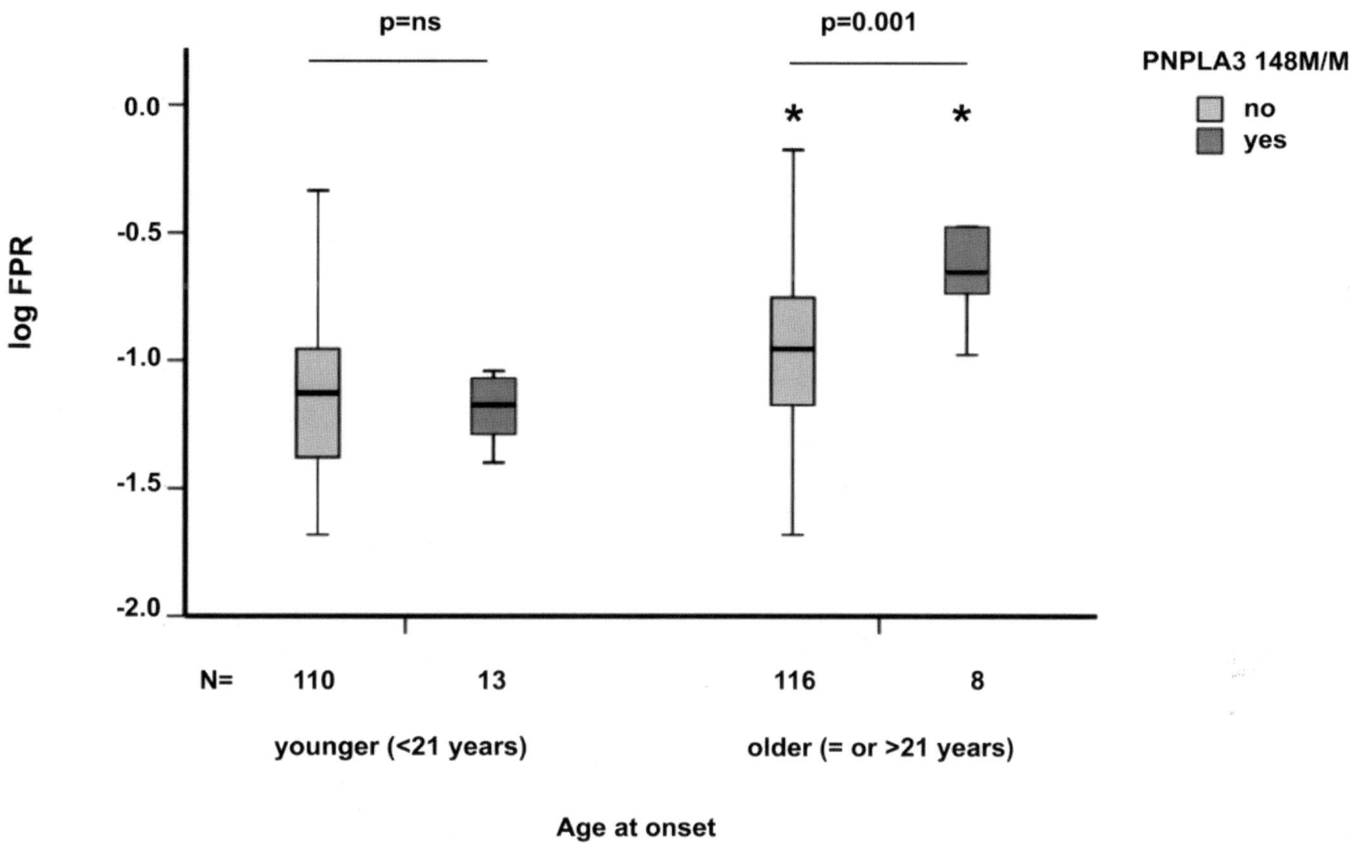

Figure 1. Fibrosis progression rate (FPR) according to age at infection (> or ≤21 years, median value) and *PNPLA3* 148M/M status in 247 patients with chronic hepatitis C. Box plots indicate median value and interquatile ranges, whiskers the 5th and 95th centiles. $p = 0.001$ for faster FPR in *PNPLA3* 148M/M positive vs. negative patients with older age at infection (>21 years). *$p < 0.0001$ vs. patients with same *PNPLA3* 148M/M status and younger age at infection (≤21 years).

Table 2. Effect of PNPLA3 148M/M on ($\log_{10}$) FPR in 247 CHC patients according to different thresholds of age at infection.

	PNPLA3		p value
	148I/I or I/M	**148M/M**	
15 years; 25th centile (±puberty)			
Younger	−1.25±0.3 (51)	−1.19±0.3 (9)	ns
Older	−0.98±0.3 (175)	−0.78±0.3 (12)	0.038
18 years; "adulthood"			
Younger	−1.25±0.3 (70)	−1.19±0.3 (9)	ns
Older	−0.99±0.3 (156)	−0.78±0.3 (12)	0.045
21 years; median			
Younger	−1.14±0.3 (110)	−1.16±0.3 (13)	ns
Older	−0.95±0.3 (116)	−0.64±0.2 (8)	0.001
27 years; 75th centile			
Younger	−1.10±0.3 (157)	−1.11±0.3 (14)	ns
Older	−0.90±0.3 (69)	−0.67±0.2 (7)	0.01

(): number of subjects; ns: not significant.

Table 3. Effect of PNPLA3 148M/M on (log_{10}) FPR in 247 CHC patients according to steatosis severity and the presence of risk factors for steatosis/altered hepatic lipid metabolism (HCV-G3 and overweight).

	PNPLA3		p value
	148I/I or I/M	148M/M	
Steatosis grade			
0–1	−1.06±0.3 (172)	−1.07±0.3 (14)	ns
2–3	−0.97±0.3 (42)	−0.67±0.2 (5)	0.024
HCV genotype			
G1, G2, G4	−1.06±0.3 (194)	−1.00±0.3 (19)	ns
G3	−0.92±0.3 (32)	−0.70±0.0 (2)	0.005
Overweight			
BMI≤25 Kg/m^2	−1.01±0.3 (116)	−1.13±0.3 (8)	ns
BMI>25 Kg/m^2	−1.07±0.3 (110)	−0.87±0.2 (13)	0.05

(): number of subjects; BMI: body mass index; ns: not significant.

estimation of steatosis, *PNPLA3* 148M/M (estimate +0.07±0.03, p = 0.033) and the interaction with older age at infection (estimate +0.07±0.03, p = 0.036) remained significantly associated with FPR.

Discussion

In this paper, we showed that in a prospective cohort with careful estimation of the date of infection and absence of major confounders the *PNPLA3* I148M sequence variant influences fibrosis progression in CHC.

Homozygosity for the I148M variant, which in line with the prevalence in the Italian population [29] was detected in about one in ten subjects, was associated an average incremental progression of fibrosis stage of as much as circa 0.8 units of Ishak score per year. The link between 148M/M status and FPR was independent of known moderators of fibrogenesis in CHC [2,3,30], and remained robust even after extensive adjustment for other potential confounders.

Our study is the first to show that the effect of *PNPLA3* I148M on fibrosis progression in CHC is modulated by the age at infection. The negative impact of 148M/M on FPR in individuals infected at older age was confirmed in sensitivity analyses with lower age cut-offs, and was prominent in individuals infected in adulthood. Previous studies suggested that *PNPLA3* I148M modulates liver damage progression in an age-dependent fashion. However, despite older age at onset was associated with faster progression of liver damage in alcoholic liver disease, the effect size of 148M/M was larger in younger patients [19]. Similarly, the reported effect size of the *PNPLA3* I148M variant on liver damage in nonalcoholic fatty liver disease was larger in pediatric case series [14–16].

The reason underlying the opposite direction of modulation by age of the effect of *PNPLA3* I148M on fibrosis progression in CHC is presently unknown. It could be speculated that the pattern of activation of the immune system towards HCV is different depending on the age at infection. According to this hypothesis, HCV infection after the developmental age would lead to immune-mediated hepatic damage, exerting a permissive role on *PNPLA3* I148M-related fibrogenesis [31]. Alternatively, older age may synergize with *PNPLA3* I148M in determining hepatic steatosis, which would favor viral replication during the acute infection [32], thus setting the stage for faster disease progression.

Indeed, evidence is accumulating that *PNPLA3* I148M synergizes with host features and environmental triggers in determining liver damage associated with altered hepatic lipid metabolism [33]. In line with these data, we found that the effect of *PNPLA3* 148M/M on fibrogenesis was more evident in subjects with grade 2–3 steatosis, and in those with other conditions favoring hepatocellular lipid accumulation, such as infection with genotype 3 and overweight.

Of note, we reported for the first time an effect of 148M/M on fibrosis progression in genotype 3 patients, even if previous studies did not detect an association between *PNPLA3* and steatosis in this subgroup [34,35]. However, since this finding was based on FPR assessment in only two 148M/M patients infected with HCV G3, it will require confirmation in future studies. Most importantly, the effect of 148M/M on fibrogenesis was independent of the histological severity of steatosis. These data are in line with results of cross-sectional studies in nonalcoholic fatty liver disease [33], and suggest that *PNPLA3* I148M may promote fibrogenesis by directly altering hepatic stellate cells lipid metabolism and trans-activation [36].

Therefore, given the independent association of the *PNPLA3* I148M variant with fibrosis progression and hepatocellular carcinoma risk [24], *PNPLA3* I148M genotyping may help refining treatment prioritization to novel therapeutic regimens based on direct antiviral agents [37], and patients follow-up.

Limitations of this study include the assumption of the absence of liver fibrosis at the time of infection, which is likely given the absence of cofactors of liver damage, the young age at infection and low risk profile. Furthermore, the model tested assumes the consistency and linearity of FPR during time, and of fibrosis progression across Ishak score stages, which are approximations of a more complex reality [38]. Notwithstanding, the present results are corroborated by the fact that our approach was able to validate the association of FPR with the major risk factors for fibrosis progression in CHC [3], and by independent findings linking *PNPLA3* 148M/M with fibrogenesis in CHC [25,33].

Conclusions

In conclusion, homozygosity for the *PNPLA3* I148M variant is associated with FPR in CHC. There is a significant interaction between age at infection and *PNPLA3* genotype in determining fibrosis progression, but the association between *PNPLA3* and

Table 4. Independent determinants of (log_{10}) FPR at multivariate generalized linear models in 247 CHC patients.

	Model 1			Model 2			Model 3		
	estimate	**SE**	**p value**	**estimate**	**SE**	**p value**	**estimate**	**SE**	**p value**
Sex F	−0.05	0.02	0.005	−0.05	0.02	0.006	−0.05	0.02	0.01
Older age at infection	+0.21	0.03	<0.0001	+0.21	0.03	<0.0001	+0.21	0.04	<0.0001
HCV genotype									
G1	ref			ref			ref		
G2	−0.10	0.04	0.004	−0.11	0.03	0.003	−0.10	0.04	0.008
G3	+0.13	0.04	0.002	+0.13	0.04	0.004	+0.11	0.05	0.02
G4	0.00	0.06	>0.1	0.02	0.06	>0.1	0.02	0.07	>0.1
PNPLA3 148M/M	+0.08	0.03	0.022	+0.08	0.03	0.018	+0.07	0.03	0.032
PNPLA3 148M/M * older age at infection	+0.07	0.03	0.025	+0.07	0.03	0.021	+0.07	0.03	0.045
Age at biopsy	NA			−0.003	0.002	0.06	−0.003	0.002	0.06
BMI>25 Kg/m^2	NA			−0.02	0.02	>0.1	−0.02	0.02	>0.1
IVDU	NA			−0.02	0.05	>0.1	−0.01	0.05	>0.1
Steatosis grade 2–3 vs. 0–1	NA			NA			+0.04	0.02	0.03

NA: not addressed; F: female; BMI: body mass index; IVDU: intravenous drug use.
Model 1: minimal model considering previously identified risk factors for FPR in the present cohort [3], plus 148M/M and the interaction between 148M/M and age infection. Model 2: extended model further corrected for potential confounding factors. Model 3: extended model with additional correction for histological severity of steatosis. P values are shown for ≤0.1.

FPR is independent of the histological severity of steatosis. These findings further establish the *PNPLA3* I148M variant as a moderator of CHC natural history, and have possible relevance for treatment prioritization and follow-up of CHC patients.

Acknowledgments

We thank all the members of the Metabolic Liver Diseases lab for helpful comments and discussion.

Author Contributions

Conceived and designed the experiments: LV RDF. Performed the experiments: PD CC RDA MP FM LD MM. Analyzed the data: LV SDN PD AA. Contributed reagents/materials/analysis tools: MC SF RDF. Contributed to the writing of the manuscript: LV SDN RDF AA CC.

References

1. Maasoumy B, Wedemeyer H (2012) Natural history of acute and chronic hepatitis C. Best Pract Res Clin Gastroenterol 26: 401–412.
2. Poynard T, Bedossa P, Opolon P (1997) Natural history of liver fibrosis progression in patients with chronic hepatitis C. The OBSVIRC, METAVIR, CLINIVIR, and DOSVIRC groups. Lancet 349: 825–832.
3. Marabita F, Aghemo A, De Nicola S, Rumi MG, Cheroni C, et al. (2011) Genetic variation in the Interleukin-28B gene is not associated with fibrosis progression in patients with chronic hepatitis C and known date of infection. Hepatology 54: 1127–1134.
4. Leandro G, Mangia A, Hui J, Fabris P, Rubbia-Brandt L, et al. (2006) Relationship between steatosis, inflammation, and fibrosis in chronic hepatitis C: a meta-analysis of individual patient data. Gastroenterology 130: 1636–1642.
5. Adinolfi LE, Gambardella M, Andreana A, Tripodi MF, Utili R, et al. (2001) Steatosis accelerates the progression of liver damage of chronic hepatitis C patients and correlates with specific HCV genotype and visceral obesity. Hepatology 33: 1358–1364.
6. Powell EE, Edwards-Smith CJ, Hay JL, Clouston AD, Crawford DH, et al. (2000) Host genetic factors influence disease progression in chronic hepatitis C. Hepatology 31: 828–833.
7. Trepo E, Potthoff A, Pradat P, Bakshi R, Young B, et al. (2011) Role of a cirrhosis risk score for the early prediction of fibrosis progression in hepatitis C patients with minimal liver disease. J Hepatol 55: 38–44.
8. Romeo S, Kozlitina J, Xing C, Pertsemlidis A, Cox D, et al. (2008) Genetic variation in PNPLA3 confers susceptibility to nonalcoholic fatty liver disease. Nat Genet 40: 1461–1465.
9. Pirazzi C, Adiels M, Burza MA, Mancina RM, Levin M, et al. (2012) Patatin-like phospholipase domain-containing 3 (PNPLA3) I148M (rs738409) affects hepatic VLDL secretion in humans and in vitro. J Hepatol 57: 1257–1262.
10. Hyysalo J, Gopalacharyulu P, Bian H, Hyotylainen T, Leivonen M, et al. (2013) Circulating Triacylglycerol Signatures in Nonalcoholic Fatty Liver Disease Associated With the I148M Variant in PNPLA3 and With Obesity. Diabetes 63: 312–322.
11. Ruhanen H, Perttila JD, Holtta-Vuori MD, Zhou YD, Yki-Jarvinen HP, et al. (2014) PNPLA3 mediates hepatocyte triacylglycerol remodelling. J Lipid Res.
12. He S, McPhaul C, Li JZ, Garuti R, Kinch L, et al. (2010) A sequence variation (I148M) in PNPLA3 associated with nonalcoholic fatty liver disease disrupts triglyceride hydrolysis. J Biol Chem 285: 6706–6715.
13. Kumari M, Schoiswohl G, Chitraju C, Paar M, Cornaciu I, et al. (2012) Adiponutrin functions as a nutritionally regulated lysophosphatidic Acid acyltransferase. Cell Metab 15: 691–702.
14. Valenti L, Al-Serri A, Daly AK, Galmozzi E, Rametta R, et al. (2010) Homozygosity for the PNPLA3/adiponutrin I148M polymorphism influences liver fibrosis in patients with nonalcoholic fatty liver disease. Hepatology 51: 1209–1217.
15. Valenti L, Alisi A, Galmozzi E, Bartuli A, Del Menico B, et al. (2010) I148M patatin-like phospholipase domain-containing 3 gene variant and severity of pediatric nonalcoholic fatty liver disease. Hepatology 52: 1274–1280.
16. Sookoian S, Pirola CJ (2011) Meta-analysis of the influence of I148M variant of patatin-like phospholipase domain containing 3 gene (PNPLA3) on the susceptibility and histological severity of nonalcoholic fatty liver disease. Hepatology 53: 1883–1894.
17. Tian C, Stokowski RP, Kershenobich D, Ballinger DG, Hinds DA (2009) Variant in PNPLA3 is associated with alcoholic liver disease. Nat Genet 42: 21–23.
18. Stickel F, Buch S, Lau K, Zu Schwabedissen HM, Berg T, et al. (2011) Genetic variation in the PNPLA3 gene is associated with alcoholic liver injury in caucasians. Hepatology 53: 86–95.
19. Burza MA, Molinaro A, Attilia ML, Rotondo C, Attilia F, et al. (2014) PNPLA3 I148M (rs738409) genetic variant and age at onset of at-risk alcohol consumption are independent risk factors for alcoholic cirrhosis. Liv Int 34: 514–520.
20. Valenti L, Aghemo A, Stattermayer AF, Maggioni P, De Nicola S, et al. (2012) Implications of PNPLA3 polymorphism in chronic hepatitis C patients receiving peginterferon plus ribavirin. Aliment Pharmacol Ther 35: 1434–1442.
21. Valenti L, Rumi M, Galmozzi E, Aghemo A, Del Menico B, et al. (2011) Patatin-Like phospholipase domain-containing 3 I148M polymorphism, steatosis, and liver damage in chronic hepatitis C. Hepatology 53: 791–799.
22. Muller T, Buch S, Berg T, Hampe J, Stickel F (2011) Distinct, alcohol-modulated effects of PNPLA3 genotype on progression of chronic hepatitis C. J Hepatol 55: 732–733.
23. Trepo E, Pradat P, Potthoff A, Momozawa Y, Quertinmont E, et al. (2011) Impact of PNPLA3 (rs738409 C>G) polymorphism on fibrosis progression and steatosis in chronic hepatitis C. Hepatology 54: 60–69.
24. Trepo E, Nahon P, Bontempi G, Valenti L, Falleti E, et al. (2013) Association between the PNPLA3 (rs738409 C>G) variant and hepatocellular carcinoma: evidence from a meta-analysis of individual participant data. Hepatology.
25. Singal AG, Manjunath H, Yopp AC, Beg MS, Marrero JA, et al. (2014) The Effect of PNPLA3 on Fibrosis Progression and Development of Hepatocellular Carcinoma: A Meta-analysis. Am J Gastroenterol 109: 325–334.
26. Ishak K, Baptista A, Bianchi L, Callea F, De Groote J, et al. (1995) Histological grading and staging of chronic hepatitis. J Hepatol 22: 696–699.
27. Kleiner DE, Brunt EM, Van Natta M, Behling C, Contos MJ, et al. (2005) Design and validation of a histological scoring system for nonalcoholic fatty liver disease. Hepatology 41: 1313–1321.
28. Hamaguchi M, Kojima T, Itoh Y, Harano Y, Fujii K, et al. (2007) The severity of ultrasonographic findings in nonalcoholic fatty liver disease reflects the metabolic syndrome and visceral fat accumulation. Am J Gastroenterol 102: 2708–2715.
29. Valenti L, Rametta R, Ruscica M, Dongiovanni P, Steffani L, et al. (2012) The i148m Pnpla3 polymorphism influences serum adiponectin in patients with fatty liver and healthy controls. BMC Gastroenterol 12: 111.
30. Reggiardo MV, Fay F, Tanno M, Garcia-Camacho G, Bottaso O, et al. (2012) Natural history of hepatitis C virus infection in a cohort of asymptomatic post-transfused subjects. Ann Hepatol 11: 658–666.
31. Knolle PA, Thimme R (2014) Hepatic Immune Regulation and its Involvement in Viral Hepatitis Infection. Gastroenterology.
32. Bassendine MF, Sheridan DA, Felmlee DJ, Bridge SH, Toms GL, et al. (2011) HCV and the hepatic lipid pathway as a potential treatment target. J Hepatol 55: 1428–1440.
33. Dongiovanni P, Donati B, Fares R, Lombardi R, Mancina RM, et al. (2013) PNPLA3 I148M polymorphism and progressive liver disease. World J Gastroenterol 19: 6969–6978.
34. Cai T, Dufour JF, Muellhaupt B, Gerlach T, Heim M, et al. (2011) Viral Genotype-Specific Role of PNPLA3, PPARG, MTTP and IL28B in Hepatitis C Virus-Associated Steatosis. J Hepatol 55: 529–535.
35. Valenti L, Aghemo A, Stattermayer AF (2012) Interaction between IL28B and PNPLA3 genotypes in the pathogenesis of steatosis in chronic hepatitis C non genotype-3 patients. J Hepatol 56: 1209–1210.
36. Pirazzi C, Valenti L, Motta BM, Pingitore P, Hedfalk K, et al. (2014) PNPLA3 has retinyl-palmitate lipase activity in human hepatic stellate cells. Hum Mol Genet.
37. Aghemo A, De Francesco R (2013) New horizons in hepatitis C antiviral therapy with direct-acting antivirals. Hepatology 58: 428–438.
38. Rosselli M, MacNaughtan J, Jalan R, Pinzani M (2013) Beyond scoring: a modern interpretation of disease progression in chronic liver disease. Gut 62: 1234–1241.

19

Impaired Expression of Type I and Type II Interferon Receptors in HCV-Associated Chronic Liver Disease and Liver Cirrhosis

Partha K. Chandra[1], Feyza Gunduz[1], Sidhartha Hazari[1], Ramazan Kurt[2], Rajesh Panigrahi[1], Bret Poat[1], David Bruce[3], Ari J. Cohen[3], Humberto E. Behorquez[3], Ian Carmody[3], George Loss[3], Luis A. Balart[2], Tong Wu[1], Srikanta Dash[1,2]*

1 Pathology and Laboratory Medicine, Tulane University Health Sciences Center, New Orleans, Louisiana, United States of America, **2** Department of Medicine, Gastroenterology and Hepatology, Tulane University Health Sciences Center, New Orleans, Louisiana, United States of America, **3** Transplant Surgery Section, Ochsner Medical Center, New Orleans, Louisiana, United States of America

Abstract

Purpose: Chronic Hepatitis C Virus (HCV)-infected patients with liver cirrhosis (LC) respond poorly to interferon-alpha (IFN-α) and ribavirin (RBV) combination therapy, but the reason for this is unclear. We previously reported that HCV-infection induces endoplasmic reticulum (ER) stress and autophagy response that selectively down regulates the type I IFN-α receptor-1 (IFNAR1) and RBV transporters (CNT1 and ENT1), leading to IFN-α/RBV resistance. The goal of this study is to verify whether an increase in ER stress and autophagy response is also associated with the reduced expression of IFNAR1 and RBV transporters in chronic HCV-infected patients.

Methods: Primary human hepatocytes (PHH) were infected with cell culture grown HCV particles (JFH-ΔV3-Rluc). HCV replication was confirmed by the detection of viral RNA by RT-qPCR and HCV-core protein by Western blotting. The ER stress and autophagy response and expression of IFN receptors and RBV transporters in HCV infected PHH and liver tissues derived from patients were measured by Western blotting.

Result: HCV infection of PHH showed impaired expression of IFNAR1, IFNγR1 (Type II IFN receptor) and RBV transporters but not IL10Rβ (Type III IFN-λ receptor). ER stress markers (BiP, IRE1α and peIF2α) and autophagy response (LC3II, Beclin 1 and ATG5) were induced in HCV infected chronic liver disease (CLD) and LC patients. Liver biopsies (CLD) show a 50% reduced expression of IFNAR1 and RBV transporters. Furthermore, the expression of IFNAR1 and RBV transporters was impaired in almost all LC patients.

Conclusion: HCV infection induces ER stress and autophagy response in infected PHH and chronically infected liver tissues. The expression of IFNAR1, IFNγR1 and RBV transporters were significantly impaired in CLD and cirrhotic livers. Our study provides a potential explanation for the reduced response rate of IFN-α and RBV combination therapy in HCV infected patients with liver cirrhosis.

Editor: Ranjit Ray, Saint Louis University, United States of America

Funding: The work was supported by the following: NIH grants: CA127481, CA089121, AI103106; and bridge funding: Tulane University Health Sciences Center. The funders had no role in study design, data collection and analysis, decision to publish, or preparation of the manuscript.

* Email: sdash@tulane.edu

Introduction

Hepatitis C virus (HCV) infection affects 150–200 million individuals worldwide [1,2] and leads to a high rate of chronic liver diseases (CLD), which often progresses to liver cirrhosis (LC) and hepatocellular carcinoma (HCC). This infection is the leading cause of liver transplantation in the United States [3]. Antiviral therapy that clears HCV infection has improved patient quality of life and has reduced incidence of liver disease progression and HCC [4,5]. Combination therapy of interferon (IFN)-α and ribavirin (RBV) with either a protease or polymerase inhibitor is now the prevalent treatment option for chronic HCV infection. Although this newly-approved therapy has improved HCV clearance rate, the treatment response has not improved among individuals who are initially non-responders to IFN-α and RBV [6,7] therapy. However, this therapy is still the standard of care for HCV infection in many parts of the world with no access to newly-approved antiviral drugs. Viral and host factors have been implicated in the failure of IFN-α and RBV treatment for chronic HCV infection and disease progression [8]. We propose that a better understanding of IFN-α and RBV resistance mechanisms would help us improve viral clearance and reduce the risk of HCV-associated liver disease.

A recent review describes the viral factors that influence response to IFN-α and RBV treatment, including HCV genotype and the patient's baseline viral load [9]. Clinical studies have reported that a low baseline viral load is an independent predictive factor for sustained virological response (SVR) [8]. Age, gender, race, obesity, insulin resistance, pre-activation of IFN-inducible genes, degree of liver fibrosis, and IL-28B genetic polymorphisms are host-related factors associated with poor treatment performance [8]. Single nucleotide polymorphisms near the type III IFN-λ gene are strongly correlated with the level of treatment response [10]. Liver cirrhosis is another host-related factor affecting the success of IFN-α and RBV combination therapy of chronic HCV infection [11–13]. Although many clinical studies have confirmed the association of host and viral-related factors with viral clearance by IFN-α and RBV therapy, the molecular mechanisms of how these factors affect HCV treatment outcomes are not well understood.

Binding of IFN-α to type I IFN-receptors (IFNAR1 and IFNAR2) expressed on hepatocytes activates receptor-associated JAK kinases, leading to the phosphorylation of STAT1 and STAT2. This phosphorylated protein complex and IFN regulatory factor 9 enter the nucleus and initiate antiviral gene transcription. The activation of JAK-STAT signaling in infected hepatocytes is critical for IFN-α to induce antiviral clearance [14]. Another recent review described the modulation of HCV infection by JAK-STAT signaling via multiple mechanisms [15]. The importance of cellular JAK-STAT signaling in the IFN-α antiviral response has also been confirmed in our laboratory using stable sub-genomic HCV replicon cell lines, as well as an infectious HCV cell culture system [16–18]. We demonstrated that HCV replication in a replicon cell line expressing a truncated IFNAR1 remained resistant to IFN-α treatment. Overexpression of wild type IFNAR1 in the same resistant cell line restored IFN-sensitivity and induced HCV clearance [17]. Recently, we reported that HCV replication in persistently-infected Huh-7.5 cells induced endoplasmic reticulum (ER) stress and autophagy response and remains resistant to IFN-α and RBV combination treatment, whereas type III IFN-λ causes a strong and sustained antiviral response that leads to viral clearance [18]. Mechanisms of IFN-α and RBV resistance in HCV cell culture models were related to reduced expression of IFNAR1 and RBV transporters. The significance of these cell culture studies needs further confirmation using tissues from chronic HCV-induced liver diseases and an infected primary human hepatocyte-based cell culture model.

The primary aim of this study was to determine if increased ER stress and autophagy response are related to impaired expression of type I and type II IFN signaling in HCV-infected human liver tissue. Our results show ER stress and autophagy marker expression are induced in HCV-infected primary human hepatocytes and liver tissues of patients with CLD. Compared to normal human liver tissues, ER stress and autophagy response are increased during CLD, but IFNAR1 expression is significantly reduced in HCV-induced CLD with or without cirrhosis. These data verify the results of our previous cell culture studies indicating impaired type I IFN signaling during CLD and provide an explanation for the reduced viral clearance in cirrhotic patients receiving IFN-α and RBV combination therapy.

Materials and Methods

Reagents

A rabbit anti-human IFNAR1 (Abcam Inc., Cambridge, MA), a mouse anti-human IL-10Rβ (IFNλR, R&D Systems Inc., Minneapolis, MN), rabbit anti-human BiP, IRE1α, peIF2α, CHOP, Beclin 1, ATG5, LC3B, and GAPDH (Cell signaling Technology, Beverly, MA), IFNAR2, IFNγR1, CNT1 (Santa Cruz Biotechnology Inc., Santa Cruz, CA), HCV-core (Thermo Fisher Scientific, Waltham, MA), HCV-NS3 (Virogen, Watertown, MA), ENT1 (Abgent, San Diego, CA). A horseradish peroxidase-coupled antirabbit or antimouse IgG was used as secondary antibodies obtained from Cell Signaling Technology, Beverly, MA. Control siRNA (siIRR) and siRNAs against PERK and ATG7 (Life Technologies, Carlsbad, CA) were as described previously [18].

Primary human hepatocytes (PHH) culture

Primary human hepatocytes obtained from a commercial source (XenoTech, LLC, Kansas City, MO) were cultured with a hepatocyte culture media with 10% human serum. After 24 hours of incubation in the CO_2 incubator, cells were infected with the cell culture derived JFH-ΔV3-Rluc virus (HCV genotype 2a) with a MOI (multiplicity of infection) of 0.1. The chimera JFH-ΔV3-Rluc virus used in the development of HCV cell culture system in Huh-7.5 cells was obtained from Curt Hagedern laboratory [19]. After 18 hours of infection, hepatocytes were replaced with fresh hepatocyte culture media (XenoTech, LLC, Kansas City, MO) supplemented with 10% human serum (Invitrogen, Brown deer, WI). Uninfected or infected PHH were harvested every 2 days and cell pellets were used for RNA isolation and Western blot analysis.

Ethics Statement

The study was conducted after IRB approval from the office of the senior Vice-President of Tulane University Health Sciences Center, New Orleans, LA, USA. The study was also received IRB approval from Ochsner Medical Center, New Orleans in order to collect explant liver tissues. All the patients were informed about the purpose of this study. Informed written consent was obtained from each patient.

Patients and liver samples

A total of twelve liver biopsy specimens from HCV infected chronic liver disease patients (CLD) were included in this study collected from Tulane Medical Center, New Orleans, LA. A total of eighteen explant livers (nine HCV infected with liver cirrhosis and nine HCV negative, HBV negative explants liver with cirrhosis) were collected from Ochsner Medical Center, New Orleans, LA were also included in this study. A serum antibody to HCV was detected by an enzyme linked immunosorbent assay (ELISA) and a serum HCV RNA level was quantified by quantitative RT-qPCR assay. The liver tissues derived from HCV negative and HBV negative patients with a history of alcohol intake, Laennec's and cryptogenic cirrhosis as well as non-alcoholic steatohepatitis (NASH). These patients had no history of other viral infection (HCV, HBV or HIV). Nine normal liver tissues obtained from National Disease Research Interchange (NDRI), Philadelphia, PA were included as control.

RT-qPCR for quantification of HCV RNA

The HCV-RNA level in infected human hepatocytes was determined using real-time RT-qPCR as described previously [20]. Briefly, one microgram of cellular RNA was used to amplify the 5′-untranslated region (UTR) of the HCV genome using sense (5′-TCTTCACGCAGAAAGCGTCTA-3′) and anti-sense (5′-CGGTTCCG CAGACCACTATG-3′) primers. The probe (5′-/56-FAM/TGAGTGTCG/ZEN/TG CAGCCTC CAGGA/3IBκFQ/-3′) labeled at the 5′ ends with a 6-carboxyfluorescein (FAM) fluorophore reporter molecule and ZEN-Iowa Black FQ (IBFQ) double quenchers were used to reduce the background and increase the signal (Integrated DNA Technologies Inc, Coralville, Iowa). The RT-qPCR assay was carried out in 20 µL containing 10 µL of iQ supermix (Bio-Rad Laboratories Inc., Hercules, CA), 0.25 µM of each primers, probe, and 4 µL of cDNA product obtained from the RT reaction. The amplification was carried out using a standard program (48°C for 30 minutes, 95°C for 10 minutes, followed by 44 additional cycles); each cycle includes a denaturation step at 95°C for 15 seconds, then an annealing and extension step at 60°C for 1 minute. Amplification, data acquisition, and analysis were carried out using a CFX96 Real-Time instrument using CFX manager software (Bio-Rad Laboratories Inc. Hercules, CA).

Detection of HCV RNA by reverse transcription (RT)-nested PCR

Detection of HCV RNA in infected human hepatocytes was carried out by RT-nested PCR [21]. Briefly, cDNA synthesis was carried out using one microgram of total RNA along with outer antisense primer 5′- CACTACTCGGCTAGCAGT-3′ (0.25 µM) utilizing the same protocol for Real-Time PCR. Amplification of cDNA was performed in 50 µL reaction mixture containing 8 µL of 5× PCR buffer, 2.4 µL $MgCl_2$ (25 mM), 2 U Taq DNA polymerase (Promega, Madison, WI), 0.25 µM outer sense primer (5′-CTGTGAGGAACTACTGTC-3′), and 10 µL of cDNA mixture as template. This was carried out for 40 cycles using the following program: denaturation for 30 sec at 95°C, annealing for 30 sec at 55°C, and extension for 1 min at 72°C. A second PCR was performed with a set of nested inner primers (sense: 5′-CACGCAGAAAGCGCCTAG-3′ and antisense: 5′- TTTATC-CAAGAAAGGACCC-3′) by utilizing one-tenth volume of the first PCR product as a DNA template. The amplification cycles were identical to the first one. The nested-PCR products were migrated in a 1.5% agarose gel to visualize the amplification of positive strand HCV-RNA. Amplification of GAPDH mRNA served as an internal control.

Western blot analysis

Western blotting was performed using our published protocol [18]. Infected primary hepatocytes were lysed in ice-cold RIPA buffer. Total protein content of the extract was quantified using a Bio-Rad protein assay kit (Bio-Rad, Hercules, CA). Hepatocytes were isolated from liver biopsies and lysed using an RIPA buffer described in a previous study [22]. Explant liver tissues were immediately collected in the RNase/DNase-free tubes containing Williams' media with 10% (v/v) FBS (Life Technologies, Carlsbad, CA). For the tissue samples, total liver protein was obtained by homogenizing liver tissue in 1 mL tissue grinders containing 1× PBS, 1% NP-40, 0.5% (v/v) Deoxycholate, 0.1% (v/v) SDS, 50 µg/mL PMSF, 5 µg/mL Aprotinin, 5 µg/mL Leupeptin, 1 µg/mL Pepstatin, and PhoSTOP phosphatase inhibitor (Roche Diagnostics Corporation, Indianapolis, IN). The sonicated protein lysates were then clarified by centrifugation at 12,000 rpm for ten minutes at 4°C. The clear supernatant was then transferred to new tubes, quantified, and stored at −20°C until used. An equal amount of protein from each sample was mixed in SDS-loading buffer, separated using NuPAGE (4–12%) gels and then transferred onto a nitrocellulose membrane (GE Healthcare, Buckinghamshire, UK). The membrane was soaked with a blocking solution for 2 h (at room temperature) and incubated with the diluted primary antibody (according to the manufacturer's instructions) at 4°C overnight. The next day, the membrane was washed and incubated with HRP-conjugated secondary antibody. The ECL detection reagent (GE Healthcare Life Sciences, Piscataway, NJ) was then added to the membrane according to the manufacturer's instructions. The membrane was then exposed to chemiluminescence film (GE Healthcare Life Sciences, Piscataway, NJ).

Statistical analysis

All results were expressed as mean ± SD (standard deviation). Comparison between two groups was performed with a Student's t-test. To compare means within groups we performed one factor analysis of variance (ANOVA) using the GraphPad Prism software. We assumed that all measurements have normal probability distributions, which is expected for these types of data. P-value for statistical analysis was significant when $p<0.05$.

Results

HCV infection of PHH-induced ER stress, autophagy response, and downregulated IFNAR1 and IFNγR1 receptors and RBV transporters

We initiated this study to verify ER stress and autophagy response seen in HCV-infected Huh-7.5 cells were also induced in primary human hepatocytes after HCV infection [18]. Prior studies reported that replication of HCV in a PHH is not as high when compared to the infected Huh-7.5 cells [23,24]. A recent report showed HCV replication in PHH is induced 1000-fold when cultured in the presence of human serum instead of fetal bovine serum. The authors observed PHH cultured with human serum showed increased expression of hepatocyte differentiation markers [25], which encouraged us to establish a replication model in PHH by using cell-cultured HCV [18]. Infected PHH were collected at 0, 2, 4, 6, 8 and 10 days and examined to see if they supported HCV replication after infection. Initially, we measured Renilla luciferase activity of the protein lysate to quantify HCV replication in infected PHH, but the assay was not sensitive enough to detect luciferase signals above background levels. This result also indicated HCV replication may be low in infected PHH. Therefore, a more sensitive real-time RT-qPCR method was used to quantify HCV positive-strand RNA in PHH nucleic acid extracts, which was sensitive enough to detect HCV replication in PHH. We also observed HCV replication was significantly higher ($P<0.001$) when cells were cultured with human serum compared to cells cultured with fetal bovine serum (**Figure S1**). Using real-time RT-qPCR assays, we found the HCV RNA level in the infected human hepatocytes gradually increased to 2.5×10^4 copies/1 µg total RNA from 0 to 10 days post-infection (**Figure 1A**). Viral titers of the infected PHH were comparable with HCV RNA levels in infected human liver [26]. Specificity of the RT-nested PCR amplified products was visualized with ethidium bromide staining of agarose gels following amplicon electrophoresis (**Figure 1B**). Viral core protein expression in the infected hepatocytes from 0 to 10 days was measured by Western blot analysis (**Figure 1C**). To confirm that a known antiviral molecule inhibits HCV replication in the infected PHH, one set of infected PHH culture was treated with IFN-α for 72 hours, and core protein was measured by Western blotting (**Figure 1D**). The increase in viral RNA levels and core protein expression over 10 days indicated that PHH cultured with human serum promoted HCV replication.

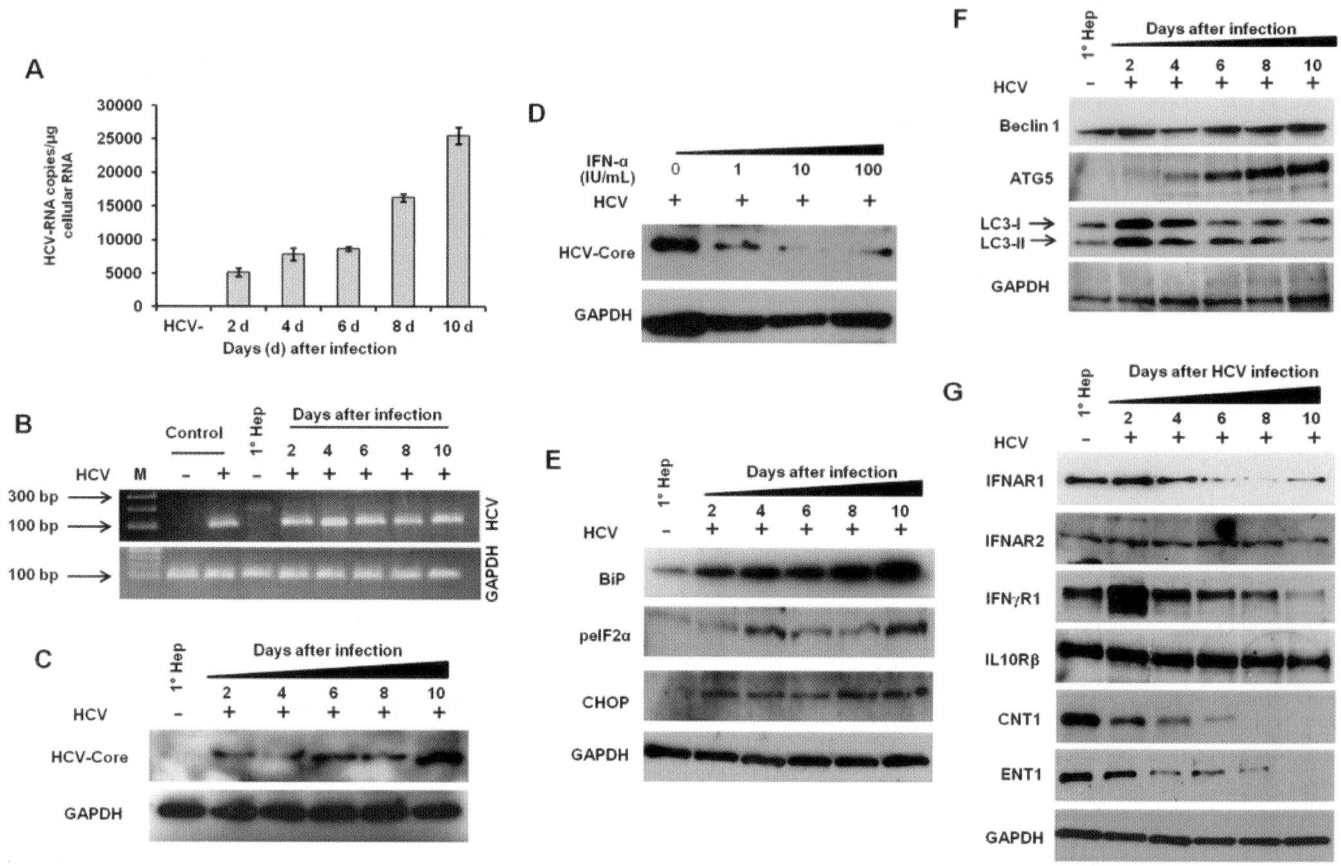

Figure 1. HCV replication in primary human hepatocytes (PHH) culture induces ER-stress and autophagy response and downregulates type I and type II IFN receptors and RBV transporters. Primary human hepatocytes were infected with cell culture derived JFH-ΔV3-Rluc HCV at a MOI = 0.1 for 18 hours. The infected cells were cultured in growth media supplemented with 10% (v/v) human serum. (**A**) HCV-RNA level measured by real-time RT-qPCR at different indicated time points. Uninfected PHH (HCV−) served as a negative control. (**B**) Ethidium bromide stained agarose gel electrophoresis picture showing the positive strand HCV-RNA was detected by RT-nested PCR. RNA from Huh-7.5 cells and *in vitro* transcribed HCV-RNA were used as negative (−) and positive (+) controls respectively. M: DNA ladder; 1° Hep: Uninfected primary human hepatocytes. (**C**) HCV-core protein level in infected primary hepatocytes was detected by Western blotting. GAPDH was used as a control. (**D**) IFN-α inhibits HCV core protein level in infected PHH. PHH were infected with JFH-ΔV3-Rluc virus for 18 hours, and after infection, cells were washed with PBS and cultured with hepatocyte culture media supplemented with 10% (v/v) human serum. After three days of infection, cells were treated with indicated concentrations of IFN-α for an additional three days. Finally, cells were harvested, lysed in RIPA buffer and HCV-core protein level was measured by Western blotting. (**E**) HCV infection induces ER stress. The level of ER-stress markers (BiP, peIF2α and CHOP) were induced in the PHH due to HCV infection. (**F**) Western blot shows expression of autophagy-related proteins (Beclin 1, ATG5 and LC3-II) in the infected hepatocytes. (**G**) The level of IFN receptors and RBV transporters were altered with HCV replication. The receptor expression of IFNAR1, IFNγR1, CNT1 and ENT1 gradually decreased with increasing time of infection. GAPDH was used as an internal control. 1° Hep: Uninfected primary human hepatocytes.

Next, protein extracts from infected human hepatocytes were used to measure expression levels of selected ER stress indicators, autophagy markers, IFN receptors, and RBV transporters by Western blotting. Expression levels of ER stress indicators, including the binding immunoglobulin protein (BiP), phosphorylation of eIF2α (peIF2α) and the C/EBP homology protein (CHOP), gradually increased throughout the duration of HCV infection (**Figure 1E**). We found the autophagy response in infected human hepatocytes was increased, and levels of Beclin 1, autophagy protein 5 (ATG5), and microtubule-associated protein 1A/1B-light chain 3 (LC3-II) correlated with the course of HCV infection (**Figure 1F**). We then examined if increased ER stress and autophagy response in the infected human hepatocyte model also correlated with decreased expression of IFNAR1. Expression levels of IFNAR1 (type I IFN) and IFNγR1 (type II IFN) receptors and RBV transporters (CNT1 and ENT1) in this model gradually decreased after HCV infection. Interestingly, levels of IFNAR2 (type I IFN receptor) and IL10Rβ (type III IFN receptor) were unaffected (**Figure 1G**). These Western blot results supported our cell culture studies of Huh-7.5 cells persistently infected with HCV [18]. To exclude the possibility that long-term culture of PHH *in vitro* could modulate the expression of IFNAR1, IFNAγR1, and RBV transporters, their expression was measured using uninfected primary human hepatocytes cultured at different time points. The expression levels of IFNAR1, IFNγR1, and RBV transporters did not change due to long-term culture of PHH (**Figure S2**). To confirm the association between induced ER stress and autophagy response with impaired expression of IFNAR1 and RBV transporters, one of the ER stress sensors (PERK) and autophagy gene (ATG7) were silenced by siRNAs in persistently HCV-infected Huh-7.5 cells. The expression level of IFNAR1 and RBV transporters (CNT1 and ENT1) were rescued after silencing PERK and ATG7 genes with siRNAs (**Figure S6**).

Liver biopsies from chronic HCV patients show increased ER stress and autophagy response and decreased expression of IFNAR1, IFNγR1, and RBV transporters

Combination therapy of IFN-α and RBV produced a sustained antiviral response in 40–50% of patients infected with the HCV genotype 1 [27,28]. These findings have been reproduced in many clinical studies, but the nature of this association has not been established. We tested if ER stress and autophagy response could also affect surface expression of IFNAR1 by examining liver biopsies from patients chronically infected with HCV. Hepatocytes were isolated from pretreatment liver biopsy samples using a standard protocol described previously [29]. Liver tissues from nine normal donor livers with no viral infection were used as controls. The clinical parameters of the HCV-infected patients and their serum viral titers are presented in **Figure S3**. Protein extracts of hepatocytes isolated from liver biopsies and normal liver tissues were examined for ER stress markers by Western blot analysis. Replication of HCV takes place in the ER-associated membranes and may induce an ER stress response due to increased accumulation of viral protein and sustained viral replication. This stress interferes with ER function. In this study, the ER stress marker expression was measured using protein extracts from liver biopsy hepatocytes using antibodies against inositol requiring 1 alpha (IRE1α), BiP, and peIF2α. Compared to normal donor liver tissues (**Figure 2A**), expression levels of ER stress markers IRE1α, BiP and peIF2α in HCV-infected CLD patients were significantly increased (**P<0.001, ***P<0.0001, and, *P<0.01 respectively) (**Figure 2B and 2C**). Western blot results were quantified by measuring band intensities, which indicated ER stress response was significantly higher in CLD patients (**Figure 2C**). Levels of GAPDH were the similar in all samples, indicating the observed differences were not due to unequal amounts of proteins in the extracts.

Induction of autophagy response secondary to ER stress has been seen in liver disease with accompanying chronic HCV infection, steatohepatitis, alcoholic liver disease, and HCC. To determine if autophagy was induced or impaired in CLD and LC patients, we investigated hallmark autophagy genes such as Beclin 1 and ATG5 and found their protein levels were induced in HCV-infected CLD patients compared to controls (**Figure 2B and 2C**). We were unable to test all ER stress and autophagy markers due to a limited amount of protein extract available from the liver biopsies. Because ER stress and autophagy markers are induced in chronic HCV patients, we also measured expression levels of IFNAR1 and RBV transporters (ENT1 and CNT1) by Western blotting and compared normal liver and CLD samples (**Figure 3A**). The expression of IFNAR1 was detectable in 40% of chronic HCV patients by Western blot analysis (**Figure 3B**), and expression of ENT1, the major transporter for RBV uptake, was detectable in 50% of chronic HCV patients (**Figure 3B**). Interestingly, the expression of the type II IFN-γ receptor-chain 1 (IFNγR1) was also impaired in chronically-infected livers. The expression level of IL10Rβ (type III IFN) was detectable in all of the infected livers (**Figure 3B**). Expression levels of IFNAR1, IFNγR1 and RBV transporters were detectable in all normal uninfected liver samples, and GAPDH levels were comparable in all samples, indicating variations were not due to differences in the amount of proteins used in our assays.

Lack of expression of IFNAR1 and RBV transporter in the explant liver tissues from patients with LC

Liver cirrhosis is an end-stage disease with both viral and non-viral causes. Without successful antiviral therapy, the majority of liver cirrhotic patients will die due to liver- related complications, such as HCC and liver failure [5]. Standard IFN-α and RBV therapy induces a sustained antiviral response from only 25% of HCV genotype 1-infected patients with LC [29]. The reason for the low treatment response to this HCV therapy in cirrhotic patients is unknown. To verify the contribution of ER stress- and autophagy-related impaired expression of IFNAR1 and RBV transporters, we measured their expression levels using nine explant livers with HCV infection and nine explant livers without HCV infection. All explant livers used in our study were cirrhotic, as confirmed by histological examination by a pathologist. The demographic characteristics of patients with or without HCV are shown in **Figure S4**. Liver tissue from nine normal donor livers with no viral infection was used as a control. The expression of ER stress and autophagy markers was examined by subjecting protein extracts to Western blot analysis. The ER stress markers (BiP, IRE1α, and peIF2α) were induced in LC patients with or without HCV infection (**Figure 4A and 4B**). Autophagy marker Beclin1 was detected in two HCV-infected LC patients (25%, 2/8) and one uninfected LC patient (12%, 1/8). The level of ATG5 was unchanged in both HCV-infected and uninfected LC patients.

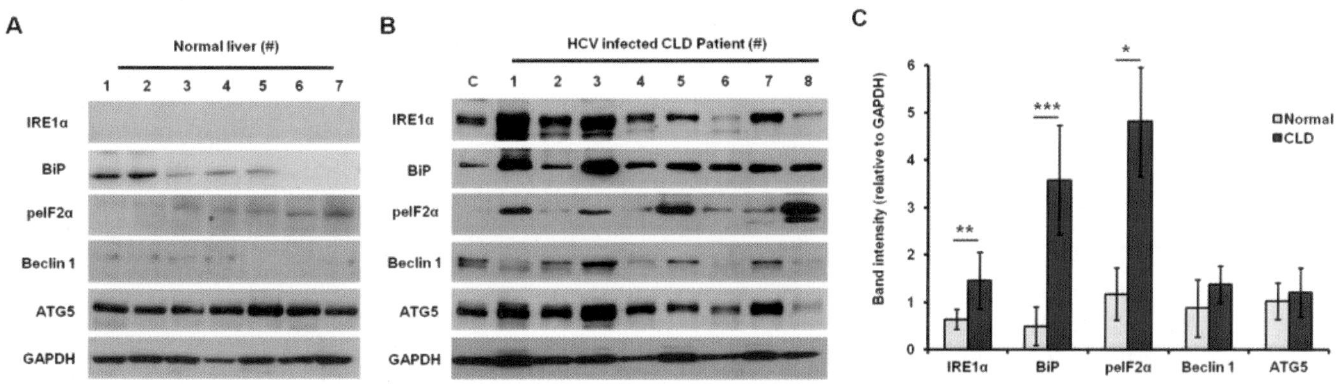

Figure 2. ER stress and autophagy response in HCV-infected liver biopsies from CLD patients. ER stress-related proteins (IRE1α, BiP, and peIF2α) and autophagy-related proteins (Beclin 1 and ATG5) were measured in the lysates prepared from liver biopsies by Western blotting (**A**) normal liver, and (**B**) HCV-infected CLD patients. (**C**) The relative band intensities of Western blot of HCV-infected CLD patients and normal liver samples were compared side-by-side by using Image J software. The relative values were reported as mean ± SD. *P<0.01, **P<0.0001, ***P< 0.0001. C: Uninfected PHH.

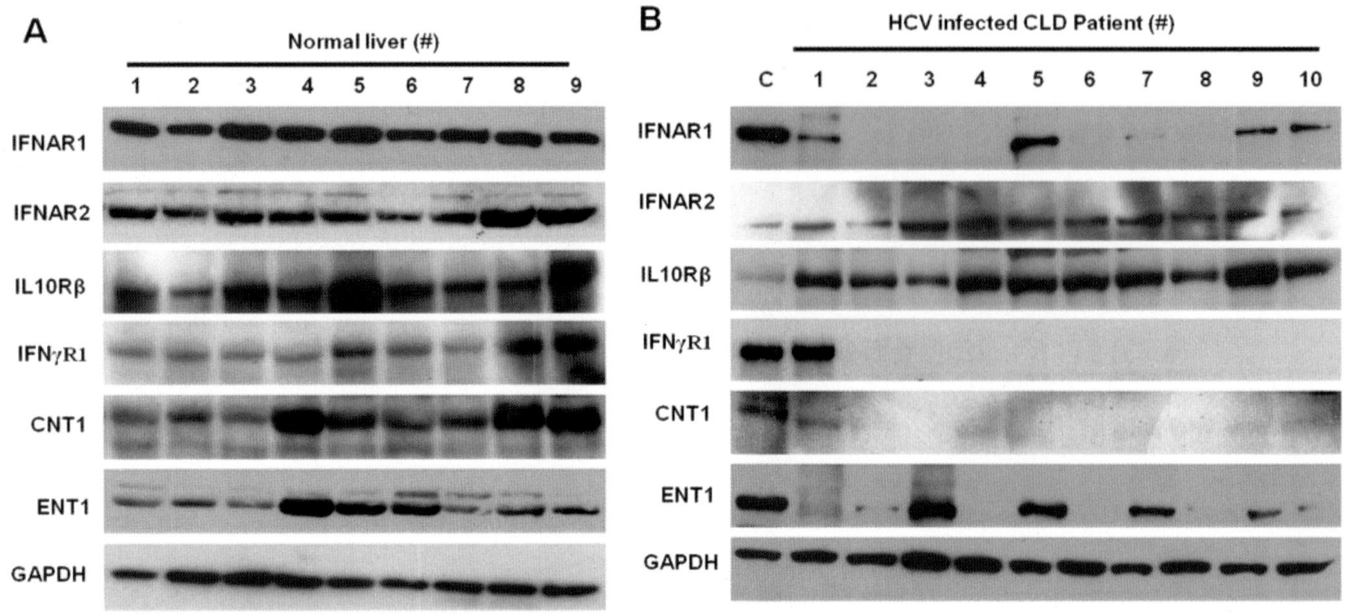

Figure 3. Expression of IFN receptors and RBV transporters in normal uninfected liver and HCV-infected liver samples. The levels of different type I (IFNAR1 and IFNAR2), type II (IFNγR1) and type III (IL10Rβ) IFN receptors and RBV transporters (CNT1 and ENT1) were measured by Western blotting using equal amounts of protein lysates from normal liver and biopsy specimens. (**A**) Nine normal liver tissues with no history of viral infection (HIV, HBV or HCV) were used as control. (**B**) Liver biopsies from ten HCV-infected CLD patients were examined. GAPDH was used as an internal control. C: Uninfected PHH.

Autophagy markers were downregulated in explant livers as compared to the expression levels of ER stress markers (**Figure 4C**). We then tested the expression levels of IFN receptors and RBV transporters in the same extracts using Western blotting. Surprisingly, IFNAR1 and IFNγR1 expression was undetectable in the majority of cirrhotic livers with or without HCV infection (**Figure 5A and 5B**). The expression of ENT1 was impaired in all cirrhotic livers with or without HCV infection (**Figure 5C and 5D**). All non-HCV cirrhotic livers showed undetectable IFNAR1 (100%) and ENT1 (100%) expression by Western blot analysis, and the IFNγR1 expression band was detectable in only two out of nine tissues (22%). These results suggest the expression of IFNAR1 and RBV transporters was severely impaired in patients with LC. However, the negative results of the Western blots are not due to low amounts of protein in the tissue extracts, as we saw stable expression of GAPDH levels in all samples.

The activity of ER stress in cirrhotic livers was higher than that of autophagy markers. The downregulation of IFNAR1 without significant autophagy suggests IFNAR1 downregulation could occur due to ER stress. The ER stress inducer downregulates IFNAR1 expression [18,30]. Because IFNAR1 expression was severely impaired compared to chronically-infected liver tissues, the mRNA level of IFNAR1 was examined using RT-PCR followed by Southern blotting. Interestingly, full-length mRNA of IFNAR1 was not detected in most of the cirrhotic livers (**Figure S5**). The primers and probes used to amplify full-length IFNAR1 are shown in **Table S1**. Liver cirrhosis also occurs due to chronic alcoholic and non-alcoholic liver disease. The non-HCV explant cirrhotic liver tissues used in our study were diagnosed as alcoholic liver disease and non-alcoholic steatohepatitis. The ER stress and autophagy response plays a role in viral- and non-viral-induced CLDs [31–38]. To understand why reduced expression of IFNAR1 occurs in non-viral liver diseases, we investigated the effect of ethanol and free fatty acids (FFA) alone or in combination on the expression levels of IFN receptors and RBV transporter proteins in Huh-7.5 cells. The induction of ER stress and autophagy markers were upregulated in Huh7.5 cell cultures treated with ethanol alone, FFA alone, and the combination ethanol plus FFA (**Figure 6**). Protein levels of peIF2α and CHOP were induced in Huh-7.5 cells by ethanol or FFA treatment, indicating induction of ER stress (**Figure 6A**). Autophagy response was not induced significantly after 24 hours of ethanol treatment, as protein levels of both Beclin 1 and ATG5 did not increase with higher concentrations of ethanol or FFA (**Figure 6A**). Interestingly, expression of IFNAR1, IFNAR2 (type I IFN receptor), and IFNγR1 (type II IFN receptor) was decreased with higher concentrations of ethanol or FFA and in a combination-treated culture. Similarly, expression levels of RBV transporters (both ENT1 and CNT1) were decreased with higher concentration of ethanol or FFA or when treated in combination (**Figure 6B**). We also measured the induction of ER stress, autophagy response, and levels of IFN receptors in HCV-infected cultures treated with ethanol and FFA (**Figures 6C–E**). The presence of HCV infection was confirmed by detecting HCV core and NS3 protein expression by Western blotting (**Figure 6C**). Interestingly, the protein levels of peIF2α and CHOP were induced when alcohol and FFA were added to the HCV-infected culture (**Figure 6D**). In addition, expression levels of IFNAR1 and the RBV transporter ENT1 were severely impaired in HCV-infected cells treated with ethanol and FFA (**Figure 6E**).

Discussion

In this study, we validated the results of previous HCV cell culture findings by confirming ER stress and autophagy responses are induced in chronic viral infection of human hepatocytes, leading to impaired expression of IFNAR1, IFNγR1, and RBV transporters. We also established an HCV replication model using

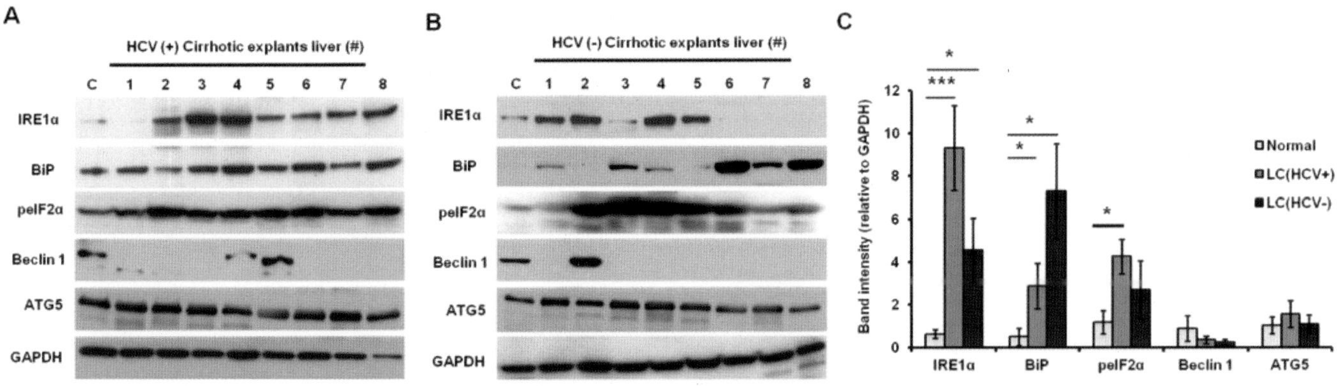

Figure 4. ER stress and autophagy response in LC patients (explant liver tissues) with or without the etiology of HCV infection. The ER stress-related proteins (IRE1α, BiP, and peIF2α) and autophagy-related proteins (Beclin 1 and ATG5) were detected by Western blot in (**A**) HCV infected (HCV+) LC patients, and (**B**) HCV uninfected (HCV−) LC patients. (**C**) The relative band intensity of each marker between normal and HCV-infected and –uninfected was compared using Image J software. The relative values were reported as mean ± SD and *P<0.01, ***P<0.0001. C: uninfected PHH.

PHH and found HCV replication in PHH can be inhibited by IFN-α. Using this system, we verified HCV replication in PHH induced ER stress and autophagy response but impaired expression of IFNAR1, IFNγR1, and RBV transporters. Expression of the IFN-λ receptor was not affected by ER stress and autophagy response.

The ER stress- and autophagy-mediated degradation of IFNAR1 and RBV transporter expression was verified using liver biopsy samples from chronic HCV patients. We show ER stress and autophagy markers are induced in chronic HCV-infected liver tissues. Our results confirm other related studies [33–35]. For example, Asselah et al. [33] observed abnormally-dilated ER, indicative of ER stress, due to viral protein accumulation in liver biopsies of patients with chronic HCV and Hepatitis B infection. Ait-Goughoulte et al. [34] showed HCV genotype 1a infection of immortalized primary human hepatocytes induced autophagy response, expression of ATG5, and LC3 accumulation. Shuda et al. [35] examined the expression of ER stress markers (ATF6, XBP1, and GRP78) using 13 surgically-resected human HCC liver tissues and normal liver tissues by Northern blot analysis. They

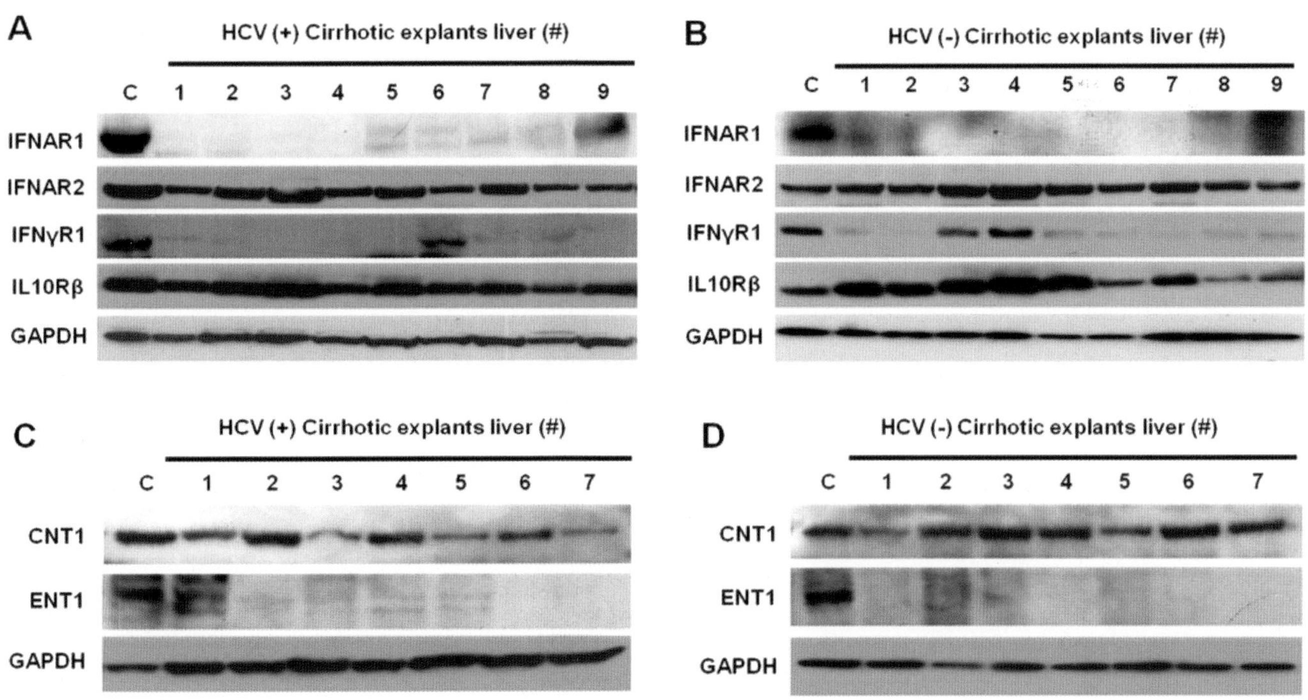

Figure 5. Expression of IFN receptors and RBV transporters in explant livers with cirrhosis. Equal amounts of protein lysates prepared from explant liver tissues and separated in 4–12% NuPAGE gels and the protein levels of different IFN receptors and RBV transporters were measured by Western blotting. Expression of type I, type II and Type III IFN-receptors were presented in (**A**) HCV infected (HCV+) explant livers and (**B**) HCV uninfected (HCV−) explant livers. Expression of RBV transporters presented in (**C**) HCV infected (HCV+) explant livers and (**D**) HCV uninfected (HCV−) explant livers. We were unable to measure RBV transporters in all samples. C: Uninfected PHH.

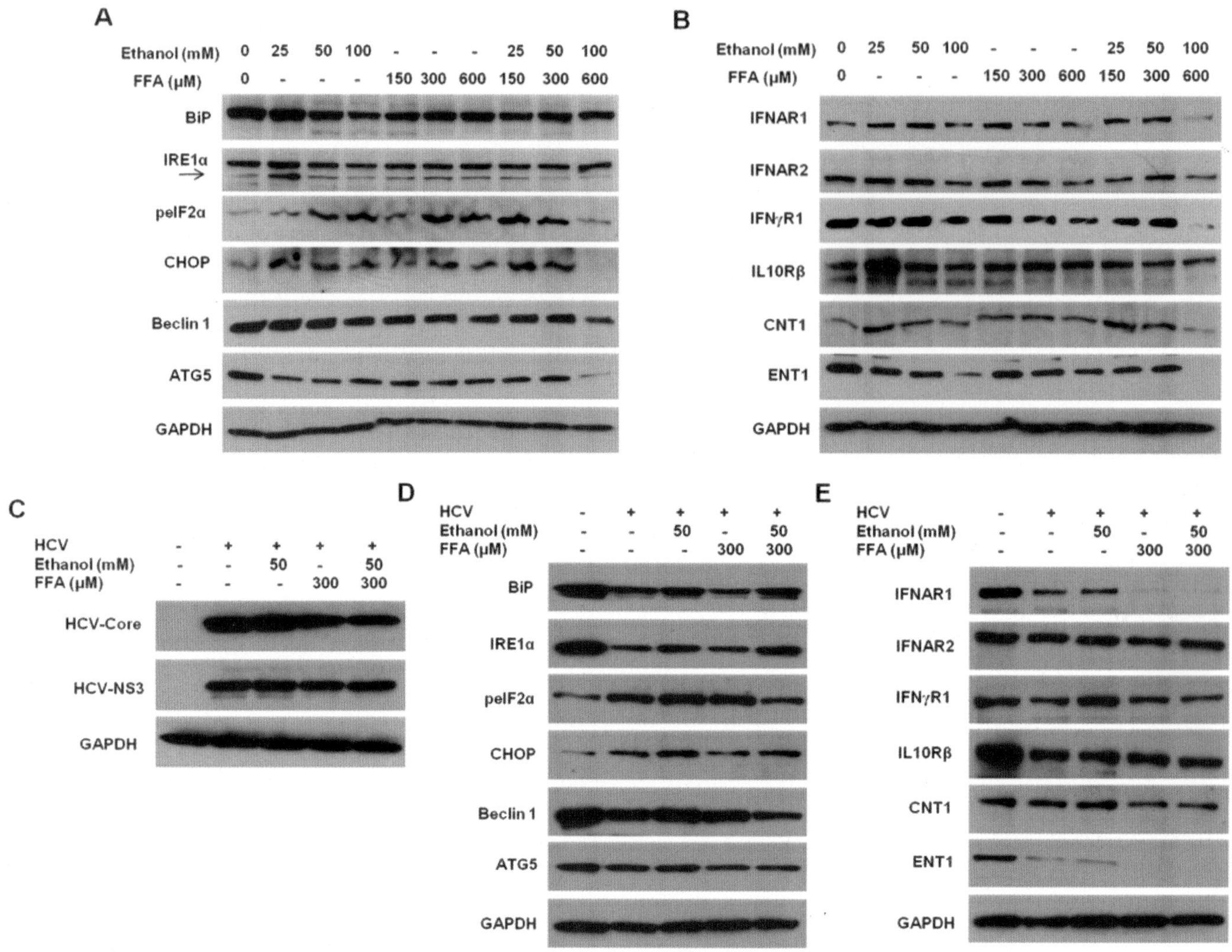

Figure 6. Ethanol and free fatty acid (FFA) induces ER stress. Huh-7.5 cells were treated with indicated concentrations of ethanol and FFA for 24 h. (**A**) ER stress-related proteins (BiP, IRE1α, peIF2α, and CHOP) and autophagy-related proteins (Beclin 1 and ATG5) were detected by Western blotting. (**B**) The expression level of IFN-receptors and RBV transporters was measured in ethanol and FFA treated cells. The effect on ER stress, autophagy response, the level IFN-receptors and RBV transporters in ethanol and FFA treated HCV-infected culture was also studied. (**C**) Persistently HCV infected Huh-7.5 cells were treated with indicated concentrations of ethanol and FFA for 24 h. HCV-core and HCV-NS3 protein levels were detected by Western blotting. (**D**) ER stress and autophagy-related proteins were detected by Western blotting. (**E**) The expression level of IFN-receptors and RBV transporters in ethanol and FFA treated HCV-infected culture was also measured by Western blotting. GAPDH was used as an internal control in all of the panels.

observed increased levels of ER stress markers in HCV infection and HCC samples. The expression of IFNAR1 and RBV transporters was absent in 40–50% of chronic HCV patients, which correlates with clinical studies explaining why only 50% of chronic HCV patients respond to peginterferon and RBV combination therapy. Interferon-γ is not an effective treatment of chronic HCV patients who are non-responders to IFN-α [39], but the reason is unknown. Impaired expression of IFNγR1 in chronic HCV infection may provide an explanation why IFN-γ therapy alone is not effective in chronic HCV patients. The results from liver biopsy assays are also consistent with our previous cell culture study, indicating chronic ER stress and autophagy response is associated with impaired expression of IFNAR1 and RBV transporters.

The sustained viral response of IFN-α and RBV combination therapy only occurs in 25% of chronic HCV patients with LC, which could be the result of several viral- and host-related factors [40]. Evidence for viral factor contribution is limited because viral strains with mutations causing IFN-α and RBV resistance has not been developed. The mechanism of IFN-α and RBV resistance is likely connected to host-related factors, which is supported by numerous studies [40]. Liver cirrhosis in chronic HCV infection is an independent predictor of poor response to IFN-α and RBV therapy [40], but there is no explanation why cirrhotic patients show less viral clearance with IFN-α and RBV combination therapy. We investigated the expression of ER stress indicators, autophagy markers, and IFNAR1 and RBV transporters using cirrhotic livers obtained during liver transplantation. The ER stress markers are upregulated in cirrhotic livers compared to autophagy markers, but the expression of IFNAR1 and RBV transporter ENT1 was severely impaired in the explant liver samples with or without HCV infection. Our results support the findings of other investigators who have shown ER stress and autophagy responses are induced in CLD of viral and non-viral etiology [37,38].

Several studies have demonstrated autophagy in chronic HCV and CLD patients due to alcohol and FFA accumulation [37]. The lack of IFNAR1 and RBV transporter expression provides a potential explanation why cirrhotic patients are less responsive to the combination therapy of IFN-α and RBV. These results verify our hypothesis that IFNAR1 expression is impaired due to ER stress and autophagy responses in HCV cell culture, as well as in CLD and LC tissues, although autophagy responses are much lower in during LC compared to CLD. The reasons for IFNAR1 and RBV transporter degradation, even during impaired autophagy, are unknown. We examined the stability of IFNAR1 mRNA in explant livers by RT-PCR, followed by Southern blotting. Full-length mRNA for IFNAR1 was not detected in the explant livers. The IRE1α RNase activity due to ER stress was also implicated in the degradation of several cellular mRNAs, including proinsulin mRNA [41]. In addition, IRE1α may be an endonuclease that plays a role in regulating the decay of numerous cellular mRNA, including IFNAR1, in response to cellular ER stress as a cell survival defense mechanism. The contribution of IRE1α-mediated gene expression in the cirrhotic liver should be examined in the future. In our study, we observed Beclin 1 was induced in HCV-infected CLD patients (**Figure 2B and C**) but was undetectable in most of the cirrhotic explant livers with or without HCV infection (**Figure 4**). However ATG5, a well-known marker for macroautophagy, is expressed in all cirrhotic livers, which indicates autophagy in the cirrhotic liver may be Beclin 1-independent. This possibility is supported by a recent study showing the autophagy process can be induced without Beclin 1 [42]. However, we observed ER stress markers are induced more in cirrhotic livers. A recent review article discusses various stress-responsive transcription factors that regulate autophagy responses in mammalian cells [43]. We suspect stress-responsive transcription factors, induced secondarily to ER stress, could also regulate autophagy processes that downregulate IFNAR1 and RBV transporter expression in cirrhotic livers.

In conclusion, we present evidence that HCV-induced ER stress and autophagy degrades IFNAR1, IFNγR1, and RBV transporters by using an HCV cell culture model, primary human hepatocytes, and HCV-infected livers. However, the significance of reduced expression of type I and type II IFN receptors in CLD and LC is not clear. Chronic liver disease, whether due to viral or non-viral causes, reduces expression of IFNAR1 and suggests suppression of host innate immunity and liver disease progression. Suppression of host immunity favors carcinogenesis, which may be why LC is a potential risk factor for HCC development. Interestingly, expression of the IFN-λ receptor is not affected by ER stress and autophagy mechanisms influenced by HCV. We propose IFN-λ treatment can be used to circumvent the IFN-α and RBV resistance mechanisms of HCV infection. Understanding how ER stress and autophagy responses play a role in chronic HCV infection and IFN resistance could help reduce HCV-associated liver diseases in humans.

Supporting Information

Figure S1 Real-time RT-PCR showing HCV-RNA levels in PHH culture in presence of human serum (HS+) and fetal bovine serum (HS−). Cells were infected with JFH-ΔV3-Rluc virus (MOI = 0.1) for 18 hours. The infected cells were washed with PBS and cultured with hepatocyte culture media supplemented with either 10% (v/v) human serum (HS+) or 10% (v/v) fetal bovine serum (HS−). HCV replication was measured by real-time RT-qPCR at different indicated time points. HCV replication was compared in the presence (HS+) or absence (HS−) of human serum. **$P<0.001$, ***$P<0.0001$.

Figure S2 The expression of different IFN receptors and RBV transporters did not change due to the long-term PHH culture. Cells were cultured in hepatocyte culture media supplemented with 10% (v/v) human serum and the levels of different indicated proteins were measured at different indicated time points by Western blotting. GAPDH was used as an internal control.

Figure S3 Characteristics of all 12 HCV-infected CLD patients. Viral titer in serum was measured by RT-qPCR to amplify a specific portion of the 5′-untranslated region (5′-UTR) of the HCV genome. HCV genotype and sub-type were determined by direct sequencing. The amplified nucleic acid was sequenced bi-directionally using dye-terminator chemistry. Results were obtained based on comparison with a database derived from GenBank sequences. Histopathology for fibrosis and steatosis were determined by the Pathologist from H&E staining of biopsy specimens. $_{\#}$c: primary human hepatocytes as control.

Figure S4 Characteristics of HCV-infected LC patients. HCV-RNA level in serum was measured by RT-qPCR. HCV genotype and sub-type were determined by direct sequencing. NR: non-responder, PR: partial-responder.

Figure S5 RT-nested PCR amplification and Southern Blotting of IFNAR1 mRNA from explant livers. Total RNA was isolated from the explant liver. The first round PCR amplification of the 3′ end of IFNAR1 was performed using the S/901 and AS/1926 primer set listed in **Table S1**. The second round, hemi-nested PCR amplification was conducted using the S/1345 and AS/1926 primer set listed in **Table S1**. The hemi-nested PCR products were then loaded onto a 2% agarose gel. The DNA was then transferred to a membrane (Bio-Rad, Hercules, CA). The membrane was then washed, air dried, and hybridized in hybridization solution (5× SSC, 20 mM NaH_2PO_4, 7%SDS, 10× Denhardt, salmon sperm DNA) for three hours at 50°C. Probe S/1633 (**Table S1**) was then added directly to the hybridization solution. The membrane and probe were then hybridized for 14 hours at 50°C. Following hybridization, the membrane was washed (3× SSC, 25 mM NaH_2PO_4, 5%SDS, 10× Denhardt, salmon sperm DNA) and finally exposed in XAR film (Kodak, Rochester, NY). The 5′ end of IFNAR1 was PCR amplified using the S/241 and AS/402 primer set and probes S/253 (**Table S1**) utilizing the method described above. (**A**) Schematic presentation for amplification of IFNAR1 gene. aa: amino acids; nt: nucleotides; S: sense primer; AS: anti-sense primer. RT-nested PCR amplification and Southern blotting of 5′ and 3′ region of IFNAR1 in (**B**) non-HCV (HCV−) LC patients, and (**C**) HCV infected (HCV+) LC patients. SB: Southern blotting.

Figure S6 Inhibition of ER stress and autophagy response rescued IFNAR1 and RBV transporters. Persistently HCV-infected Huh-7.5 cells were transfected with 100 picomole concentrations of control siRNA (siIRR) and siRNAs against PERK (ER stress sensor) and ATG7 (autophagy gene) for 72 h. The expression of IFN-α receptor 1 (IFNAR1) IFN-γ receptor 1

(IFNγR1) and RBV transporters (CNT1 and ENT1) was detected by Western blotting. GAPDH was used as an internal control.

Table S1 Nucleotide sequences of primers and probes used to demonstrate IFNAR1 mRNA by RT-PCR and Southern blotting.

Acknowledgments

We thank Daniel Hoskins for critically reviewing this manuscript.

Author Contributions

Conceived and designed the experiments: PKC SH TW SD. Performed the experiments: PKC FG SH RK RP BP. Analyzed the data: PKC TW SD. Contributed reagents/materials/analysis tools: PKC DB AJC HEB IC GL LAB. Wrote the paper: PKC LAB SD. Liver biopsy specimens: FG RK LAB. Explant liver tissues: DB AJC HEB IC GL.

References

1. Lemoine M, Thursz M (2014) Hepatitis C, a global issue: Access to care and new therapeutic and preventive approaches in resource-constrained areas. Seminar Liver Dis 34: 89–97.
2. Shepard CW, Finelli L, Alter MJ (2005) Global epidemiology of hepatitis C virus infection. Lancer Infect Dis 5: 558–567.
3. Thomas DL, Seeff LB (2005) Natural history of hepatitis C. Clin Liver Dis 9: 383–398.
4. Morgan RL, Baack B, Smith BD, Yartel A, Pitasi M, et al. (2013) Eradication of hepatitis C virus infection and the development of hepatocellular carcinoma: a meta-analysis of observational studies. Ann Intern Med 158: 329–337.
5. Toshikuni N, Arisawa T, Tsutsumi M (2014) Hepatitis C-related liver cirrhosis-stretegies for the prevention of hepatic decompensation, hepatocarcinogenesis and mortality. World J Gastroenterol 20: 2876–2887.
6. Forestier N, Zeuzem S (2012) Triple therapy with telaprevir: results in hepatitis C virus-genotype 1 infected relapsers and non-responders. Liver Int 32: 44–50.
7. Zeuzem S, Andreone P, Pol S, Lawitz E, Diago S, et al. (2011) Telaprevir for retreatment of HCV infection. N Eng J Med 364: 2417–2428.
8. Asselah T, Estrabaud E, Bieche I, lapalus M, De Muynck S, et al. (2010) Hepatitis C: viral and host factors associated with non-response to pegylated interferon plus ribavirin. Liver International 30: 1259–1269.
9. Zhu Y, Chen S (2013) Antiviral treatment of hepatitis C virus infection and factors affecting efficacy. World J Gastroenterol 19: 8963–8973.
10. Booth DR, Ahlenstiel G, George J (2012) Pharmacogenomics of hepatitis C infections: personalizing therapy. Genome Med 4: 99.
11. Bota S, Sporea I, Sirli R, Popescu A, Neghina AM, et al. (2013) Severe adverse events during antiviral therapy in hepatitis C virus cirrhotic patients: A systematic review. World J Hepatol 5: 120–126.
12. Wright TL (2002) Treatment of patients with hepatitis C and cirrhosis. Hepatology 36: S185–S192.
13. Veldt BJ, Heathcote EJ, Wedemeyer H, Reichen J, Hoffmann WP, et al. (2007) Sustained virologic response and clinical outcomes in patients with chronic hepatitis C and advanced fibrosis. Ann Intern Med 147: 677–684.
14. Darnell JE Jr., Kerr IM, Stark GR (1994) Jak-STAT pathways and transcriptional activation in response to IFNs and other extracellular signaling proteins. Science 264: 1415–1421.
15. Lemon SM (2010) Induction and evasion of innate antiviral responses by hepatitis C virus. J Biol Chem 285: 22741–22747.
16. Hazari S, Chandra PK, Poat B, Datta S, Garry RF, et al. (2010) Impaired antiviral activity of interferon alpha against hepatitis C virus 2a in Huh-7 cells with a defective Jak-Stat pathway. Virology J 7: 36–52.
17. Datta S, Hazari S, Chandra PK, Samara M, Poat B, et al. (2011) Mechanisms of HCV's resistance to IFN-alpha in cell culture involves expression of functional IFN-alpha receptor 1. Virology J 8: 351–369.
18. Chandra PK, Bao L, Song K, Aboulnasr FM, Baker DP, et al. (2014) HCV infection selectively impairs Type I but not the Type III IFN signaling. Am J Pathol 184: 214–229.
19. Liu S, Nelson CA, Xiao L, Lu L, Davis DR, et al (2011) Measuring antiviral activity of benzimidazole molecules that alters IRES RNA structure with an infectious hepatitis C virus chimera expressing *Renilla* Luciferase. Antiviral Res 89: 54–63.
20. Chandra PK, Kundu AK, Hazari S, Chandra S, Bao L, et al. (2012) Inhibition of hepatitis C virus replication by intracellular delivery of multiple siRNAs by nanosomes. Mol Ther 20: 1724–1736.
21. Gerber MA, Sheih C, Shim K-S, Thung SN, Demetris AJ, et al. (1992) Detection of replicative hepatitis C virus sequences in hepatocellular carcinoma. Am J Pathol 141: 1271–1277.
22. Gunduz F, Mallikarjun C, Balart LA, Dash S (2014) Interferon alpha induced intrahepatic pSTAT1 inversely correlates with serum HCV RNA levels in chronic HCV infection. Exp Mol Pathol 96: 36–41.
23. Bukh M (2008) Direct infection and replication of naturally occurring hepatitis C virus genotypes 1, 2, 3 and 4 in normal human hepatocyte cultures. PLoS One 3: e2660.
24. Gondeau C, Briolotti P, Razafy F, Duret C, Rubbo PA, et al. (2013) In vitro infection of primary human hepatocytes by HCV-positive sera: insight on a highly relevant model. Gut 0: 1–11.
25. Steenbergen RHG, Joyce MA, Thomas BS, Jones D, Law J, et al. (2013) Human serum leads to differentiation of human hepatoma cells, restoration of very-low-density lipoprotein secretion, and a 1000-fold increase in HCV JFH type 1 titers. Hepatology 58:1907–1917.
26. Dash S, Rege TA, Tsuji H, Gaglio P, Garry RF, et al. (2000) HCV RNA levels in hepatocellular carcinomas and adjacent non-tumorous livers. J Virol Methods 90: 15–23.
27. Manns MP, McHutchison JG, Gordon SC, Rustgi VK, Shiffman M, et al. (2001) Peginterferon alfa-2b plus ribavirin compared with interferon alfa-2b plus ribavirin for initial treatment of chronic hepatitis C: a randomized trial. Lancet 358: 958–965.
28. Fried MW, Shiffman ML, Reddy KR, Smith C, Marinos G, et al. (2002) Peginterferon alfa-2a plus ribavirin for chronic hepatitis C virus infection. N Eng J Med 347: 975–82.
29. Roffi L, Colloredo G, Pioltelli P, Bellati G, Pozzpi M, et al. (2008) Peginterferon alfa-2b plus ribavirin: an efficacious and well tolerated regimen for patients with hepatitis C virus related histologically proven cirrhosis. Antiviral Ther 13: 663–673.
30. Liu J, HuangFu WC, Kumar KG, Qian J, Casey JP, et al. (2009) Virus-induced unfolded protein response attenuates anti-viral defenses via phosphorylation-dependent degradation of Type I interferon receptor. Cell Host Microbe 5: 72–83.
31. Malhi H, Kaufman RJ (2011) Endoplasmic reticulum stress in liver disease. J Hepatol 54:795–809.
32. Czaja MJ, Ding W-X, Donohue TM (2013) Functions of autophagy in normal and diseased liver. Autophagy 9: 1131–1158.
33. Asselah T, Bieche I, Mansouri A, laurendeau I, Cazals-Hatem D, et al. (2010) In vivo hepatic endoplasmic stress in patients with chronic hepatitis C. J Pathol 221: 264–274.
34. Ait-Goughoulte M, Kanda T, Meyer K, Ryerse JS, Ray RB, et al. (2008) Hepatitis C Virus genotype 1a growth and induction of autophagy. J Virol 82: 2241–2249.
35. Shuda M, Kondoh N, Imazeki N, Tanaka K, Okada T, et al. (2003) Activation of the ATG6, XBP1 and GRP78 genes in human hepatocellular carcinoma: a possible involvement of the ER-stress pathway in hepatocarcinogenesis. J Hepatol 38: 605–614.
36. Su IJ, Wang HC, Wu HC, Huang WY (2008) Ground glass hepatocytes contain pre-S mutants and represent preneoplastic lesions in chronic HBV infection. J Gastroenterol Hepatol 23:1169–1174.
37. Rautou PE, Cazals-Hatem D, Feldmann G, Mansouri A, Grodet A, et al. (2011) Changes in autophagy response in patients with chronic hepatitis C virus infection. Am J Pathol 178: 2708–2715.
38. Lin JH, Walter P, Benedict Yen TS (2008) Endoplasmic Reticulum Stress in Disease Pathogenesis. Annu Rev Path Mech Dis 3: 399–425.
39. Soza A, Heller T, Ghany M, Lutchman G, Liang TJ, et al. (2005) Pilot study of interferon gamma for hepatitis C. J Hepatol 43: 67–71.
40. Zeuzem S (2004) Heterogeneous virologic response rates to interferon-based therapy in patients with chronic hepatitis C: who responds less well? Ann Intern Med 140:370–381.
41. Han D, Lerner AG, Vande Walle L, Upton JP, et al. (2009) IRE1 alpha kinase activation modes control alternate endoribonuclease outputs to determine divergent cell fates. Cell 138: 562–575.
42. Li X, Yan J, Wang L, Xiao F, Yang Y, et al. (2013) Beclin1 inhibition promotes autophagy and decreases gemcitabine-induced apoptosis in Miapaca2 pancreatic cancer cells. Cancer Cell Int 13: 13–26.
43. Pietrocola F, Izzo V, Niso-Santano M, Vacchelli E, Gulluzzi L, et al. (2013) Regulation of autophagy by stress-responsive transcription factors. Semin Cancer Biol 23: 310–322.

20

Hepatic HMOX1 Expression Positively Correlates with Bach-1 and miR-122 in Patients with HCV Mono and HIV/HCV Coinfection

Elżbieta Jabłonowska[1]*, Kamila Wójcik[1], Bożena Szymańska[2], Aleksandra Omulecka[3], Hanna Ćwiklińska[4], Anna Piekarska[1]

1 Department of Infectious Diseases and Hepatology, Medical University of Lodz, Łódź, Poland, **2** Central Laboratory, Medical University of Lodz, Łódź, Poland, **3** Department of Pathology, Biegański Provincial Specialistic Hospital, Łódź, Poland, **4** Laboratory of Neuroimmunology, Department of Neurology, Medical University of Łódź, Poland

Abstract

Aim: To analyze the expression of HMOX1 and miR-122 in liver biopsy samples obtained from HCV mono-and HIV/HCV co-infected patients in relation to selected clinical parameters, histological examination and IL-28B polymorphism as well as to determine whether HMOX1 expression is dependent on Bach-1.

Materials and Methods: The study group consisted of 90 patients with CHC: 69 with HCV mono and 21 with HIV/HCV co-infection. RT-PCR was used in the analysis of HMOX1, Bach-1 and miR-122 expression in liver biopsy samples and in the assessment of IL-28B single-nucleotide polymorphism C/T (rs12979860) in the blood. Moreover in liver biopsy samples an analysis of HO-1 and Bach-1 protein level by Western Blot was performed.

Results: HCV mono-infected patients, with lower grading score ($G<2$) and higher HCV viral load (>600000 IU/mL) demonstrated higher expression of HMOX1. In patients with HIV/HCV co-infection, the expression of HMOX1 was lower in patients with lower lymphocyte CD4 count and higher HIV viral load. IL28B polymorphism did not affect the expression of either HMOX1 or miR-122. Higher HMOX1 expression correlated with higher expression of Bach-1 (Spearman's $\rho = 0.586$, $p = 0.000001$) and miR-122 (Spearman's $\rho = 0.270$, $p = 0.014059$).

Conclusions: HMOX1 and miR-122 play an important role in the pathogenesis of CHC in HCV mono-and HIV/HCV co-infected patients. Reduced expression of HMOX1 in patients with HIV/HCV co-infection may indicate a worse prognosis in this group. Our results do not support the importance of Bach-1 in repression of HMOX1 in patients with chronic hepatitis C.

Editor: Jean-Pierre Vartanian, Institut Pasteur, France

Funding: The authors have no support or funding to report.

Competing Interests: The authors have declared that no competing interests exist.

* E-mail: elajablonowska@gmail.com

Introduction

Hepatitis C virus infection (HCV) remains a worldwide health problem with about 3–4 million cases reported each year [1]. Approximately 80% of patients become chronically infected after acute infection, 20% of whom progress to cirrhosis [2–3]. The annual rate of hepatocellular carcinoma (HCC) in cirrhosis patients is about 3–8% [4].

Current therapy based on pegylated interferon, ribavirin and protease inhibitors like boceprevir or telaprevir is effective in no more than 70% of patients with CHC [5,6].

Reactive oxygen species (ROS) production can suppress HCV replication [7]. However, excessive production may cause hepatocyte damage [8–11]. Hence, antioxidant enzymes, such as Heme oxygenase-1 (HO-1), induced in response to "stressful stimuli", play a crucial role by suppressing inflammation and protecting against oxidative stress [12,13].

However, the effect of HO-1 on HCV replication is unclear. While several experimental studies indicate that it plays an important role in the inhibition of HCV replication [14,15], others indicate the contrary [16]. Moreover, experimental studies describing the increase of HCV replication under the influence of microRNA-122 (miR-122) are not always confirmed *in vitro* [17]. Interestingly, the antagomir of miR-122 has been found to increase HO-1 mRNA levels in CNS3 and NS3–5B Huh-7 cells [15].

The aim of this present study is to examine the expression of heme oxygenase-1 gene (HMOX1), BTB and CNC homology 1 (Bach-1) as well as miR-122 in liver biopsy specimens obtained from patients with CHC in relation to selected clinical parameters, histological examination and IL-28B polymorphism. In addition, Western-Blot analysis was used to investigate the levels of Bach-1 and HO-1 proteins in liver biopsy specimens.

Table 1. Selected demographic, laboratory and histo-pathological features of subjects.

	HIV/HCV co-infection		HCV mono-infection		P
	LQ-UQ	**MEDIAN**	**LQ-UQ**	**MEDIAN**	
Age years	29–34	32	21–48	29	>0.05
ALT U/L	44–83	54	39–83	54	>0.05
HCV viremia $\times 10^6$ IU/mL	0.39–4.56	1.68	0.39–6.23	2.19	>0.05
	Number of patients	**fraction**	**Number of patients**	**fraction**	**P**
age≥40 years	2	9.52	20	28.99	>0.05
age<40 years	19	90.48	49	71.01	
Women	7	33.33	20	28.99	>0.05
Men	14	66.67	49	71.01	
HCV viremia >600 000 IU/mL	13	61.90	45	65.22	>0.05
HCV viremia ≤600 000 IU/mL	8	38.10	24	34.78	
IL28 B genotypes:					
CC	6	28.57	22	31.88	>0.05
TT	3	14.29	12	17.39	>0.05
CT	12	57.14	35	50.72	>0.05
ALT≥50 U/L	13	61.90	39	56.52	>0.05
ALT<50 U/L	8	38.10	30	43.48	
G≥2	3	14.29	20	28.99	>0.05
G<2	18	85.71	49	71.01	
S≥2	15	71.43	50	72.46	>0.05
S<2	6	28.57	19	27.54	
HCV genotype 1	6	0.29	63	0.91	= 0.00000
HCV genotype 3	6	0.29	6	0.09	= 0.018973
HCV genotype 4	9	0.42	0	0.00	= 0.00000

ALT - alanine aminotransferase, in liver biopsy: G- grade of inflammation and necrosis, S-stage of fibrosis.

Materials and Methods

The study was approved by the Ethical Committee of the Medical University of Lodz. Informed written consent was obtained from all patients.

Liver biopsies were performed as part of routine standard of care for the subjects studied. The study group consisted of 90 patients: 69 with HCV mono-and 21 with HIV/HCV co-infection. The diagnosis of chronic hepatitis was based on the results of liver biopsy specimen examination. Patients with other systemic or inflammatory diseases, other causes of liver disease, previous immunosuppressive or anti HCV treatment and pregnant women were excluded from this study. Grade of inflammation and necrotic changes (grading-G) as well as stage of fibrosis (staging-S) were assessed according to the Batt and Ludwig scale [18]. RNA analyses were performed by use of 2-mm sections of liver that were excised from the core liver biopsy samples immediately after the biopsy procedure. These sections were immediately submerged in RNA later solution and stored at $-70^{\circ}C$ until use.

Plasma HCV viral load was measured within 3 months of liver biopsy and was determined by reverse transcription polymerase chain reaction (RT-PCR method; Cobas AmpliPrep/Cobas TaqMan HCV Test, Roche Diagnostics), HCV genotypes were determined by VERSANT HCV Genotype 2.0 Assay, LiPA test. Alanine aminotransferase (ALT) activity was measured 1–3 days before the liver biopsy, reference ranges for men and women were 0–41 U/L and 0–31 U/L, respectively. To diagnose HIV infection, an enzyme linked immunosorbent assay (ELISA test) and confirmatory W-Blot were used. In patients with HIV/HCV co-infection, HIV viral load (RT-PCR method, Cobas Ampli-Prep/Cobas TaqMan HIV-1 Test, Roche Diagnostics) and lymphocytes CD4 count (using flow cytometry) were measured.

Analysis of IL-28B Single-nucleotide Polymorphism C/T (rs12979860)

Genomic DNA was isolated from 200 μL of blood using the QIAamp DNA Blood Mini Kit (Qiagen) according to the manufacturer's protocol. DNA was quantified using a PicoDrop spectrophotometer (Picodrop Limited). IL-28B single-nucleotide polymorphism C/T (rs12979860) was analyzed by means of Custom® SNP Genotyping Assays (Applied Biosystems). Primer and probe sequences were Forward Primer 5′GCCTGTCGTGTACTGAACCA, Reverse Primer 5′-GCGCGGAGTGCAATTCAAC, Probe (C allele) 5′-VIC-TGGTTCGCGCCTTC, Probe (T allele) 5′-FAM-CTGGTTCACGCCTTC. Genotyping was performed using the ABI7900HT Real-Time PCR System (Applied Biosystems) in 25 μL reaction volume containing 10 ng DNA, 12.5 μL TaqMan® Universal PCR Master Mix and 1.25 μL (40×) Custom® SNP Genotyping Assays and analyzed by means of Sequence Detection System 2.3 Software.

Table 2. HMOX1 expression depending on the studied parameters.

HMOX1 Median N = 82		**P**
Women	53.78	>0.05
Men	72.63	
Co-infection	27.74	= 0.0204
No co-infection	78.65	
Age≥40 years	61.35	= 0.05
Age<40 years	102.04	
HCV viremia >600 000 IU/mL	111.69	= 0.0006
HCV viremia ≤600 000 IU/mL	35.80	
IL-28B CC	81.10	>0.05
IL-28B not CC	65.97	
ALT≥50 U/L	62.16	>0.05
ALT<50 U/L	84.66	
G≥2	53.78	= 0.0495
G<2	106.98	
S≥2	72.55	>0.05
S<2	45.90	
HCV genotype 1	91.68	= 0.0274*
HCV genotype 3	26.36	
HCV genotype 4	17.50	

ALT - alanine aminotransferase, genotypes of IL28B: CC and not CC (CT and TT). In liverbiopsy: G- grade of inflammation and necrosis, S-stage of fibrosis.*Genotype 1 versus 3 p = 0.0501, genotype 1 versus 4 p = 0.0344, genotype 3 versus 4 p>0.05.

Total RNA Isolation

Total RNA was extracted using the mirVana™ miRNA isolation kit (Ambion) according to the manufacturer's instructions. Briefly, frozen samples were homogenized in 300 µl of Lysis/Binding Solution using a TissueRuptor homogenizer (Qiagen). RNA was eluted in 100 µl RNase-free water and quantified using PicoDrop spectrophotometer. The quality of RNA samples was analyzed by measuring the ratio of absorptions at 260/280 nm. The purified total RNA was immediately used for cDNA synthesis or stored at −80°C.

miRNA-122 Expression

Reverse transcription was carried out on 10 ng of total RNA in 15 µl reactions using the TaqMan® MicroRNA Reverse Transcription Kit (Applied Biosystems) according to the manufacturer's instructions. The RT reaction was diluted 10 times in nuclease-free water and 9 µL of aliquots were subsequently used for PCR amplification using TaqMan® MicroRNA Assays (miR-122 -Assay ID 002130, RNU 24 -Assay ID 001001), according to the manufacturer's instructions (Applied Biosystems). RNU 24 (SNORD24 small nucleolar RNA, C/D box 24) was used as an endogenous control.

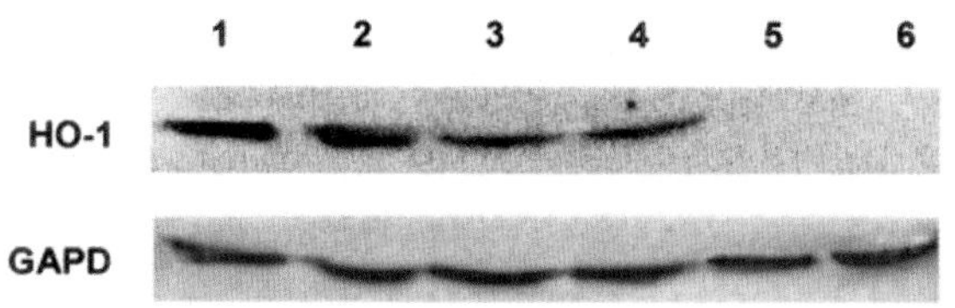

Figure 1. Presence of HO-1 protein levels for representative patients (Western Blot analysis).

mRNA Expression

Homo sapiens-specific TaqMan Gene Expression Assays (Applied Biosystems) for heme oxygenase (HMOX1, Hs01110250_m1), BTB and CNC homology 1 (Bach-1, Hs154276 _XX) were used. cDNA generation was performed using 250 ng of total RNA with High Capacity cDNA Reverse Transcription Kits according to the manufacturer's protocols (Applied Biosystems). First-strand cDNA was subsequently diluted 10 times in nuclease-free water before addition to the RT-PCR reaction mixture. mRNA expression levels were analyzed using beta actin (ACTB) as an endogenous control.

Real Time PCR Analysis

TaqMan PCR assays were performed in 96-well optical plates on 7900HT Fast Real-Time PCR System (Applied Biosystems) and were analyzed using Sequence Detection System 2.0 Software. Fold induction values were calculated according to the equation 2ΔΔCt, where ΔCt represents the differences in cycle threshold numbers between the target gene and endogenous control, and ΔΔCt represents the relative change in these differences between examined and control groups.

Western Blot Analysis

W-Blot analysis was performed in 32 out of 90 patients. Samples were chosen based on the RT-PCR analysis performed previously. W-Blot was carried out in 10 patients with HCV monoinfection among whom 5 patients were found to have viremia higher than 600 000 IU/ml and HO-1 expression closest to the median for this group (the result obtained by RT-PCR). The remaining 5 patients had viremia below 600 000 IU/ml and HO-1 expression closest to the median for this group (the result obtained by RT-PCR). In the group with HIV/HCV coinfection W-Blot analysis was performed in 15 patients. In this group selection criteria for W-B analysis included CD4 count and HIV viremia.

Total homogenates of biopsy samples were resolved on SDS electrophoresis gels by standard procedures. Immunoblotting was performed with anti-HO-1 rabbit polyclonal antibody, ADISPA-896 (Enzo Life Sciences, Germany) or with anti-Bach1 goat polyclonal antibody, sc-14700 (Santa Cruz Biotechnology, INC). Final detection was achieved with the appropriate secondary antibody coupled to HRP (anti-rabbit IgG-HRP or anti-goat IgG-HRP, Santa Cruz Biotechnology, INC), followed by Western Lightning ECL Pro substrate (Perkin Elmer), and visualized by gel imaging system for chemiluminescence G:Box Chemi XR5 (Syngene).

Equal loading of proteins was checked by immunodetection of glyceraldehyde 3-phosphate dehydrogenase (GAPDH) mouse monoclonal Ab, MAB 374 (Millipore) and anti-mouse IgG-HRP as a secondary antibody (Santa Cruz Biotechnology, INC).

Statistical Methods

Average values and standard deviation of quantitative traits were calculated for parameters with normal distribution. Variables that were not normally distributed were expressed as median, lower -upper quartiles (LQ-UQ). These variables were compared using the Mann-Whitney test for two groups and the Kruskal-Wallis test with post-hoc Conover-Inman test for more than two groups. The Chi-square distribution, Yates' correction for continuity or Fisher's exact test were used to compare categorical variables between groups, based on the size of the studied group. Spearman's rank correlation coefficient was applied to determine the association between two quantities which were not normally distributed.

Results

Characteristics of the Study Group

The study group consisted of 90 patients: 69 with HCV mono- and 21 with HIV/HCV coinfection, of whom 27 were women and 63 were men. The median age of patients was 30 years (LQ 29 years-UQ34 years).

Among subjects with HIV/HCV co-infection 16 were receiving antiretroviral treatment, while 5 were not. The median CD4 cell count was 405 cells/µL (LQ 339 cells/µL–UQ 469 cells/µL). All patients had CD4 cell count >200 cells/µL, 14 patients had CD4 cell count >350 cells/µL. Fifteen patients demonstrated an HIV viral load below 50 copies/mL. The highest HIV viral load amounted to 385 000 copies/mL.

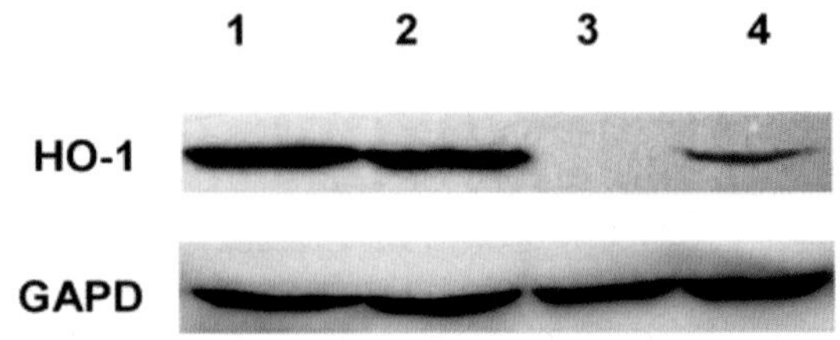

Figure 2. HO-1 protein levels in selected patients with HIV/HCV co-infection (Western Blot analysis).

The comparison between patients with and without HIV/HCV co-infection is depicted in table 1. In the group of co-infected patients, a higher incidence of infection with HCV genotypes 3 and 4, and a lower incidence of infection with genotype 1, was observed compared to the group with HCV mono–infection.

HMOX1

HMOX1 expression was analyzed in 90 liver biopsy samples. Eight specimens were rejected because of the insufficient RNA amount or quality (A260/A280<1.8).

A lower expression of HMOX1 was observed in patients co-infected with HIV/HCV. Expression of this gene was also lower in patients with lower HCV viral load (table 2). As regards the studied genotypes, a lower expression of HMOX1 was detected in patients infected with HCV genotype 4 in comparison with patients infected with HCV genotype 1. Results of the W-Blot confirm the described correlations (figure 1). While a strong band for HO-1 was observed in 4 out of 5 subjects with HCV viremia higher than 600 000 IU/ml, a weak band for HO-1 was observed in 3 out of 5 patients with HCV viremia below 600 000 IU/ml.

Figure 1 depicts the results of selected patients Only in some patients with co-infection no visible bands of HO-1 were seen (lane 5,6). Anti GAPDH antibody was used to confirm equal presence of cellular material in each sample.

Subgroup of Patients with Co-infection

Higher expression of HO-1 was found in patients with CD4 count >350 cells/µl and HIV viral load <50 copies/ml (table 3). The presented results of the W-Blot confirmed this correlation on the protein level.

All nine patients who had both CD4 count higher than 350 cells/ul and undetectable HIV viremia as well as all 6 patients with detectable HIV viremia were qualified for the W-Blot analysis.

Table 3. HMOX1 depending on HIV viral load and CD4 count.

	HMOX1 Median N = 21	P
HIV viremia<50 copies/mL	52.59	= 0.046
HIV viremia≥50 copies/mL	3.29	
Lymphocytes CD4>350 cells/µL	77.32	= 0.05
Lymphocytes CD4≤350 cells/µL	8.13	

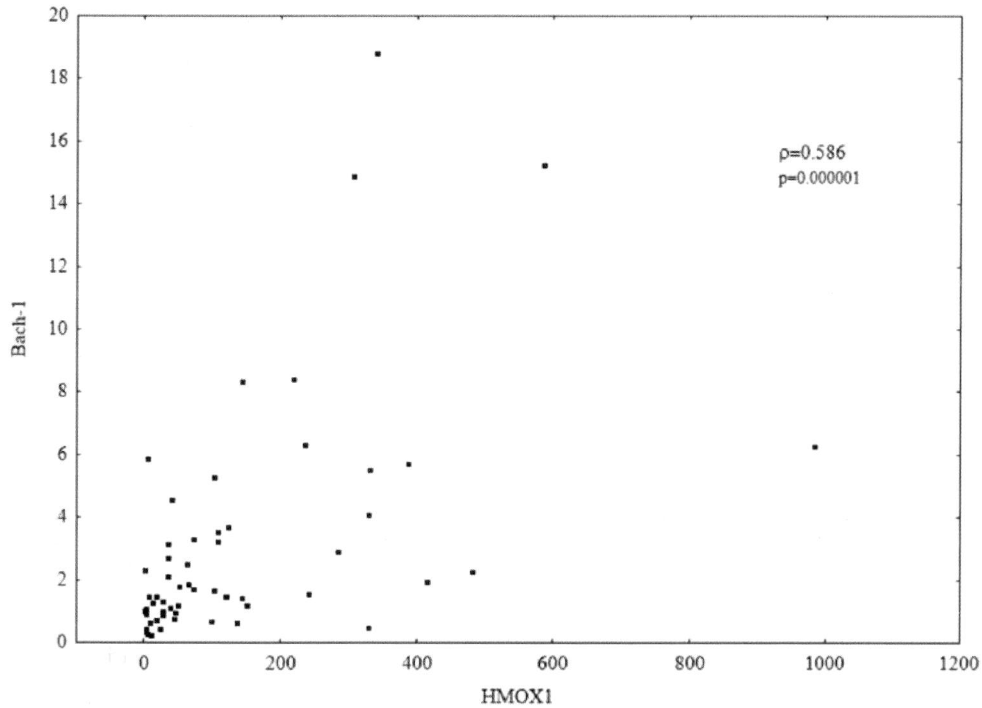

Figure 3. Correlation between the expression of HMOX1 and Bach-1. Gene expression was analyzed by relative quantitative (RQ) real-time PCR. mRNA levels were normalized to ACTB. Higher HMOX1 expression correlated with a higher expression of Bach-1 (Spearman's rank correlation coefficient; $\rho = 0.586$, $p = 0.000001$).

In the First Subgroup a Band for HO-1 was Observed in 8 out of 9 Patients

No band was observed in patients with CD4 count below 350 cells/ul and detectable HIV viremia.

Figure 2 depicts the results of selected patients with HIV/HCV co-infection, but different CD4 counts and HIV viral loads. Bach-1 has not been confirmed to have any inhibitory effect of on HO-1 expression.

Bach-1 expression was analyzed in first 60 liver biopsy samples. Two specimens were rejected because of the insufficient RNA amount or quality (A260/A280<1.8).

The results of gene expression indicate a positive correlation between HO-1 and Bach-1. Higher HMOX1 expression correlated with a higher expression of Bach-1(Spearman's $\rho = 0.586$, $p = 0.000001$) figure 3. Such a correlation was also confirmed by the W-Blot analysis, and selected results are presented in figure 4. Both in patients with mono- and coinfection, a weak band for Bach-1 was associated with a weak band for HO-1, and a strong band for Bach-1 was observed in the presence of a strong band for HO-1. Similarly, in coinfected patients in whom no band for HO-1 was observed, no band for Bach-1 was found.

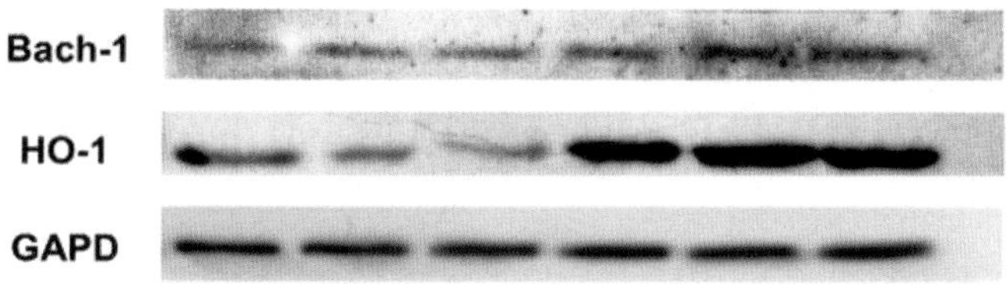

Figure 4. Positive correlation between HO-1 and Bach-1 protein level (Western Blot analysis).

miR-122

The expression was found to be higher in patients with ALT <50 U/L than those with higher ALT activity (table 4). Higher HMOX1 expression correlated with a higher expression of miR-122 ($\rho = -0.336$, $p = 0.001196$) figure 5. Higher ALT activity was associated with a lower expression of miR-122 ($\rho = -0.336$, $p = 0.001196$) figure 6. No correlation between HCV viral load and miR-122 expression was observed.

Discussion

The HCV core protein is considered to cause increased production of ROS by altering mitochondrial function [19]. Controlled ROS production might be beneficial because it supports the elimination of HCV [7]. On the other hand, excessive production of ROS can result in hepatocyte injury. Therefore it is crucial to maintain a balance between pro-and antioxidative processes. HO-1 is one of the principal antioxidative enzymes. It is a cytoprotective enzyme which catalyzes the degradation of heme to bilirubin, carbon monoxide and iron and is induced by its substrate, heme, and by other stress-induced molecules [13,20,21].

Some authors suggested that different HCV proteins induce different antioxidant defense responses in hepatocytes. Abdalla et al [22,23] showed that the expression of HO-1 was reduced in cell lines that stably expressed HCV core protein but increased in cell lines over-expressing HCV-NS proteins. On the contrary, Ghazini [16] demonstrates that HO-1 is up-regulated in hepatoma cells expressing not only HCV core protein but also additional structural and nonstructural proteins.

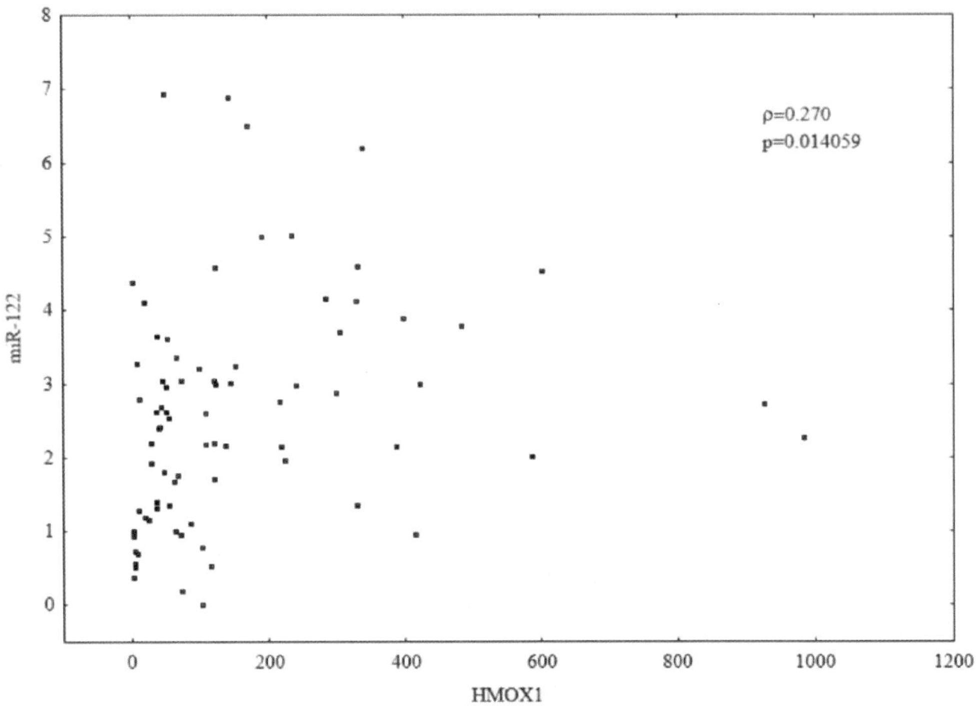

Figure 5. Correlation between the expression of HMOX1 and miR-122. Gene expression was analyzed by relative quantitative (RQ) real-time PCR. mRNA levels were normalized to ACTB for HMOX1 and to RNU24 for miR-122. Higher HMOX1 expression correlated with higher expression of miR-122. (Spearman's rank correlation coefficient; ρ = 0.270, p = 0.014059).

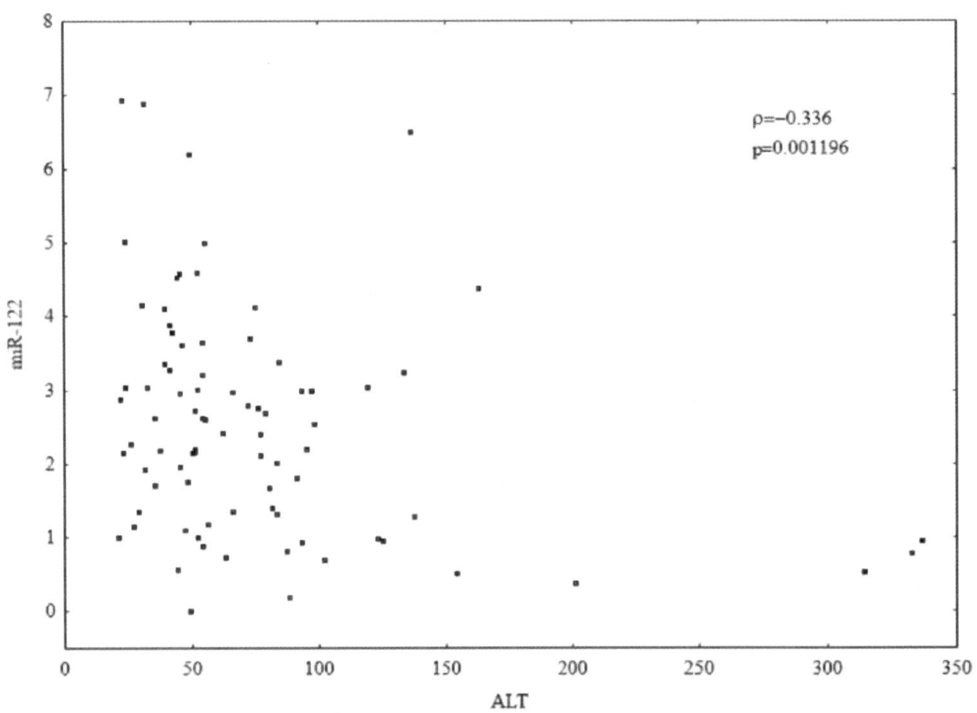

Figure 6. Correlation between ALT activity (U/L) and miR-122 expression. Gene expression was analyzed by relative quantitative (RQ) real-time PCR. mRNA levels were normalized to RNU24 for miR-122. Higher ALT activity correlated with a lower expression of miR-122 (Spearman's rank correlation coefficient; ρ = −0.336, p = 0.001196).

Table 4. MiR-122 expression depending on the studied parameters.

MiR-122 Median N = 90		**P**
Women	3.22	>0.05
Men	2.20	
Co-infection	2.19	>0.05
No co-infection	2.73	
Age≥40 years	1.97	>0.05
Age<40 years	2.80	
Viral load>600 000 IU/mL	2.61	>0.05
Viral load ≤600 000 IU/mL	2.66	
IL-28B CC	2.84	>0.05
IL-28B not CC	2.52	
ALT≥50 U/L	2.41	= 0.0453
ALT<50 U/L	3.00	
G≥2	2.41	>0.05
G<2	2.69	
S≥2	2.76	>0.05
S<2	2.20	
HCV genotype 1	2.63	>0.05
HCVgenotype 3	2.71	
HCV genotype 4	2.19	

ALT - alanine aminotransferase, genotypes of IL28B: CC and not CC (CT and TT). In liver biopsy: G- grade of inflammation and necrosis, S-stage of fibrosis.

HO-1 has been shown to interfere with HCV replication but this connection is not yet clear. Several studies indicate that HO-1 induction or overexpression in replicons inhibit HCV replication [14,15], while others have specified that it might be the products of the reaction catalyzed by HO-1 that are responsible for this process. It has been demonstrated that both iron and biliverdin display antiviral activity [24–27]. However, on the contrary, Kakizaki et al [28] note that iron enhances hepatitis C virus replication in cultured human hepatocytes. The present study demonstrates that HMOX1 expression positively correlated with HCV viremia in patients with CHC, and that expression was higher in patients with HCV viremia values greater than 600 000 IU/mL than in those with lower levels.

The mechanism of HMOX1 up-regulation in HCV infection is not precisely known, although it may be the result of a protective antioxidant response to excessive ROS production. One of the models explaining the increased expression of HMOX1 in patients with CHC was presented by Ghazani et al [16], who postulate that during HCV infection, the expression of Bach-1 gene is decreased, which causes de-repression of HMOX1. Bach-1 downregulation might be connected with oxidative stress, and HMOX1 induction could be a part of the response that hepatocytes use to protect themselves against oxidative stress.

However, the results of the present study do not indicate that a higher expression of Bach-1 is associated with a lower expression of HMOX1. On the contrary, Bach-1 positively correlated with HO-1. The W-Blot analysis provided similar results: patients in whom no band for HO-1 was observed also had a weak or absent band for Bach-1 and conversely, in those who had a strong band for HO-1, a band for Bach-1 was also found. Hence Bach-1 does not seem to play a role in the repression of HMOX1 in patients infected with HCV.

MiRNAs are post-transcriptional regulators which bind to complementary sequences on target messenger RNA transcripts. Several hundred miRNAs have already been distinguished and each of them is considered to regulate hundreds of target mRNAs. MiR-122, the most abundant miRNA in the liver, is known to positively regulate replication of the HCV in cell culture [29,30]. However, no correlation between the expression of miR-122 and HCV viremia in patients with CHC was identified in the present study. Similarly, Sarasin-Filipowicz [17] report no positive correlation between miR-122 expression and intrahepatic and serum viral load in patients with CHC.

Some papers suggest that the antiviral effects of IFN in treatment of patients with CHC may be connected with the influence of IFN on miR-122. Pedersen [31] confirms that IFN-beta stimulation of Huh7 cells leads to a significant reduction in the expression of the liver-specific miR-122. However, Sarasin-Filipowicz [17] reports that the level of miR-122 in liver biopsies did not change significantly between before starting pegylated IFN-α treatment and 4 h afterwards. Interestingly, a study by Sarasin-Filipowicz [17] suggests that the role of miR-122 in controlling the HCV replication might be less important *in vivo* than *in vitro*.

It is worthy of note that miRNAs can also be involved in the regulation of HO-1. In our study, a positive correlation between miR-122 and HMOX1 was observed. Higher HMOX1 correlated with higher miR-122 expression. Additionally, it can be seen that a higher expression of HMOX1 implies a higher HCV viremia. Our results may suggest that in patients with CHC, miR-122 can regulate HCV replication partly through modulation of HMOX1 expression. Another possible explanation of the correlation between miR-122 and HMOX1 is that miR-122 indirectly increases oxidative stress and consequently leads to a protective increase of HMOX1 expression by affecting HCV replication. However, a fuller investigation of these correlations should be the subject of later studies.

The expression of HMOX1 was found to be higher in patients with lower gradings in liver biopsy specimens (G<2), which may suggest that the enzyme plays a protective, anti-inflammatory role. Conversely, HMOX1 expression was lowest in patients with HIV/HCV co-infection, especially those with lower CD4 lymphocyte counts and higher HIV viral loads, which is disadvantageous.

Lower expression of HMOX1 in patients with HIV/HCV co-infection can indicate a weaker antioxidative response to oxidative stress in this group of patients. Some authors suggest that HO-1 induction may counteract the effects of lipopolysaccharides (LPS) and proinflammatory cytokines in HIV infection [32].

Conclusion

Reduced expression of HMOX1 in patients with HIV/HCV co-infection may indicate a worse prognosis in this group. Our results do not support the importance of Bach-1 in repression of HMOX1 in patients infected with HCV.

Acknowledgments

We gratefully acknowledge the assistance of Grażyna Lipowczan M.D., Ph.D, for HCV and HIV viral load and HCV genotype assessment.

Author Contributions

Conceived and designed the experiments: EJ KW AP AO BS HĆ. Performed the experiments: EJ KW AP AO BS HĆ. Analyzed the data: EJ KW AP AO BS HĆ. Contributed reagents/materials/analysis tools: EJ KW AP AO BS HĆ. Wrote the paper: EJ KW BS HĆ.

References

1. Chen SL, Morgan TR (2006) The natural history of hepatitis C virus (HCV) infection. Int J Med Sci 3: 47–52.
2. Lauer GM, Walker BD (2001) Hepatitis C virus infection. N Engl J Med 345: 41–52.
3. Koziel MJ, Peters MG (2007) Viral hepatitis in HIV infection. N Engl J Med 356: 1445–1454.
4. Caballeria L, Pares A, Castells A, Gines A, Bru C, et al. (2001) Hepatocellular carcinoma in primary biliary cirrhosis: similar incidence to that in hepatitis C virus-related cirrhosis. Am J Gastroenterol 96: 1160–1163.
5. Jacobson IM, McHutchison JG, Dusheiko G, Di Bisceglie AM, Reddy KR, et al. (2011) Telaprevir for previously untreated chronic hepatitis C virus infection. N Engl J Med 364: 2405–2416.
6. Poordad F, McCone J, Jr., Bacon BR, Bruno S, Manns MP, et al. (2011) Boceprevir foruntreated chronic HCV genotype 1 infection. N Engl J Med 364: 1195–1206.
7. Choi J, Lee KJ, Zheng Y, Yamaga AK, Lai MM, et al. (2004) Reactive oxygen species suppress hepatitis C virus RNA replication in human hepatoma cells. Hepatology 39: 81–89.
8. Mutlu-Turkoglu U, Ademoglu E, Turkoglu S, Badur S, Uysal M, et al. (1997) The effects of interferonalpha on serum lipid peroxidation and total thiol content in patients with chronic active hepatitis-C. Res Commun Mol Pathol Pharmacol 96: 357–361.
9. De Maria N, Colantoni A, Fagiuoli S, Liu GJ, Rogers BK, et al. (1996) Association between reactive oxygen species and disease activity in chronic hepatitis C. Free Radic Biol Med 21: 291–295.
10. Farinati F, Cardin R, De Maria N, Della Libera G, Marafin C, et al. (1995) Iron storage, lipid peroxidation and glutathione turnover in chronic anti-HCV positive hepatitis. J Hepatol 22: 449–456.
11. Shimoda R, Nagashima M, Sakamoto M, Yamaguchi N, Hirohashi S, et al. (1994) Increased formation of oxidative DNA damage, 8-hydroxydeoxyguanosine, in human livers with chronic hepatitis. Cancer Res 54: 3171–3172.
12. Wen T, Zhao JY, Mei S, Guan L, Zhang YL (2006) [Protective effect of heme oxygenase-1 and its reaction product, carbon monoxide on acute liver injury induced by carbon tetrachloride in rats]. Beijing Da Xue Xue Bao 38: 618–622.
13. Abraham NG, Kappas A (2008) Pharmacological and clinical aspects of heme oxygenase. Pharmacol Rev 60: 79–127.
14. Zhu Z, Wilson AT, Mathahs MM, Wen F, Brown KE, et al. (2008) Heme oxygenase-1 suppresses hepatitis C virus replication and increases resistance of hepatocytes to oxidant injury. Hepatology 48: 1430–1439.
15. Shan Y, Zheng J, Lambrecht RW, Bonkovsky HL (2007) Reciprocal effects of micro-RNA-122 on expression of heme oxygenase-1 and hepatitis C virus genes in human hepatocytes. Gastroenterology 133: 1166–1174.
16. Ghaziani T, Shan Y, Lambrecht RW, Donohue SE, Pietschmann T, et al. (2006) HCV proteins increase expression of heme oxygenase-1 (HO-1) and decrease expression of Bach1 in human hepatoma cells. J Hepatol 45: 5–12.
17. Sarasin-Filipowicz M, Krol J, Markiewicz I, Heim MH, Filipowicz W (2009) Decreased levels of microRNA miR-122 in individuals with hepatitis C responding poorly to interferon therapy. Nat Med 15: 31–33.
18. Batts KP, Ludwig J (1995) Chronic hepatitis. An update on terminology and reporting. Am J Surg Pathol 19: 1409–1417.
19. Korenaga M, Wang T, Li Y, Showalter LA, Chan T, et al. (2005) Hepatitis C virus core protein inhibits mitochondrial electron transport and increases reactive oxygen species (ROS) production. J Biol Chem 280: 37481–37488.
20. Elbirt KK, Bonkovsky HL (1999) Heme oxygenase: recent advances in understanding its regulation and role. Proc Assoc Am Physicians 111: 438–447.
21. Takahashi T, Shimizu H, Morimatsu H, Inoue K, Akagi R, et al. (2007) Heme oxygenase-1: a fundamental guardian against oxidative tissue injuries in acute inflammation. Mini Rev Med Chem 7: 745–753.
22. Abdalla MY, Ahmad IM, Spitz DR, Schmidt WN, Britigan BE (2005) Hepatitis C virus-core and non structural proteins lead to different effects on cellular antioxidant defenses. J Med Virol 76: 489–497.
23. Abdalla MY, Britigan BE, Wen F, Icardi M, McCormick ML, et al. (2004) Down-regulation of heme oxygenase-1 by hepatitis C virus infection in vivo and by the in vitro expression of hepatitis C core protein. J Infect Dis 190: 1109–1118.
24. Hou WH, Rossi L, Shan Y, Zheng JY, Lambrecht RW, et al. (2009) Iron increases HMOX1 and decreases hepatitis C viral expression in HCV-expressing cells. World J Gastroenterol 15: 4499–4510.
25. Zhu Z, Wilson AT, Luxon BA, Brown KE, Mathahs MM, et al. (2010) Biliverdin inhibits hepatitis C virus nonstructural 3/4A protease activity: mechanism for the antiviral effects of heme oxygenase? Hepatology 52: 1897–1905.
26. Fillebeen C, Pantopoulos K (2010) Iron inhibits replication of infectious hepatitis C virus in permissive Huh7.5.1 cells. J Hepatol 53: 995–999.
27. Lehmann E, El-Tantawy WH, Ocker M, Bartenschlager R, Lohmann V, et al. (2010) The heme oxygenase 1 product biliverdin interferes with hepatitis C virus replication by increasing antiviral interferon response. Hepatology 51: 398–404.
28. Kakizaki S, Takagi H, Horiguchi N, Toyoda M, Takayama H, et al. (2000) Iron enhances hepatitis C virus replication in cultured human hepatocytes. Liver 20: 125–128.
29. Jopling CL, Norman KL, Sarnow P (2006) Positive and negative modulation of viral and cellular mRNAs by liver-specific microRNA miR-122. Cold Spring Harb Symp Quant Biol 71: 369–376.
30. Roberts AP, Lewis AP, Jopling CL (2011) miR-122 activates hepatitis C virus translation by a specialized mechanism requiring particular RNA components. Nucleic Acids Res 39: 7716–7729.
31. Pedersen IM, Cheng G, Wieland S, Volinia S, Croce CM, et al. (2007) Interferon modulation of cellular microRNAs as an antiviral mechanism. Nature 449: 919–922.
32. Devadas K, Dhawan S (2006) Hemin activation ameliorates HIV-1 infection via heme oxygenase-1 induction. J Immunol 176: 4252–4257.

A Novel Fibrosis Index Comprising a Non-Cholesterol Sterol Accurately Predicts HCV-Related Liver Cirrhosis

Magdalena Ydreborg[1], Vera Lisovskaja[2], Martin Lagging[1], Peer Brehm Christensen[3], Nina Langeland[4], Mads Rauning Buhl[5], Court Pedersen[3], Kristine Mørch[4], Rune Wejstål[1], Gunnar Norkrans[1], Magnus Lindh[1], Martti Färkkilä[6]❡, Johan Westin[1]*❡

1 Department of Infectious Diseases/Virology, Institute of Biomedicine, University of Gothenburg, Gothenburg, Sweden, **2** Department of Mathematical Sciences, Chalmers University of Technology and University of Gothenburg, Gothenburg, Sweden, **3** Department of Infectious Diseases, Odense University Hospital, Odense, Denmark, **4** Department of Clinical Science, University of Bergen, Bergen, Norway, **5** Department of Infectious Diseases, Aarhus University, Aarhus, Denmark, **6** Institute of Clinical Medicine, Department of Gastroenterology, Helsinki University, Helsinki, Finland

Abstract

Diagnosis of liver cirrhosis is essential in the management of chronic hepatitis C virus (HCV) infection. Liver biopsy is invasive and thus entails a risk of complications as well as a potential risk of sampling error. Therefore, non-invasive diagnostic tools are preferential. The aim of the present study was to create a model for accurate prediction of liver cirrhosis based on patient characteristics and biomarkers of liver fibrosis, including a panel of non-cholesterol sterols reflecting cholesterol synthesis and absorption and secretion. We evaluated variables with potential predictive significance for liver fibrosis in 278 patients originally included in a multicenter phase III treatment trial for chronic HCV infection. A stepwise multivariate logistic model selection was performed with liver cirrhosis, defined as Ishak fibrosis stage 5–6, as the outcome variable. A new index, referred to as Nordic Liver Index (NoLI) in the paper, was based on the model: Log-odds (predicting cirrhosis) = −12.17+ (age $\times$0.11) + (BMI (kg/m^2)$\times$0.23) + (D$_7$-lathosterol (μg/100 mg cholesterol)$\times$(−0.013)) + (Platelet count (x10^9/L)$\times$(−0.018)) + (Prothrombin-INR$\times$3.69). The area under the ROC curve (AUROC) for prediction of cirrhosis was 0.91 (95% CI 0.86–0.96). The index was validated in a separate cohort of 83 patients and the AUROC for this cohort was similar (0.90; 95% CI: 0.82–0.98). In conclusion, the new index may complement other methods in diagnosing cirrhosis in patients with chronic HCV infection.

Editor: Gulam Waris, Rosalind Franklin University of Medicine and Science, United States of America

Funding: ALF Funds at Sahlgrenska University Hospital and The Gothenburg Society of Medicine supported this study. Unrestricted grants from Roche affiliates in the Nordic region and MSD Sweden also supported this study. The funders had no role in study design, data collection and analysis, decision to publish, or preparation of the manuscript.

* E-mail: johan.westin@gu.se

❡ These authors contributed equally to this work.

Introduction

Morbidity and mortality in Hepatitis C virus (HCV) infection results mainly from the development of complications of cirrhosis, or hepatocellular carcinoma (HCC) [1]. Thus, the assessment of liver fibrosis is of pivotal importance. Although the development of new, highly efficacious treatment regimens will likely lessen the significance of fibrosis staging for prognostication of treatment outcome, it may remain central for tailoring of choice and duration of therapy. Additionally, the diagnosis of cirrhosis will continue to be vital to establish the need for HCC surveillance.

Liver biopsy remains the gold standard for the assessment of liver fibrosis [2]. However, due to the potential risk of complications [3] as well as other limitations, e.g. the risk of sampling error and inter-observer variability [4,5] associated with liver biopsy, several non-invasive methods for fibrosis assessment previously have been proposed. Studies evaluating potential serum biomarkers of fibrosis have been reported, either alone or combined in indices [6–16]. Transient elastography has been thoroughly evaluated among HCV infected patients [17–20] with a high diagnostic accuracy for cirrhosis [21] but it may often be difficult to obtain a valid examination, especially in obese patients. In recent years algorithms combining different non-invasive methods has improved the diagnostic accuracy for staging of fibrosis [22,23]. For identification of cirrhosis, transient elastography appears to be the most accurate method when compared with currently available biomarkers [14,21], but a freely available biochemical index that could complement to liver elastography measurement for the diagnosis of cirrhosis is desirable.

Cholesterol synthesis is a process involving several steps. Lathosterol and desmosterol are intermediates in the cholesterol synthesis pathway and their serum concentration reflects cholesterol synthesis ([24,25]. Sitosterol, avenasterol and campesterol are plant sterols (phytosterols) derived from ingested food reflecting intestinal absorption, while cholestanol is produced by enzymatic cleavage of endogenous cholesterol. Cholestanol as well as plant sterols reflects biliary secretion, and cholestanol is a marker of chronic cholestasis [26,27]. In line with this, plasma levels of non-

Table 1. Baseline characteristics in the (A) exploratory set and (B) the validation set according to presence of cirrhosis in liver biopsy.

A. Exploratory set	**Cirrhosis**	**Non cirrhosis**	**P value**
	n = 36	**n = 242**	
Sex female/male (%)	28/72	42/58	n.s
Age (years)	51(46–56)	41 (32–49)	<0.0001
BMI (kg/m$^{2)}$	27 (24–32)	25 (22–28)	0.001
Duration of infection (years)	28.5 (20–35)[a]	11 (6–23)[b]	<0.0001
AST (/ULN)	2.05 (1.53–3.34)	1.23 (0.89–1.94)	<0.0001
ALT (/ULN)	2.32 (1.45–2.83)	1.43 (0.82–2.37)	0.001
Platelet count (10^9/L)	150 (97–206)	227 (196–266)	<0.0001
Prothrombin index INR	1.1 (1.0–1.2)	1.0 (1.0–1.1)	<0.0001
D7-lathosterol (μg/100 mg cholesterol)	97 (57–127)	118 (87–150)	0.008
Genotype 2/3	33/67	30/70	n.s
Ishak fibrosis stage 0/1/2/3/4 (%)		4/17/35/28/16	NA
Ishak fibrosis stage 5/6 (%)	42/58		NA
B. Validation set	**n = 8**	**n = 75**	
Sex female/male (%)	25/75	48/52	n.s
Age (years)	52(44–64)	51(44–55)	n.s
BMI (kg/m2)	27 (25–29)	25(23–28)	n.s
Duration of infection (years)	30(26–40)[c]	30(24–34)[d]	n.s
AST (/ULN)	2.0(1.8– 3.0)	1.1 (0.9–1.8)	0.003
ALT (/ULN)	2.1(1.7–3.6)	1.1 (0.9–1.6)	0.001
Platelets (10^9/L)	141(109–213)	256(201–299)	0.001
Prothrombin-INR	1.1(1.0–1.2)	1.0(1.0–1.1)	0.02
D7-lathosterol (μg/100 mg cholesterol)	77(47–117)	117(85–155)	0.02
HCV genotype 1/2/3/4/mixed (%)	75/0/12.5/0/12.5	73/1/24/1/1	n.s
Ishak fibrosis stage 0/1/2/3/4 (%)		5/21/40/19/15	NA
Ishak fibrosis stage 5/6 (%)	38/62		NA

All values are presented as median (interquartile range; IQR) or percentage.
[a]n = 28.
[b]n = 166.
[c]n = 6.
[d]n = 60.

cholesterol sterols have been associated with either chronic cholestasis or hepatocyte function, particularly in the setting of primary biliary cirrhosis (PBC) [28]. Thus, it may be hypothesized that concentrations of such non-cholesterol sterols potentially could serve as biomarkers of disease progression, also in the presence of HCV infection.

The aim of the present study thus was to evaluate a broad range of non-invasive biomarkers for liver fibrosis, including a panel of non-cholesterol sterols (cholestanol, desmosterol, lathosterol, sitosterol and campesterol) in order to create a predictive model for HCV-related cirrhosis. This was done within the framework of a phase III treatment trial, with a well-defined cohort of treatment-naïve patients and where pre-treatment liver biopsies were mandatory.

Materials and Methods

Exploratory Set

The exploratory set cohort was derived from a phase III multicenter, investigator initiated, treatment trial for treatment-naïve HCV genotype 2 or 3 infected patients (the NORDynamIC study, n = 382) conducted at 31 centers in Denmark, Finland, Norway and Sweden. Details regarding trial design and outcome have been published previously [29]. The main outcome of the trial was sustained viral response. Evaluation of biomarkers for non-invasive diagnosis of cirrhosis was included among the secondary aims of the trial in the study protocol. All patients included were adults with detectable plasma HCV-RNA of genotype 2 or 3 had compensated liver disease and were seronegative for hepatitis B surface antigen and for antibodies to human immunodeficiency virus (HIV). A liver biopsy within 24 months of entry was required. Body Mass Index (BMI kg/m^2), alcohol consumption during the previous year (g/week) and duration of infection were recorded. Of the 382 patients enrolled, 298 patients had a liver biopsy that fulfilled the criteria for staging and grading and had serum samples analyzed for potential fibrosis markers in accordance with the study protocol. When all patients with missing data in any of the parameters were excluded 278 patients remained. These patients constituted the exploratory set.

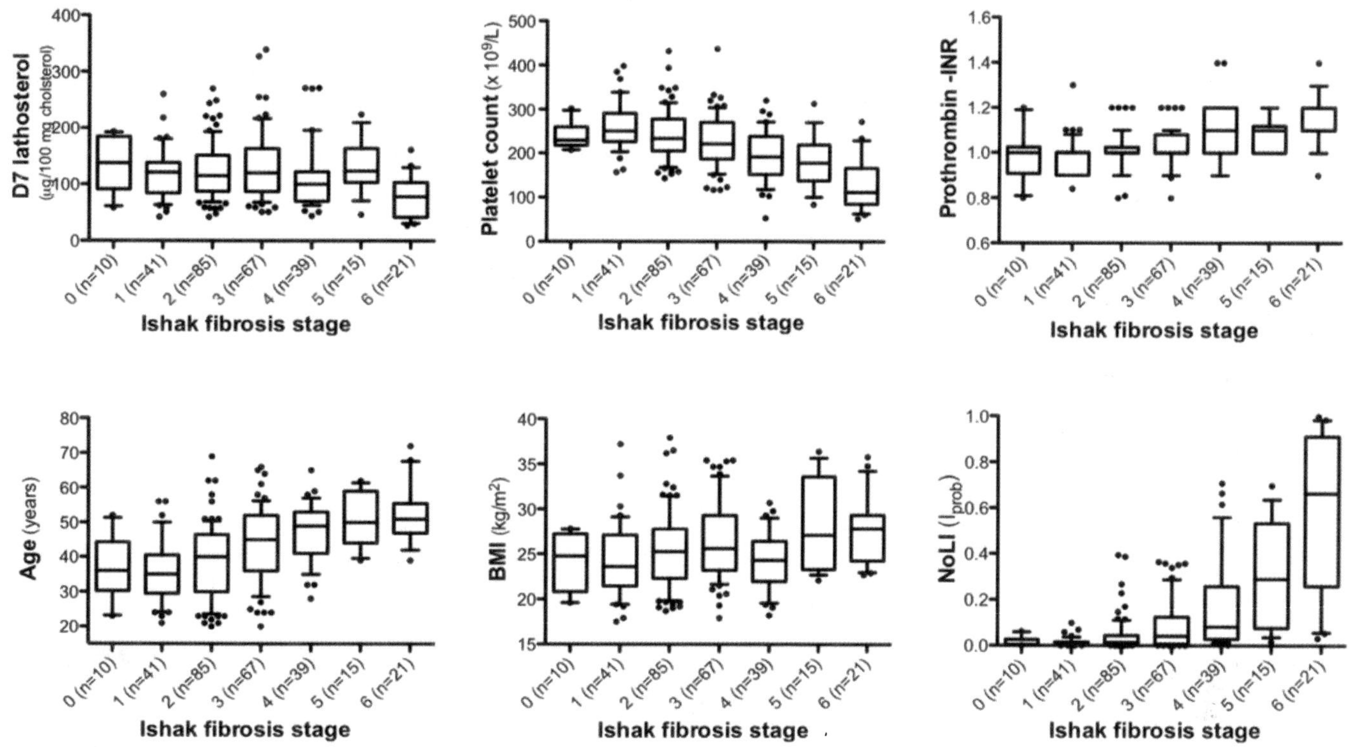

Figure 1. Box-plots displaying the different components of the NoLI index (D_7 lathosterol, platelet count, Prothrombin complex-INR, age and BMI) and the NoLI index in relation to Ishak fibrosis stage.

Validation Set

The validation set was derived from a cohort of 100 chronic HCV infected patients enrolled in a study evaluating the use of liver biopsy, serum fibrosis markers and transient elastography by use of the Fibroscan device [30], performed at the Department of Infectious Diseases at Sahlgrenska University Hospital in Gothenburg in 2008–2010. All consecutive patients referred for a liver biopsy during an eighteen months period were asked to participate. Blood tests for analysis of serum fibrosis markers, transient elastography examination and liver biopsy were performed in the fasting state at the same day. All patients included were HCV-RNA positive, HBsAg negative and anti-HIV negative adults and had signed an informed consent.

Patients with missing data for any of the relevant parameters were excluded from the present study, leaving 83 patients in the validation set.

Ethical Considerations

Exploratory set. Written informed consent was obtained from each participating patient. Ethics committees in each participating country approved the study (i.e. Regional Ethical Review Board, Gothenburg, Sweden (Regionala etikprövningsnämnden i Göteborg), Regional Committee for Ethics in Medical Research, Bergen, Norway (Regionaletisk komite for medisinsk og helsefaglig forskning i Bergen), The Scientific Ethical Committee for the Region of Middle Jutland, Viborg, Denmark (Den Videnskabsetiske Komité for Region Midtjylland), The Scientific Ethical Committee for the Region of South Denmark, Vejle, Denmark (Den Videnskabsetiske Komité for Region Syddanmark), and the Ethics Committee, Department of Medicine for the Hospital District of Helsinki and Uusimaa, Finland (Etiska kommittén för invärtesmedicin)). The study has been registered at the NIH trial registry (ClinicalTrials.gov Identifier: NCT00143000).

Validation set. Written informed consent was obtained from each participating patient. The Regional Ethical Review Board, Gothenburg, Sweden (Regionala etikprövningsnämnden i Göteborg) approved the study.

Serum Markers

In the exploratory cohort, baseline serum samples were drawn within 30 days prior to study entrance. Platelet count (x 10^9/L) and Prothrombin complex-INR were analyzed at each center. All other serum samples were stored in -70°C and subsequently analyzed at a central laboratory at Helsinki University Hospital, Finland. Liver function tests and serum fibrosis markers analyzed by standard laboratory methods included normalized AST and ALT, Gammaglutamyl-transferase (GGT) (U/L), Bilirubin (μmol/L), Haptoglobin (g/L), alfa2-macroglobulin (g/L), Hyaluronic acid (HA) (ng/ml), amino-terminal propeptide of type III procollagen (PIIINP) (ug/L), Apolipoprotein A1 (g/L) and carboxy-terminal telopeptide of type I collagen (ICTP) and serum cholesterol (mg/100 ml). The non-cholesterol sterols (cholestanol, D8-lathosterol, desmosterol, D7-lathosterol, campesterol, sitosterol, sitostanol, avenasterol and squalene) were analyzed by gas–liquid chromatography (GLC) (Agilent 6890N Network GC System, Agilent Technologies Inc., Wilmington, DE) on a 50-m long Ultra 2 capillary column (5% Phenyl-methyl siloxane) (Agilent Technologies, Wilmington, DE, USA), with 5a-cholestane as internal standard [31,32].

To correct for differences in serum levels of sterols as a consequence of varying concentrations of lipoprotein particles, the non-cholesterol sterol values are expressed as proportions of serum

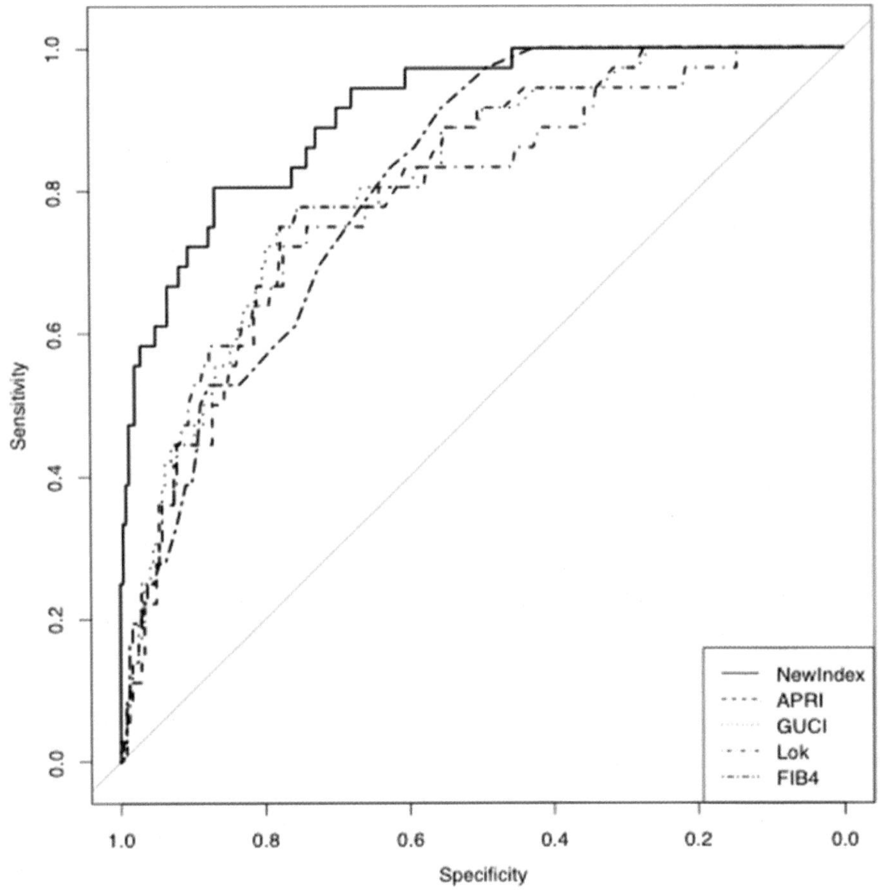

Figure 2. Receiver operator characteristics curves plotting sensitivity against specificity for prediction of cirrhosis in the exploratory set (n = 278) for the new index (NoLI) in comparison with some other biochemical indices. The AUROC for NoLI was 0.91 (95% CI 0.86–0.96). The corresponding AUROC for the other indices in the exploratory set were for FIB4 0.81 (95% CI 0.75–0.87), Lok 0.79 (95% CI 0.71–0.87), APRI 0.81 (95% CI 0.74–0.88), and for GUCI 0.81 (95% CI 0.74–0.88).

cholesterol (µg/100 mg of cholesterol) as well as absolute concentrations (µg/100 ml).

In the validation set all serum samples were drawn the same day as the liver biopsy and immediately stored in −70°C. Serum sterols were subsequently analyzed as stated above, all other analyzes were performed according to routine laboratory procedures at the Sahlgrenska University Hospital.

Histological Assessment

All liver biopsies in the exploratory and validation cohort were retrieved and re-assessed for necroinflammatory activity and fibrosis stage according to the Ishak protocol [33] by two experienced observers in a dual observer consensus fashion as previously described [29] where the two observers first independently scored all biopsies. Potential topics of disagreement were discussed, and a consensus score was agreed upon, which then was used in the analysis. Steatosis was graded as absent (score of 0), mild (score of 1, <30% of the hepatocytes involved), moderate (score of 2, 30–70%) or severe (score of 3, >70%) [34]. Biopsies with a total length of <15 mm or containing less than six portal tracts were excluded. Cirrhosis was defined as Ishak fibrosis stage 5–6.

Statistical Analysis

The following variables were analyzed in the exploratory set: age, sex, weight, BMI, genotype, platelets, PK-INR, normalized

Table 2. Diagnostic accuracy for the proposed cut-off levels regarding the NoLI score for prediction of cirrhosis in 278 HCV-infected patients.

Cut-off	Sensitivity (%)	Specificity (%)	+LR	−LR	NPV (%)	PPV (%)
0.054	94(81–99)	68(62–74)	2.9(2.4–3.6)	0.08(0.02–0.32)	99(96–100)	30(22–40)
0.37	58(41–75)	95(92–97)	10.9(6.0–19.7)	0.44(0.30–0.65)	94(90–97)	62(44–78)

Abbreviations: +LR, positive likelihood ration; −LR, negative likelihood ratio; NPV, negative predictive value; PPV, positive predictive value. All values are presented with 95% confidence interval.

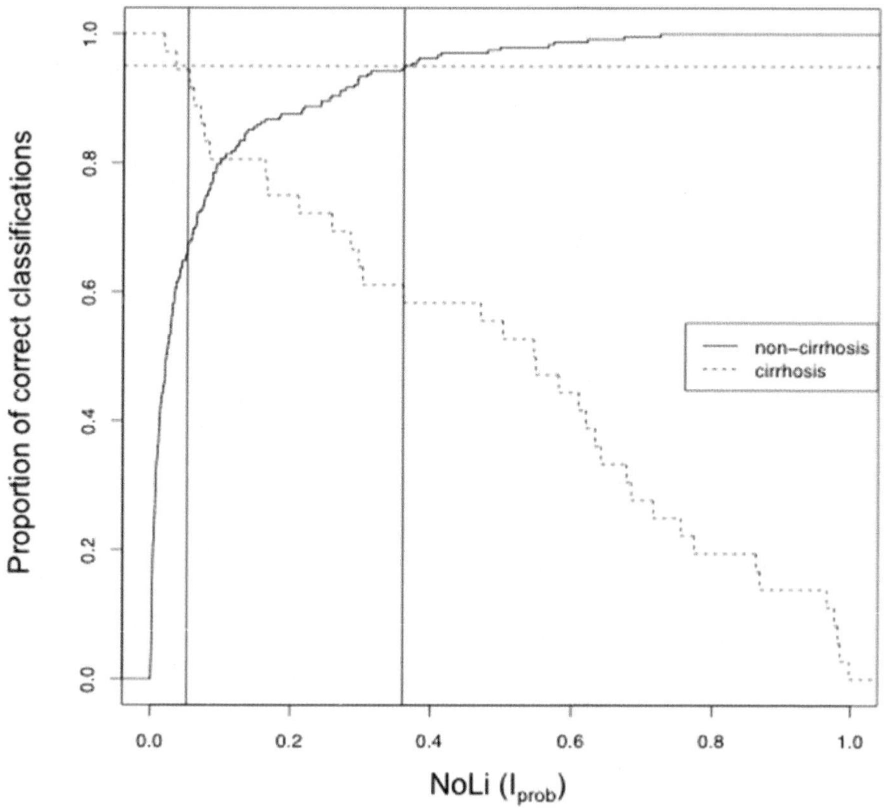

Figure 3. Proportion of correct classifications (i.e. non-cirrhotic classified as non-cirrhotic and cirrhotic classified as cirrhotic) according to different cut-off levels for NoLI. The solid vertical lines represent the chosen cut-offs 0.054 and 0.37. Using these cut-offs, the misclassification error would be approximately 5% for cirrhotic as well as non-cirrhotic patients, respectively (dotted horizontal line).

AST and ALT, GGT, Bilirubin, Haptoglobin, alfa2-macroglobulin, HA, PIIINP, Apolipoprotein A1, ICTP, total cholesterol, cholestanol, D8-lathosterol, desmosterol, D7-lathosterol, campesterol, sitosterol, sitostanol, avenasterol and squalene. Classification was made in two groups that encompassed fibrosis stages 0–4 (n = 242) and 5–6 (n = 36), respectively. The suggested classification procedure consisted of two steps: (i) an index that resulted from fitting of a model to the data and (ii) cut-off values for this index that can be used to divide the predictions into two groups.

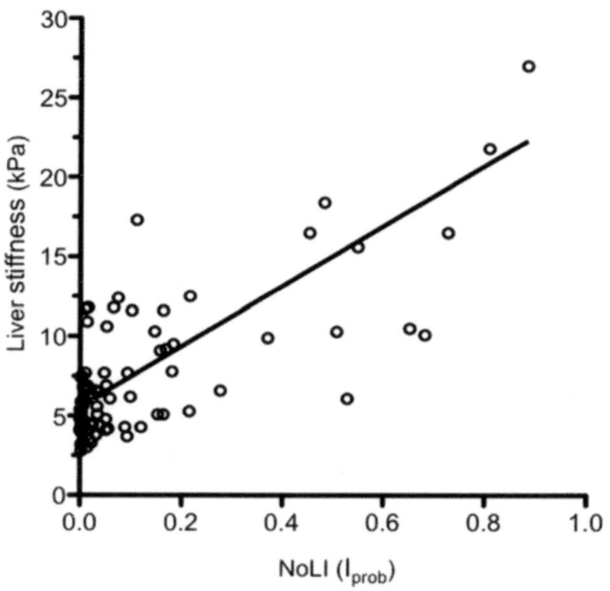

Figure 4. Scatter plot comparing the New index (NoLI) with liver stiffness measured by transient elastography. The Spearman correlation coefficient was 0.542 ($p<0.001$).

The data was modeled through logistic regression, with model selection based on Akaike information criterion (AIC). The model selection was done using goodness-of-fit criteria rather than the magnitude of the p-values for each variable. The large number of sometimes highly correlated factors leads to over fitting, i.e. a model that was too large and sensitive to small perturbations in the data. We decided to make the process of model selection more robust by constructing logistic regression for a large number of re-samples of the data and taking only those factors in the final index that appeared in many of these, re-sampled models. The final estimation of the coefficients was performed using the original dataset. The new index based on the model above can be formulated either in terms of probabilities (I_{prob}) or log-odds (I_{odds}), which are equivalent. I_{odds} uses a more natural scale while I_{prob} may be perceived as more intuitive since it reflects the probability that a certain patient has cirrhosis. I_{prob} was chosen for further calculations, hereafter referred to as the Nordic Liver Index, NoLI. Cutoff values were chosen in order to minimize the misclassification error. Rather than choosing one cut-off, we suggest applying two, C_{low} and C_{high}. If the index is below C_{low}, the observation will be classified into group 1. If it is above C_{high} it will be classified as group 2. If between C_{low} and C_{high} it will not be classified as either group and further investigations may have to be undertaken to make a correct diagnosis.

Diagnostic performance was analyzed by constructing receiver operator characteristics curves (ROC) for specificity and sensitivity with calculation of the area under the ROC curve (AUROC) and the corresponding confidence interval (CI). The R software package (Free software; www.r-project.org) version 2.15.0 was used for all calculations and the package pROC was used to calculate ROC curves and the corresponding CI. Comparisons of baseline characteristics between groups were analyzed by Mann-Whitney's U test or Chi-squared test where appropriate. Correlation between transient elastography and NoLI was assessed by Spearman's r test. These latter analyses were performed using IBM SPSS Statistics version 19.0 software package (IBM Corporation, Somers, NY). All reported p-values are two-sided, and p-values <0.05 were considered significant.

Results

Baseline Characteristics

Of the 278 patients included in the exploratory set, 36 (13%) had cirrhosis; baseline characteristics for cirrhotic and non-cirrhotic patients in the exploratory set are reported in Table 1A. Of the 83 patients included in the validation set, 8 (10%) had cirrhosis. Baseline characteristics are displayed in Table 1B.

There were no patients with clinically decompensated liver cirrhosis in either exploratory or validation set. Patients in the validation set were older than patients in the exploratory set; median age was 49 (IQR 44–55) vs. 42 years (IQR 34–50) (p< 0.001), and had a longer duration of infection; 29 (IQR 24–34) vs. 13.5 years (IQR 6,8–25) (p<0.001) in the validation and exploratory set respectively. In the exploratory set, 69% of the patients were infected with HCV genotype 3, whereas in the validation set HCV genotype 1 was most frequent, present in 72% of patients.

Model for Prediction of Fibrosis

Application of the model selection methodology described earlier lead to a final model comprising the following variables: Age ($p = 0.0002$), BMI ($p = 8.0 \times 10^{-5}$), D_7-lathosterol ($p = 0.02$), platelet count ($p = 7.0 \times 10^{-5}$) and Prothrombin-INR ($p = 0.122$). The model characteristics are summarized in table S1 and the relation between each component of the index separately and Ishak fibrosis stage is displayed in Figure 1. D7 lathosterol, was the only sterol in the panel of sterols, which was independently associated with cirrhosis.

The regression formula for this final model is: Log-odds; I_{odds} (predicting cirrhosis) $= -12.17 +$ (age $\times 0.11$) $+$ (BMI (kg/m^2)$\times 0.23$) $+$ (D_7-lathosterol (μg/100 mg cholesterol)$\times(-0.013)$) $+$ (Platelet count (x10^9/L)$\times(-0.018)$) $+$ (Prothrombin-INR$\times 3.69$).

Predicted probability; $I_{prob} = \exp(\text{log-odds})/(1+\exp(\text{log-odds}))$.

As stated above, we chose predicted probability (I_{prob}) for further calculations, referred to as the Nordic Liver Index (NoLI). The relation between NoLI and Ishak fibrosis stage is illustrated in the lower right panel of Figure 1.

Area Under ROC (AUROC)

The ROC curve formed by plotting sensitivity against specificity for the new index in prediction of cirrhosis in the exploratory set is shown in Figure 2. The area under the ROC curve (AUROC) was 0.91 (95% CI 0.86–0.96). Figure 2 also displays ROC curves for APRI [11], Lok index [10], GUCI [15] and FIB-4 [16]. Theses indices were chosen for comparison since they are all freely available non-invasive scores, evaluated and validated for the detection of cirrhosis. The corresponding AUROC for the other indices in the exploratory set were for FIB-4 0.81 (95% CI 0.75–0.87), Lok index 0.79 (95% CI 0.71–0.87), APRI 0.81 (95% CI 0.74–0.88), and for GUCI 0.81 (95% CI 0.74–0.88).

Cutoff Values

Two cut-off values were chosen that would produce a minimal misclassification error of approximately 5% for each group. Using a predicted cut-off value of <0.053 for the exclusion of cirrhosis and >0.37 for the identification of cirrhosis would misclassify 5.6% (2/36) of patients with cirrhosis as non-cirrhotic and 5.0% (12/242) of non-cirrhotic as having cirrhosis (with a cirrhosis prevalence of 13%, a misclassification rate of 5.6% is the closest to 5% we can get). Figure 3 shows the proportion of correct classifications for cirrhosis and non-cirrhosis according to different cut-offs. The sensitivity, specificity, likelihood ratios and negative and positive predictive values for the proposed cut-offs (0.053 and 0.37) are displayed in table 2. Among the 12 patients misclassified as having cirrhosis, the Ishak fibrosis stages were distributed as follows; F4 n = 7 (58%), F3 n = 3 (25%) and F2 n = 2 (17%). HCV genotypes 2 and 3 were evenly distributed.

Validation Set

Applying the new index to the validation set, the AUROC for prediction of cirrhosis was 0.90 (95% CI 0.83–0.98). In the validation set, patients were also examined by transient elastography. The Spearman correlation coefficient for the new index and liver stiffness values was 0.54 (p<0.001; Figure 4). One patient (a 66 year-old genotype-1-infected male with compensated cirrhosis and mild steatosis) with a liver stiffness value of 50 kPa was included in the calculation but not in the figure. To evaluate the diagnostic capability of the new index using transient elastography as reference, we used a cut-off of 12.5 kPa for cirrhosis [17]. The resulting Roc-curve had an AUROC for prediction of cirrhosis of 0.95 (95% CI 0.89–1.0).

Since the exploratory set included only patients infected with HCV genotypes 2 and 3 and the validation set mainly genotype 1 infected patients, we combined the exploratory and validation set to evaluate potential genotypic differences. No significant differences were detected and the AUROC for specificity vs. sensitivity for each genotype was 0.91 (95% CI 0.82–1.0), 0.86 (95% CI 0.73–0.98) and 0.93 (95% CI 0.88–0.97) for genotypes 1, 2, and 3 respectively.

Discussion

The primary aim of this study was to develop a reliable model for predicting HCV-related liver cirrhosis. The model created could confidently predict cirrhosis in both the exploratory and the validation sets, although the findings need to be confirmed in larger series. Although there is considerable overlap between adjacent fibrosis stages, this model has a good ability to exclude cirrhosis in patients with less severe stages of fibrosis (Ishak F0-4) as well as to predict cirrhosis in biopsy-verified cirrhotic patients (Ishak F5-6). Like many other biochemical indices, NoLI performs better in excluding than confirming cirrhosis.

The new index combines age, BMI, platelet count and prothrombin index, i.e. factors that previously have been consistently associated with fibrosis [6,9–11,35], along with D7-lathosterol which, to our knowledge, has not previously been evaluated in this setting. Serum D7-lathosterol is a precursor of cholesterol and its plasma concentration reflects cholesterol synthesis and correlates with 5-alfa-HMG-reductase activity, the rate-limiting enzyme of cholesterol synthesis [24,25]. With the development of liver cirrhosis, the synthetic function in the liver, including cholesterol synthesis, decreases [36]. Thus, it is plausible that the concentration of D7-lathosterol in serum would reflect liver function and that decreased levels of lathosterol could be an early sign of advanced liver fibrosis. On the other hand, the sterols primarily reflecting cholestasis did not predict cirrhosis in this setting, which is not surprising since cholestasis is not a common feature in HCV-related cirrhosis. Accordingly, none of the cirrhotics in any of the sets cohorts had elevated serum-bilirubin levels indicating cholestasis. The hepatitis C virus is known to interfere with host lipid metabolism resulting in reduced levels of s-cholesterol and hepatic steatosis [37] that resolves following successful antiviral treatment, at least in genotype 3 infected patients [38,39]. In non-genotype 3 patients, however, steatosis has been associated with insulin resistance and the metabolic syndrome [40,41]. In a recent study, Clark et al [42] demonstrated that HCV genotype 3, but not genotype 2, interferes with the distal cholesterol pathway, which resolves after successful antiviral treatment. In the same study, no significant differences in the levels of lathosterol was found between genotype 2 and 3 infected patients suggesting that this genotype-specific interaction occurs further down in the pathway. The evaluation of NoLI index according to HCV genotype in the present study showed no statistically significant differences regarding AUROC between genotypes and the level of serum lathosterol does not seem to be genotype-dependent in this setting.

Several studies on the prediction of cirrhosis have been reported during the past 10 years [7,10–13,15,16,43–45]. In a large multicenter study by Degos et al [14] evaluating the diagnostic accuracy of Fibroscan and FibroMeter, FibroTest, APRI and Hepascore for the prediction of cirrhosis, AUROC ranged from 0.77 to 0.86. FibroMeter [7], FibroTest [14] and Hepascore [12] are all validated and frequently used for the prediction of cirrhosis but they are all protected by patented formula making them less accessible. The AST-to-platelet ratio index (APRI) [11] as well as the Lok-index [10] and FIB-4 [16] are all free of cost and based on routine laboratory parameters making them easy to use in routine clinical practice. When compared in the exploratory set, our model performed slightly superior to these other non-patented scores. Unfortunately, the size of and cirrhosis prevalence in the validation set did not allow for in-depth comparison.

Our study had some potential limitations. Measurement of serum lathosterol is not a standard biochemical test. Although it is measured using gas-chromatography standard patent-free laboratory technique, commonly used for analysis of other compounds, it may be slightly cumbersome to use. Still, the presence of D7-lathosterol improves the diagnostic performance of the NoLI index why we choose to keep it in the model.

The prevalence of cirrhosis in the exploratory and validation sets was 13% and 10% respectively, which is low compared with some other studies on non-invasive fibrosis markers using liver biopsy as reference [10,21]. This lessens the ability to create a solid model for prediction. However, a cirrhosis prevalence of around 15% seems to be common in unselected Hepatitis C populations [14,46]. The limited sample size and the low prevalence of cirrhosis in the validation set is a major limitation and does not permit accurate comparison between different indices, and the diagnostic performance of the new index need to be tested also in other larger cohorts. Moreover, other studies of fibrosis markers have been validated in cohorts of similar size, e.g. AST to platelet ratio index (APRI), a very reliable and widespread fibrosis index, was created in an exploratory set of 192 patients (15 (16%) cirrhotics) and validated in a cohort of 78 subjects (13 (17%) cirrhotics) [11]. The patients in the validation set were recruited from a group of consecutive patients referred for routine liver biopsy and were thus potential candidates for non-invasive fibrosis assessment in clinical practice. The patients in the exploratory and validation sets differed regarding HCV genotypes as well as country of residency, although none of these factors were independently associated with cirrhosis when patients in the two sets were analyzed together (cirrhosis was more common in Sweden and Denmark which was due to an age effect, data not shown). Thus they would not have influenced the statistical model.

In the exploratory set, liver biopsies and serum samples were not taken at the same time point, although both were sampled prior to initiation of therapy. The index, however, performed well in the validation set where blood samples were drawn on the day of the liver biopsy. As with all non-invasive tests, the use of liver biopsy as comparison poses a problem since liver biopsy is prone to sampling error and thus can both over- and underestimate the true liver fibrosis stage [4]. As shown by Bedossa et al only 65% of biopsies relying on 15-mm samples led to correct diagnosis using METAVIR scoring system [5]. Hence, the absolute correctness of a non-invasive fibrosis marker would need to be estimated by use of other methods. Potential exclusion of cirrhotic patients due to a greater tendency towards inadequate biopsy size may have introduced a bias in the exploratory set. However, contrary to this notion, non-invasive markers (GUCI and APRI) did not differ significantly among excluded ($n = 27$) vs. included patients ($p = 0.3$). Although not the primary aim of this study, it is still interesting to note that the concordance of this index with Transient Elastography might be greater than with liver biopsy (AUC 0.95 (95% CI 0.89–1,0) vs. 0.90 (95% CI 0.83–0.98). Another perhaps more appropriate endpoint to use as gold standard would be the risk of liver related complications or death over time but that would be beyond the scope of the present study. A liver biopsy can provide much more pertinent information than serologic fibrosis markers on liver histology and may remain of importance in some cases in the future. However, we believe that serologic markers should be considered an important complement to liver biopsy.

In summary, our results indicate that an index combining well-known predictors of liver fibrosis in combination with measurement of a non-cholesterol sterol can be useful in predicting cirrhosis. These new findings could be of value as a supplement to already existing non-invasive methods and the application of our model potentially could aid clinical decision-making, e.g. on which patients require continued monitoring in spite of successful antiviral treatment.

Acknowledgments

We thank Professor Olle Nerman for statistical advice and Leena Kaipiainen, Lena Johansson, Helen Christiansen, Pia Paghold, Anna Rosnäs and Eva Karlsson for expert technical assistance.

Author Contributions

Conceived and designed the experiments: MY VL MF M. Lagging JW. Performed the experiments: MY VL MF M. Lagging JW. Analyzed the data: MY VL M. Lagging JW. Wrote the paper: MY VL M. Lagging PBC NL MRB CP KM RW GN M. Lindh MF JW. Design and performance of original treatment trial and patient management: M. Lagging PBC NL MRB CP KM RW GN M. Lindh MF.

References

1. Fattovich G, Giustina G, Degos F, Tremolada F, Diodati G, et al. (1997) Morbidity and mortality in compensated cirrhosis type C: a retrospective follow-up study of 384 patients. Gastroenterology 112: 463–472.
2. (2011) EASL Clinical Practice Guidelines: management of hepatitis C virus infection. J Hepatol 55: 245–264.
3. Perrault J, McGill DB, Ott BJ, Taylor WF (1978) Liver biopsy: complications in 1000 inpatients and outpatients. Gastroenterology 74: 103–106.
4. (1994) Intraobserver and interobserver variations in liver biopsy interpretation in patients with chronic hepatitis C. The French METAVIR Cooperative Study Group. Hepatology 20: 15–20.
5. Bedossa P, Dargere D, Paradis V (2003) Sampling variability of liver fibrosis in chronic hepatitis C. Hepatology 38: 1449–1457.
6. Pohl A, Behling C, Oliver D, Kilani M, Monson P, et al. (2001) Serum aminotransferase levels and platelet counts as predictors of degree of fibrosis in chronic hepatitis C virus infection. Am J Gastroenterol 96: 3142–3146.
7. Cales P, Oberti F, Michalak S, Hubert-Fouchard I, Rousselet MC, et al. (2005) A novel panel of blood markers to assess the degree of liver fibrosis. Hepatology 42: 1373–1381.
8. Fontana RJ, Goodman ZD, Dienstag JL, Bonkovsky HL, Naishadham D, et al. (2008) Relationship of serum fibrosis markers with liver fibrosis stage and collagen content in patients with advanced chronic hepatitis C. Hepatology 47: 789–798.
9. Poynard T, Bedossa P (1997) Age and platelet count: a simple index for predicting the presence of histological lesions in patients with antibodies to hepatitis C virus. METAVIR and CLINIVIR Cooperative Study Groups. J Viral Hepat 4: 199–208.
10. Lok AS, Ghany MG, Goodman ZD, Wright EC, Everson GT, et al. (2005) Predicting cirrhosis in patients with hepatitis C based on standard laboratory tests: results of the HALT-C cohort. Hepatology 42: 282–292.
11. Wai CT, Greenson JK, Fontana RJ, Kalbfleisch JD, Marrero JA, et al. (2003) A simple noninvasive index can predict both significant fibrosis and cirrhosis in patients with chronic hepatitis C. Hepatology 38: 518–526.
12. Adams LA, Bulsara M, Rossi E, DeBoer B, Speers D, et al. (2005) Hepascore: an accurate validated predictor of liver fibrosis in chronic hepatitis C infection. Clin Chem 51: 1867–1873.
13. Rosenberg WM, Voelker M, Thiel R, Becka M, Burt A, et al. (2004) Serum markers detect the presence of liver fibrosis: a cohort study. Gastroenterology 127: 1704–1713.
14. Degos F, Perez P, Roche B, Mahmoudi A, Asselineau J, et al. (2010) Diagnostic accuracy of FibroScan and comparison to liver fibrosis biomarkers in chronic viral hepatitis: a multicenter prospective study (the FIBROSTIC study). J Hepatol 53: 1013–1021.
15. Islam S, Antonsson L, Westin J, Lagging M (2005) Cirrhosis in hepatitis C virus-infected patients can be excluded using an index of standard biochemical serum markers. Scand J Gastroenterol 40: 867–872.
16. Vallet-Pichard A, Mallet V, Nalpas B, Verkarre V, Nalpas A, et al. (2007) FIB-4: an inexpensive and accurate marker of fibrosis in HCV infection. comparison with liver biopsy and fibrotest. Hepatology 46: 32–36.
17. Castera L, Forns X, Alberti A (2008) Non-invasive evaluation of liver fibrosis using transient elastography. J Hepatol 48: 835–847.
18. Ganne-Carrie N, Ziol M, de Ledinghen V, Douvin C, Marcellin P, et al. (2006) Accuracy of liver stiffness measurement for the diagnosis of cirrhosis in patients with chronic liver diseases. Hepatology 44: 1511–1517.
19. Ziol M, Handra-Luca A, Kettaneh A, Christidis C, Mal F, et al. (2005) Noninvasive assessment of liver fibrosis by measurement of stiffness in patients with chronic hepatitis C. Hepatology 41: 48–54.
20. Friedrich-Rust M, Ong MF, Martens S, Sarrazin C, Bojunga J, et al. (2008) Performance of transient elastography for the staging of liver fibrosis: a meta-analysis. Gastroenterology 134: 960–974.
21. Castera L, Le Bail B, Roudot-Thoraval F, Bernard PH, Foucher J, et al. (2009) Early detection in routine clinical practice of cirrhosis and oesophageal varices in chronic hepatitis C: comparison of transient elastography (FibroScan) with standard laboratory tests and non-invasive scores. J Hepatol 50: 59–68.
22. Boursier J, de Ledinghen V, Zarski JP, Rousselet MC, Sturm N, et al. (2011) A new combination of blood test and fibroscan for accurate non-invasive diagnosis of liver fibrosis stages in chronic hepatitis C. Am J Gastroenterol 106: 1255–1263.
23. Sebastiani G, Halfon P, Castera L, Pol S, Thomas DL, et al. (2009) SAFE biopsy: a validated method for large-scale staging of liver fibrosis in chronic hepatitis C. Hepatology 49: 1821–1827.
24. Bjorkhem I, Miettinen T, Reihner E, Ewerth S, Angelin B, et al. (1987) Correlation between serum levels of some cholesterol precursors and activity of HMG-CoA reductase in human liver. J Lipid Res 28: 1137–1143.
25. Miettinen TA, Tilvis RS, Kesaniemi YA (1990) Serum plant sterols and cholesterol precursors reflect cholesterol absorption and synthesis in volunteers of a randomly selected male population. Am J Epidemiol 131: 20–31.
26. Nikkila K, Hockerstedt K, Miettinen TA (1991) High cholestanol and low campesterol-to-sitosterol ratio in serum of patients with primary biliary cirrhosis before liver transplantation. Hepatology 13: 663–669.
27. Nikkila K, Hockerstedt K, Miettinen TA (1992) Serum and hepatic cholestanol, squalene and noncholesterol sterols in man: a study on liver transplantation. Hepatology 15: 863–870.
28. Nikkila K, Miettinen TA, Hockerstedt KV, Isoniemi H (2005) Sterol parameters as markers of liver function in primary biliary cirrhosis before and after liver transplantation. Transpl Int 18: 221–225.
29. Lagging M, Langeland N, Pedersen C, Farkkila M, Buhl MR, et al. (2008) Randomized comparison of 12 or 24 weeks of peginterferon alpha-2a and ribavirin in chronic hepatitis C virus genotype 2/3 infection. Hepatology 47: 1837–1845.
30. Sandrin L, Fourquet B, Hasquenoph JM, Yon S, Fournier C, et al. (2003) Transient elastography: a new noninvasive method for assessment of hepatic fibrosis. Ultrasound Med Biol 29: 1705–1713.
31. Miettinen TA (1988) Cholesterol metabolism during ketoconazole treatment in man. J Lipid Res 29: 43–51.
32. Gylling H, Hallikainen M, Simonen P, Miettinen HE, Nissinen MJ, et al. (2012) Serum and lipoprotein sitostanol and non-cholesterol sterols after an acute dose of plant stanol ester on its long-term consumption. Eur J Nutr 51: 615–622.
33. Ishak K, Baptista A, Bianchi L, Callea F, De Groote J, et al. (1995) Histological grading and staging of chronic hepatitis. J Hepatol 22: 696–699.
34. Westin J, Nordlinder H, Lagging M, Norkrans G, Wejstal R (2002) Steatosis accelerates fibrosis development over time in hepatitis C virus genotype 3 infected patients. J Hepatol 37: 837–842.
35. Adinolfi LE, Giordano MG, Andreana A, Tripodi MF, Utili R, et al. (2001) Hepatic fibrosis plays a central role in the pathogenesis of thrombocytopenia in patients with chronic viral hepatitis. Br J Haematol 113: 590–595.
36. Nikkila K, Nissinen MJ, Gylling H, Isoniemi H, Miettinen TA (2008) Serum sterols in patients with primary biliary cirrhosis and acute liver failure before and after liver transplantation. J Hepatol 49: 936–945.
37. Negro F (2010) Abnormalities of lipid metabolism in hepatitis C virus infection. Gut 59: 1279–1287.
38. Kumar D, Farrell GC, Fung C, George J (2002) Hepatitis C virus genotype 3 is cytopathic to hepatocytes: Reversal of hepatic steatosis after sustained therapeutic response. Hepatology 36: 1266–1272.
39. Poynard T, Ratziu V, McHutchison J, Manns M, Goodman Z, et al. (2003) Effect of treatment with peginterferon or interferon alfa-2b and ribavirin on steatosis in patients infected with hepatitis C. Hepatology 38: 75–85.
40. Cua IH, Hui JM, Kench JG, George J (2008) Genotype-specific interactions of insulin resistance, steatosis, and fibrosis in chronic hepatitis C. Hepatology 48: 723–731.
41. Camma C, Bruno S, Di Marco V, Di Bona D, Rumi M, et al. (2006) Insulin resistance is associated with steatosis in nondiabetic patients with genotype 1 chronic hepatitis C. Hepatology 43: 64–71.
42. Clark PJ, Thompson AJ, Vock DM, Kratz LE, Tolun AA, et al. (2012) Hepatitis C virus selectively perturbs the distal cholesterol synthesis pathway in a genotype-specific manner. Hepatology 56: 49–56.
43. Fontana RJ, Kleiner DE, Bilonick R, Terrault N, Afdhal N, et al. (2006) Modeling hepatic fibrosis in African American and Caucasian American patients with chronic hepatitis C virus infection. Hepatology 44: 925–935.
44. Imbert-Bismut F, Ratziu V, Pieroni L, Charlotte F, Benhamou Y, et al. (2001) Biochemical markers of liver fibrosis in patients with hepatitis C virus infection: a prospective study. Lancet 357: 1069–1075.
45. Parkes J, Guha IN, Roderick P, Harris S, Cross R, et al. (2011) Enhanced Liver Fibrosis (ELF) test accurately identifies liver fibrosis in patients with chronic hepatitis C. J Viral Hepat 18: 23–31.
46. Poynard T, Bedossa P, Opolon P (1997) Natural history of liver fibrosis progression in patients with chronic hepatitis C. The OBSVIRC, METAVIR, CLINIVIR, and DOSVIRC groups. Lancet 349: 825–832.

Q-FISH Measurement of Hepatocyte Telomere Lengths in Donor Liver and Graft after Pediatric Living-Donor Liver Transplantation: Donor Age Affects Telomere Length Sustainability

Youichi Kawano[1,2]*, Naoshi Ishikawa[2]*, Junko Aida[2], Yukihiro Sanada[3], Naotaka Izumiyama-Shimomura[2], Ken-ichi Nakamura[2], Steven S. S. Poon[4], Koshi Matsumoto[5], Koichi Mizuta[3], Eiji Uchida[1], Takashi Tajiri[1], Hideo Kawarasaki[3], Kaiyo Takubo[2]

1 Department of Surgery, Nippon Medical School, Tokyo, Japan, **2** Research Team for Geriatric Pathology, Tokyo Metropolitan Institute of Gerontology, Tokyo, Japan, **3** Department of Transplant Surgery, Jichi Medical University, Tochigi, Japan, **4** Terry Fox Laboratory, British Columbia Cancer Research Centre, Vancouver, British Columbia, Canada, **5** Department of Clinical Pathology, Ebina General Hospital, Kanagawa, Japan

Abstract

Along with the increasing need for living-donor liver transplantation (LDLT), the issue of organ shortage has become a serious problem. Therefore, the use of organs from elderly donors has been increasing. While the short-term results of LDLT have greatly improved, problems affecting the long-term outcome of transplant patients remain unsolved. Furthermore, since contradictory data have been reported with regard to the relationship between donor age and LT/LDLT outcome, the question of whether the use of elderly donors influences the long-term outcome of a graft after LT/LDLT remains unsettled. To address whether hepatocyte telomere length reflects the outcome of LDLT, we analyzed the telomere lengths of hepatocytes in informative biopsy samples from 12 paired donors and recipients (grafts) of pediatric LDLT more than 5 years after adult-to-child LDLT because of primary biliary atresia, using quantitative fluorescence *in situ* hybridization (Q-FISH). The telomere lengths in the paired samples showed a robust relationship between the donor and grafted hepatocytes ($r = 0.765$, $p = 0.0038$), demonstrating the feasibility of our Q-FISH method for cell-specific evaluation. While 8 pairs showed no significant difference between the telomere lengths for the donor and the recipient, the other 4 pairs showed significantly shorter telomeres in the recipient than in the donor. Multiple regression analysis revealed that the donors in the latter group were older than those in the former ($p = 0.001$). Despite the small number of subjects, this pilot study indicates that donor age is a crucial factor affecting telomere length sustainability in hepatocytes after pediatric LDLT, and that the telomeres in grafted livers may be elongated somewhat longer when the grafts are immunologically well controlled.

Editor: Gabriele Saretzki, University of Newcastle, United Kingdom

Funding: This work was supported by Japan Society for the Promotion of Science (JSPS) KAKENHI, 19790926 and 24592013 (to Y.K.), 24590468 (to N.I.). The funders had no role in study design, data collection and analysis, decision to publish, or preparation of the manuscript.

Competing Interests: The authors have declared that no competing interests exist.

* E-mail: y-kawano@nms.ac.jp (YK); naoshi@tmig.or.jp (NI)

Introduction

Liver transplantation (LT) has been carried out worldwide for patients with end-stage liver failure [1]. Since the supply of cadaveric liver grafts is far short of the number of patients awaiting transplantation, living-donor liver transplantation (LDLT) has emerged as a critical surgical option for the patients. Along with the increasing need for LDLT, the issue of organ shortage continues to extend worldwide and has become a serious problem. Therefore, the use of organs from marginal donors, such as the elderly, has been increasing [2]. The short-term results of LDLT have greatly improved because of advances in surgical techniques, antiviral therapy and, particularly, immunosuppressive regimens [3,4,5,6]. However, new problems, including recurrence of hepatitis C or hepatocellular carcinoma and development of *de novo* malignancies, have arisen as major problems affecting the long-term outcome of transplant patients [7]. Ensuring that a transplanted organ has a potentially sufficient working life remains one of the most important issues associated with LDLT [8,9,10]. In this context, a fundamental question has arisen concerning the senescence (aging process) of organs that are transplanted from elderly donors into young recipients. LDLT provides a unique and valuable means of answering this question, because it allows us to compare the characteristics of hepatocyte samples from an originally identical liver, part of which continues to be viable and functional in the donor, and another part that has functioned in a young recipient for a number of years after transplantation.

Human telomeric DNA is considered to protect chromosomes against degeneration, fusion, and loss [11]. In many human organs and tissues, including the liver [12,13], *in vivo* telomere shortening occurs with aging, and is accelerated by various environmental factors such as oxidative stress, chronic inflammation, social stress, alcohol, and transplantation [14,15,16,17,18,19,20]. The telomere hypothesis of cellular aging suggests that when telomere shortening reaches a critical level, a DNA damage checkpoint mechanism may be initiated and the cells stop dividing [21,22]. Therefore, measurement of telomere length is expected to provide information for evaluating the life span of a cell.

Since Lansdorp et al. devised the quantitative fluorescence *in situ* hybridization (Q-FISH) method [23], several studies of telomere length using various Q-FISH methods have been reported by different groups including us [16,24,25,26,18]. However there have been no reports of telomere length measurement in liver grafts after LDLT. We had an opportunity to study 12 pairs of samples obtained at the same time by needle biopsy from the donors and recipients more than after 5 years after LDLT. To address the question of whether telomere shortening is accelerated in the graft relative to the native liver remaining in the donor after pediatric LDLT, we used Q-FISH to measure the telomere length in hepatocytes.

Materials and Methods

Patients

We offered all of the LDLT patients (donors and recipients) being treated at our institution a chance to participate in this pilot study, and twelve pairs volunteered to take part. These twelve cases were considered suitable for our study protocol, which involved examination of a pair of liver biopsy specimens from both the donor and recipient after a follow-up period of more than 5 years after LDLT. No other selection criteria were adopted. These informative cases were obtained from among 134 recipients who had undergone LDLT at the Jichi Medical University Hospital between May 2001 and March 2009. The overall patient survival rate in our department was 95.0% (134/141). The ages, relationships (parent to child in all pairs) and post-LT survivals of the 12 pairs of donors and recipients are listed in Table 1. All of the patients examined in this study had end-stage biliary atresia, a condition that accounted for 73% of total LDLT operations performed at our hospital. Hepatocellular reserve capacity after Kasai portoenterostomy is usually evaluated in terms of the pediatric end-stage liver disease (PELD) score [27,28]. The PELD score is calculated on the basis of several objective values, the main components being age, growth failure (based on sex, height, and weight), albumin (g/dl), prothrombin time (international normalized ratio), and total bilirubin (mg/dl) (shown in Table S2).

The ethics committees of Jichi Medical University and Tokyo Metropolitan Institute of Gerontology approved the use of liver biopsy for this study. The participants provided written informed consent before each liver biopsy in accordance with the Declaration of Helsinki. Parental written permission was obtained when the patients were younger than 20 years old.

Surgical procedure and postoperative management

The surgical procedure (left side liver graft) and postoperative management (immunosuppression started using tacrolimus and steroid) for LDLT were basically the same as described previously [29]. The immunosuppression status of the recipients at the time of biopsy is summarized in Table 2, and the most recent status is summarized in Table S3. All of the grafted livers from donors were confirmed to be histologically normal by biopsy at the time of LDLT.

Episodes of acute cellular rejection (ACR) are summarized in Table S3. Liver biopsy was indicated when any liver function parameters (aspartate aminotransferase, alanine aminotransferase, gamma-glutamyl transpeptidase, and total bilirubin) showed abnormal values suggesting ACR. All episodes of ACR were diagnosed on the basis of liver biopsy pathology. Highly experienced pathologists evaluated the degree of portal infiltration by lymphocytes, bile duct inflammation or damage, and venous endothelial inflammation, according to the Banff scheme.

Preparation of biopsy specimens and histological assessment

The liver specimens were obtained by ultrasonography-guided core needle (16 gauge) biopsy from the donor and recipient under local anesthesia. These paired biopsies were performed within a week of each other. The donors fully approved biopsy of their liver because they expressed a desire to know the pathological state of the liver and the pathological relationship between the donor and recipient livers after receiving a full explanation about all the potential complications of the biopsy.

The liver biopsy specimens were fixed in 10% buffered formalin solution and embedded in paraffin. The specimens were then sliced into sections 3 μm thick for hematoxylin and eosin (HE) staining and into sections 2 μm thick for Q-FISH. All sections included more than 6 portal tracts. Histological findings were assessed by a histopathologist who was an expert in liver pathology (K.M), and described based on the criteria proposed by the Banff Working Group [30].

Telomere length quantification by Q-FISH

The slides were processed with the Q-FISH method, as reported previously [18,26]. In brief, the telomeres were labeled with Cy3-labeled CCCTAACCCTAACCCTAA peptide nucleic acid probe (teloC: F1002; Fasmac, Japan) and the centromeres were labeled with a FITC-labeled CTTCGTTGGAAACGGGGT peptide nucleic acid probe (CENP1: a non-specific centromere probe) (custom-made, Fasmac). The chromosome preparations were counterstained with 40, 6-diamino-2-phenylindole (DAPI, Molecular Probes, Eugene, OR, USA). Microscopical images were captured with the Image-Pro Plus software package (version 5.0, Media Cybernetics Co. Ltd., Silver Spring, MD, USA), and analyzed using our own telomere analysis software 'TissueTelo Ver. 2'. The telomere length estimate for each nucleus was defined as the ratio of the detected signal intensity of the telomere relative to that of the centromere (telomere-to-centromere ratio: TCR). At least 127 cells (median: 208 cells, range: 127–463 cells) were analyzed in each case.

TCR normalization using a cell block

As a control for variations in sample preparation, we also performed Q-FISH on a cell block-section of a cultured fibroblast strain, TIG-1 [31] (34 population doubling levels, terminal restriction fragment length determined as 8.6 kilo base pairs), placed on the same slide as each hepatic section. Every TCR for hepatocytes was divided by the median TCR for the cell block on the same slide to give the normalized TCR (NTCR) [26].

Limitation of the study

The main limitation of this study was the small number of subjects for whom NTCR values for the paired donor and graft could be determined. However, despite the limited number (12 pairs) of informative cases, the major findings were statistically significant.

Statistical analyses

The values of measured variables were expressed as mean ± standard deviation or median with a range of values. The median

Table 1. Characteristics of donors and patients.

Group	Pair No.		Age at LDLT	Relation	Biopsy Duration from LDLT	Blood type	HLA mismatch number	Median value of NTCR	*p* value
Lower NTCR Group		Donor	36y8m	Father		A+		1.51	
	1				12y6m		3		$p<0.001$
		Recipient	1y3m	Daughter		A+		1.07	
		Donor	44y10m	Father		O+		0.42	
	2				11y4m		2		$p<0.001$
		Recipient	8y4m	Son		O+		0.27	
		Donor	39y0m	Father		A+		1.04	
	3				5y6m		3		$p=0.015$
		Recipient	1y10m	Daughter		A+		0.78	
		Donor	42y3m	Mother		B+		1.13	
	4				5y6m		3		$p<0.001$
		Recipient	9m	Daughter		B+		0.73	
Comparable NTCR Group		Donor	36y7m	Father		O+		1.05	
	5				16y10m		3		$p=0.265$
		Recipient	9m	Daughter		O+		0.95	
		Donor	35y7m	Father		B+		0.57	
	6				15y3m		3		$p=0.948$
		Recipient	1y7m	Daughter		AB+		0.53	
		Donor	38y4m	Father		O+		0.99	
	7				5y4m		3		$p=0.366$
		Recipient	7y3m	Daughter		O+		0.96	
		Donor	37y9m	Stepfather		B+		0.37	
	8				13y0m		6		$p=0.065$
		Recipient	4y1m	Son		B+		0.46	
		Donor	28y7m	Mother		O+		0.56	
	9				10y6m		2		$p=0.109$
		Recipient	1y0m	Son		A+		0.77	
		Donor	32y1m	Father		A+		1.03	
	10				8y9m		3		$p=0.056$
		Recipient	2y6m	Daughter		A+		1.2	
		Donor	34y8m	Father		B+		0.88	
	11				6y7m		3		$p=0.115$
		Recipient	2y7m	Daughter		B+		1.02	
		Donor	29y5m	Father		A+		0.77	
	12				5y5m		2		$p=0.342$
		Recipient	1y5m	Daughter		A+		0.82	

NTCR: normalized telomere centromere ratio.
Lower NTCR group: Median NTCRs of the recipient hepatocyte were significantly lower than those of the donor.
Comparable NTCR group: Median NTCRs of the recipient hepatocyte were neither significantly lower nor higher than those of the donor.
Median donor age and median recipient age at the time of LDLT were 36.6 y (28.6 y to 44.8 y) and 1.7 y (0.8 y to 8.3 y), respectively.
Median donor age and median recipient age at the time of biopsy were 46.2 y (34.8 y to 56.2 y) and 12.0 y (6.3 y to 19.7 y), respectively.
The median interval from LDLT to biopsy was 9.6 y.

NTCRs of the donor and recipient hepatocytes were compared between cases using the Mann-Whitney test or Wilcoxon test. Correlations were analyzed with the Spearman correlation coefficient test and a single regression analysis using the software package Dr.SPSS II (SPSS, Chicago, IL). The relationships among NTCR values, donor age and group (lower versus comparable NTCR) were assessed by multiple regression analyses using StatView software version 5.0 (SAS Institute Inc.). Differences were considered significant at $p<0.05$.

Table 2. Clinical and pathological status of donors and recipients.

Group	Pair No.		Major complication of recipient	Pathological findings	Immunosuppression status
Lower NTCR Group		Donor		(-)	
	1	Recipient	Chronic hepatitis	Mild interface hepatitis	Tacrolimus: twice a day
			de novo HBV		Micophenolate mofetil
		Donor		(-)	
	2	Recipient		Mild interface hepatitis	Tacrolimus: twice a day
					Micophenolate mofetil
					Steroid
		Donor		(-)	
	3	Recipient			Tacrolimus: twice a day
			HV stenosis	Marked bridging fibrosis	Micophenolate mofetil
					Steroid
		Donor		(-)	
	4	Recipient	Unstable liver function	Mild lobular hepatitis	Cyclosporine: twice a day
					Micophenolate mofetil
Comparable NTCR Group		Donor		Moderate steatosis	
	5	Recipient	*de novo* HBV	(-)	Cyclosporine: twice a day
			(seroconversion)		Micophenolate mofetil
		Donor			
	6	Recipient	Liver dysfunction	Marked bridging fibrosis	Tacrolimus: twice a day
			HV stenosis		Micophenolate mofetil
					Steroid
	7	Donor		(-)	
		Recipient	None	Mild interface hepatitis	Tacrolimus: twice a day
		Donor		Moderate steatosis	
	8			(NASH suspected)	
		Recipient	Biliary stricture	Canalicular cholestasis	Cyclosporine: twice a day
		Donor		(-)	
	9	Recipient	HV stenosis	Mild interface hepatitis	Cyclosporine: twice a day
					Micophenolate mofetil
	10	Donor		(-)	
		Recipient	None	(-)	Complete cessation
	11	Donor		(-)	
		Recipient	None	(-)	Tacrolimus: once a week
		Donor		Moderate steatosis	
	12	Recipient	Unstable liver function	(-)	Tacrolimus: twice a day
					Micophenolate mofetil

HBV: hepatitis B virus, HV: hepatic vein, NTCR: normalized telomere centromere ratio, NASH: none-alcoholic steatotic hepatitis, (-): almost normal.
Lower NTCR group: Median NTCRs of the recipient hepatocyte was significantly lower than those of the donor.
Compatible NTCR group: Median NTCRs of the recipient hepatocyte was not significantly lower nor higher than those of the donor.

Results

Quantification of telomere length in liver tissue of donors and recipients using Q-FISH

Figure 1A shows a Q-FISH image of a TIG-1 cell block placed on the same slide as liver sections from the donor and recipient. Representative Q-FISH images of liver tissues from the donor and recipient are shown in Figure 1B, D (pair 4), and Figure 1C, E (pair 10), in which the telomere signals (Cy3) appear red while the centromere signals (FITC) appear green on the DAPI-stained nuclei. With reference to HE-stained serial sections (Shown in Figure 2), we were able to distinguish hepatocytes from other cell types (including ductal cells, interstitial fibroblasts and infiltrating lymphocytes). The profiles of the measured telomere:centromere ratio (TCR) are plotted in Figure 1F, G. Since the frequency of TCR values did not show a normal distribution, we chose the median values as representative. The median values of the TCR for the donor and recipient hepatocytes are divided by the TCR

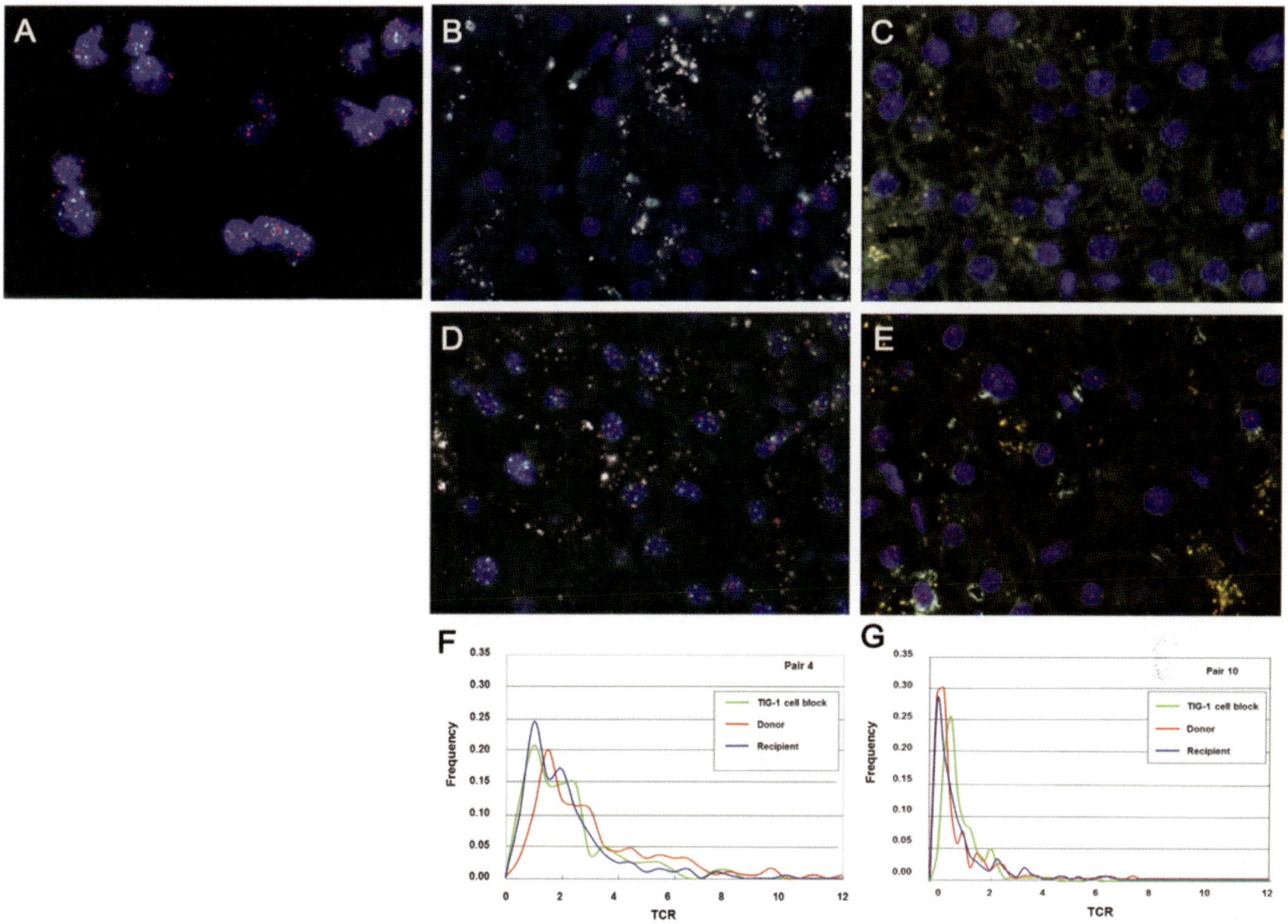

Figure 1. Representative Q-FISH images of TIG-1 and paired liver tissues (red: Cy3, telomere signals; green: FITC, centromere signals; blue: DAPI, nuclei). (A) Q-FISH image reveals the TIG-1 cell block placed on the same slide together with liver sections. Telomere (Cy3, red) and centromere (FITC, green) signals are evident (original magnification ×400). (B) Q-FISH images of pair 4 donor. Telomere and centromere signals are evident in the nuclei (original magnification ×400). (C) Q-FISH images of pair 10 donor. (original magnification ×400). (D) Q-FISH image of pair 4 recipient in the lower NTCR group reveals weaker telomere signals (red) than those in the paired donor (Figure 1B) (original magnification ×400). (E) Q-FISH images of pair 10 recipient, showing brighter telomere signals (red) than those in the paired donor (Figure 2D) (original magnification ×400). (F) Distributions of the telomere intensity given by telomere-to-centromere ratio (TCR) in TIG-1 and hepatocytes from paired liver tissues of pair 4 samples. Green: TIG-1 cells in a cell block, red: hepatocytes in donor, blue: hepatocytes in recipient grafted liver. (G) TCR distribution in TIG-1, and hepatocytes from paired liver tissues of pair 10 samples.

value for TIG-1 cells and obtained normalized TCR (NTCR) (summarized in Table 1). Among interstitial cells, strong signal intensity for Cy3 was often evident in fibroblasts.

Relationship between NTCR values for the donor and recipient

Scatter plot analysis of the median NTCR values for hepatocytes provided a robust correlation between donors and recipients ($p = 0.0038$) (Figure 3A). The slope provided by the regression analysis was less than 1, and the mean of the median NTCR value for hepatocytes from donors and that of hepatocytes from recipients (grafts) was 0.82 and 0.78, respectively. Hence, the NTCR values for recipients generally tended to be lower than those for the donors. However, in individual cases, even if the NTCR value for the grafted liver was higher or lower than that for the donor liver, the difference was not statistically significant ($p = 0.092$).

From the relationship between the hepatocyte NTCR values for the donor liver and the graft, we found 4 sample pairs in which the NTCR values for the graft hepatocytes were significantly lower than those for remaining hepatocytes in the donor (Table 1, Figure 4). In the other 8 pairs, although the NTCR values for graft hepatocytes were higher than, comparable to, or lower than the corresponding values for the hepatocytes remaining in the donor, the differences were not statistically significant (Table 1, Figure 4). Hence, we categorized the former as a lower NTCR group and the latter as a comparable NTCR group. Intriguingly, the donors were significantly older in the lower NTCR group (median age 40 y 8 m) than in the corresponding comparable NTCR group (median age 35 y 2 m) ($p = 0.017$) (Figure 3B). Conversely, the oldest one-third of the donors (pairs 2, 4, 3, 7) demonstrated decreased NTCR values in the recipient, and the youngest one-third of the donors (pairs 9, 12, 10, 11) showed increased NTCR values in the recipient.

Next, we applied a multiple regression model to assess the difference between the two groups (see Figure 3A legend). This

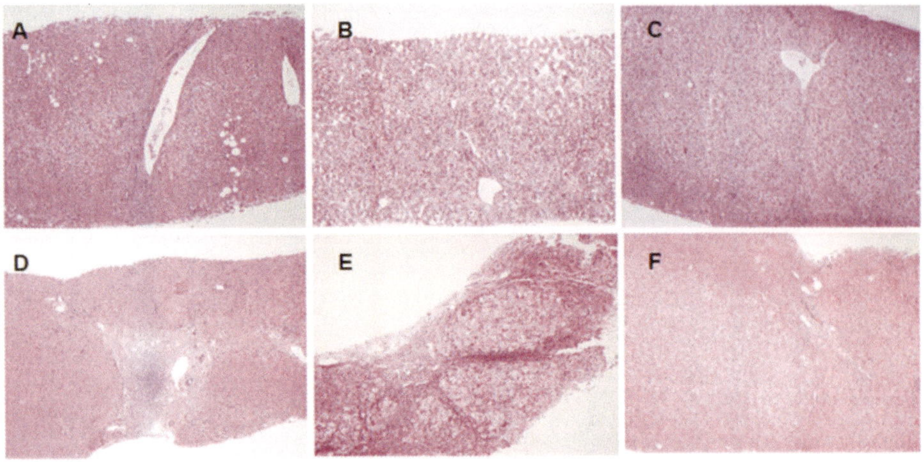

Figure 2. Representative histological and histopathological features of the livers. (A) Histological findings in pair 1 donor, showing almost normal feature (HE, original magnification ×100). (B) Histological findings in pair 3 donor, showing almost normal feature (HE, original magnification ×100). (C) Histological findings in pair 10 donor, showing almost normal feature (HE, original magnification ×100). (D) Histological findings in pair 1 recipient in the lower NTCR group, showing mild interface hepatitis due to infection with hepatitis B virus via the graft from the HBV carrier donor (HE, original magnification ×40). (E) Histological findings in pair 3 recipient in the lower NTCR group, showing marked bridging fibrosis due to repeated hepatic vein stenosis (HE, original magnification ×40). (F) Histological findings in pair 10 recipient, with good liver function and complete withdrawal of immunosuppressant, showing almost normal feature (HE, original magnification ×100).

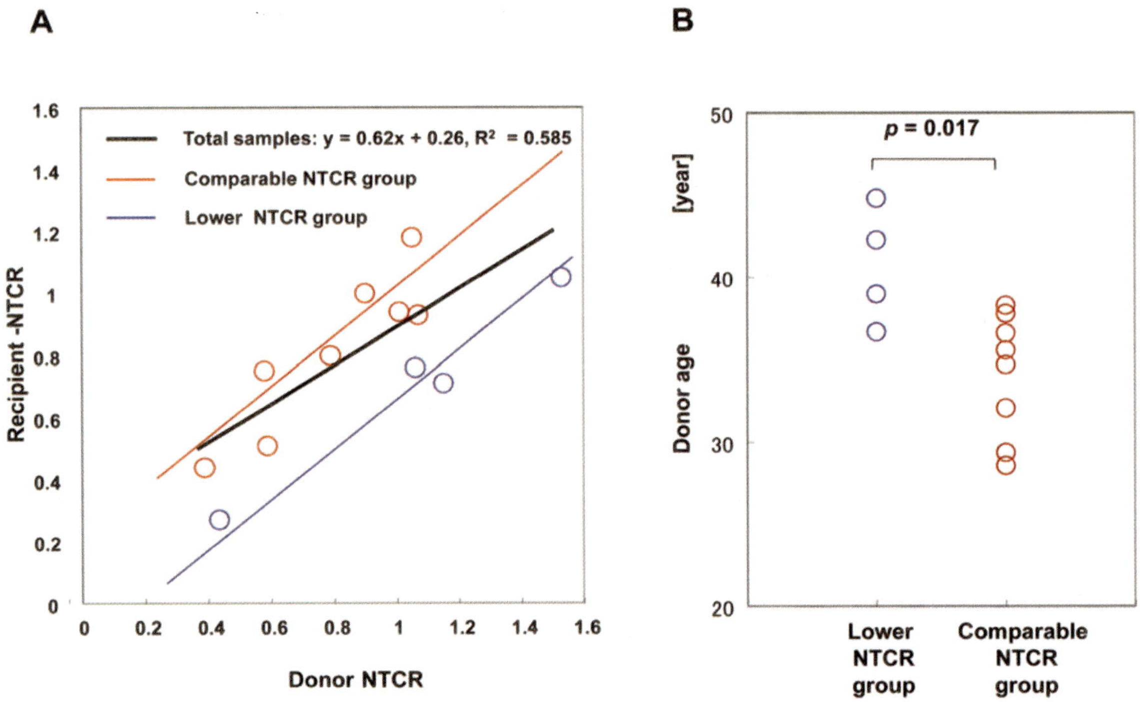

Figure 3. (**A**) Scatter plot analysis of the relationship between NTCRs in donor hepatocytes and those in recipient hepatocytes. A regression line was obtained from all of the paired subjects (n = 12), y (recipient NTCR) = 0.62x(donor NTCR)+0.26, ($r = 0.765$, $R^2 = 0.544$, $p = 0.0038$), shown by a solid black line. By using model 1: $Y = \beta_0 + \beta_1 X_1$ (age)$+\beta_2 X_2$ (group), that related Y (recipient NTCR) to X_1 (donor NTCR) and X_2 (group), given that the value for the comparable group was 1 and that for the lower group was 0. This model yielded a regression line from the comparable patient group (n = 8): Y (recipient NTCR) = −0.10+0.79X(donor NTCR) +0.32, shown by a red line; and a regression line from the lower patient group (n = 4): Y (recipient NTCR) = −0.10+0.79X (donor NTCR), shown by a blue line. The difference of recipient NTCR values between the groups was 0.32 and significant ($P = 0.001$). Red circles: the recipient-donor pair categorized as the comparable NTCR group. Blue circles: the recipient-donor pair categorized as the lower NTCR group. (**B**) Comparison between donors in the comparable group and those in the lower group by age factor. The difference of donor ages (median values) between the groups was 5 y 6 m and significant ($p = 0.017$). Red circles, the donors categorized as the comparable NTCR group. Blue circles, the donors categorized as the lower NTCR group.

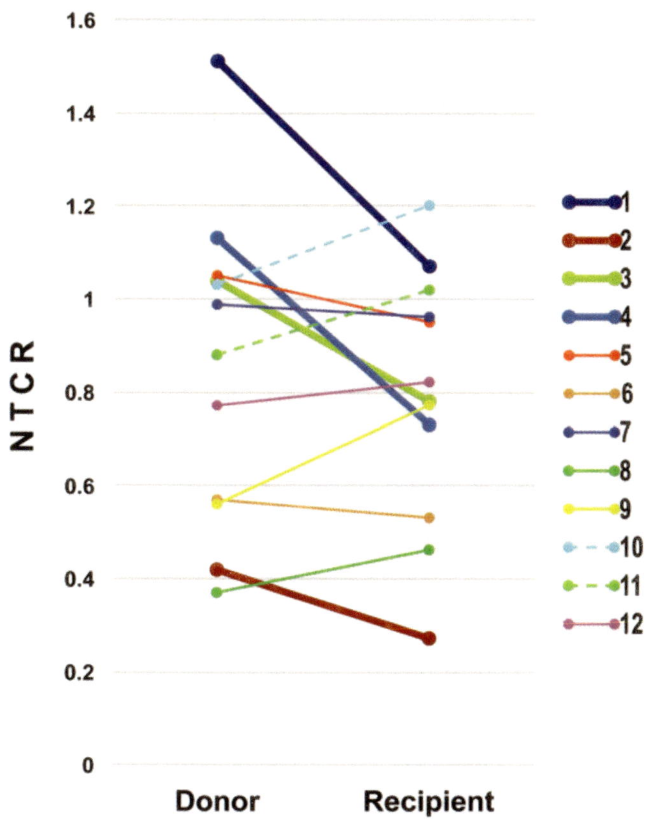

Figure 4. Comparison between donor and recipient NTCR values. Bold lines connect lower NTCR group pairs, and thin lines connect comparable NTCR group pairs. Dashed lines connect the pairs (10 and 11), who achieved complete withdrawal of immunosuppression.

model yielded a regression line indicating that the average ratio of the recipient NTCR to the donor NTCR was 0.794 ($p<0.0001$), and that the difference between the groups was significant ($p=0.001$) (Figure 3A).

With regard to other factors, the ages of the recipients at LDLT showed no significant difference between the two groups (lower NTCR group: median age 1 y 10 m, comparable NTCR group: median age 2 y 1 m, $p=0.799$). Also, neither the NTCR values for recipients nor those for the donors differed significantly between the two groups (0.73 vs. 0.89, $p=0.570$; 1.04 vs. 0.83, $p=0.241$, respectively. The period between LDLT and liver biopsy showed no significant differences between the two groups (lower NTCR group: median duration 8 y 5 m, comparable NTCR group: median period 9 y 8 m, $p=0.734$).

Histopathological findings in donors and recipients

The liver biopsy samples from all 4 donors in the lower NTCR group showed normal histological findings. On the other hand, three (pairs 5, 8, and 12) of the 8 donors in the comparable NTCR group showed moderate steatosis.

Among the liver biopsy samples from recipients, significant abnormalities were observed in all of the 4 recipients in the lower NTCR group (mild interface hepatitis in cases 1 and 2, mild lobular hepatitis in case 4, marked bridging fibrosis in case 3) and in 4 of the 8 recipients in the comparable NTCR group (marked bridging fibrosis in case 6, mild interface hepatitis in cases 7 and 9, canalicular cholestasis in case 8) (Figure 2, and summarized in Table 2).

Immunological findings in grafts

In the comparable NTCR group, 3 recipients (pairs 10, 11 and 12) showed a benign course after LDLT, and were treatable with a calcineurin inhibitor at a frequency of less than once a day, or without any immunosuppressant. In particular, the recipient in pair 10, who achieved complete withdrawal of immunosuppression, had a higher median NTCR than the donor, but the difference was of borderline statistical significance ($p=0.056$). The recipient in pair 11, who has recently achieved complete withdrawal of immunosuppression, also had a higher median NTCR than the donor. In only one recipient (pair 8) who received a graft from a non-father non-mother (stepfather) donor and was treated with a calcineurin inhibitor, the median NTCR was also higher than that of the donor, but the difference was of borderline statistical significance ($p=0.065$). While only one of 8 recipients in the comparable NTCR group (pair 6) continued to require oral maintenance steroid therapy, 2 of 4 recipients (pairs 2 and 3) in the lower NTCR group did so.

Episodes of acute cellular rejection (ACR) were observed in 2 cases in the lower NTCR group and 4 cases in the comparable NTCR group. Among the cases associated with ACR, 4 (pairs 2, 3, 5, 6; cases 2 and 3 being statistically significant) showed decreasing NTCR values in the recipients, and 2 (pairs 8, 12) showed increasing NTCR values in the recipients, but not to a significant degree. With regard to steatosis, 3 of the 4 cases in the comparable NTCR group associated with ACR in the recipient showed steatosis in the donor.

Laboratory data for donors and recipients

The laboratory data for recipients (summarized in Table S1) at liver biopsy have so far revealed no significant differences between the lower NTCR group and the comparable NTCR group. In addition, the PELD scores for recipients (summarized in Table S2) have shown no significant differences between the two groups.

Discussion

In parallel with the increasing need for LDLT, the issue of organ shortage continues to extend worldwide and has become a serious problem. Therefore, the use of organs from marginal donors, such as the elderly, has been increasing [2]. Currently, LDLT is able to ensure survival for more than 5 years, mainly because of improvements in immunosuppression regimens [4,5,6]. However, there is still insufficient knowledge of factors that would facilitate long-term or life-long viability or function of the grafted liver after LDLT. Accumulated studies have demonstrated that higher donor age is a risk factor for early relaparotomy and poor outcome [32,33]; however, some reports have suggested that liver grafts from elderly donors can yield a favorable outcome [34,35]. Thus, the question of whether the use of grafts from elderly donors may influence the long-term outcome of the graft after LT/LDLT remains unsettled. In addressing possible factors that might have a crucial impact on long-term prognosis, we speculated that hepatocyte telomere length in the recipient might be an indicator of long-term survival potential, as telomere length reportedly reflects not only cellular senescence but also possibly organ aging [36,37,13,38].

The present study represents the first attempt to provide statistical support of telomere length differences in hepatocytes obtained by liver biopsy at almost the same time from both donors and recipients followed up for more than 5 years after pediatric

LDLT using the Q-FISH method. The main findings were as follows: Firstly, based on the relationship between the NTCR of the recipient and that of the donor, recipients were classifiable into two groups: a comparable group (showing no significant difference in NTCR) and a lower group (showing a significantly lower NTCR in the recipient than in the donor). However, in 5 of the 8 cases in the comparable group, hepatocyte NTCR values for recipients were larger than those for the donors. Secondly, donors in the lower NTCR group were significantly older than those in the comparable NTCR group, and there was no relationship between the absolute NTCR values *per se* in the two groups, nor with any of the recipient conditions examined.

With regard to the methodology used for telomere length measurement, numerous approaches have been adopted, including Southern blotting, PCR-based methods, and Q-FISH. Previous studies using Southern blotting have shown that fibrosis or hepatitis can accelerate telomere shortening in the liver [15,39,40] in recipients with immune-mediated injury and/or pathological abnormalities of the liver, where the telomere length might be shorter than that of donors [41]. This approach has an underlying problem in that hepatic tissue includes a variety of cell types, such as hepatocytes, macrophages, and fibroblasts, whose telomere lengths are measured simultaneously. On the other hand, Q-FISH makes it possible to analyze the length of hepatocellular telomeres in a cell type-specific manner, although precise calibration is required. We have measured telomere lengths in various human organs and tissues by the Q-FISH method utilizing the centromere signal as an internal control and the terminal restriction fragment length defined fibroblasts as an external control [26,18,42]. Recently, we have demonstrated telomere length shortening in the hepatocytes of biliary atresia with severe inflammatory changes and fibrosis using the present Q-FISH method, but failed to reproduce our findings by authentic Southern blotting [43]. The robust correlation between the paired values found in the present study further demonstrated that our Q-FISH method was reliable for cell type-specific analysis.

Our previous population studies demonstrated that telomeres in the liver shorten most rapidly with age among those in the major organs. The telomere shortening in liver is especially rapid in infants, and then the rate of shortening slows from adolescence to middle age; no significant decrease is evident from forties to centenarian age [12,13,38]. Hence, from the viewpoint of telomere dynamics, the most critical period for liver aging is assumed to be from birth to forties. Our present data, based on a donor population ranging in age from 28 y 7 m to 44 y 10 m, indicated that donors in the lower NTCR group were significantly older than those in the comparable NTCR group. Taken together, the data strongly suggest that the mechanisms for maintenance of telomere length in the grafts were affected by aging-related changes during early adulthood.

The regeneration of a liver graft in a recipient suggests that the structure and function of the graft might be largely controlled by the host environment [44], organ chimerism, or cell migration from the host to the transplanted liver [45], and that telomerase may play a pivotal role in maintaining telomere length and chromosomal stability in proliferating cells [46]. In relation to LT/LDLT and telomere shortening, several candidate causative factors have been examined, including chronic inflammation, fibrosis, and steatosis. Nakajima *et al.* have reported that non-alcoholic fatty liver disease with steatosis causes prominent telomere shortening in hepatocytes [47], and therefore steatosis in a grafted liver might potentially accelerate telomere shortening. In the present study, 3 of 12 donors had moderate steatosis (pairs 5, 8, and 12), and all were categorized in the lower NTCR group. Hence, these cases would require careful attention. Liver fibrosis is another histopathological feature of liver disease, and has been reported to be a significant indicator of prognosis after LDLT [48]. In the present study, 2 of the 12 recipients showed marked fibrosis (pairs 3 and 6); both were treated with continuous steroid, but were separated into different groups. Hence, to date, we have been unable to confirm the relationship between fibrosis and telomere length. Hepatitis after LT/LDLT is another critical complication. Three of the lower NTCR group (cases 1, 2, 4) and two of the comparable NTCR group (cases 7, 9) suffered mild hepatitis, and all of them showed a decrease of hepatocyte NTCR in the recipient. These findings are comparable to previous studies [15,39,40,41], and suggest that livers from younger donors may have higher resistance to hepatitis.

With regard to immunological findings, we recently assessed the association of ACR with several factors in 114 LDLTs performed at our institute, including the cases analyzed in the present study. We found that paternal grafts with gender mismatch were associated with a higher incidence of ACR than maternal grafts with gender match, and that there was no significant difference between the donor age groups [49]. Since all of the donors except one in the present study were male, it was not possible to examine any influence of donor gender. However, the latter conclusion is compatible with our present findings. Intriguingly, some graft hepatocytes, including those in pairs 10 and 11, where complete withdrawal of immunosuppression was possible, showed a larger NTCR than those of the donor. Although the difference was not statistically significant, our findings strongly suggest that the telomeres in grafted livers might be elongated somewhat longer when the grafts are immunologically well controlled. Human leukocyte antigen (HLA) compatibility matching is indisputably important in kidney, heart, and bone marrow transplantation, but is not largely considered to have a clinically significant impact in liver transplantation [50,51]. In the present study, we were unable to demonstrate any significant effect of HLA compatibility on telomere dynamics.

With regard to the relationship between recipient status and LT/LDLT outcome, some studies have demonstrated a correlation between the PELD score before LT and outcome after LT [6,21]. However, we were unable to find any significant relationship between NTCR dynamics and host status, including PELD score, in this series.

Major arguments concerning the clinical impact of donor age on LT/LDTP outcome have focused mainly on the elderly (60~65 years of age or more). However, aging phenomena have been observed not only in the elderly but also in young adult or middle-aged individuals [33]. For example, concentrations of growth-hormone/insulin-like growth factor reportedly begin to decline from early adulthood (~20 years of age), and muscle area/strength from 30 years of age [52,53]. Our previous population studies of telomere length have demonstrate that telomeres in the skin start to shorten at around 30 years of age [54]; on the other hand, those in the liver shorten rapidly during young age, and continue to do so at 30 to 40 years of age, and then reach a stationary state [12,13]. The present data provide further evidence for the aging process that occurs during youth and middle age, and shed more light on the importance of the aging process during this earlier period before old age.

Notwithstanding our retrospective study design and the limited number of samples analyzed, our findings lend additional support to the validity of LDLT, because telomere lengths in the majority of the recipients were statistically comparable to those in the native liver of the donor. Furthermore, telomere lengths showed a tendency to be elongated in well-controlled grafted livers. Our data also provide essential clues to the relationship between hepatocyte aging and LDLT outcome, particularly with regard to young/middle-aged individuals. Further studies will undoubtedly reveal other factors that affect hepatocyte telomere length in the grafted liver and their long-term effects on the graft after pediatric LDLT.

Supporting Information

Table S1 Laboratory data of recipients and donors at biopsy. Lower NTCR group: Median NTCRs of the recipient hepatocyte was significantly lower than those of the donor. Comparable NTCR group: Median NTCRs of the recipient hepatocyte was neither significantly lower nor higher than those of the donor. AST: aspartate aminotransferase, ALT: serum alanine aminotransferase, γ-GTP: γ-glutamyl transpeptidase, Alb: albumin, T-bil: total bilirubin, PT-INR: international normalized ratio of prothrombin time.

Table S2 Pediatric End-stage Liver Disease (PELD) score of patients. Alb: albumin, T-bil: total bilirubin, PT-INR: international normalized ratio of prothrombin time.

Table S3 Acute cellular rejection episodes and Immunosuppression status. ACR: Acute Cellular Rejection.

Acknowledgments

We thank Sachiko Nishimura and Jun Nishimura for technical assistance, Dr. Shunzaburo Iwatsuki for helpful discussions, and Dr. David Douglas for language editing.

Author Contributions

Conceived and designed the experiments: YK KT NI. Performed the experiments: JA YS NI-S KN K. Matsumoto K. Mizuta EU TT HK. Analyzed the data: YK NI JA YS NI-S KN. Wrote the paper: YK NI. Participated in contributing to the discussion on analyzing software: SP. Participated in collecting materials: K. Matsumoto K. Mizuta EU TT HK. Discussion: JA YS NI-S KN SP K. Matsumoto K. Mizuta EU TT HK KT.

References

1. Starzl TE, Groth CG, Brettschneider L, Penn I, Fulginiti VA, et al. (1968) Orthotopic homotransplantation of the human liver. Ann Surg 168: 392–415.
2. Attia M, Silva MA, Mirza DF (2008) The marginal liver donor—an update. Transpl Int 21: 713–724.
3. Jain A, Reyes J, Kashyap R, Dodson SF, Demetris AJ, et al. (2000) Long-term survival after liver transplantation in 4,000 consecutive patients at a single center. Ann Surg 232: 490–500.
4. Starzl TE, Klintman GBG, Porter KA, Iwatsuki S, Schroter GP (1981) Liver transplantation with use of cyclosporine A and prednisone. N Engl J Med 305: 266–269.
5. Starzl TE, Fung J, Venkataramman R, Todo S, Demetris AJ, et al. (1989) FK506 for human liver, kidney and pancreas transplantation. Lancet 334: 1000–1004.
6. Calne RY, Rolles K, White DJ, Thiru S, Evans DB, et al. (1979) Cyclosporin A initially as the only immunosuppressant in 34 recipients of cadaveric organs: 32 kidneys, 2 pancreas, and 2 livers. Lancet 314: 1033–1036.
7. Abbasoglu O (2008) Liver transplantation: yesterday, today and tomorrow. World J Gastroenterol 14: 3117–3122.
8. Mehrabi A, Fonouni H, Muller SA, Schmidt J (2008) Current concepts in transplant surgery: liver transplantation today. Langenbecks Arch Surg 393: 245–260.
9. Evans HM, Kelly DA, McKiernan PJ, Hubscher S (2006) Progressive histological damage in liver allografts following pediatric liver transplantation. Hepatology 43: 1109–1117.
10. Barber K, Blackwell J, Collett D, Neuberger J (2007) Life expectancy of adult liver allograft recipients in the UK. Gut 56: 279–282.
11. Blackburn EH (2000) Telomere states and cell fate. Nature 408: 53–56.
12. Takubo K, Nakamura K, Izumiyama N, Furugori E, Sawabe M, et al. (2000) Telomere shortening with aging in human liver. J Gerontol A Biol Sci Med Sci 55: B533–536.
13. Takubo K, Izumiyama-Shimomura N, Honma N, Sawabe M, Arai T, et al. (2002) Telomere lengths are characteristic in each human individual. Exp Gerontol 37: 523–531.
14. Saretzki G, von Zglinicki T (2002) Replicative aging, telomeres, and oxidative stress. Ann N Y Acad Sci 959: 24–29.
15. Aikata H, Takaishi H, Kawakami Y, Takahashi S, Kitamoto M, et al. (2000) Telomere reduction in human liver tissues with age and chronic inflammation. Exp Cell Res 256: 578–582.
16. O'Sullivan JN, Bronner MP, Brentnall TA, Finley JC, Shen WT, et al. (2002) Chromosomal instability in ulcerative colitis is related to telomere shortening. Nat Genet 32: 280–284.
17. Epel ES, Blackburn EH, Lin J, Dhabhar FS, Adler NE, et al. (2004) Accelerated telomere shortening in response to life stress. Proc Natl Acad Sci U S A 101: 17312–17315.
18. Aida J, Yokoyama A, Izumiyama-Shimomura N, Nakamura K, Ishikawa N, et al. (2011) Alcoholics show reduced telomere length in the oesophagus. J Pathol 223:410–416.
19. Chkhotua A, Shohat M, Tobar A, Magal N, Kaganovski E, et al. (2002) Replicative senescence in organ transplantation-mechanisms and significance. Transpl Immunol 9: 165–171.
20. Baerlocher GM, Rovo A, Muller A, Matthqy S, Stern M, et al. (2009) Cellular senescence of white blood cells in very long-term survivors after allogeneic hematopoietic stem cell transplantation: the role of chronic graft-versus-host disease and female donor sex. Blood 114: 219–222.
21. Harley CB, Futcher AB, Greider CW (1990) Telomeres shorten during ageing of human fibroblasts. Nature 345: 458–460.
22. Allsopp RC, Vaziri H, Patterson C, Goldstein S, Younglai EV, et al. (1992) Telomere length predicts replicative capacity of human fibroblasts. Proc Natl Acad Sci U S A 89: 10114–10118.
23. Lansdorp PM, Verwoerd NP, van de Rijke FM, Dragowska V, Little MT, et al. (1996) Heterogeneity in telomere length of human chromosomes. Hum Mol Genet 5: 685–691.
24. Meeker AK, Gage WR, Hicks JL, Simon I, Coffman JR, et al. (2002) Telomere length assessment in human archival tissues: combined telomere fluorescence in situ hybridization and immunostaining. Am J Pathol 160: 1259–1268.
25. Ferlicot S, Youssef N, Feneux D, Delhommeau F, Paradis V, et al. (2003) Measurement of telomere length on tissue sections using quantitative fluorescence in situ hybridization (Q-FISH). J Pathol 200: 661–666.
26. Aida J, Izumiyama-Shimomura N, Nakamura K, Ishikawa N, Poon SS, et al. (2008) Basal cells have longest telomeres measured by tissue Q-FISH method in lingual epithelium. Exp Gerontol 43: 833–839.
27. McDiarmid SV, Merion RM, Dykstra DM, Harper AM (2004) Selection of pediatric candidates under the PELD system. Liver Transpl 10:S23–30.
28. Cowles RA, Lobritto SJ, Ventura KA, Harren PA, Gelbard R, et al. (2008) Timing of liver transplantation in biliary atresia – results in 71 children managed by a multidisciplinary team. J Pediatr Surg 43:1605–1609.
29. Sugawara Y, Makuuchi M (1999) Technical advances in living-related liver transplantation. J Hepatobiliary Pancreat Surg 6: 245–253.
30. Demetris AJ, Adeyi O, Bellamy CO, Clouston A, Charlotte F, et al. (2006) Liver biopsy interpretation for causes of late liver allograft dysfunction. Hepatology 44: 489–501.
31. Takubo K, Aida J, Izumiyama N, Ishikawa N, Fujiwara M, et al. (2010) Chromosomal instability and telomere lengths of each chromosomal arm measured by Q-FISH in human fibroblast strains prior to replicative senescence. Mech Age Dev 131: 614–624.
32. Yoshiya S, Shirabe K, Kimura K, Yoshizumi T, Ikegami T, et al. (2012) The causes, risk factors, and outcomes of early relaparotomy after living-donor liver transplantation. Transplantation 94:947–952.
33. Floreani A (2007) Liver Diseases in the Elderly: An Update. Dig Dis. 25: 138–143.
34. Borchert D, Glanemann M, Mogl M, Langrehr JM, Neuhaus P (2005) Older liver graft transplantation, cholestasis and synthetic graft function. Transpl Int 18: 709–715.
35. Singhal A, Sezginsoy B, Ghuloom AE, Hutchinson IV, Cho YW, et al. (2010) Orthotopic liver transplant using allografts from geriatric population in the United States: is there any age limit? Exp Clin Transplant 8:196–201.
36. Campisi J (2001) From cells to organisms: can we learn about aging from cells in culture? Exp Gerontl 36: 607–618.
37. Hornsby PJ (2002) Cellular senescence and tissue aging in vivo. J Gerontol A Biol Sci Med Sci 57: B251–256.
38. Ishikawa N, Nakamura KI, Izumiyama N, Aida J, Sawabe M, et al. (2012) Telomere length dynamics in the human pituitary gland: robust preservation throughout adult life to centenarian age. Age 34: 795–804.

39. Paradis V, Youssef N, Dargere D, Ba N, Bonvoust F, et al. (2001) Replicative senescence in normal liver, chronic hepatitis C, and hepatocellular carcinomas. Hum Pathol 32:327–332.
40. Wiemann SU, Satyanarayana A, Tsahuridu M, Tillmann HL, Zender L, et al. (2002) Hepatocyte telomere shortening and senescence are general markers of human liver cirrhosis. Faseb J 16:935–942.
41. Aini W, Miyagawa-Hayashino A, Tsuruyama T, Hashimoto S, Sumiyoshi S, et al. (2012) Telomere shortening and karyotypic alterations in hepatocytes in long-term transplanted human liver allografts. Transpl Int 25: 956–966.
42. Takubo K, Fujita M, Izumiyama N, Nakamura K, Ishikawa N, et al. (2010) Q-FISH analysis of telomere and chromosome instability in the oesophagus with and without squamous cell carcinoma in situ. J Pathol 221:201–209.
43. Sanada Y, Aida J, Kawano Y, Nakamura K, Shimomura N, et al. (2012) Hepatocellular Telomere Length in Biliary Atresia Measured by Q-FISH. World Journal of Surgery 36: 908–916.
44. Nobori S, Shimizu A, Okumi M, Samelson-Jones E, Griesemer A, et al. (2006) Thymic rejuvenation and the induction of tolerance by adult thymic grafts. Proc Natl Acad Sci U S A 103:19081–19086.
45. Starzl TE, Murase N, Ildstad S, Ricordi C, Demetris AJ, et al. (1992) Cell migration, chimerism, and graft acceptance. Lancet 339: 1579–1582.
46. Wege H, Brummendorf TH (2007) Telomerase activation in liver regeneration and hepatocarcinogenesis: Dr. Jekyll or Mr. Hyde? Curr Stem Cell Res Ther 2: 31–38.
47. Nakajima T, Moriguchi M, Katagishi T, Sekoguchi S, Nishikawa T, et al. (2006) Premature telomere shortening and impaired regenerative response in hepatocytes of individuals with NAFLD. Liver Int 26: 23–31.
48. Ohe H, Li Y, Nafady-Hego H, Kayo W, Sakaguchi S, et al. (2011) Minimal but essential doses of immunosuppression: a more realistic approach to improve long-term outcomes for pediatric living-donor liver transplantation. Transplantation 91: 808–810.
49. Sanada Y, Kawano Y, Miki A, Aida J, Nakamura KI, et al. (2014) Maternal grafts protect daughter recipients from acute cellular rejection after pediatric living donor liver transplantation for biliary atresia. Transpl Int. doi: 10.1111/tri.12273. [Epub ahead of print]
50. Markus BH, Duquesnoy RJ, Gordon RD, Fung JJ, Vanek M, et al. (1988) Histocompatibility and liver transplant outcome. Does HLA exert a dualistic effect? Transplantation 46: 372–377.
51. Navarro V, Herrine S, Katopes C, Colombe B, Spain CV (2006) The effect of HLA class I (A and B) and class II (DR) compatibility on liver transplantation outcomes: an analysis of the OPTN database.Liver Transpl 12: 652–658.
52. Veldhuis JD (2008) Aging and hormones of the hypothalamo-pituitary axis: gonadotropic axis in men and somatotropic axes in men and women. Ageing Res Rev. 7:189–208.
53. Nair KS (2005) Aging muscle. Am J Clin Nutr. 81:953–63.
54. Nakamura K, Izumiyama-Shimomura N, Sawabe M, Arai T, Aoyagi Y, et al. (2002) Comparative analysis of telomere lengths and erosion with age in human epidermis and lingual epithelium. J Invest Dermatol. 119:1014–9.

23

The Performance of Enhanced Liver Fibrosis (ELF) Test for the Staging of Liver Fibrosis: A Meta-Analysis

Qingsong Xie[1,2,3], Xiaohu Zhou[1,2,3], Pengfei Huang[1,2,3], Jianfeng Wei[1,2,3], Weilin Wang[1,2,3]*, Shusen Zheng[1,2,3]*

1 Division of Hepatobilitary and Pancreatic Surgery, Department of Surgery, First Affiliated Hospital, School of Medicine, Zhejiang University, Hangzhou, Zhejiang Province, China, **2** Key Laboratory of Combined Multi- Organ Transplantation, Ministry of Public Health, Zhejiang Province, Hangzhou, China, **3** Key laboratory of Organ Transplantation, Zhejiang Province, Hangzhou, China

Abstract

Background: The enhanced liver fibrosis test (ELF) has been shown to accurately predict significant liver fibrosis in several liver diseases.

Aims: To perform a meta-analysis to assess the performance of the ELF test for the assessment of liver fibrosis.

Study: Electronic and manual searches were performed to identify studies of the ELF test. After methodological quality assessment and data extraction, pooled estimates of the sensitivity, specificity, area under the receiver operating characteristic curve (AUROC), positive likelihood ratio (PLR), negative likelihood ratio (NLR), diagnostic odds ratio (DOR) and summary receiver operating characteristics (sROC) were assessed systematically. The extent of heterogeneity and reasons for it were assessed.

Results: Nine studies were identified for analysis. The pooled sensitivity, specificity, positive LR, negative LR, and DOR values of ELF test, for assessment of significant liver fibrosis, were 83% (95% CI = 0.80–0.86), 73% (95% CI = 0.69–0.77), 4.00 (95% CI = 2.50–6.39), 0.24 (95% CI = 0.17–0.34), and 16.10 (95% CI = 8.27–31.34), respectively; and, for evaluation of severe liver fibrosis, were 78% (95% CI = 0.74–0.81), 76% (95% CI = 0.73–0.78), 4.39 (95% CI = 2.76–6.97), 0.27 (95% CI = 0.16–0.46), and 16.01 (95% CI: 7.15–35.82), respectively; and, for estimation of cirrhosis, were 80% (95% CI = 0.75–0.85), 71% (95% CI = 0.68–0.74), 3.13 (95% CI = 2.01–4.87), 0.29 (95% CI = 0.19–0.44), and 14.09 (95% CI: 5.43–36.59), respectively.

Conclusions: The ELF test shows good performance and considerable diagnostic value for the prediction of histological fibrosis stage.

Editor: James Fung, The University of Hong Kong, Hong Kong

Funding: This work was supported by grants from the National Natural Science Foundation of China (No. 81172315/H1617) and the research Special Fund For public welfare industry of health and the translational research of early diagnosis and comprehensive treatment in pancreatic cancer (201202007). The funders had no role in study design, data collection and analysis, decision to publish, or preparation of the manuscript.

Competing Interests: The authors have declared that no competing interests exist.

* E-mail: shusenzheng@zju.edu.cn (SZ); wam@zju.edu.cn (WW)

Introduction

Liver fibrosis is a consequence of various chronic liver diseases, often caused by viruses, alcohol, and fat deposition, and can result in liver cirrhosis. Cirrhosis is the main cause of morbidity and mortality in chronic liver disease, but is often asymptomatic until the synthetic and filtering functions of the liver are finally compromised or portal hypertension develops. In addition, for chronic viral hepatitis, the degree of liver fibrosis is an important parameter for decisions on antiviral therapy [1], so the early detection of fibrosis progression and the development of cirrhosis are important in the management of patients with chronic liver disease.

Presently, a liver biopsy remains the reference standard for evaluating liver fibrosis. However, it is limited by sampling error and the risk of complications [2,3]. Intra- and interobserver variability may lead to misinterpretation of the fibrosis stage [4–7]. One reason for the difficulty in correctly assessing the fibrosis stages may be simply that a biopsy specimen represents only 1/50,000th of the total liver mass [2]. Even with adequate biopsy samples (≥15 mm in length with five or more portal tracts), cirrhosis can be understaged in 10–30% of cases [8]. Moreover, it is usually difficult to undertake biopsies on a repeated basis, because of their invasive nature and complications, such as pain and bleeding.

Thus, much attention has been focused on the development of non-invasive methods, including radiological and biochemical tests, to detect liver fibrosis. Transient elastography for assessing liver stiffness has become available for the evaluation of liver fibrosis as a rapid, non-invasive method. However, this technique is cost-intensive and its availability is largely limited to specialist liver centres. Moreover, liver stiffness measurements can be difficult or impossible in obese patients, in those with narrow

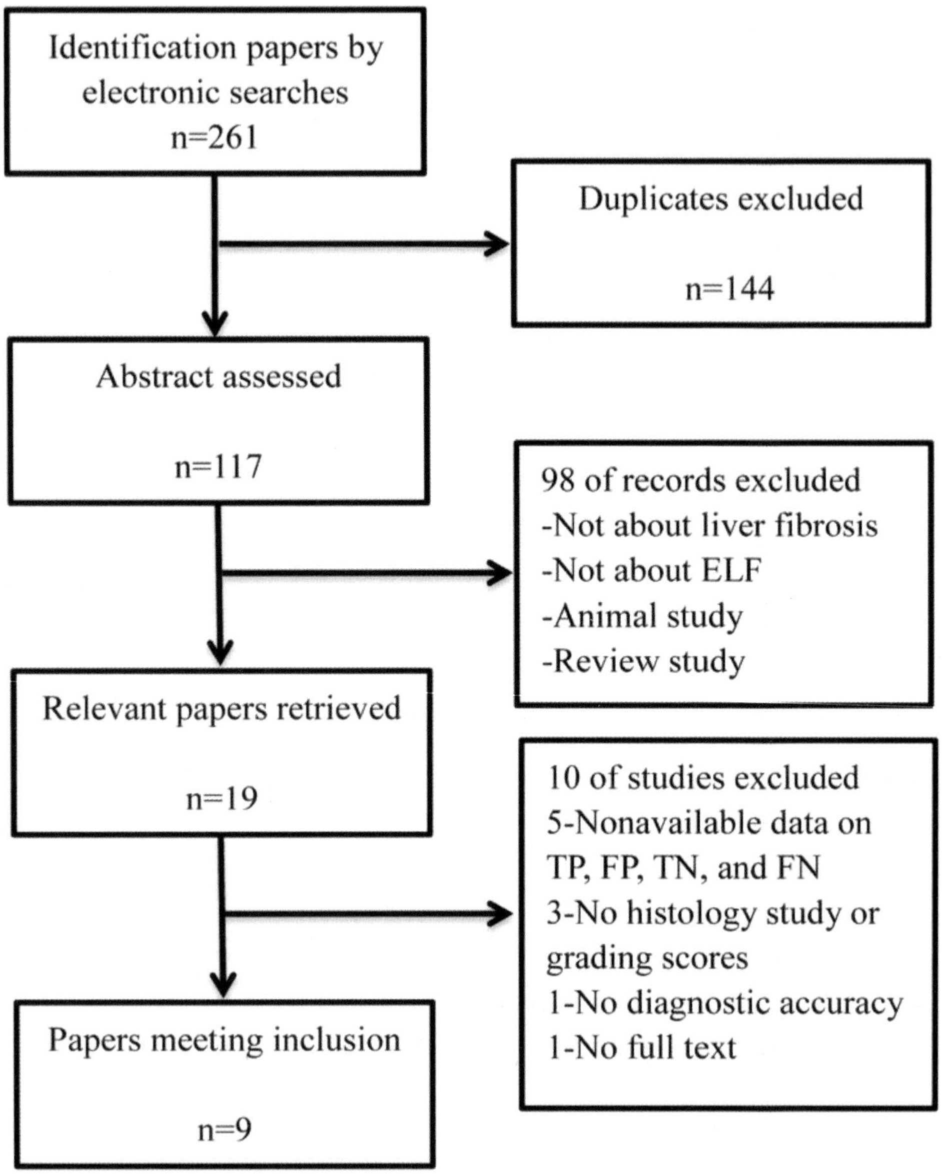

Figure 1. Flowchart for the literature search.

intercostal space, and in patients with ascites [9], and a failure rate up to 18.9% has been reported [10].

Alternative method assessing the degree of liver fibrosis focused on serum biomarkers. The combined use of three serum biomarkers of hyaluronic acid (HA) [11], which is a component of the extracellular matrix (ECM) and is primarily cleared from the bloodstream by the hepatic sinusoids, tissue inhibitors of metalloproteinases (TIMP-1) [12–16] inhibiting the activities of matrix metalloproteinases (MMPs) and amino-terminal propeptide of procollagen type III (PIIINP) [17–20] reflecting collagen synthesis at the site of disease has recently been proposed for the detection of fibrosis. In clinical practice, serum samples were analysed for levels of HA, TIMP-1 and PIIINP. Results were entered into the established algorithm and expressed as discriminant scores. This simplified version of panel was called enhanced liver fibrosis (ELF) score. In other word, a higher concentration of individual biomarkers leads to a higher ELF score and indicates a greater likelihood of more severe fibrosis. The ELF test has several strengths such as better automaticity, high reproducibility, less invasiveness and proven considerable diagnostic performance in the assessment of the degree of liver fibrosis [21–23]. The ELF test has received the Conformité Européénne mark in May 2007 [24].

The aim of this study was to perform a meta-analysis to evaluate the diagnostic accuracy of ELF, with histopathology as a reference standard.

Methods

Search Strategy

A computerised search was performed in PubMed/Medline, EMBASE, the Cochrane Library, and Google Scholar to identify relevant articles published from 2003 to 2013. The literature search was performed with the following terms: cirrhosis, liver fibrosis, and enhanced liver fibrosis test or ELF test. The research was limited to articles concerning humans with an abstract in English. The complete search yielded 260 articles from databases.

Table 1. Characteristic of patients of included studies.

Study	Date	Country	Range time of study	Patients N	Male (%)	Age (mean±SD)	Disease spectrum	Fibrosis stage (%)
Guha, I.N. *et al*	2008	UK	2003–2006	192	64	50±13	CHC, CHB, PBC	F0:41, F1:19, F2:17, F3:13, F4:10
Nobili, V. *et al*	2009	UK	2004–2006	112	56.2	14.1±3.7	NAFLD	F0:33, F1:51.8,F2:8, F3–4:7.2
Friedrich-Rust, M. *et al*	2010	Germany	2005–2008	74	41.9	50±13	CHC, CHB, PBC	F0:5.4,F1:28.4,F2:24.3,F3:27, F4:14.9
Parkes, J. *et al*	2011	UK	1999–2001	347	61	43(19–75)§	CHC	F0:13.3,F1:26.8,F2:31.1,F3–4:28.8
Kim, B.K. *et al*	2012	Korea	2010–1011	170	60	45.3±15.1	CHB	F0:5.9,F1:22.9,F2:21.2,F3:22.4, F4:27.6
Wahl, K *et al*	2012	Germany	NR	102	52	46.6±1.3	VH, AIH, Wilson's diseases, NALFLD, others	F0–1:66.7,F2–4:22.5,F5–6:10.8
Guechot, J. *et al*	2012	France	2007–2008	512	59.8	50(18–79)§	CHB, ALD, CHC, other	F0:6.6,F1:45.1,F2:18,F3:15.4, F4:14.9
Lichtinghagen, R. *et al*	2013	Germany	NR	NR	NR	NR	CHC	F0:26.6,F1–2:24.1,F3–4:12.7,F5–6:36.7
Wong GL	2014	Hong Kong	2006–2009	238	80	50±11	CHB	F0:6, F1:24, F2:29, F3:16, F4:24

§Values are median age and range of age of patients. Abbreviations: NR, not reported; CHC, chronic hepatitis C; CHB, chronic hepatitis B; PBC, primary biliary cirrhosis; NAFLD, Non-Alcoholic Fatty Liver Disease; VH, viral hepatitis; AIH, autoimmune hepatitis; ALD, alcoholic liver disease.

Study Selection and Quality Assessment

Two reviewers (W-L.W. and Q-S.X.) read the titles and abstracts of original articles that addressed the diagnostic accuracy of ELF for staging liver fibrosis in humans to select potentially relevant articles. All of the selected articles were collected and reviewed independently by the same reviewers to determine their eligibility for detailed analysis. The inclusion criteria were as follows: patients with suspected cirrhosis, ELF scores as the index test, defined optimal cut-off values or a threshold of ELF, histopathology as the reference test, and raw data (i.e., true-positive (TP), false-positive (FP), true-negative (TN), and false-negative (FN) results could be found or calculated). Exclusion criteria were duplicate publication (based on the same primary study) and sample size of less than 20. Disagreements between the two reviewers regarding study inclusion were resolved by consensus after a face-to-face discussion. Investigators in the primary research were approached for additional information as necessary.

The methodological quality of each study was assessed using a checklist based on the Quality Assessment for Studies of Diagnostic Accuracy (QUADAS) tool [25], which enables reviewers to evaluate the quality of studies, especially investigations of diagnostic accuracy [26,27].

Data Extraction

Data were extracted from primary studies by the two reviewers (W-L.W. and Q-S.X.) independently. In cases of discrepancies between the first two reviewers, a senior surgeon (S-S.Z.), with more than 20 years of experience in hepatic disease, was consulted and a consensus was reached. We defined significant fibrosis as a fibrosis stage ≥ 2 for studies using grading systems with five stages (F0–F4; i.e., the METAVIR, Brunt, Batts-Ludwig systems) or as a fibrosis stage ≥ 3 for studies using the Ishak scoring system (S0–S6). For grading systems using five stages or the Ishak scoring system, severe fibrosis was defined as a fibrosis stage ≥ 3 or ≥ 4, and cirrhosis was defined as a fibrosis stage = 4 or ≥ 5, respectively [28]. We extracted available data on TPs, FNs, FPs, and TNs for staging liver fibrosis to construct a 2×2 contingency table.

Data Synthesis and Statistical Analysis

From the extracted data, arranged in 2×2 contingency tables, we computed sensitivity, specificity, and diagnostic odds ratios (DORS) to estimate the diagnostic performance of each test modality to assess each stage of liver fibrosis. All statistics are reported as point values with 95% confidence intervals (CIs). Sensitivity was defined by the TP rate and was calculated as TP/(TP+FN). Specificity was defined by the TN rate and was calculated as TN/(FP+TN). The DOR is a single overall indicator of diagnostic performance and is the ratio of the odds of positivity in disease subjects relative to the odds of positivity in non-diseased subjects [29]. The DOR was calculated as $(TP\times TN)/(FP\times FN)$.

The performance was summarised using a bivariate binomial model [30]. This model assumed a binomial distribution for the number of patients with TP and TN results and allowed the inclusion of covariates and random effects. The inherent association between sensitivity and specificity was modelled in a bivariate normal distribution by assuming random effects [31].

The heterogeneity of all diagnostic test parameters was evaluated initially with a graphic examination of forest plots for each parameter. A statistical assessment was then made of the inconsistency index (I^2). The I^2 statistic is defined as the percentage of variability due to heterogeneity beyond that from chance; values greater than 50% represent the possibility of substantial heterogeneity. The pooled summary statistics for the sensitivities,

Table 2. Test characteristics and histological scoring system of included studies of ELF for the assessment of fibrosis.

Study	Reference test	Histological scoring system	Liver biopsy length(mm)	Fibrosis Stage	Cut-off Value	Sensitivity	Specificity	Positive predictive value	Negative predictive Value	AUROC value (95%CI)
Guha, I.N. ***et al***	liver biopsy	NIDDKD	NR	≥F2	−0.11	0.7	0.8	0.7	0.8	0.82(0.75–0.88)
				≥F3	0.357§	0.8	0.9	0.71	0.94	0.9(0.84–0.96)
Nobili, V. ***et al***	liver biopsy	Modified Brunt	20.7±2.3	≥F2	10.18	0.94	0.93	0.7	0.99	0.98(0.96–1)
				≥F3	10.51	1	0.98	0.8	1	0.99(0.97–1)
Friedrich-Rust, M. ***et al***	liver biopsy	METAVIR	22.3±9.3	≥F2	9.78	0.78	0.8	0.88	0.65	0.78(0.67–0.89)
				≥F3	10.22	0.74	0.7	0.64	0.79	0.79(0.67–0.91)
				= F4	10.31	0.91	0.62	0.29	0.98	0.92(0.83–1)
Parkes, J. ***et al***	liver biopsy	METAVIR/Ishak	NR	= F5–6	10.48§	0.62	0.89	0.73	0.83	0.86(0.83–0.89)
Kim, B.K. ***et al***	liver biopsy	Batts-Ludwig	21.3±0.7	≥F2	8.5	0.86	0.857	0.937	0.712	0.901(0.849–0.953)
				≥F3	9.4	0.835	0.777	0.789	0.825	0.86(0.805–0.915)
				= F4	10.1	0.702	0.789	0.559	0.874	0.862(0.809–0.915)
Wahl, K. ***et al***	liver biopsy	Ishak	18.9±2.1	≥F2	8.99	0.86	0.7	NR	NR	0.87(0.78–0.96)
				= F5–6	9.39	1	0.77	NR	NR	0.93(0.88–0.99)
Guechot, J. ***et al***	liver biopsy	METAVIR	25.1±8.8	≥F2	9	0.86	0.62	0.8	0.7	0.78(0.74–0.82)
				≥F3	9.33	0.9	0.63	0.73	0.85	0.82(0.78–0.86)
				= F4	9.35	0.83	0.75	0.44	0.95	0.85(0.81–0.9)
Lichtinghagen, R. ***et al***	liver biopsy	Ishak	NR	≥F3	9.8	0.846	0.75	NR	NR	0.95(NR)
				= F5–6	11.3	0.828	0.96	NR	NR	0.9(NR)
Wong GL. ***et§al***	liver biopsy	METAVIR	NR	≥F3	9.8	0.62	0.66	0.55	0.72	0.69(0.63–0.75)
				= F4	9.5	0.78	0.47	0.31	0.88	0.68(0.61–0.75)

§Values are diagnostic threshold. Abbreviations: NR, not reported; NIDDKD, National Institute of Diabetes and Digestive and Kidney Diseases.

Table 3. Characteristics and performance of three studies comparing ELF test with transient elastography (TE).

Study	Patient N	Fibrosis stage (%)	Methods	Fibrosis Stage	Cut-off Value	Sensitivity	Specificity	Positive predictive value	Negative predictive Value	AUROC value (95%CI)
Friedrich-Rust, M. *et al* 2010	102	F0:5.4,F1:28.4, F2:24.3,F3:27, F4:14.9	ELF	≥F2	9.78	0.78	0.8	0.88	0.65	0.78(0.67–0.89)
				≥F3	10.22	0.74	0.7	0.64	0.79	0.79(0.67–0.91)
				=F4	10.31	0.91	0.62	0.29	0.98	0.92(0.83–1)
			TE	≥F2	7.2 kPa	0.64	0.76	0.85	0.5	0.8(0.69–0.91)
				≥F3	12.5 kPa	0.5	0.87	0.74	0.76	0.66(0.51–0.82)
				=F4	17.6 kPa	0.82	0.91	0.64	0.78	0.94(0.86–1)
Kim, B.K. *et al* 2012	170	F0:5.9,F1:22.9, F2:21.2,F3:22.4, F4:27.6	ELF	≥F2	8.5	0.86	0.857	0.937	0.712	0.901(0.849–0.953)
				≥F3	9.4	0.835	0.777	0.789	0.825	0.86(0.805–0.915)
				=F4	10.1	0.702	0.789	0.559	0.874	0.862(0.809–0.915)
			TE	≥F2	8 kPa	0.777	0.959	9.979	0.635	0.937(0.903–0.971)
				≥F3	10.1 kPa	0.906	0.965	0.962	0.911	0.956(0.929–0.983)
				=F4	14 kPa	0.872	0.91	0.788	0.949	0.963(0.937–0.989)
Wahl, K *et al* 2012	102	F0–1:66.7,F2–4:22.5, F5–6:10.8	ELF	≥F2	8.99	0.86	0.7	NR	NR	0.87(0.78–0.96)
				≥F5	9.39	1	0.77	NR	NR	0.93(0.88–0.99)
			TE	≥F2	8.5 kPa	0.86	0.73	NR	NR	0.92(0.85–0.98)
				≥F5	17.45	0.91	1	NR	NR	0.95(0.87–1)
Wong GL *et§al* 2014	238	F0:6,F1:24, F2:29,F3:16, F4:24	ELF	≥F3	9.8	0.62	0.66	0.55	0.72	0.69(0.63–0.75)
				=F4	9.5	0.78	0.47	0.31	0.88	0.68(0.61–0.75)
			TE	≥F3	9 kPa	0.64	0.84	0.69	0.76	0.83(0.76–0.91)
				=F4	10 kPa	0.78	0.81	0.56	0.93	0.9(0.84–0.96)

Abbreviations: ELF, enhanced liver fibrosis; TE, transient elastography.

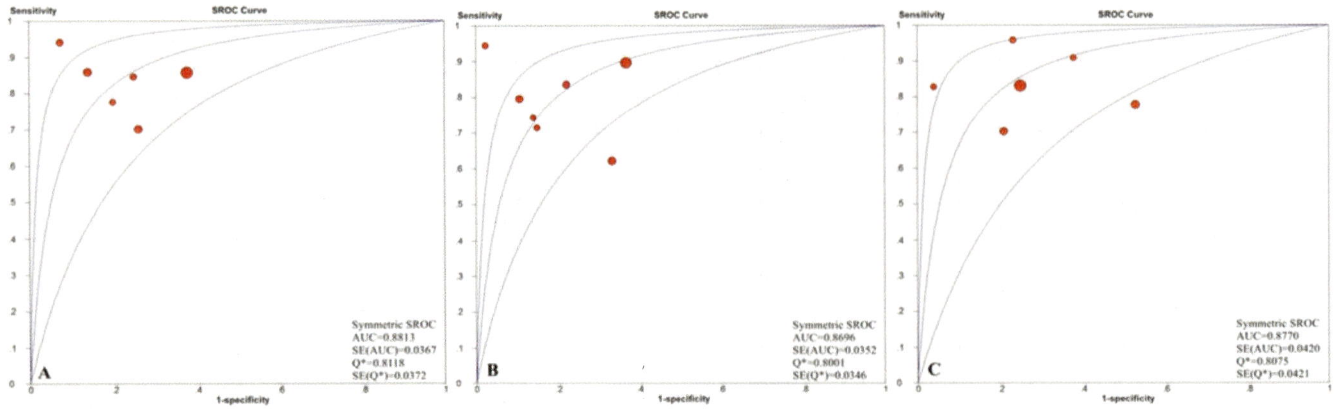

Figure 2. The SROC curves for the studies examining ELF test versus liver biopsy for the assessment of (A) significant liver fibrosis, (B) severe liver fibrosis and (C) cirrhosis.

specificities, likelihood ratios, and diagnostic odds ratios of the individual studies are reported.

Summary receiver operating characteristic (SROC) curves were also constructed to express the test parameter results as the diagnostic odds ratios. These curves were also used to assess the presence of a diagnostic threshold (cut-off) bias as a cause of between-study heterogeneity. Analyses were performed using the Meta-Disc 1.4 statistical software (Unit of the Clinical Biostatistics team of the Ramón y Cajal Hospital in Madrid, Spain).

Results

Study Characteristics

Figure 1 depicts the flow of our search results. In total, 261 studies were identified using electronic searches. Without duplicates, 117 abstracts were assessed. Of them, 19 seemed relevant and the full studies were assessed. Ultimately, nine investigations were identified for inclusion in this study [32–40]. Quality assessment scores for the diagnostic studies were above 10 of the 14 QUADAS items describing methodological quality.

The nine studies evaluated involved 1826 patients from Asian and European medical centres. In four trials, the disease spectrum was restricted to chronic viral hepatitis, in one trial to non-alcoholic fatty liver disease (NAFLD), and in four trials, there was no restriction (Table 1).

Five studies reported quality criteria for liver biopsy specimens [32,34,36–38], and three investigations reported a minimum length of 15 mm [33,35,39]. The Ishak histological scoring system was used in three studies [35,38,39], the National Institute of Diabetes and Digestive and Kidney Diseases system was used in one study [33], the modified Brunt system was used in one study [32], the Batts-Ludwig system was used in one study [37], and the METAVIR system was used in four studies [34–36,40] (Table 2). Moreover, there are four studies [34,37,38,40] comparing the performance of ELF test with transient elastograhpy (TE) for staging liver fibrosis (Table 3).

The demographic and clinical features of the patients in the studies analysed are listed in Table 1. The median sample size of the studies assessing the presence of significant liver fibrosis was 141 (range, 74–512) [32–34,36,37,39], the median sample size of

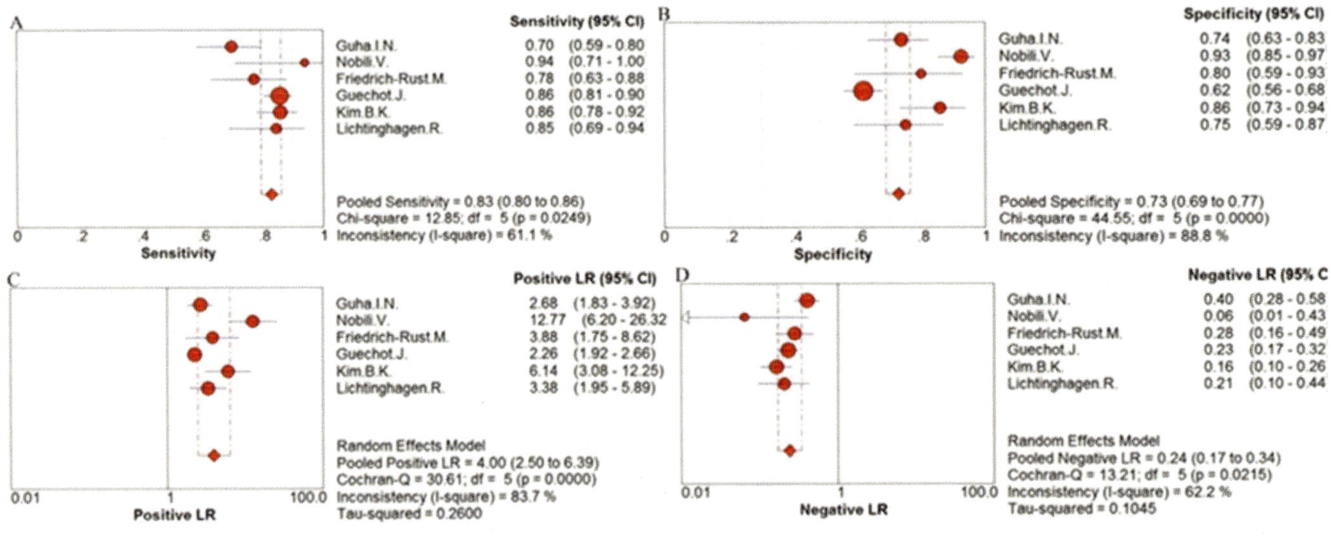

Figure 3. Forest plot and meta-analysis of studies assessing (A) the sensitivity, (B) the specificity, (C) the positive LR and (D) the negative LR of ELF test versus biopsy for the detection of significant liver fibrosis.

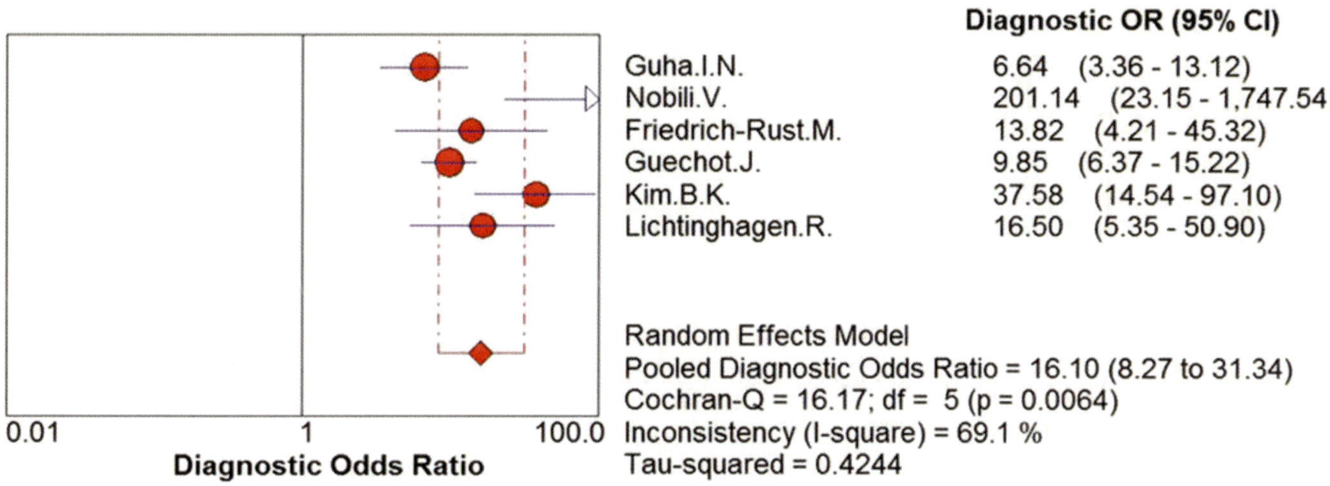

Figure 4. Forest plot and meta-analysis of studies appraising the diagnostic odds ratio of ELF test versus liver biopsy for the assessment of significant liver fibrosis.

the studies assessing the presence of severe liver fibrosis was 181 (range, 74–512) [32–37,40], and the median sample size of the studies assessing the presence of cirrhosis was 102 (range, 74–512) [34,36–39,40].

In the studies analysed, the median proportion of individuals with cirrhosis was 14.9% (range, 10–36.7%). The diagnostic cut-off values ranged from 8.5 to 10.18 for significant liver fibrosis [32–34,36,37,39], from 9.33 to 10.51 for severe liver fibrosis [32–37,40], and from 9.35 to 11.3 [32,34–37,40] for cirrhosis.

Diagnostic Threshold Bias and Meta-Regression Assessment

To assess the diagnostic threshold (cut-off) bias as a cause of heterogeneity in test performance, we prepared an ROC plot of the sensitivity versus 1-the specificity. Among the six primary studies providing data for the detection of significant liver fibrosis, the diagnostic threshold (cut-off) yielded an area under receiver operating characteristic (AUROC) of 0.8813, among another seven primary studies providing data for the assessment of severe liver fibrosis, the diagnostic threshold (cut-off) yielded an AUROC of 0.8696, among another six primary studies providing data for the prediction of cirrhosis, the diagnostic threshold (cut-off) yielded an AUROC of 0.8770, and they all revealed evidence supporting the diagnostic threshold (cut-off) bias as a major cause of heterogeneity(Fig. 2).

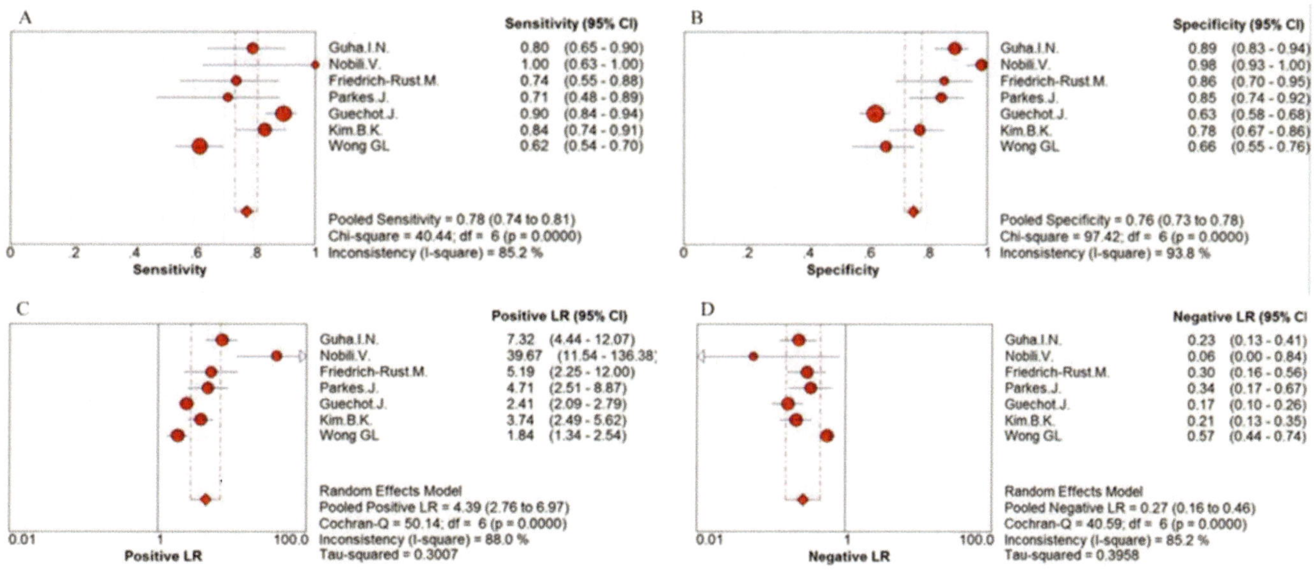

Figure 5. Forest plot and meta-analysis of studies estimating (A) the sensitivity, (B) the specificity, (C) the positive LR and (D) the negative LR of ELF test versus liver biopsy for the detection of severe liver fibrosis.

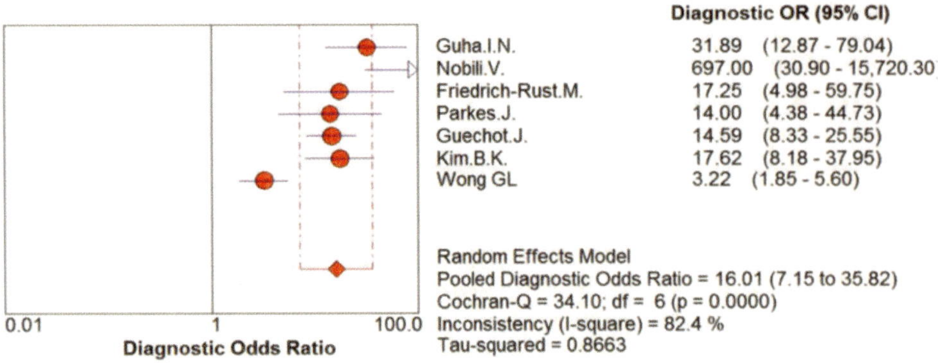

Figure 6. Forest plot and meta-analysis of studies assessing the diagnostic odds ratio of ELF test versus liver biopsy for the measurement of severe liver fibrosis.

Summary Estimates of Primary Studies

For the assessment of significant liver fibrosis, the sensitivity values of ELF ranged from 70% to 94%, and the pooled sensitivity value was 83% (95% CI = 0.8–0.86, P = 0.0249, I^2 = 61.1%). The specificity values ranged from 62% to 93%, and the pooled specificity value was 73% (95% CI = 0.69–0.77, P<0.0001, I^2 = 88.8%). The pooled positive likelihood ratio was 4.00 (95% CI = 2.03–6.39, P<0.0001, I^2 = 83.7), and the pooled negative likelihood ratio was 0.24 (95% CI = 0.17–0.34, P = 0.0215, I^2 = 62.2%) (Fig. 3) The summary diagnostic odds ratio was 16.10 (95% CI = 8.27–31.34, P = 0.0064, I^2 = 69.1%) (Fig. 4).

For the prediction of severe liver fibrosis, the sensitivity values of ELF test ranged from 62% to 100%, and the pooled sensitivity value was 78% (95% CI = 0.74–0.81, P<0.0001, I^2 = 85.2%). The specificity values ranged from 66% to 98%, and the pooled specificity value was 76% (95% CI = 0.73–0.78, P<0.0001, I^2 = 93.8%). The pooled positive likelihood ratio was 4.39 (95% CI = 2.76–6.97, P<0.0001, I^2 = 88.0%), and the pooled negative likelihood ratio was 0.27 (95% CI = 0.16–0.46, P<0.0001, I^2 = 85.2%) (Fig. 5) The summary diagnostic odds ratio was 16.01 (95% CI = 7.15–35.82, P<0.0001, I^2 = 82.4%) (Fig. 6).

For the evaluation of cirrhosis, the sensitivity values of ELF test ranged from 70% to 100%, and the pooled sensitivity value was 80% (95% CI = 0.75–0.85, P = 0.0987, I^2 = 46.1%). The specificity values ranged from 47% to 95%, and the pooled specificity value was 71% (95% CI: 0.68–0.74, P<0.0001, I^2 = 99.3%). The pooled positive likelihood ratio was 3.13 (95% CI = 2.01–4.87, P< 0.0001, I^2 = 91.4%), and the pooled negative likelihood ratio was 0.29 (95% CI = 0.19–0.44, P = 0.0646, I^2 = 51.9%) (Fig. 7) The summary diagnostic odds ratio was 14.09 (95% CI = 5.43–36.59, P = 0.0002, I^2 = 79.3%) (Fig. 8).

Two [34,38] of the 4 studies [34,37,38,40] comparing the performance of ELF test with TE for assessment of cirrhosis reported that ELF test has a higher sensitivity, while the all 3 studies [34,37,38,40] uncovered TE has a preferable performance of specificity. More specifically, compared to ELF test that revealed a pooled sensitivity of 78% (95% CI = 0.70–0.85, P = 0.0401, I^2 = 63.9%), a specificity of 64% (95% CI = 0.59–0.69, P<0.0001, I^2 = 92.5%) and an AUROC of 0.7947, the

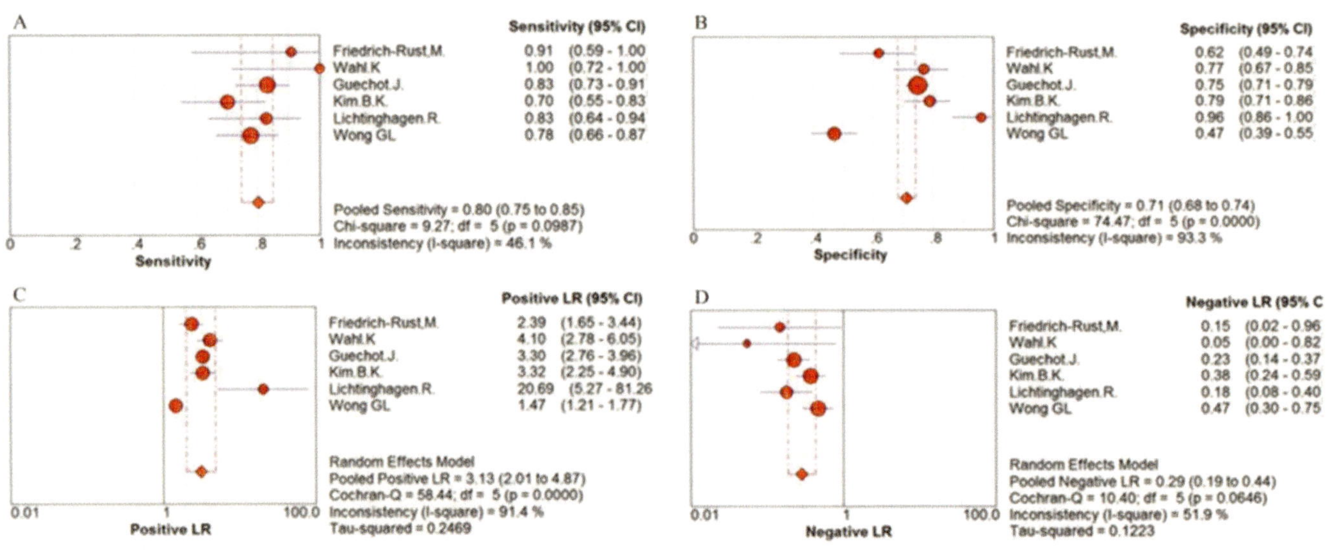

Figure 7. Forest plot and meta-analysis of studies evaluating (A) the sensitivity, (B) the specificity, (C) the positive LR and (D) the negative LR of ELF test versus liver biopsy for the detection of cirrhosis.

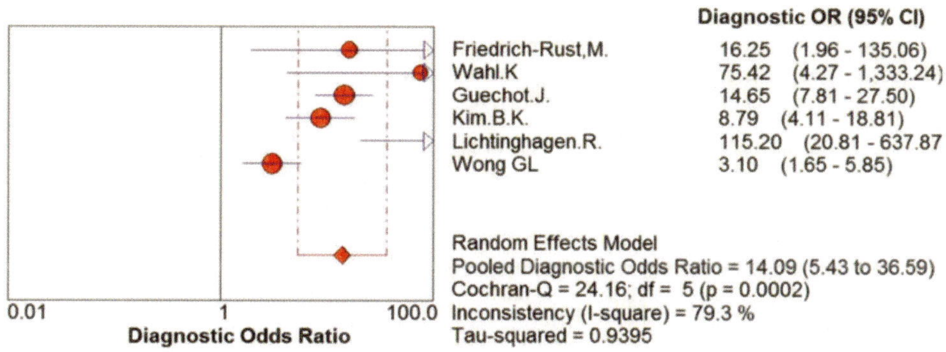

Figure 8. Forest plot and meta-analysis of studies assessing the diagnostic odds ratio of ELF test versus liver biopsy for the prediction of cirrhosis.

transient elastography showed a higher pooled sensitivity 82% (95% CI = 0.75–0.88, P = 0.4820, $I^2 = 0.0\%$), a higher pooled specificity 89% (95% CI = 0.86–0.92, P<0.0001, $I^2 = 90.5\%$) and a higher AUROC (0.8812) for detection of cirrhosis(Fig. 9, Fig. 10, Fig. 11).

Discussion

Information on the presence and degree of liver fibrosis is pivotal for making therapeutic decisions and predicting disease outcomes [41]. For example, the ultimate goal of treatment at the stage of significant liver fibrosis is to prevent the potential pathogenesis of liver disease [41,42]. In contrast, given that the severe liver fibrosis or cirrhosis may have a risk of progression to hypertension and HCC, discrimination of severe liver fibrosis and cirrhosis is important [42]. The increasing awareness of the limitations of liver biopsies [43,44] has stimulated the development and refinement of non-invasive techniques for the assessment of liver fibrosis. Theoretically, non-invasive techniques for the assessment of liver fibrosis should possess the advantages of liver specificity, easy execution, and high diagnostic performance, in terms of sensitivity, specificity, DOR, PLR, NLR, and AUROC. The most studied non-invasive detection method for liver fibrosis is transient elastography, but it has shown less accuracy in discriminating lower fibrosis stages [45,46] and restricted by narrow intercostal space and ascites.

Studies have confirmed that the ELF test can accurately determine the degree of liver fibrosis [32,47–49] and revealed a lower significance for discrimination of low and moderate fibrosis stages and a broad overlapping range for those stages [38]. In the three subgroups of this meta-analysis, the pooled sensitivity, pooled specificity, and summary DOR of the ELF test were greater than 80%, 74%, and 17, respectively. That indicates that at least 74% of patients could reasonably avoid a liver biopsy. With summary AUROCs of 0.8813, 0.8696, and 0.8770 for significant and severe liver fibrosis and cirrhosis, respectively, the results of this meta-analysis demonstrate that ELF has good diagnostic performance for assessing liver fibrosis.

A diagnostic tool is deemed perfect if the AUROC is 100%, excellent if the AUROC is greater than 90%, and good if the

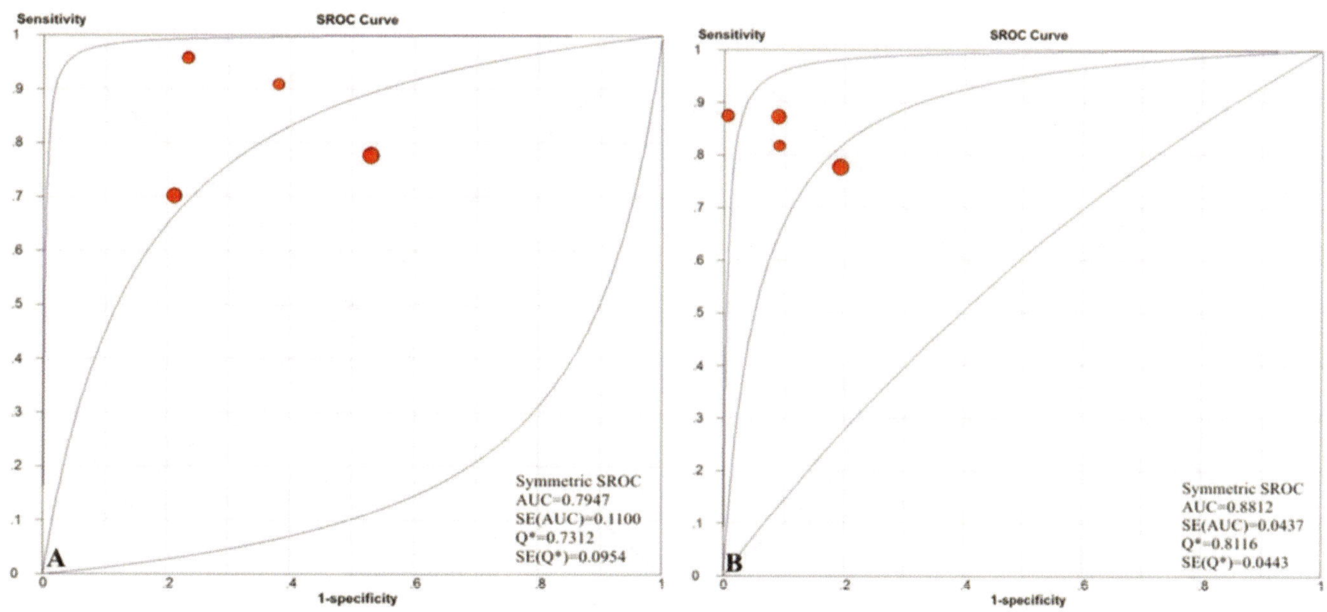

Figure 9. The comparison of SROC curves between (A) ELF test and (B) transient elastogrphy for assessment of cirrhosis.

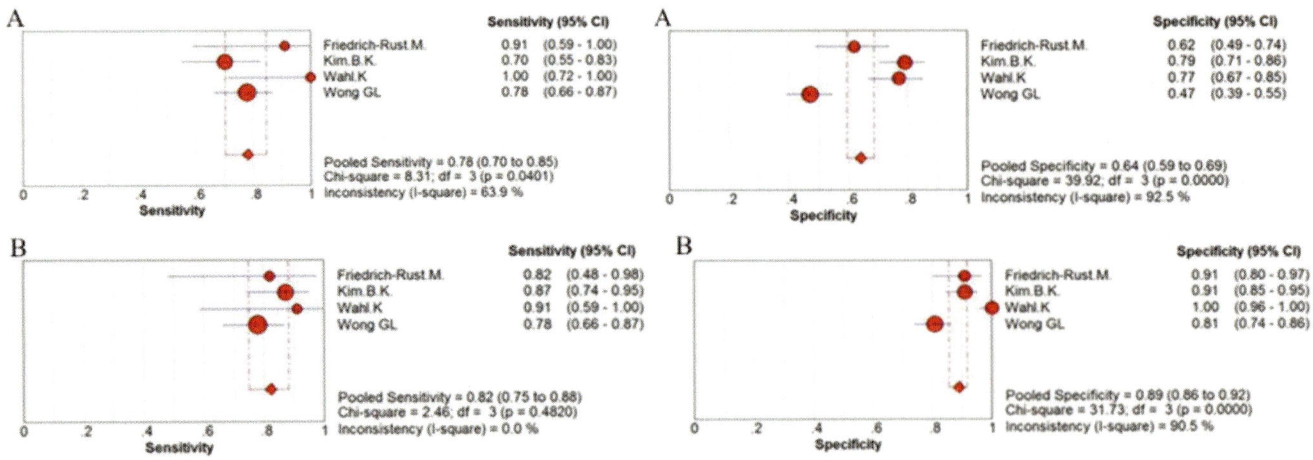

Figure 10. The comparison of sensitivity and specificity between (A) ELF test and (B) transient elastography for assessment of cirrhosis.

AUROC is greater than 80% [50]. According to these results, coupled with its reproducibility, the ELF test can be used in clinical practice as a good tool for the staging of cirrhosis. The fine performance of the ELF test may result from the fact that serum markers reflect fibrosis in the whole liver rather than $1/50{,}000^{\text{th}}$ of the organ, as does a biopsy sample, or, alternatively, that the ELF test evaluates the impact of liver fibrosis on liver function as well as the architectural damage associated with histological fibrosis and cirrhosis.

It is worth noting that the ELF test showed a high correlation with aminotransferase levels and revealed a significantly high correlation with inflammation [38]. One study [47] found that the ELF test, reflecting on-going pathophysiological processes and functions that a biopsy cannot capture, had prognostic value. The ELF test, an index of HA, PIIINP, and TIMP-1, exhibited prognostic ability even in the early stages of the disease process (AUROC = 0.737–0.863 at all times points) [48], because, probably, the above indices are expressed during the early stages of collagen deposition in the liver. In further analysis of ELF test performance in predicting all-cause mortality, it was found that the AUROC of the ELF test at 6 years was significantly greater than that of a biopsy [47].

In future, the ELF test may be used to evaluate the impact of treatment directed at the underlying causes, such as viral hepatitis,

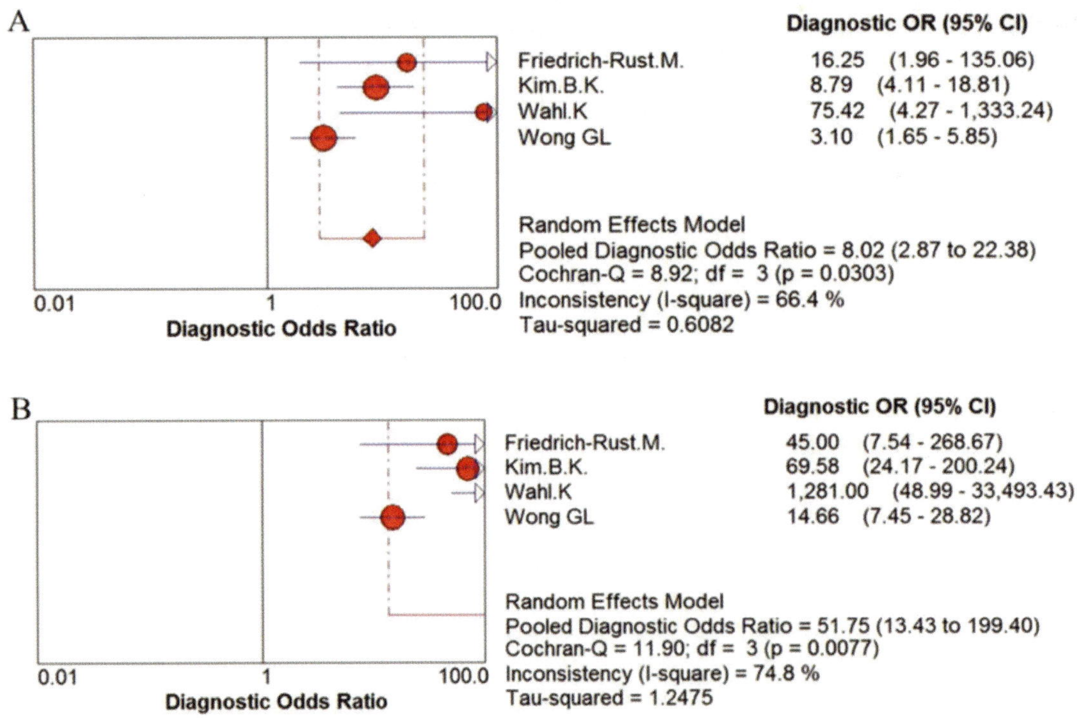

Figure 11. The comparison of diagnostic odds ratio between (A) ELF test and (B) transient elastography for assessment of cirrhosis.

and in the development of new treatments, such as anti-fibrotic drugs.

Indeed, there was significant heterogeneity in this meta-analysis, which may be due to the following reasons. First, differences in study methodologies are well-recognised causes of heterogeneity in meta-analyses of diagnostic tests. Second, subtle variations in the algorithm of the ELF score and liver biopsy may also contribute to between-study variation. Third, the use of different histological scoring systems may result in discrepancies in the findings of the studies. The studies included in this meta-analysis used five histological scoring systems. Although the histological staging system is complex, it is relevant for the assessment, follow-up, and definition of the rate of fibrosis progression, and is also categorical in nature. The current reliance on histological staging using categorical scores for liver biopsy samples is recognised as suboptimal for assessing efficacy, and this may be a source of heterogeneity [51]. Fourth, the size of liver biopsy tissue cores may impact the accuracy of liver fibrosis staging. Criteria for liver biopsy specimens (≥20 mm in length and/or 11 portal tracts) have been described previously [8]. However, in practice, it is difficult for biopsy samples to achieve these criteria. In this meta-analysis, the mean length of specimens ranged from 18.9 to 25.1 mm, so no study reported liver biopsy samples meeting the criteria, and only two studies [32,36] described liver biopsy specimens with 11 complete portal tracts. Thus, the observed heterogeneity may be secondary to intrinsic errors in liver biopsy measurements, which limit the diagnostic accuracy of non-invasive evaluations [52,53]. Fifth, a diagnostic threshold (or cut-off value) bias was identified as an important cause of heterogeneity in the pooled results for the three patient groups. In this meta-analysis, there was no consistent cut-off value, which would also generate heterogeneity. Finally, publication bias may also have resulted in heterogeneity in this meta-analysis because we excluded some studies having no full text and published in languages other than English.

In summary, the ELF test showed good performance and considerable diagnostic value for the prediction of histological fibrosis stage and can be deemed a 'good' diagnostic tool in clinical practice for the staging of cirrhosis.

Acknowledgments

This manuscript has been edited and proofread by Textcheck and the certificate can beacquired from the following link. http://www.textcheck.com/login.

Author Contributions

Conceived and designed the experiments: SZ WW QX. Performed the experiments: QX XZ PH. Analyzed the data: QX JW. Wrote the paper: SZ WW QX.

References

1. National Institutes of Health Consensus Development Conference (2002) National Institutes of Health Consensus Development Conference Statement: Management of hepatitis C: 2002; June 10–12, 2002; Hepatology 36: S3–20.
2. Bravo AA, Sheth SG, Chopra S (2001) Liver biopsy. N Engl J Med 344: 495–500.
3. Castera L, Negre I, Samii K, Buffet C (1999) Pain experienced during percutaneous liver biopsy. Hepatology 30: 1529–1530.
4. Bedossa P, Dargere D, Paradis V (2003) Sampling variability of liver fibrosis in chronic hepatitis C. Hepatology 38: 1449–1457.
5. Rousselet MC, Michalak S, Dupre F, Croue A, Bedossa P, et al. (2005) Sources of variability in histological scoring of chronic viral hepatitis. Hepatology 41: 257–264.
6. Afdhal NH (2003) Diagnosing fibrosis in hepatitis C: is the pendulum swinging from biopsy to blood tests? Hepatology 37: 972–974.
7. Regev A, Berho M, Jeffers LJ, Milikowski C, Molina EG, et al. (2002) Sampling error and intraobserver variation in liver biopsy in patients with chronic HCV infection. Am J Gastroenterol 97: 2614–2618.
8. Afdhal NH, Nunes D (2004) Evaluation of liver fibrosis: a concise review. Am J Gastroenterol 99: 1160–1174.
9. Sandrin L, Fourquet B, Hasquenoph JM, Yon S, Fournier C, et al. (2003) Transient elastography: a new noninvasive method for assessment of hepatic fibrosis. Ultrasound Med Biol 29: 1705–1713.
10. Castera L, Foucher J, Bernard PH, Carvalho F, Allaix D, et al. (2010) Pitfalls of liver stiffness measurement: a 5-year prospective study of 13,369 examinations. Hepatology 51: 828–835.
11. Eriksson S, Fraser JR, Laurent TC, Pertoft H, Smedsrod B (1983) Endothelial cells are a site of uptake and degradation of hyaluronic acid in the liver. Exp Cell Res 144: 223–228.
12. Gomez DE, Alonso DF, Yoshiji H, Thorgeirsson UP (1997) Tissue inhibitors of metalloproteinases: structure, regulation and biological functions. Eur J Cell Biol 74: 111–122.
13. Arthur MJ, Mann DA, Iredale JP (1998) Tissue inhibitors of metalloproteinases, hepatic stellate cells and liver fibrosis. J Gastroenterol Hepatol 13 Suppl: S33–38.
14. Prakobwong S, Pinlaor S, Yongvanit P, Sithithaworn P, Pairojkul C, et al. (2009) Time profiles of the expression of metalloproteinases, tissue inhibitors of metalloproteases, cytokines and collagens in hamsters infected with Opisthorchis viverrini with special reference to peribiliary fibrosis and liver injury. Int J Parasitol 39: 825–835.
15. Kossakowska AE, Edwards DR, Lee SS, Urbanski LS, Stabbler AL, et al. (1998) Altered balance between matrix metalloproteinases and their inhibitors in experimental biliary fibrosis. Am J Pathol 153: 1895–1902.
16. Herbst H, Wege T, Milani S, Pellegrini G, Orzechowski HD, et al. (1997) Tissue inhibitor of metalloproteinase-1 and -2 RNA expression in rat and human liver fibrosis. Am J Pathol 150: 1647–1659.
17. Kivirikko KI, Myllyla R (1985) Post-translational processing of procollagens. Ann N Y Acad Sci 460: 187–201.
18. Horslev-Petersen K (1990) Circulating extracellular matrix components as markers for connective tissue response to inflammation. A clinical and experimental study with special emphasis on serum aminoterminal type III procollagen peptide in rheumatic diseases. Dan Med Bull 37: 308–329.
19. Entzian P, Huckstadt A, Kreipe H, Barth J (1990) Determination of serum concentrations of type III procollagen peptide in mechanically ventilated patients. Pronounced augmented concentrations in the adult respiratory distress syndrome. Am Rev Respir Dis 142: 1079–1082.
20. Waydhas C, Nast-Kolb D, Trupka A, Lenk S, Duswald KH, et al. (1993) Increased serum concentrations of procollagen type III peptide in severely injured patients: an indicator of fibrosing activity? Crit Care Med 21: 240–247.
21. Zarski JP, Sturm N, Guechot J, Zafrani ES, Vaubourdolle M, et al. (2013) Contribution of the ELFG test in algorithms of non-invasive markers towards the diagnosis of significant fibrosis in chronic hepatitis C. PLoS One 8: e59088.
22. Yoo EJ, Kim BK, Kim SU, Park JY, Kim do Y, et al. (2013) Normal enhanced liver fibrosis (ELF) values in apparently healthy subjects undergoing a health check-up and in living liver donors in South Korea. Liver Int 33: 706–713.
23. Janciauskiene S, Wallmark A, Piitulainen E, Kohnlein T, Welted T, et al. (2011) Performance of enhanced liver fibrosis plasma markers in asymptomatic individuals with ZZ alpha1-antitrypsin deficiency. Eur J Gastroenterol Hepatol 23: 716–720.
24. National Institute for Health Research National Horizon Scanning Centre (2008) Enhanced Liver Fibrosis Test (ELF) for evaluating liver fibrosis. Birmingham: National Horizon Scanning Centre 2008.
25. Whiting P, Rotes AW, Reitman JB, Bossuet PM, Keenen J (2003) The development of QUADAS: a tool for the quality assessment of studies of diagnostic accuracy included in systematic reviews. BMC Med Res Methodol 3: 25.
26. Hollingworth W, Medina LS, Lenkinski RE, Shibata DK, Bernal B, et al. (2006) Interrater reliability in assessing quality of diagnostic accuracy studies using the QUADAS tool. A preliminary assessment. Acad Radiol 13: 803–810.
27. Whiting P, Harbord R, de Salis I, Egger M, Sterne J (2008) Evidence-based diagnosis. J Health Serv Res Policy 13 Suppl 3: 57–63.
28. Ishak K, Baptista A, Bianchi L, Callea F, De Groote J, et al. (1995) Histological grading and staging of chronic hepatitis. J Hepatol 22: 696–699.
29. Glas AS, Lijmer JG, Prins MH, Bonsel GJ, Bossuet PM (2003) The diagnostic odds ratio: a single indicator of test performance. J Clin Epidemiol 56: 1129–1135.
30. Reitman JB, Glas AS, Rotes AW, Scholten RJ, Bossuet PM, et al. (2005) Bivariate analysis of sensitivity and specificity produces informative summary measures in diagnostic reviews. J Clin Epidemiol 58: 982–990.

31. Chu H, Cole SR (2006) Bivariate meta-analysis of sensitivity and specificity with sparse data: a generalized linear mixed model approach. J Clin Epidemiol 59: 1331–1332; author reply 1332–1333.
32. Nobili V, Parkes J, Bottazzo G, Marcellini M, Cross R, et al. (2009) Performance of ELF serum markers in predicting fibrosis stage in pediatric non-alcoholic fatty liver disease. Gastroenterology 136: 160–167.
33. Guha IN, Parkes J, Roderick P, Chattopadhyay D, Cross R, et al. (2008) Noninvasive markers of fibrosis in nonalcoholic fatty liver disease: Validating the European Liver Fibrosis Panel and exploring simple markers. Hepatology 47: 455–460.
34. Friedrich-Rust M, Rosenberg W, Parkes J, Herrmann E, Zeuzem S, et al. (2010) Comparison of ELF, FibroTest and FibroScan for the non-invasive assessment of liver fibrosis. BMC Gastroenterol 10: 103.
35. Parkes J, Guha IN, Roderick P, Harris S, Cross R, et al. (2011) Enhanced Liver Fibrosis (ELF) test accurately identifies liver fibrosis in patients with chronic hepatitis C. J Viral Hepat 18: 23–31.
36. Guechot J, Trocme C, Renversez JC, Sturm N, Zarski JP (2012) Independent validation of the Enhanced Liver Fibrosis (ELF) score in the ANRS HC EP 23 Fibrostar cohort of patients with chronic hepatitis C. Clin Chem Lab Med 50: 693–699.
37. Kim BK, Kim HS, Park JY, Kim do Y, Ahn SH, et al. (2012) Prospective validation of ELF test in comparison with Fibroscan and FibroTest to predict liver fibrosis in Asian subjects with chronic hepatitis B. PLoS One 7: e41964.
38. Wahl K, Rosenberg W, Vaske B, Manns MP, Schulze-Osthoff K, et al. (2012) Biopsy-controlled liver fibrosis staging using the enhanced liver fibrosis (ELF) score compared to transient elastography. PLoS One 7: e51906.
39. Lichtinghagen R, Pietsch D, Bantel H, Manns MP, Brand K, et al. (2013) The Enhanced Liver Fibrosis (ELF) score: Normal values, influence factors and proposed cut-off values. J Hepatol 59: 236–242.
40. Wong GL, Chan HL, Choi PC, Chan AW, Yu Z, et al. (2014) Non-invasive algorithm of enhanced liver fibrosis and liver stiffness measurement with transient elastography for advanced liver fibrosis in chronic hepatitis B. Aliment Pharmacol Ther. 39: 197–208.
41. Ghany MG, Strader DB, Thomas DL, Seeff LB (2009) Diagnosis, management, and treatment of hepatitis C: an update. Hepatology 49: 1335–1374.
42. Friedrich-Rust M, Ong MF, Martens S, Sarrazin C, Bojunga J, et al. (2008) Performance of transient elastography for the staging of liver fibrosis: a meta-analysis. Gastroenterology 134: 960–974.
43. Berenguer M (2009) Non-invasive biomarkers of liver fibrosis in liver transplant patients with hepatitis C: can we avoid liver biopsies? Dig Liver Dis 41: 226–228.
44. Kamphues C, Lotz K, Rocken C, Berg T, Eurich D, et al. (2010) Chances and limitations of non-invasive tests in the assessment of liver fibrosis in liver transplant patients. Clin Transplant 24: 652–659.
45. Foucher J, Chanteloup E, Vergniol J, Castera L, Le Bail B, et al. (2006) Diagnosis of cirrhosis by transient elastography (FibroScan): a prospective study. Gut 55: 403–408.
46. The French METAVIR Cooperative Study Group (1994) Intraobserver and interobserver variations in liver biopsy interpretation in patients with chronic hepatitis C. Hepatology 20: 15–20.
47. Parkes J, Roderick P, Harris S, Day C, Mutimer D, et al. (2010) Enhanced liver fibrosis test can predict clinical outcomes in patients with chronic liver disease. Gut 59: 1245–1251.
48. Mayo MJ, Parkes J, Adams-Huet B, Combes B, Mills AS, et al. (2008) Prediction of clinical outcomes in primary biliary cirrhosis by serum enhanced liver fibrosis assay. Hepatology 48: 1549–1557.
49. Trepo E, Potthoff A, Pradat P, Bakshi R, Young B, et al. (2011) Role of a cirrhosis risk score for the early prediction of fibrosis progression in hepatitis C patients with minimal liver disease. J Hepatol 55: 38–44.
50. Swets JA (1988) Measuring the accuracy of diagnostic systems. Science 240: 1285–1293.
51. Guha IN, Myers RP, Patel K, Talwalkar JA (2011) Biomarkers of liver fibrosis: what lies beneath the receiver operating characteristic curve? Hepatology 54: 1454–1462.
52. Mehta SH, Lau B, Afdhal NH, Thomas DL (2009) Exceeding the limits of liver histology markers. J Hepatol 50: 36–41.
53. Cholongitas E, Quaglia A, Samonakis D, Senzolo M, Triantos C, et al. (2006) Transjugular liver biopsy: how good is it for accurate histological interpretation? Gut 55: 1789–1794.

Plasma Sphingolipids as Potential Indicators of Hepatic Necroinflammation in Patients with Chronic Hepatitis C and Normal Alanine Aminotransferase Level

Jun-Feng Li[1,2❡], Feng Qu[3❡], Su-Jun Zheng[2❡], Jin-Yu Ren[4], Hui-Li Wu[2], Mei Liu[2], Hui Liu[5], Feng Ren[2], Yu Chen[2], Jin-Lan Zhang[3]*, Zhong-Ping Duan[2]*

1 The First Clinical Medical School, Lanzhou University, Lanzhou, China, **2** Artificial Liver Center, Beijing YouAn Hospital, Capital Medical University, Beijing, China, **3** State Key Laboratory of Bioactive Substance and Function of Natural Medicines, Institute of Materia Medica, Chinese Academy of Medical Sciences & Peking Union Medical College, Beijing, China, **4** Evergreen Wellness Center, Kansas College of Chinese Medicine, Wichita, Kansas, United States of America, **5** Department of Pathology, Beijing YouAn Hospital, Capital Medical University, Beijing, China

Abstract

Accurate estimation of hepatic necroinflammation caused by chronic hepatitis C (CHC) is crucial for prediction of prognosis and design of therapeutic strategy, which is particularly true for CHC patients with normal alanine aminotransferase (ALT) level. Recent studies have shown that sphingolipids have a close relationship with hepatitis C virus infection. The present study aimed to identify plasma sphingolipids related to hepatic necroinflammation. We included 120 treatment-naïve CHC patients and 64/120 had normal ALT levels (<40 U/L). CHC patients who underwent liver biopsies were subjected to Scheuer scoring analysis for scope of hepatic inflammation. Plasma sphingolipids were detected by high-performance liquid chromatography tandem mass spectrometry. Our results showed 44 plasma sphingolipids were detected altogether. Of all detected sphingolipids, hexosylceramide (HexCer) (d18:1/22:0) and HexCer (d18:1/24:0) showed a significant difference among G0/G1, G2, and G3/G4 ($P<0.05$). For identifying hepatic necroinflammation (G≥2), after adjusting other factors, the odds ratio (OR) of HexCer (d18:1/22:0) reached 1.01 (95% confidence interval [CI]: 1.00–1.02). Furthermore, the area under the curve (AUC) of HexCer (d18:1/22:0) was 0.7 ($P=0.01$) and approached that of ALT (AUC = 0.78). However, in CHC patients with normal ALT, HexCer (d18:1/22:0) was an independent factor (OR: 1.02, 95% CI: 1.01–1.03) to identify the hepatic necroinflammation (G≥2). HexCer (d18:1/22:0) not only showed the largest AUC (0.78, $P=0.001$), but also exhibited the highest specificity of all indicators. These results indicate that plasma HexCer (d18:1/22:0) is a potential indicator to distinguish hepatic necroinflammation in CHC patients. For CHC with normal ALT, the ability of HexCer (d18:1/22:0) to distinguish hepatic necroinflammation might be superior to conventional serum indicators.

Editor: Ratna B. Ray, Saint Louis University, United States of America

Funding: This study is supported by the National Science and Technology Key Project on "Major Infectious Diseases such as HIV/AIDS, Viral Hepatitis Prevention and Treatment" (2012ZX10002004-006, 2012ZX10004904-003-001, 2013ZX10002002-006); Ministry of Science and Technology of People's Republic of China (2012ZX09301002-006); the High Technical Personnel Training Item in Beijing Health System (2011-3-083); the Beijing Municipal Science & Technology Commission (No. Z131107002213019); the Special Scientific Research Fund for Beijing Health Development (2011-2018-04); and YouAn Scientific Research Fund for Liver Disease and HIV/AIDS (BJYAH-2011-045). The funders had no role in study design, data collection and analysis, decision to publish, or preparation of the manuscript.

Competing Interests: The authors have declared that no competing interests exist.

* E-mail: duan2517@163.com (ZPD); zhjl@imm.ac.cn (JLZ)

❡ These authors contributed equally to this work.

Introduction

Hepatitis C is a major public health problem, affecting over 2% of the global population who are at risk of cirrhosis or hepatocellular carcinoma [1,2]. Persistent hepatitis C virus (HCV) infection triggers hepatic necroinflammation, which may eventually contribute to liver fibrogenesis [3]. It has been confirmed that chronic hepatitis C (CHC) patients with extensive periportal hepatocellular necrosis and inflammation have higher rates of fibrosis progression [4]. Therefore, the necroinflammatory activity should be regarded as a major clue for deciding therapy [5]. As the gold criterion for estimating hepatic necroinflammation, liver biopsies are recommended in treatment guidelines worldwide. Nevertheless, these biopsies are not undertaken widely nowadays because of the invasive procedures with potential complications [6]. Serum aminotransferases are used to evaluate hepatic injury indirectly, but are limited because 15–30% of CHC patients have consistently normal alanine aminotransferase (ALT) despite the presence of liver inflammation [7,8]. Furthermore, through long-term follow-up, liver histological injury can also be found in CHC patients with normal serial ALT [9]. There is an urgent need to find novel noninvasive biomarkers to evaluate accurately hepatic necroinflammation in CHC patients, especially those with normal ALT, to identify candidates for antiviral therapy.

Sphingolipids are enriched in lipid rafts of biological membranes and provide a distribution platform for different signal processes including proliferation, differentiation and apoptosis

[10,11]. During infection, pathogens are able to exploit lipid rafts composed of sphingolipids and others to gain entry to their target host cells [12]. For HCV infection, it has been reported that, in HCV-infected chimeric mice, inhibition of serine palmitoyltransferase, which is a first-step enzyme in the sphingolipid biosynthetic pathway, could suppress replication of HCV [13]. Moreover, inhibitors of HCV replication can prevent the *de novo* synthesis of sphingolipids *in vitro* [14]. After persistent infection in CHC patients, altered plasma sphingosine 1-phosphate, as a bioactive sphingolipid, has also been found recently to be involved in liver fibrosis [15]. Thus, sphingolipids have a close relationship with CHC, especially for the metabolites ceramide, which have been implicated in apoptosis and necrosis of hepatic cells and contribute to progression of liver diseases [16,17,18].

We have previously established a mature high-performance liquid chromatography–tandem mass spectrometry (HPLC-MS/MS) method to quantify sphingolipids in other diseases [19]. Based on that improved quantitative high-throughput lipidomic platform, we initially found a relationship between plasma sphingolipids and hepatic inflammation in CHC [20]. However, the relationship between plasma sphingolipids and hepatic necroinflammation has only rarely been studied before, especially for CHC patients with normal ALT.

Therefore, in the present study, based on our previous improved HPLC-MS/MS methods and liver biopsy, we aimed to evaluate the diagnostic ability of plasma sphingolipids to identify hepatic necroinflammation (G≥2) among patients with CHC and the subgroup of patients with normal ALT levels, respectively.

Materials and Methods

Patients

A group of 122 CHC patients with long-term follow-up, from Dingxi City, Gansu Province, China, were enrolled from July 2010 to June 2011. All the patients had a history of paid plasma donations with blood cell re-transfusions between 1992 and 1995, and did not receive antiviral treatment before being recruited into the present study. CHC diagnosis was made in accordance with established criteria [21,22]. Patients with co-infections with other viruses or who were ineligible for liver biopsy were excluded. Two patients who were ineligible for liver biopsy, one due to ascites, the other due to the small size of the liver biopsy specimen, were excluded. One hundred and twenty patients were eligible for the study. To seek potential biomarkers among plasma sphingolipids for patients with normal ALT levels (<40 U/L), 64 patients were rescreened for analysis (Figure 1).

Fasting blood samples were collected on the day of the liver biopsy. Liver function and coagulation function tests were performed in all patients. Each patient gave signed informed consent at the beginning of the study. The study protocol was conducted in accordance with the provisions of the Declaration of Helsinki, 1975 and approved by the Institutional Review Board of Beijing YouAn Hospital, Capital Medical University, Beijing, China.

Liver Biopsy

Liver biopsies were obtained from CHC patients under ultrasound guidance. Specimens were fixed in formalin and embedded in paraffin. Specimens longer than 1.5 cm, containing at least six complete portal areas, were reviewed by two senior pathologists who were unaware of the patients' clinical data. The Scheuer scoring system was used to assess hepatic necroinflammatory activity, and G≥2 was considered to show the presence of necrosis [23]. Also, with fewer samples from G0 and G4 patients, G0 and G1, and G3 and G4 were respectively merged into G0/G1 or G3/G4 groups for statistical analysis.

HPLC-MS/MS

Blood was collected into cold lithium heparin used as an anticoagulant and immediately centrifuged at 4°C at 8000 × *g*.

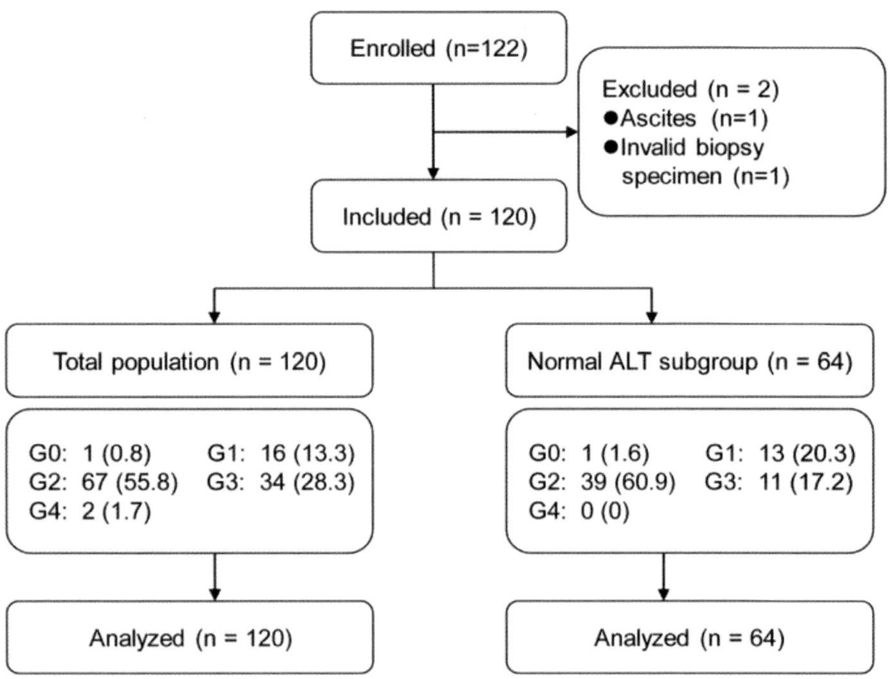

Figure 1. Flowchart of patient selection and study design. Serum ALT level <40 U/L was considered normal. Data are number of patients (%).

Table 1. Characteristics of patients included and univariate analysis of routine indicators according to hepatic inflammation grade.

Variable	Total patients (n = 120)	G0/G1 (n = 17)	G2 (n = 67)	G3/G4 (n = 36)	*P* value
Age, yrs	51.33±7.33	50.41±8.42	50.88±7.07	52.58±7.33	0.36
Male, n (%)	57(47.50)	3 (17.65)	35 (52.24)	19 (52.78)	0.03
ALT (U/L)	60.42±70.88	29.34±17.66	48.37±33.78	97.52±112.35	<0.001
AST (U/L)	47.94±44.30	27.49±10.18	40.33±18.78	71.76±71.16	<0.001
TBIL (μmol/L)	16.51±7.25	13.40±4.47	17.06±7.42	16.96±7.75	0.13
DBIL (μmol/L)	3.26±1.36	2.89±1.14	3.23±1.23	3.50±1.65	0.43
TP (g/L)	70.93±4.95	69.84±3.65	71.23±5.27	70.89±4.89	0.59
Albumin (g/L)	43.21±2.36	44.34±1.84	43.19±2.38	42.72±2.43	0.06
Globulin (g/L)	29.19±17.29	26.08±3.57	30.50±22.84	28.23±4.19	0.09
GGT (U/L)	22.04±16.50	16.49±10.89	18.00±8.00	32.17±24.46	<0.001
ALP (U/L)	76.29±20.91	75.35±18.52	72.57±17.25	83.64±26.19	0.11
TBA (μmol/L)	11.24±46.76	4.57±2.75	13.70±62.44	9.80±6.61	0.004
Cholinesterase (U/L)	6957.09±1442.44	7541.44±2140.99	6882.53±1350.68	6819.92±1158.74	0.09
PTA (%)	92.41±9.11	98.47±6.30	92.96±9.39	88.50±7.99	<0.001

Data are means ± SD or number of patients (%).
P values are acquired by one-way analysis of variance or the nonparametric Kruskal-Wallis test for continuous variables depending on the data distribution, and by Pearson χ^2 for categoric variables.
ALT: alanine aminotransferase; AST: aspartate aminotransferase; TBIL: total bilirubin; DBIL: direct bilirubin; TP: total protein; GGT: γ-glutamyl transpeptidase; ALP, alkaline phosphatase; TBA: total bile acid; PTA: prothrombin activity.

The samples were stored at −80°C. All lipid standards were from Avanti Polar Lipids (Alabaster, AL, USA). Ultra Resi-analyzed grade methanol and HPLC grade methyl-tert-butyl ether (MTBE) were purchased from Mallinckrodt Baker (Phillipsburg, NJ, USA). Formic acid of analytical grade was obtained from TEDIA (Fairfield, OH, USA). Ammonium formate (purity >99.99%) was purchased from Sigma–Aldrich (St. Louis, MO, USA). Ultrapure water was prepared using a Milli-Q purification system (Millipore, Bedford, MA, USA). HPLC-MS/MS was performed on an Agilent 6410B Triple Quad mass spectrometer (QQQ; Agilent Technologies Santa Clara, CA, USA) comprising a triple quadrupole MS analyzer with an electrospray ionization interface and an Agilent 1200 RRLC system. Sphingolipidomic assays were performed at the Institute of Materia Medica, Peking Union Medical College (Beijing, China) as previously described [19].

Statistical Analysis

Data were expressed as mean ± standard deviation (SD). In univariate analysis, depending on the data distribution according to the Kolmogorov–Smirnov test, continuous variables among multiple groups were analyzed by one-way analysis of variance or the nonparametric Kruskal–Wallis test. Comparisons between pairs of groups subsequently were analyzed by the least significant difference *t* test or Mann–Whitney test. Additionally, the independent-samples *t* test or Mann–Whitney test was used to compare G<2 against G≥2. Categoric variables were analyzed by Pearson χ^2 test. Correlation analysis between plasma sphingolipids and inflammation grades was performed by Spearman's rank correlation. Moving forward, the (LR) multivariate logistic regression analysis was performed, and the *P* values of entry and removal were respectively set to 0.05 and 0.1. The diagnostic value of each indicator with significant difference in univariate analysis was assessed by the area under the receiver operating characteristic (ROC) curve. Statistical analysis was performed using SPSS version 19.0 (Chicago, IL, USA), while a two-sided *P* value <0.05 was considered statistically significant.

Results

Clinical Characteristics of Patients

The characteristics of the 120 patients who underwent a liver biopsy are summarized in Figure 1 and Table 1. The patient group comprised 57 (47.5%) male and 63 (52.5%) female patients with a mean age of 51.33 years. According to the Scheuer inflammation score, G2 was present in 67 patients, which accounted for the largest proportion (55.8%). This was followed by G3 (28.3%, 34/120) and G1 (13.3%, 16/120). G0 and G4 were found in 0.8% (1/120) and 1.7% (2/120) of the patients, respectively. In the subgroup of patients (n = 64) with normal ALT levels (<40 U/L), G2 predominated (39/64, 60.9%), followed by G1 (13/64, 20.3%) and G3 (11/64, 17.2%) (Figures 1 and 2). In univariate analysis of routine serological indicators in all patients, ALT ($P<0.001$), aspartate aminotransferase (AST) ($P<0.001$), γ-glutamyl transpeptidase (GGT) ($P<0.001$), total bile acid (TBA) ($P<0.05$), and prothrombin activity (PTA) ($P<0.001$) showed a significant difference among G0/G1, G2, and G3/G4 (Table 1).

Relationship between Plasma Sphingolipids and Hepatic Inflammation Grades in CHC Patients

Plasma sphingolipids in the 120 patients were analyzed by HPLC-MS/MS, and 44 sphingolipids were identified and quantified (Table S1). Two plasma sphingolipids showed a significant difference among G0/G1, G2, and G3/G4 ($P<0.05$). hexosylceramide (HexCer) (d18:1/22:0), which differed significantly between G0/G1 and G2 ($P=0.02$), also showed a significant difference between G0/G1 and G3/G4 ($P=0.01$). Similarly, another sphingolipid HexCer (d18:1/24:0) showed a significant difference in both G2 versus G0/G1 ($P=0.02$) and G3/G4 versus G0/G1 ($P=0.02$) (Figure 3). To analyze further the correlation between these two sphingolipids and hepatic inflammation grades, Spearman's correlation analysis was performed. The results revealed that HexCer (d18:1/22:0) correlated with

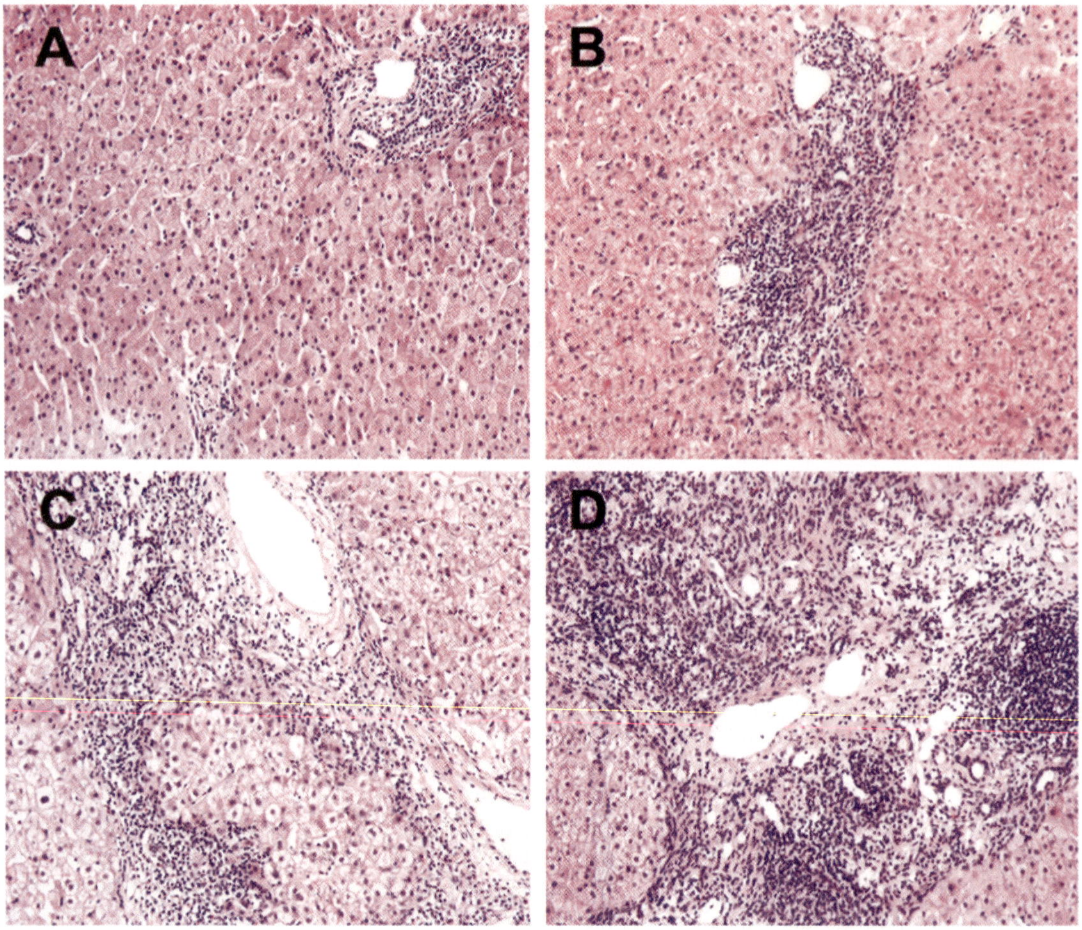

Figure 2. Liver histopathology of patients with G0/G1, G2 and G3/G4 according to the Scheuer scoring system. (A) G1, portal inflammation (HE ×200); (B) G2, mild piecemeal necrosis (HE ×200); (C) G3, moderate piecemeal necrosis (HE ×200); (D), G4, severe piecemeal necrosis and bridging necrosis (HE ×200).

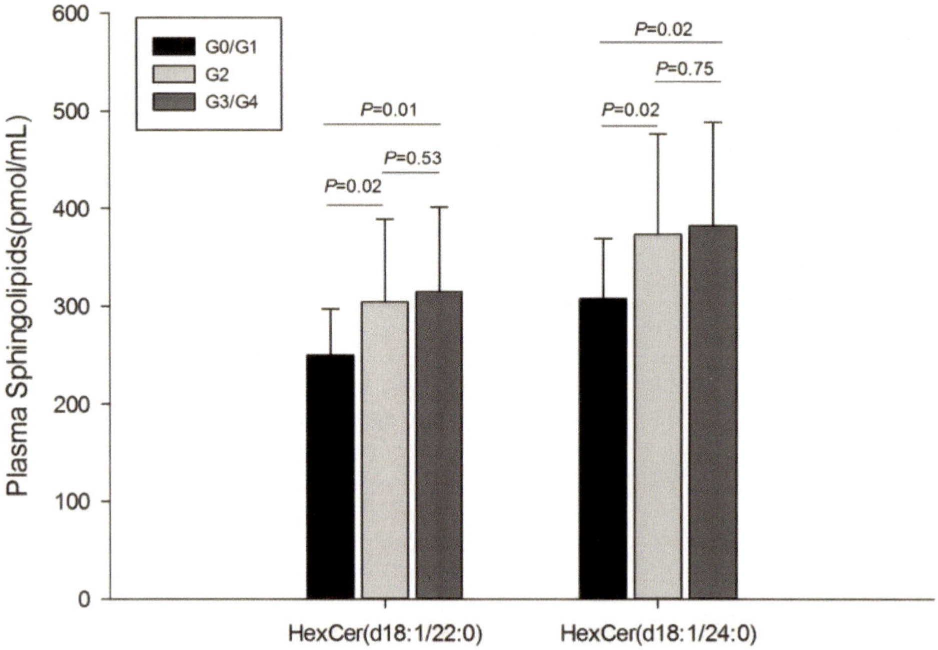

Figure 3. Plasma sphingolipids with significant difference by hepatic inflammation grades in patients with CHC.

Table 2. Indicators related to necroinflammation in CHC patients in univariate and multivariate analyses.

Variable	G<2 (n = 17)	G≥2 (n = 103)	*P* value	OR (95% CI)
Age, yrs	50.41±8.42	51.48±7.17	0.83	
Male, n (%)	3 (17.65)	54 (52.43)	0.01	
ALT (U/L)	29.34±17.66	65.55±75.00	<0.001	
AST (U/L)	27.49±10.18	51.32±46.83	<0.001	1.07 (1.01–1.13)
TBIL (μmol/L)	13.40±4.47	17.02±7.50	0.05	
DBIL (μmol/L)	2.89±1.14	3.32±1.39	0.21	
TP (g/L)	69.84±3.65	71.11±5.12	0.33	
Albumin (g/L)	44.34±1.84	43.02±2.40	0.03	
Globulin (g/L)	26.08±3.57	29.70±18.57	0.03	
GGT (U/L)	16.49±10.89	22.95±17.12	0.01	
ALP (U/L)	75.35±18.52	76.44±21.36	0.58	
TBA (μmol/L)	4.57±2.75	12.34±50.41	0.04	
Cholinesterase (U/L)	7541.44±2140.99	6860.64±1281.44	0.03	
PTA (%)	98.47±6.30	91.40±9.14	0.002	0.89 (0.81–0.98)
Cer(d18:1/18:1) (pmol/mL)	3.85±1.11	3.30±1.33	0.03	
HexCer(d18:1/16:0) (pmol/mL)	1131.87±525.58	1324.62±493.48	0.03	
HexCer(d18:1/22:0) (pmol/mL)	250.11±46.82	308.01±85.18	0.01	1.01 (1.00–1.02)
HexCer(d18:1/24:1) (pmol/mL)	372.25±106.73	483.20±175.46	0.001	
HexCer(d18:1/24:0) (pmol/mL)	307.86±61.45	376.58±103.94	0.01	

Data are means ± SD or number of patients (%).
P values are acquired by independent-samples *t* test or the Mann-Whitney test for continuous variables depending on the data distribution, and by Pearson χ^2 for categoric variables.
OR: odds ratio; CI: confidence interval; ALT: alanine aminotransferase; AST: aspartate aminotransferase; TBIL: total bilirubin; DBIL: direct bilirubin; TP: total protein; GGT: γ-glutamyl transpeptidase; ALP, alkaline phosphatase; TBA: total bile acid; PTA: prothrombin activity; Cer: ceramide; HexCer: hexosylceramide.

inflammation grades, and the correlation coefficient (r) was 0.21 (P = 0.02). HexCer (d18:1/24:0) also showed a correlation with inflammation grade (r = 0.19, P = 0.04).

Distinction of Hepatic Necroinflammation (G≥2) in CHC Patients

Hepatic necroinflammatory activity is one of the most important predictors of fibrosis progression in CHC patients [4,5,24]. Likewise, the identification of hepatic necroinflammation (G≥2) is essential for assessment of disease status in CHC patients. We analyzed plasma sphingolipids and routine clinical indicators to establish better noninvasive markers. Of all plasma sphingolipids, ceramide (Cer) (d18:1/18:1), HexCer (d18:1/16:0), HexCer (d18:1/22:0), HexCer (d18:1/24:1), and HexCer (d18:1/24:0) showed a significant difference between G<2 and G≥2 (P<0.05) in univariate analysis. Routine serological indicators such as ALT, AST, albumin, globulin, GGT, TBA, cholinesterase, and PTA also showed significant differences between G<2 and G≥2 (P< 0.05). To determine independent factors for the absence or presence of necroinflammation (G<2 versus. G≥2), the multivariate logistic regression analysis was performed. Sex, ALT, AST, GGT, cholinesterase, PTA, Cer (d18:1/18:1), HexCer (d18:1/16:0), HexCer (d18:1/22:0), HexCer (d18:1/24:1), and HexCer (d18:1/24:0) were initially included in multivariate analysis. The final results showed that the odds ratio (OR) for HexCer (d18:1/22:0) reached 1.01 [95% confidence interval (CI): 1.0–1.02]. In addition, the OR of AST and PTA was 1.07 (95% CI: 1.01–1.13) and 0.89 (95% CI: 0.81–0.98), respectively (Table 2).

Subsequently, the ROC analysis was performed to determine the diagnostic value of these significantly altered indicators. The area under curve (AUC) of HexCer (d18:1/22:0) reached 0.7 (P = 0.01). Although it was lower than that of ALT (AUC = 0.78, P<0.001), the specificity and positive likelihood ratio of HexCer (d18:1/22:0) (0.82 and 3.30, respectively) were higher than the routine serological indicators, including ALT. The AUC value of the other plasma sphingolipids HexCer (d18:1/24:0), HexCer (d18:1/24:1) ranged from 0.69 to 0.70 (all P<0.05); both of which were larger than that of globulin, cholinesterase, albumin, and TBA (Table S2).

Identification of Hepatic Necroinflammation (G≥2) in the Subgroup of CHC Patients with Normal ALT levels

In order to evaluate whether sphingolipids could differentiate the hepatic necroinflammation (G≥2) in the subgroup of CHC patients with normal ALT levels, we also performed a univariate and multivariate analysis (Table 3). Routine serological indicators AST, total bilirubin, albumin, GGT, and PTA were significantly different between G<2 and G≥2 (P<0.05). HexCer (d18:1/22:0), HexCer (d18:1/24:1), and HexCer (d18:1/24:0) showed significant differences between G<2 and G≥2 (P<0.05) among all the plasma sphingolipids. During the logistic regression analysis, sex, AST, total bilirubin, GGT, PTA, HexCer (d18:1/22:0), HexCer (d18:1/24:1), and HexCer (d18:1/24:0) were included. The final multivariate results revealed that HexCer (d18:1/22:0) was independent of other factors and its OR value was 1.02 (95% CI: 1.01–1.03).

Table 3. Indicators related to necroinflammation (G≥2) in CHC patients with normal ALT in univariate and multivariate analyses.

Variable	G<2 (n = 14)	G≥2 (n = 50)	*P* value	OR (95% CI)
Age, yrs	49.29±8.84	51.84±6.97	0.26	
Male, n (%)	1(7.14)	18(36.00)	0.08	
AST (U/L)	24.13±7.44	30.86±8.61	0.01	
TBIL (μmol/L)	12.53±4.15	17.48±8.40	0.02	
DBIL (μmol/L)	2.67±1.10	3.24±1.36	0.11	
TP (g/L)	70.24±3.32	71.10±5.39	0.58	
Albumin (g/L)	44.60±1.83	43.17±2.36	0.04	
Globulin (g/L)	26.35±3.53	27.98±4.23	0.19	
GGT (U/L)	12.97±4.27	16.61±7.31	0.03	
ALP (U/L)	74.98±20.09	71.10±13.91	0.41	
TBA (μmol/L)	4.21±2.43	6.54±4.72	0.10	
Cholinesterase (U/L)	7546.39±2232.91	6884.89±1437.77	0.19	
PTA (%)	99.59±6.18	93.39±10.04	0.02	
HexCer(d18:1/16:0) (pmol/mL)	1079.01±495.41	1271.33±390.77	0.05	
HexCer(d18:1/22:0) (pmol/mL)	236.83±40.12	315.53±90.33	<0.001	1.02(1.01–1.03)
HexCer(d18:1/24:1) (pmol/mL)	340.53±86.46	490.90±189.20	<0.001	
HexCer(d18:1/24:0) (pmol/mL)	291.15±50.55	377.49±102.57	<0.001	
dhCer(d18:0/24:1) (pmol/mL)	35.10±11.78	48.48±22.56	0.05	

Data are means ± SD or number of patients (%).
P values are acquired by independent-samples *t* test or the Mann-Whitney test for continuous variables, and by Pearson χ^2 for categoric variables.
OR: odds ratio; CI: confidence interval; AST: aspartate aminotransferase; TBIL: total bilirubin; DBIL: direct bilirubin; TP: total protein; GGT: γ-glutamyl transpeptidase; ALP, alkaline phosphatase; TBA: total bile acid; PTA: prothrombin activity; Cer: ceramide; HexCer: hexosylceramide; dhCer: dihydroceramide.

In the ROC analysis, two plasma sphingolipids demonstrated larger AUCs than those of routine serological indicators. Of concern was the fact that HexCer (d18:1/22:0) with the largest AUC (0.78, $P = 0.001$) exhibited the highest specificity (1.0) when the optimal cutoff value was set to 281.37 pmol/mL. The AUC of HexCer (d18:1/24:1) followed closely, which reached 0.75 (95% CI: 0.62–0.87, $P<0.05$) and was the same as AST. The AUCs of total bilirubin, PTA, and GGT fluctuated from 0.69 to 0.71 (Table 4).

Discussion

In our cohort, all CHC patients had definite histories of plasma donation with blood cell re-transfusion and did not receive antiviral treatment before enrollment. Therefore, in this context of an interferon-naïve state of disease, we were able to obtain true results of sphingolipids changes after eliminating the influence of interferon therapy on hepatic inflammation. From our data, for the first time, we reported that HexCer (d18:1/22:0) might be a surrogate marker for assessing hepatic necroinflammation in patients with CHC, especially, for those with normal ALT level.

Currently, although increasing evidence confirms the close relationship between sphingolipids and liver diseases [18], for example, ceramides which interact with several pathways involved in oxidative stress, inflammation and apoptosis, can promote the progress of nonalcoholic fatty liver disease [25], the role of sphingolipids in hepatic inflammation in CHC patients remains to be elucidated. In our study, the univariate and multivariate analyses showed that HexCer (d18:1/22:0) correlated with alteration of hepatic inflammation grade in CHC, and verified that HexCer (d18:1/22:0) had an independent relationship with hepatic necroinflammation (G≥2) after adjusting for other factors, especially in CHC patients with normal ALT level. Our results show that HexCer (d18:1/22:0), which was elevated in CHC patients with hepatic necroinflammation, might contribute uniquely to the pathogenesis of hepatic necroinflammation in CHC. Although there is no direct evidence of the role of HexCer (d18:1/22:0) in hepatic necroinflammation caused by CHC, there are several possible mechanisms that may be involved in the relationship between this specific sphingolipid and hepatic necroinflammation. One *in vivo* study has reported that α-galactosylceramide induces pronounced cytokine responses that could contribute to hepatic inflammation, by activating natural killer T cells [26]. In addition, α-galactosylceramide can also lead to hepatic injury through tumor necrosis factor, which increased Fas-ligand expression of natural killer T cells in an animal model [27]. However, experimental studies are needed to determine the exact underlying mechanisms responsible for the association of HexCer (d18:1/22:0) with hepatic necroinflammation in CHC.

Furthermore, we focused on the potential of plasma sphingolipids to identify the presence of hepatic necroinflammation (G≥2) in CHC. Another interesting finding in our study was that, although the AUC value of these sphingolipids to identify hepatic necroinflammation (G≥2) was not larger than that of routine serological indicators in the total patient population, others such as negative likelihood ratio and positive likelihood ratio of some sphingolipids were better indicators than routine serological indicators. This indicated that plasma sphingolipids, especially HexCer (d18:1/22:0), which was independently linked to hepatic necroinflammation with the largest AUC of all sphingolipids, had a certain superiority in identifying hepatic necroinflammation in CHC patients.

Table 4. ROC analysis of indicators related to identification of necroinflammation (G≥2) in CHC patients with normal ALT levels.

Variable	AUC(95%CI)	*P* value	Cut-off value	Se	Sp	PLR	NLR
HexCer(d18:1/22:0)	0.78(0.67–0.90)	0.001	281.37	0.62	1.00	–	0.38
HexCer(d18:1/24:1)	0.75(0.62–0.87)	0.01	452.10	0.56	1.00	–	0.44
AST	0.75(0.60–0.91)	0.004	27.15	0.74	0.79	3.52	0.33
HexCer(d18:1/24:0)	0.74(0.62–0.87)	0.01	371.63	0.52	1.00	–	0.48
TBIL	0.71(0.56–0.87)	0.02	11.55	0.80	0.64	2.24	0.31
PTA	0.71(0.56–0.86)	0.02	96.10	0.64	0.79	2.99	0.46
GGT	0.69(0.54–0.84)	0.03	14.20	0.52	0.86	3.64	0.56

The indicators whose *P* values of AUC were less than 0.05 were listed in the Table.
AUC: area under curve; CI: confidence interval; Se: sensitivity; Sp: specificity; PLR: positive likelihood ratio; NLR: negative likelihood ratio; HexCer: hexosylceramide; AST: aspartate aminotransferase; TBIL: total bilirubin; PTA: prothrombin activity; GGT: γ-glutamyl transpeptidase.

We also verified the superiority of plasma sphingolipids compared with routine serological indicators to reflect the presence of necroinflammation (G≥2) in CHC patients with normal ALT levels. At present, elevated ALT level, as an indirect surrogate marker for hepatic necrosis, still has poor ability to identify hepatic inflammation in CHC patients [28], which is particularly true for CHC patients with normal ALT and liver inflammation [7,8]. Thus, it is more meaningful to find new markers for hepatic necroinflammation in CHC patients with normal ALT for deciding therapeutic strategy. Our results revealed that plasma HexCer (d18:1/22:0) exhibited the largest AUC (0.78, $P = 0.001$) and the highest specificity (1.0) of all the indicators including plasma sphingolipids and routine serological indicators. This suggests that HexCer (d18:1/22:0) might become a potential marker for identifying hepatic necroinflammation in CHC patients with normal ALT.

Although HexCer (d18:1/24:0) showed that its AUC approached that of HexCer (d18:1/22:0) in ROC analysis, HexCer (d18:1/24:0) was not an independent factor to identify hepatic necroinflammation in CHC in multivariate analysis. However, we speculated that the association with small samples and poor statistical power could not be ruled out. We confirmed the superior diagnostic value of HexCer (d18:1/22:0) to identify hepatic necroinflammation in patients with CHC and normal ALT level.

There were some limitations in our study. We analyzed the relationship between the plasma sphingolipids and hepatic necroinflammation based on a long-term (~20 years) follow-up in a cohort of interferon-naïve CHC patients, and the actual number of cases was not large, and the different inflammation groups were not matched exactly for sex. However, by adjusting for sex, the multivariate analysis showed that sex had minimal effects on plasma sphingolipid level.

In summary, based on liver biopsies and HPLC-MS/MS, we have found for the first time that plasma sphingolipid HexCer (d18:1/22:0) has a positive diagnostic value to distinguish hepatic necroinflammation in CHC, especially in patients with normal ALT levels. Meanwhile, our discovery of plasma sphingolipids has opened new directions of research to identify novel noninvasive markers for progression of CHC.

Supporting Information

Table S1 Plasma sphingolipids profile of untreated chronic hepatitis C patients with G0/G1, G2, G3/G4. Data are expressed as mean ± standard deviation, *P* values were calculated by one-way analysis of variance or the nonparametric Kruskal-Wallis test.

Table S2 Performance of indicators for identification of liver necroinflammation (G≥2) in ROC analysis. The indicators whose *P* values of AUC were less than 0.05 are listed in the Table.

Acknowledgments

We thank all the patients involved in this study.

Author Contributions

Conceived and designed the experiments: S-JZ J-YR J-LZ Z-PD. Performed the experiments: FQ S-JZ J-FL H-LW ML HL FR YC. Analyzed the data: J-FL. Contributed reagents/materials/analysis tools: FQ J-LZ. Wrote the paper: J-FL.

References

1. Shepard CW, Finelli L, Alter MJ (2005) Global epidemiology of hepatitis C virus infection. Lancet Infect Dis 5: 558–567.
2. Lavanchy D (2009) The global burden of hepatitis C. Liver Int 29 Suppl 1: 74–81.
3. Ascione A, Tartaglione T, Di Costanzo GG (2007) Natural history of chronic hepatitis C virus infection. Dig Liver Dis 39 Suppl 1: S4–7.
4. Ghany MG, Kleiner DE, Alter H, Doo E, Khokar F, et al. (2003) Progression of fibrosis in chronic hepatitis C. Gastroenterology 124: 97–104.
5. Fontaine H, Nalpas B, Poulet B, Carnot F, Zylberberg H, et al. (2001) Hepatitis activity index is a key factor in determining the natural history of chronic hepatitis C. Hum Pathol 32: 904–909.
6. Bravo AA, Sheth SG, Chopra S (2001) Liver biopsy. N Engl J Med 344: 495–500.
7. Marcellin P, Levy S, Erlinger S (1997) Therapy of hepatitis C: patients with normal aminotransferase levels. Hepatology 26: 133S–136S.
8. Tassopoulos NC (1999) Treatment of patients with chronic hepatitis C and normal ALT levels. J Hepatol 31 Suppl 1: 193–196.
9. Okanoue T, Makiyama A, Nakayama M, Sumida Y, Mitsuyoshi H, et al. (2005) A follow-up study to determine the value of liver biopsy and need for antiviral therapy for hepatitis C virus carriers with persistently normal serum aminotransferase. J Hepatol 43: 599–605.
10. Bartke N, Hannun YA (2009) Bioactive sphingolipids: metabolism and function. J Lipid Res 50 Suppl: S91–96.
11. Lingwood D, Simons K (2010) Lipid rafts as a membrane-organizing principle. Science 327: 46–50.
12. Hawkes DJ, Mak J (2006) Lipid membrane; a novel target for viral and bacterial pathogens. Curr Drug Targets 7: 1615–1621.
13. Umehara T, Sudoh M, Yasui F, Matsuda C, Hayashi Y, et al. (2006) Serine palmitoyltransferase inhibitor suppresses HCV replication in a mouse model. Biochem Biophys Res Commun 346: 67–73.
14. Sakamoto H, Okamoto K, Aoki M, Kato H, Katsume A, et al. (2005) Host sphingolipid biosynthesis as a target for hepatitis C virus therapy. Nat Chem Biol 1: 333–337.
15. Ikeda H, Ohkawa R, Watanabe N, Nakamura K, Kume Y, et al. (2010) Plasma concentration of bioactive lipid mediator sphingosine 1-phosphate is reduced in patients with chronic hepatitis C. Clin Chim Acta 411: 765–770.
16. Jones BE, Lo CR, Srinivasan A, Valentino KL, Czaja MJ (1999) Ceramide induces caspase-independent apoptosis in rat hepatocytes sensitized by inhibition of RNA synthesis. Hepatology 30: 215–222.
17. Arora AS, Jones BJ, Patel TC, Bronk SF, Gores GJ (1997) Ceramide induces hepatocyte cell death through disruption of mitochondrial function in the rat. Hepatology 25: 958–963.
18. Mari M, Fernandez-Checa JC (2007) Sphingolipid signalling and liver diseases. Liver Int 27: 440–450.
19. Qu F, Wu CS, Hou JF, Jin Y, Zhang JL (2012) Sphingolipids as new biomarkers for assessment of delayed-type hypersensitivity and response to triptolide. PLoS One 7: e52454.
20. Qu F, Zheng SJ, Wu CS, Jia ZX, Zhang JL, et al. (2014) Lipidomic profiling of plasma in patients with chronic hepatitis C infection. Anal Bioanal Chem 406: 555–564.
21. Ghany MG, Strader DB, Thomas DL, Seeff LB (2009) Diagnosis, management, and treatment of hepatitis C: an update. Hepatology 49: 1335–1374.
22. Hepatotogy Branch, Infectious and Parasitology branch, Chinese Medical Association(2004) Guideline of prevention and treatment of hepatitis C. Zhonghua Yu Fang Yi Xue Za Zhi 38: 210–215.
23. Scheuer PJ (1991) Classification of chronic viral hepatitis: a need for reassessment. J Hepatol 13: 372–374.
24. Lagging LM, Westin J, Svensson E, Aires N, Dhillon AP, et al. (2002) Progression of fibrosis in untreated patients with hepatitis C virus infection. Liver 22: 136–144.
25. Pagadala M, Kasumov T, McCullough AJ, Zein NN, Kirwan JP (2012) Role of ceramides in nonalcoholic fatty liver disease. Trends Endocrinol Metab 23: 365–371.
26. Biburger M, Tiegs G (2005) Alpha-galactosylceramide-induced liver injury in mice is mediated by TNF-alpha but independent of Kupffer cells. J Immunol 175: 1540–1550.
27. Inui T, Nakashima H, Habu Y, Nakagawa R, Fukasawa M, et al. (2005) Neutralization of tumor necrosis factor abrogates hepatic failure induced by alpha-galactosylceramide without attenuating its antitumor effect in aged mice. J Hepatol 43: 670–678.
28. Sanai FM, Benmousa A, Al-Hussaini H, Ashraf S, Alhafi O, et al. (2008) Is serum alanine transaminase level a reliable marker of histological disease in chronic hepatitis C infection? Liver Int 28: 1011–1018.

HCV Viral Decline at Week 2 of Peg-IFN-Alpha-2a/RBV Therapy as a Predictive Tool for Tailoring Treatment in HIV/HCV Genotype 1 Co-Infected Patients

Antonio Rivero-Juarez[1], Luis F. López-Cortés[2], Angela Camacho[1], Almudena Torres-Cornejo[2], Ana Gordon[1], Rosa Ruiz-Valderas[2], Julian Torre-Cisneros[1], Juan A. Pineda[3], Pompeyo Viciana[2], Antonio Rivero[1]*

1 Unidad de Enfermedades Infecciosas, Instituto Maimonides de Investigación Biomédica de Córdoba (IMIBIC), Hospital Universitario Reina Sofía de Córdoba, Córdoba, Spain, **2** Unidad Clínica de Enfermedades Infecciosas, Microbiología y Medicina Preventiva, Instituto de Biomedicina de Sevilla (IBiS), Hospital Universitario Virgen del Rocío/CSIC/Universidad de Sevilla, Seville, Spain, **3** Unidad de Enfermedades Infecciosas y Microbiología Clínica, Instituto de Biomedicina de Sevilla (IBiS), Hospital Universitario de Valme, Seville, Spain

Abstract

Background: Optimizing HCV genotype 1 therapy in terms of response prediction and tailoring treatment is undoubtedly the cornerstone of treating HIV co-infected patients in clinical practice. Accordingly, our aim was to analyze the predictive value of HCV viral decline for sustained virological response (SVR), measured at a time point as early as week 2 of therapy with pegylated interferon alpha-2a plus ribavirin (Peg-IFN/RBV).

Methods: Previously untreated HIV/HCV genotype 1 co-infected patients were included in this study. The HCV RNA titer was measured at week 2 after starting treatment with Peg-IFN/RBV. The likelihood of reaching SVR when HCV RNA viral titers declined at week 2 was evaluated relative to predictive baseline factors.

Results: A total of 192 HIV/HCV genotype-1 co-infected patients were enrolled in the study and began therapy. One hundred and sixty-three patients completed a full course of Peg-IFN/RBV treatment for 2 weeks and 59 of these (36.2%) reached SVR. An HCV RNA viral load decline of $\geq$1.5 log IU/mL at week 2 had the maximum positive predictive value for SVR (83.3%; 95% CI: 68.5%–92.9%) and was identified as the strongest independent predictive factor for reaching SVR across all baseline predictive factors.

Conclusions: HCV viral decline at week 2 had a high predictive value for identifying patients with a high and low likelihood of reaching SVR using dual therapy, regardless of strong predictive baseline factors. This finding may be useful for developing a predictive tool to help tailor HCV genotype 1 therapy in HIV co-infected patients.

Editor: Yue Wang, National Institute for Viral Disease Control and Prevention, CDC, China, China

Funding: This work was partly supported by grants from the Fundación Progreso y Salud, Consejería de Salud de la Junta de Andalucía (grants for health research projects; refs. 0036-2010, 0157-2011, 0430-2012). A.R. was the recipient of a research extension grant from the Fundación Progreso y Salud, Consejería de Salud de la Junta de Andalucía (ref. AI-0021). A.R.-J. is the recipient of a Post-Doctoral Research Grant from the Fundación Progreso y Salud, Consejería de Salud de la Junta de Andalucía. The funders had no role in study design, data collection and analysis, decision to publish, or preparation of the manuscript.

Competing Interests: Neither the authors nor their institution have received payment or services at any time from a third party for any aspect of the submitted work (e.g., data monitoring board, study design, manuscript preparation, statistical analysis, etc.). Apart from the submitted work, A.R. and J.A.P. have received consulting fees from Bristol-Myers Squibb, Abbott, Gilead, Roche, Boehringer Ingelheim, GlaxoSmithKline, Merck Sharp & Dohme, and Janssen-Cilag. They have received lecture fees from GlaxoSmithKline, Roche, Abbott, Bristol-Myers Squibb, Boehringer Ingelheim and Schering-Plough. The remaining authors have no conflicts of interest to declare.

* Email: ariveror@gmail.com

Introduction

Adding a direct-acting antiviral (DAA) drug for the treatment of hepatitis C (HCV) to pegylated-interferon plus ribavirin therapy (Peg-IFN/RBV) substantially improves the sustained virological response (SVR) rate in HCV genotype 1 patients co-infected with the human immunodeficiency virus (HIV) [1]. HCV DAAs are currently available in routine clinical practice. The results obtained from using these new drugs in previously untreated co-infected HIV/HCV genotype 1 patients show significantly enhanced SVR rates in this subset of patients [1]. Nevertheless, there are several limitations to the addition of these drugs that could limit their use in those patients who are starting their first anti-HCV treatment. Perhaps the most important limitation worldwide is the substantial increase in therapy costs [2]. Therefore, even though DAAs increase the chances of reaching SVR, the use of Peg-IFN/RBV alone in HCV genotype 1 patients may remain the first-line therapeutic option in most countries according to World Health Organization (WHO) HCV treatment guidelines [1]. So, optimizing HCV genotype 1 therapy, in terms of response prediction and tailoring the treatment, is unquestionably the cornerstone for treating HIV co-infected patients in clinical practice.

Host genetic patterns are excellent clinical tools for estimating patient treatment outcomes after a full course of therapy with Peg-IFN/RBV [3–7]. However, achieving on-treatment virological milestones is the critical factor for determining outcome across all baseline factors [8–11]. Those patients who achieve a rapid virological response (RVR) even if they harbor theoretically unfavorable baseline factors have a high chance of achieving SVR [8,9].

Bringing forward the predictive treatment time points could be an important aspect of clinical practice for providing each patient with the best treatment regimen earlier. The aim of this study therefore was to analyze the predictive value of HCV viral decline for SVR, as measured at the early time point of week 2 of therapy with Peg-IFN/RBV, relative to well-known predictive factors.

Materials and Methods

Selection of Patients

HIV-infected patients with previously untreated chronic hepatitis C caused by viral genotype 1 were included in the study. Those patients who were positive for the hepatitis B surface antigen (HBsAg) were excluded. Patients were prospectively followed-up in two reference hospitals in southern Spain. The criteria used to determine hepatitis C therapy followed the American Association for the Study of Liver Diseases (AASLD) guidelines [12]. Host, clinical and virological characteristics were collected. The liver fibrosis stage was determined by liver biopsy using METAVIR fibrosis scores. Transient liver elastography (FibroScan, Echosens, Paris) was used to measure the liver stiffness values of those patients who had not undergone a pre-treatment liver biopsy. Liver stiffness measurements were taken by a single experienced operator at each participating hospital, following a routine described elsewhere. Advanced liver fibrosis was defined as a liver fibrosis stage of F3 or higher in patients who had undergone a pre-treatment liver biopsy or as a baseline liver stiffness value of ≥11kPa [13]. IL28B genotyping assays are described elsewhere [3].

Treatment Regimens, Virological Evaluation and Outcomes

All individuals were treated with Peg-IFN-alpha-2a at doses of 180 μg per week, in combination with a weight-adjusted dose of oral ribavirin (1000 mg/day for patients <75 kg and 1200 mg/day for patients ≥75 kg) for 48 or 72 weeks, following AASLD guidelines [12].

Plasma HCV RNA titers were measured using a quantitative RT-PCR assay (Cobas Taq Man, Roche Diagnostic Systems Inc., Pleasanton, CA, USA), with a detection limit set at 15 IU/mL. In addition to routine treatment point measurements of plasma HCV RNA, for the purpose of this study, HCV RNA titers were measured 2 weeks after starting treatment.

HCV genotypes were determined using a hybridization assay (INNO-LiPa HCV, Bayer Corp., Tarrytown, NY, USA). HCV genotype 1was defined as 1a or 1b.

RVR was defined as a serum HCV RNA titer below the 15 IU/mL detection limit at day 28 after start of treatment. Patients with HCV RNA viral decline lower than 2 log UI/mL at week 12 after starting treatment were classified as null responders (NRs). An end-of-treatment response (ETR) was defined as a serum HCV RNA concentration below the 15 IU/mL detection limit upon the completion of therapy. SVR was defined as a serum HCV RNA titer below the 15 IU/mL detection limit 24 weeks after completion of therapy. Viral relapse (REL) was defined as detectable serum HCV RNA after having reached ETR.

Statistical Analyses

Continuous variables were expressed as the mean ± standard deviation and were analyzed using the Student's *t*-test, the Mann-Whitney *U*-test or the Kruskal-Wallis test. Categorical variables were expressed as number of cases (percentage). Frequencies were compared using the χ^2 test or Fisher's exact test. Significance was defined as a *p*-value of less than 0.05. For the purpose of this study, analyses were assessed using an on-treatment approach, excluding those who voluntarily dropped out or discontinued therapy due to adverse events. Patients were stratified according to the magnitude of HCV RNA viral decline 2 weeks after starting therapy. The likelihood of reaching SVR based on HCV RNA viral decline at week 2 was evaluated. Positive predictive value (PPV) was defined as the probability of achieving SVR based on HCV RNA reduction at week 2. For the PPV, a two-sided 95% confidence interval (95% CI) was calculated using the exact binomial distribution. Predictive accuracy was assessed by comparing area under the receiver operating characteristic (AUROC) curves. Variables associated with SVR were entered into logistic regression models. The analysis was carried out using the SPSS statistical software package, version 18.0 (IBM Corporation, Somers, NY, USA).

Ethical Statement

The study was designed and performed according to the Helsinki Declaration and approved by the ethics committee of the Reina Sofia University Hospital, Cordoba, Spain. All patients provided a written informed consent form before participating in the study and gave permission for biological samples from routine diagnostic processes to be stored and processed in the Biobanco del Hospital Universitario Reina Sofía de Córdoba [biobank of the University Hospital Reina Sofia, Cordoba] (ISCIII reference: B.0000419), which forms part of the Biobanco del Sistema Sanitario Público de Andalucía [biobank of the Public Health System of Andalusia]. The CEIC [Clinical Trial and Ethical Committee] of the Hospital Universitario Reina Sofía de Córdoba approved the study protocol.

Results

Study Population

A total of 192 HIV/HCV genotype 1 co-infected patients started therapy and were enrolled in the study. Twenty-nine patients (15.1%) withdrew from therapy: 12 (6.2%) voluntarily dropped out and 17 (8.8%) discontinued therapy due to adverse events. Consequently, the on-treatment population that completed a full-course of therapy consisted of 163 patients. The most relevant demographic, virological and clinical characteristics of the on-treatment population are shown in Table 1.

Virological Response

The overall SVR was 30.7% (95% CI: 24.5%–37.5%). Among the 163 on-treatment patients, 59 reached SVR (36.2%; 95% CI: 29.1%–43.8%). Sixteen patients (9.8%; 95% CI: 5.9%–15.1%) experienced REL. Fifty-two patients (31.9%; CI 95%: 25.1%–39.3%) dropped below 2 log IU/mL at week 12 of treatment and were classified as NRs.

Eighteen patients (11.04%; 95% CI: 6.9%–16.5%) achieved RVR, and all but 1 of these achieved SVR (PPV 94.4%; 95% CI: 75.5%–99.7%). Seven patients (4.3%; CI 95%: 1.9%–8.6%)

Table 1. Demographic, virological and clinical characteristics of the on-treatment population.

Characteristic	On-treatment approach (N = 163)
Gender male, n (%)	133 (81.6)
Age (years), mean (SD)	41.5 (5.9)
BMI (kg/m^2), mean (SD)	24.1 (4.2)
Previous AIDS-defining criteria, n (%)*	46 (28.2)
IDU, n (%)	132 (80.9)
Nadir CD4 cell count (cells/mL), mean (SD)	167 (132)
Baseline CD4 cell count (cells/mL), mean (SD)	554 (273)
HAART use, n (%)	150 (92.02)
Unquantifiable HIV RNA viral load, n (%)†	138 (84.6)
HCV genotype, n (%)	
1a	89 (54.6)
1b	62 (38)
1a/1b	6 (3.7)
Not genotyped	6 (3.7)
Liver fibrosis stage F3–F4, n (%)‡	83 (50.9)
ALT (IU/L), mean (SD)	79.03 (57.7)
LDL cholesterol (mg/dL), mean (SD)	84.6 (31.3)
IL28B genotype, n (%)§	
TT	11 (7.4)
CT	84 (56.7)
CC	53 (35.9)

Legend: number of cases (N); standard deviation (SD); Body mass index (BMI); kilograms (kg); meters (m); acquired immunodeficiency syndrome (AIDS); injecting drugs user (IDU); highly active antiretroviral treatment (HAART); human immunodeficiency virus (HIV); hepatitis C virus (HCV); alanine aminotransferase (ALT); low-density lipoprotein (LDL); interleukin 28B (IL28B); cytosine (C); thymine (T).

*Classified on the basis of Center for Disease Control and Prevention (CDC) recommendations *(Revised surveillance case definitions for HIV infection among adults, adolescents, and children aged <18 years and for HIV infection and AIDS among children aged 18 months to <13 years-United States, 2008. MMWR 2008; 57 (No RR-10): 1–14).*

†HIV viral load was measured by PCR (CobasTaqMan, Roche Diagnostic Systems Inc., Pleasanton, CA, USA), detection limit set at 20 IU/mL.

‡Fibrosis stage was determined by liver biopsy according to METAVIR fibrosis score staging or using liver transient elastography (FibroScan, Echosens, Paris).

§Available in 148 (90.8%) patients.

reached unquantifiable HCV RNA at week 2, and all of these patients reached SVR (PPV 100%; 95% CI: 65.2%–100%).

SVR Rate According to HCV RNA Viral Decline during the First Two Weeks of Therapy

The AUROC curve value for HCV RNA decline at week 2 for SVR was 0.788 (0.703–0.869). When patients were sorted according to HCV RNA viral decline at week 2, 36 patients (22.09%; 95% CI: 16.2%–28.9%) experienced a ≥1.5 log IU/mL decline. Of these, 30 achieved SVR (PPV 83.3%; 95% CI: 68.5%–92.9%) (Table 2).

PPV for SVR of HCV RNA Viral Decline at Week 2 According to Baseline Factors

The PPV for SVR of an HCV RNA viral decline of ≥1.5 log IU/mL at week 2 was analyzed relative to IL28B genotype (Figure 1A), liver fibrosis stage (Figure 1B), HCV genotype (Figure 1C), and baseline HCV RNA viral load (Figure 1D). Among those patients who reached an HCV viral decline of ≥1.5 log IU/mL at week 2, no differences in SVR rates were found across all the baseline predictive factors analyzed (Figure 1).

Two multiple logistic regression analyses for SVR were performed (Figure 2). Both RVR (Figure 2A) and HCV viral decline of ≥1.5 log IU/mL at week 2 (Figure 2B) were identified as the strongest independent predictive factors for reaching SVR in both models, independent of baseline predictive factors.

Table 3 shows the PPV for SVR of HCV viral decline at week 2, baseline HCV RNA viral loads and IL28B genotypes. The combination of these three factors had a PPV for SVR of 100% (95% CI: 60.7%–100%), whereas in patients who lacked these three predictive factors, the SVR rate was 15.1% (95% CI: 7.9%–25.3%). Furthermore, in patients carrying the IL28B CC genotype and having a low baseline HCV viral load, the chance of achieving SVR varied significantly according to whether they reached an HCV viral decline of ≥1.5 log IU/mL by week 2 (100%; 95% CI: 60.7%–100%) or not (50%; 95% CI: 18.4%–81.6%) ($p = 0.085$) (Table 3). Similarly, in patients carrying the unfavorable IL28B genotype and having higher baseline HCV viral loads, the likelihood of reaching SVR varied according to whether HCV viral decline of ≥1.5 log IU/mL was reached (77.8%; 95% CI: 43.8%–96.1%) or not (15.1%; 95% CI: 7.9%–25.3%) ($p<0.001$) (Table 3).

Discussion

Our study shows that HCV viral decline at week 2 of treatment exhibits a high PPV for SVR using Peg-IFN/RBV therapy. This finding could have important clinical applications since this

Table 2. Positive predictive value of HCV RNA viral decline at week 2 after starting therapy for sustained virological response (on-treatment approach, N = 163).

HCV viral decline at week 2	N	SVR	PPV (%)	95% CI
≥0.25 log IU/mL	123	54	43.9	35.3–52.7
≥0.5 log IU/mL	87	47	54.02	43.5–64.3
≥1 log IU/mL	56	39	69.6	56.7–80.6
≥1.5 log IU/mL	36	30	83.3	68.5–92.9
≥2 log IU/mL	25	21	84	65.7–94.7
≥2.5 log IU/mL	21	17	80.9	60.2–93.6
≥3 log IU/mL	13	10	76.9	49.1–93.7

Legend: Hepatitis C virus (HCV); number of patients (N); Sustained Virological Response (SVR); Positive predictive value (PPV), sustained virological response (SVR); 95% confidence interval (95% CI), international unit per milliliter (IU/mL).

strategy could enable the clinician to identify earlier those patients with a high likelihood of reaching SVR using dual therapy, with undoubted cost savings.

The use of HCV viral decline at week 4 of therapy for optimizing HCV treatment has been widely described [8,12]. With respect to previously untreated HCV genotype 1 patients, achievement of RVR is the best treatment time point [8]. This has also been demonstrated in the DAA scenario [14]. In this context, patients on Peg-IFN/RBV therapy in a clinical trial who reached RVR had the same probability of achieving SVR as patients with Peg-IFN/RBV plus boceprevir [15]. Accordingly, the authors suggested that all patients initiating treatment against HCV genotype 1 should start therapy with two drugs, then use HCV viral kinetics to determine whether a third drug should be added during week 4 of therapy [15]. Nevertheless, even though RVR was the strongest predictive factor for SVR, only a small

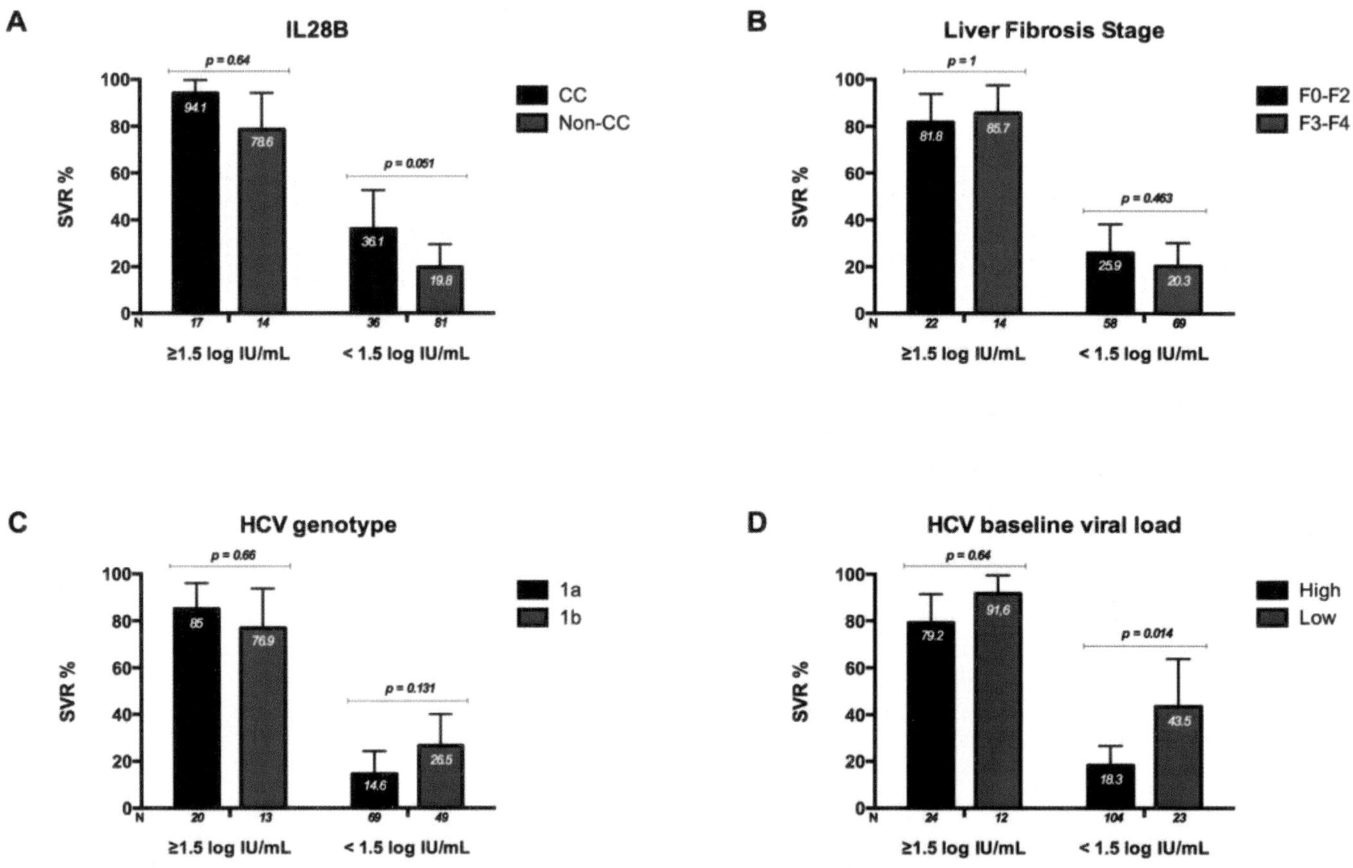

Figure 1. Comparison of Positive Predictive Value (PPV) for Sustained Virological Response (SVR) of viral decline of ≥ or < than 1.5 log IU/mL at week 2 after start of therapy relative to IL28B genotype (CC *versus* non-CC) (Figure 1A), liver fibrosis stage (F0–F2 *versus* F3–F4) (Figure 1B), HCV genotype (1a *versus* 1b) (Figure 1C), and baseline HCV viral load (≥600,000 IU/mL *versus* <600,000 IU/mL) (Figure 1D). *P* value was obtained using Fisher's exact test or the chi-square test.

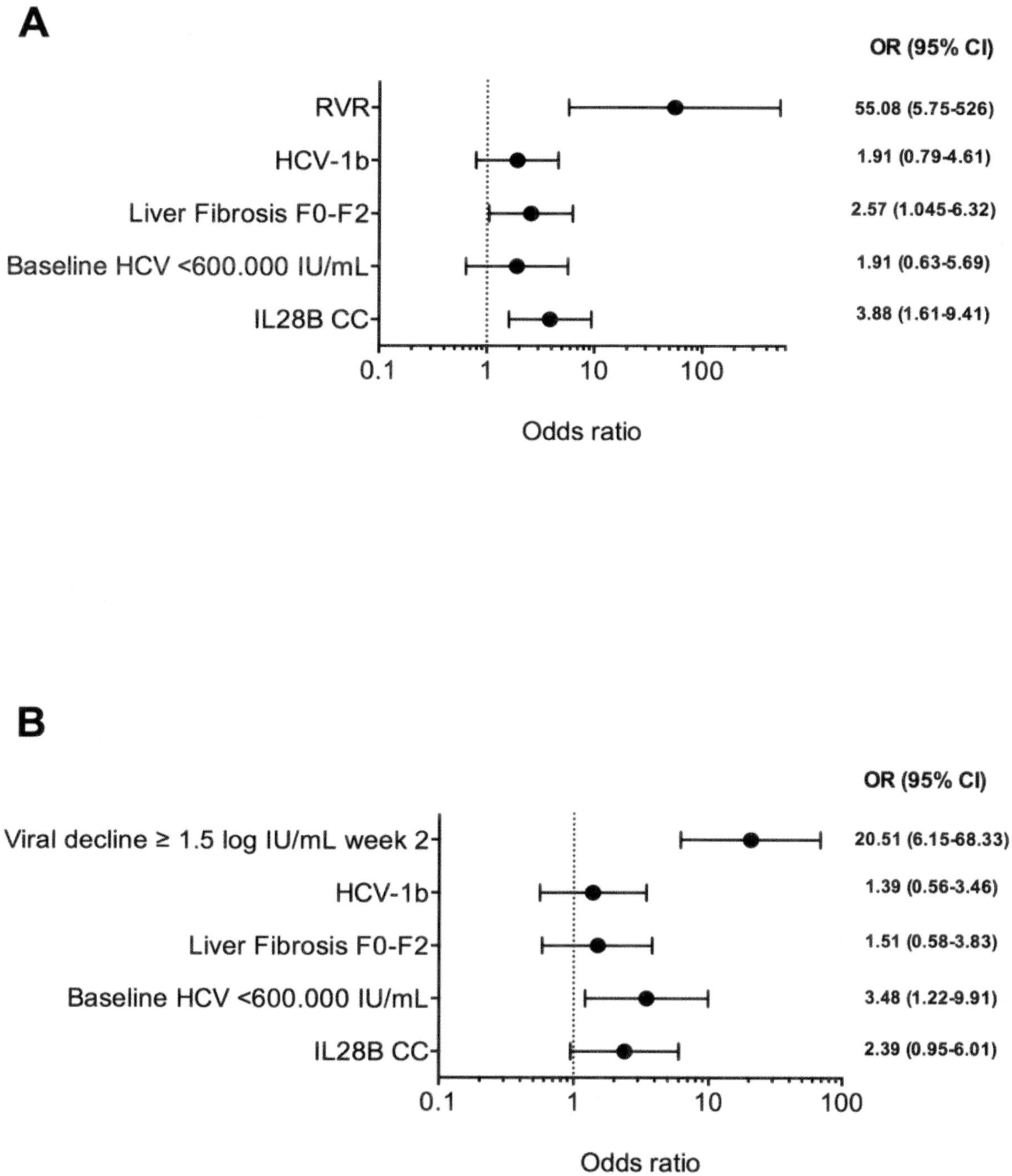

Figure 2. Multivariate logistic regression analysis for sustained virological response (SVR) including rapid virological response (RVR) (2A) and HCV viral decline of ≥1.5 log IU/mL at week 2 (2B). Odds Ratios (OR) and 95% Confidence Interval (95% CI) of each variable are shown to the right of the figure.

proportion of patients actually reached it, so limiting the benefit of the strategy [9,10]. By increasing the number of classified patients and maintaining the PPV, evaluating the magnitude of HCV viral decline at week 4 considerably improved the clinical value, relative to the single criterion of RVR [9–11]. A recent study performed by our group described how including an evaluation of HCV viral decline at week 4 (≥2.5 log IU/mL) identified a higher number of potential SVR patients than the single criterion of RVR [9].

Our study shows that it is possible to predict a successful treatment outcome as early as 2 weeks after starting therapy. Based on our results, previously untreated HIV/HCV genotype 1 patients who experience an HCV viral decline of ≥1.5 log IU/mL at week 2 have a high chance of achieving SVR with a treatment based on Peg-IFN/RBV, and so allow us to identify a higher proportion of patients than when a prediction of RVR is used (22.1% and 11.04%, respectively). This suggests that the applicability of week 4 in predicting a successful treatment outcome could be brought forward to week 2 after start of therapy. Accordingly, clinicians could use an initial treatment phase of just 2 weeks with Peg-IFN/RBV, after which, depending

Table 3. Positive predictive value of HCV RNA viral decline at week 2 after starting therapy, HCV baseline viral load and IL28B genotype for Sustained Virological Response.

HCV decline ≥1.5 log IU/mL	Viral load <600,000 IU/mL	IL28B CC	N*	SVR	PPV (%)	95% CI
+	+	+	6	6	100	60.7–100
+	–	+	11	10	90.9	62.6–99.5
+	+	–	5	4	80	33.4–99
+	–	–	9	7	77.8	43.8–96.1
–	+	+	8	4	50	18.4–81.6
–	+	–	15	6	40	18.1–65.4
–	–	+	28	9	32.1	16.9–50.8
–	–	–	66	10	15.1	7.9–25.3

Legend: Hepatitis C virus (HCV); international unit per milliliter (IU/mL); Interleukin 28B (IL28B); number of patients (N); Sustained Virological Response (SVR); Positive predictive value (PPV); 95% Confidence Interval (95% CI); Matched condition (+); Unmatched condition (–). The negative condition refers to: HCV decline of <1.5 log IU/mL, baseline viral load ≥600,000 IU/mL, and IL28B Non-CC genotype.
*Total population included = 148.

on HCV viral decline, the treatment strategy could be personalized on a cost/benefit basis.

Our data provided one interesting finding concerning the clinical value of predicting the success of Peg-IFN/RBV therapy in co-infected HIV/HCV genotype1 patients. Among patients carrying both favorable baseline predictive factors (namely, the IL28B CC genotype and a low baseline HCV viral load), the likelihood of achieving SVR varied strongly according to viral decline at week 2 (Table 3). Similarly, among patients harboring both unfavorable factors (namely, the Il28B non-CC genotype and a high baseline HCV viral load), the likelihood of achieving SVR varied according to whether viral decline was higher or lower than 1.5 log IU/mL. Consequently, applying a treatment strategy to a therapy whose success is based only on baseline host factors has limited power for accurately predicting SVR because the early response to therapy matters more for prognosis than baseline host factors. This finding is consistent with a recent study published by our group, in which the likelihood of IL28 CC patients with a slow HCV viral decline at week 4 of treatment of reaching a successful treatment outcome using dual therapy was small [16]. Therefore, regardless of the patient's baseline "prognosis profile", the strategy of an initial 2-week phase of treatment with dual therapy might be an excellent tool for identifying those with a high chance of achieving SVR.

However, our study has several drawbacks. First, the number of patients was relatively small, which may have prevented us from detecting differences between baseline groups according to HCV viral decline at week 2. Second, the impact of using our findings on HIV/HCV genotype 1 patients is unknown, because we did not carry out a study of response-guided therapy. Third, we determined the IL28B genotype in 90.8% of patients; however, because it was not available for the entire study population, the impact of this host factor on statistical analysis may be limited. Finally, our results may not be generalizable to types of pegylated interferon preparation other than alpha-2a, although differences in treatment response and HCV viral decline using, for example, peg-interferon alpha-2b, would not be expected.

In conclusion, our findings show that HCV viral decline at week 2 after start of therapy could be used to predict the treatment outcome of Peg-IFN/RBV in HIV/HCV genotype 1 co-infected patients. The cut-off value of 1.5 log IU/mL yielded a high predictive value for identifying patients with a high and low likelihood of reaching SVR using dual therapy, regardless of whether strong predictive baseline factors were present. This finding may be useful for developing a predictive tool that may help in tailoring HCV genotype 1 therapy in HIV co-infected patients, so avoiding unnecessary costs and without compromising the chance of achieving SVR. Before applying our results to clinical practice, a response-guided therapy study is mandatory.

Author Contributions

Conceived and designed the experiments: ARJ LFLC AR. Performed the experiments: ARJ LFLC AC AG ATC RRV AR. Analyzed the data: ARJ LFLC AR. Contributed reagents/materials/analysis tools: ARJ AC AG ATC RRV. Wrote the paper: ARJ AR. Critical discussion of the manuscript: ARJ LFLC AC ATC AG RRV JTC JAP PV AR.

References

1. World Health Organization (2014) Guidelines for the screening, care and treatment of persons with hepatitis C infection. Available: http://www.who.int/hiv/pub/hepatitis/hepatitis-c-guidelines. Accessed 2014 Apr 28.
2. Ahmed F (2013) What about us? Recent advances in the treatment of chronic hepatitis C threaten to leave some parts of the world behind. J Viral Hepat 20: 367–8.
3. Pineda JA, Caruz A, Rivero A, Neukam K, Salas I, et al. (2010) Prediction of response to pegylated interferon plus ribavirin by IL28B gene variation in patients coinfected with HIV and hepatitis C virus. ClinInfectDis 51: 788–95.
4. Pineda JA, Caruz A, Di Lello FA, Camacho A, Mesa P, et al. (2011) Low-density lipoprotein receptor genotyping enhances the predictive value of IL28B genotype in HIV/hepatitis C virus coinfected patients. AIDS 25: 1415–20.
5. Rivero-Juarez A, Gonzalez R, Camacho A, Manzanares-Martin B, Caruz A, et al. (2013) Natural killer KIR3DS1 is closely associated with HCV viral clearance and sustained virological response in HIV/HCV patients. PLoSOne 8: e61992.
6. Neukam K, Caruz A, Rivero-Juárez A, Barreiro P, Merino D, et al. (2013) Variations at multiple genes improve interleukin 28b genotype predictive capacity for response to therapy against hepatitis c genotype 1 or 4 infection. AIDS 27: 2715–24.
7. Andriulli A, Marco VD, Margaglione M, Ippolito AM, Fattovich G, et al. (2014) Identification of Naïve Hcv-1 Patients with Chronic Hepatitis who may Benefit from Dual Therapy with Peg-Interferon and Ribavirin. J Hepatol 60: 16–21.
8. Marcellin P, Cheinquer H, Curescu M, Dusheiko GM, Ferenci P, et al. (2012) High sustained virologic response rates in rapid virologic response patients in the large real-world PROPHESYS cohort confirm results from randomized clinical trials. Hepatology 56: 2039–50.
9. Rivero-Juarez A, Neukam K, Labarga P, Camacho A, Macias J, et al. (2014) Sustained virological response in HIV/HCV co-infected patients treated with pegylated interferon/ribavirin can be predicted from the overall rate of viral load decline over the first 4 weeks of therapy. J Infection 68: 372–7.

10. Marcellin P, Reau N, Ferenci P, Hadziyannis S, Messinger D, et al. (2012) Refined prediction of week 12 response and SVR based on week 4 response in HCV genotype 1 patients treated with peginterferon alfa-2a (40KD) and ribavirin. J Hepatol 56: 1276–1282.
11. Dogan UB, Akın MS, Yalaki S (2013) Sustained virological response based on the week 4 response in hepatitis C virus genotype 1 patients treated with peginterferons α-2a and α-2b, plus ribavirin. Eur J Gastroenterol Hepatol 25: 1317–1320.
12. Ghany MG, Strader DB, Thomas DL, Seeff LB (2009) Diagnosis, Management and Treatment of Hepatitis C: An update. AASLD PracticeGuidelines. Hepatology 49: 1335–1374.
13. Vergara S, Macías J, Rivero A, Gutiérrez-Valencia A, González-Serrano M, et al. (2007) The use of transient elastometry for assessing liver fibrosis in patients with HIV and hepatitis C virus coinfection. Clin Infect Dis 45: 969–74.
14. Pascale A, Serfaty L (2013) Triple therapy with first generation HCV protease inhibitors: lead-in or no lead-in phase? J Hepatol 58: 391–4.
15. Pearlman BL, Ehleben C (2014) Hepatitis C genotype 1 virus with low viral load and rapid virologic response to peginterferon/ribavirin obviates a protease inhibitor.Hepatology 59: 71–77.
16. Neukam K, Barreiro P, Rivero-Juárez A, Caruz A, Mira JA, et al. (2013) Pegylated interferon plus ribavirin is suboptimal in IL28B CC carriers without rapid response. J Infect 67: 59–64.

26

Cannabinoid Receptor 2-63 QQ Variant Is Associated with Persistently Normal Aminotransferase Serum Levels in Chronic Hepatitis C

Nicola Coppola[1]*, Rosa Zampino[2], Caterina Sagnelli[3], Giulia Bellini[4], Aldo Marrone[2], Maria Stanzione[3], Nicolina Capoluongo[1], Adriana Boemio[2], Carmine Minichini[1], Luigi Elio Adinolfi[2], Sabatino Maione[4], Emanuele Miraglia Del Giudice[5], Evangelista Sagnelli[1], Francesca Rossi[5]

1 Department of Mental Health and Public Medicine, Second University of Naples, Naples, Italy, **2** Internal Medicine and Hepatology, Second University of Naples, Naples, Italy, **3** Department of Clinical and Experimental Medicine and Surgery, Second University of Naples, Naples, Italy, **4** Department of Experimental Medicine, Second University of Naples, Naples, Italy, **5** Department of Pediatrics, Second University of Naples, Naples, Italy

Abstract

Background and Aim: To evaluate in anti-HCV-positive patients the clinical impact of the rs35761398 variant of the *CNR2* gene leading to the substitution of Gln (Q) of codon 63 of the cannabinoid receptor 2 (CB2) with Arg (R).

Patients and Methods: 253 consecutive anti-HCV-/HCV-RNA-positive patients were enrolled, of whom 53 were HCV carriers with persistently normal ALT (PNALT group) and 200 had a history of steadily abnormal serum ALT values (abnormal ALT group). All patients were naive for antiviral therapy and were screened for the CNR2 rs35761398 polymorphism by a TaqMan assay.

Results: Subjects in the PNALT group, compared with those in the abnormal ALT group were older (58.5 ± 12 vs. 50.7 ± 12.4 years, $p=0.001$), more frequently female (66% vs. 42%, $p=0.003$), with lower body massindex (BMI) (24.5 ± 3.1 vs. 26.6 ± 4.6, $p=0.003$), and more frequently with HCV genotype 2 (43.1% vs 17.7%, $p=0.0002$) and CB2-63 QQ variant (34% vs. 11%, $p=0.0001$). Considering all 253 patients, no difference in the demographic, biochemical, or virological data was observed between patients in the different CB2-63 variants. The logistic regression analysis identified CB2-63 QQ, HCV genotype 2, older age and lower BMI as independent predictors of PNALT ($p<0.00001$).

Discussion: The CB2-63 QQ variant in HCV patients was independently associated with the PNALT status.

Editor: Yury E. Khudyakov, Centers for Disease Control and Prevention, United States of America

Funding: This study was supported by a grant from PRIN 2008, M.I.U.R., Rome, Italy "OTTIMIZZAZIONE DELLA DIAGNOSI EZIOLOGICA DELL'EPATITE ACUTA C E STUDIO DEI FATTORI VIRO-IMMUNOLOGICI DI GUARIGIONE, DI CRONICIZZAZIONE E DI RISPOSTA ALLA TERAPIA CON INTERFERONE" and in part by a grant from Regione Campania "Progetti per il miglioramento della qualità dell'assistenza, diagnosi e terapia del paziente affetto da AIDS nei settori: immunologia, coinfezioni, informazione e prevenzione", 2008. The funders had no role in study design, data collection and analysis, decision to publish, or preparation of the manuscript.

Competing Interests: The authors have declared that no competing interests exist.

* E-mail: nicola.coppola@unina2.it

Introduction

The Cannabinoid (CB) receptors are seven membrane domain receptors of the G-coupled receptor superfamily that are activated by endogenous (endo) or exogenous (phyto and synthetic) cannabinoids [1,2]. Among the endocannabinoids, anandamide (AEA) was the first discovered, followed by 2-arachidonoylglycerol (2-AG) [1,2]. Two types of CB receptors are known, type 1 (CB1) and type 2 (CB2): CB1 is predominantly expressed in the central nervous system but also in the lung, liver and kidney, and CB2 in the immune and immune-derived cells (lymphocyte T and B cells, etc.) [3,4] .CB2 is also highly expressed in Kupffer cells, resident macrophages in the liver, which, due to their phagocytic activity, play an essential role in the acute and chronic responses of the liver to toxic and infectious agents [5].

A polymorphism at codon 63 of the Cannabinoid Receptor 2 gene (CNR2) leads to the substitution of glutamine, Gln (Q), with arginine, Arg (R), causing a different polarization state of the protein; the CB2 variants have been demonstrated to affect differently the ability of the CB2 receptor to exert its inhibitory function[5,6]. Specifically, *in-vitro* T lymphocytes from CB2-63 RR homozygotes showed an approximately two-fold reduction in the endocannabinoid-induced inhibition of proliferation compared to cells from CB2-63 QQ homozygotes [6,7].

The hepatitis C virus (HCV) infects over 170 million people worldwide and is a leading cause of cirrhosis and hepatocellular carcinoma [8]. The severity of chronic hepatitis C (CHC) is highly variable among patients and over time. Some individuals show a mild indolent clinical course for decades, others rapidly progress to end-stage liver disease [9], whereas about 20–30% of cases remain asymptomatic with normal serum alanine aminotransferase (ALT) levels lifelong. According to the Italian guidelines, the definition of an anti-HCV carrier with persistently normal ALT (PNALT) serum values applies to a subject with at least 9 consecutive ALT normal values observed at two-monthly intervals over an 18-month observation period[10]and identifies a subclinical form of CHC. The majority of carriers with PNALT show histological evidence of necroinflammation and fibrosis, but the liver lesions are clearly less severe than those observed in subjects with abnormal ALT [11,12]. Most of them show a slow fibrosis progression [13], but liver cirrhosis may develop after an ALT flare-up has occurred [14].

Several factors have been found to be linked to the progression and severity of CHC, including virus-related (duration of infection) and host factors (interleukin-28B polymorphism), co-morbidities (coinfection with human immunodeficiency virus, HIV, or hepatitis B virus, HBV, insulin-resistance, high body mass index, immunosuppression), and lifestyle factors (alcohol intake, cannabis use) [15–20]. Moreover, the data from a recent study suggested the involvement in CHC of the rs35761398 variant of the CNR2 gene encoding for CB2, since the CB2-63 QQ variant was associated with more severe necroinflammation in anti-HCV-positive patients with abnormal ALT [21]. Instead, only a few published data on factors possibly associated with the subclinical form of chronic HCV infection are available at present.

The present paper analyzes the role of CB2 variants in 53 consecutive HCV carriers with PNALT in comparison with 200 consecutive patients with abnormal ALT.

Patients and Methods

Patients

Two Liver Units in the Campania region (southern Italy) participated in the study. These two centers have cooperated in several clinical investigations using the same clinical approach and the same laboratory methods [21–23].

Two hundred and fifty-three consecutive Italian patients with chronic HCV infection (anti-HCV- and HCV-RNA-positive) for 18–36 months were included in the study. The patients were first observed from July 2009 to December 2012 and were naive for antiviral therapy at that time. Of the 253 patients enrolled, 53 (20.9%) were HCV carriers with PNALT (PNALT group) and 200 (79.1%) had a history of steadily abnormal serum ALT values (abnormal ALT group).

All 253 cases underwent complete physical examination, liver ultrasound scan, liver function tests, assessment of triglycerides, cholesterol, blood cell counts, alpha-fetoprotein and HBV, HCV, hepatitis delta virus (HDV) and HIV serum markers. All patients enrolled were asymptomatic, negative for anti-HIV, HBsAg and anti-HDV. On a specific home-made questionnaire none stated ongoing intravenous drug addiction at admission. Alcohol abuse was defined as the consumption of alcohol exceeding 30 g per day for females and 40 g per day for males in the last 6 months; the patient's statements regarding intravenous drug addiction and alcohol abuse were corroborated by the patient's family and by serum/urine tests in uncertain cases.

Liver biopsy was performed for 186 (73.5%) patients. The liver biopsy was proposed for all patients in the abnormal ALT group, but it was not performed for 29 (11.5%) because of refusal in 20 cases and contraindication in 9. In the PNALT group the liver biopsy was advised for the 18 patients aged 50 to 65 years with genotype 1 and was performed only for 15 of these because of refusal by the remaining 3 patients. Liver specimens were fixed in formalin, embedded in paraffin and stained with hematoxylin-eosin and Masson's trichrome stain. In each case, the liver specimens were more than 2 cm in length and had more than 11 portal tracts. Liver biopsies were examined by a pathologist who, unaware of the clinical and laboratory data, used the Ishak's scoring system to grade necroinflammation and fibrosis [24]. To assess liver steatosis we used a home-made scoring system obtained with a partial modification of Kleiner's scoring system for non-alcoholic fatty liver diseases [25], extensively reported in previously published papers [12,21,23]. Briefly, score 1 identifies the presence of fatty deposition in 1–10% of hepatocytes, score 2 in 11–31%, score 3 in 31–60% and score 4 in >60%. Samples of serum and whole blood were obtained for each patient at the time of enrolment and stored at −80°C until used for this investigation.

As a control group, six hundred normal subjects were evaluated for the CB2-63 polymorphism and ALT serum value.

Ethics Statement

All procedures used were in accordance with the international guidelines and with the Helsinki Declaration of 1975 and revised in 1983. The study was approved by the Ethics Committee of the Azienda Ospedaliera Universitaria of the Second University of Naples. All patients provided written informed consent for the collection and storage of biological samples and for the anonymous use of their data in clinical research.

Routine Analysis

HBV and HDV serum markers were sought using commercial immunoenzymatic assays (Abbott Laboratories, North Chicago, IL, USA, for HBsAg, anti-HBs and anti-HBc, and DiaSorin, Saluggia, VC, Italy, for anti-HDV). The anti-HCV antibody was sought using a 3rd generation commercial immunoenzymatic assay (Ortho Diagnostic Systems, Neckargemund, Germany). Antibodies to HIV 1 and 2 were sought using a commercial ELISA (Abbott Lab., North Chicago, Ill, USA). Liver function tests (ALT; aspartate aminotransferase; γ-glutamyltransferase, etc.) were performed by the routine serological methodsin Cobas Modular 6,000 automated analyzer using c501 biochemistry modules (Roche Diagnostics Ltd, Rotkreuz, Switzerland).

HCV Genotype and Viral Load

HCV genotype was determined using HCV genotype assay Lipa (Bayer, France), following the manufacturer's instructions.

Viral RNA was extracted from 140 μl of plasma samples using a microspin column (QIAamp RNA viral kit, Qiagen GmbH, Hilden, Germany). The HCV RNA was quantified by performing a real-time polymerase chain reaction (PCR) in a Light cycler 1.5 (Roche Diagnostics, Branchburg, NJ, USA), as reported in a previous paper [26]; by this method, the detection limit in plasma samples is estimated at around 40 IU/mL.

Genetic Analysis

Genomic DNA was extracted from peripheral whole blood with a DNA extraction kit (Roche Diagnostics, Branchburg, NJ, USA) after written informed consent. Molecular screening for the CNR2 rs35761398 polymorphism (CAA/CGG) underlying the CB2 Q63R substitution was performed using a TaqMan Assay (Real Master Mix Probe, 5 PRIME, Germany). Primers and probes were the following: sense primer 5′-GTGCTCTATCT-GATCCTGTC-3′ and anti-sense primer 5′-TAGT-CACGCTGCCAATC-3′; AA-probe 5′-CCCAC-CAACTCCGC-3′ and GG-probe 5′-CCCACCGGCTCCG-3′ (PRIMM, Milan, Italy). Both PCR and post-PCR allelic discrimination were carried out on an ABI PRISM 9600 apparatus (Applied Biosystems, Foster City, CA). Random samples were confirmed by direct PCR sequencing consisting of 94°C for 4 min followed by 31 cycles of 94°C for 30 s, 60°C for 30 s and 72°C for

Table 1. Demographic, genetic, virological, biochemical and histological data according to clinical condition.

	PNALT group	Abnormal ALT group	P-value
No. of patients	53	200	
Males, no. (%)	18 (33.9)	116 (58)	0.003
Age, years (M ± SD)	58.50±12.04	50.70±12.38	0.0001
BMI, (M ± SD)	24.51±3.14	26.56±4.63	0.003
AST, × n.v. (M ± SD)	0.58±0.27	1.84±1.36	0.0001
ALT, × n.v. (M ± SD)	0.58±0.29	2.38±1.62	0.0001
gGT, IU/ml (M ± SD)	39±54	53±45	0.055
Glucose, mg/dl (M ± SD)	102±33	95.37±21,72	0.067
Iron, ug/dl (M ± SD)	106±32	112±50	0.408
Ferritin, ng/ml (M ± SD)	132±106	157±127	0.189
Transferrin, (M ± SD)	290±45	287±46	0.552
Triglycerides, mg/dl (M ± SD)	96±49	106±58	0.251
Total cholesterol, mg/dl, (M ± SD)	173±23	177±42	0.506
HCV RNA, IU×10^3 (M ± SD)	3,559±5,087	2,367±5,746	0.171
HCV genotype, no. (%):			
1	28 (54.9)	131 (68.2)	2 vs non-2: 0.0002
2	22 (43.1)	34 (17.7)	
3	1 (1.96)	21 (10.9)	
4	0	4 (2.1)	
Missing	2	0	
IL28-B, no. (%):			
CC	20 (37.7)	53 (26.5)	CC vs. non CC: 0.151
CT	27 (50.1)	121 (60.5)	
TT	6 (11.3)	26 (13)	
CB2-63, no. (%):			
QQ	18 (34)	22 (11)	QQ vs non-QQ: 0.0001
QR	19 (35.8)	110 (55)	
RR	16 (30.2)	68 (34)	
Patients with LB, no. (%):	15 (28.3)	171 (88.5)	////
HAI score, (M ± SD)	3.47±2.47	6.04±3.50	0.0001
Fibrosis score, (M ± SD)	1.27±0.59	2.39±1.44	0.0001
Steatosis score, (M ± SD)	0.33±0.62	1.21±1.26	0.0001

M: mean; SD: standard deviation; BMI: body mass index; AST: aspartate-aminotransferase; x n.v.: times normal value; ALT: alanine aminotransferase; gGT: g-glutamyltransferase; LB: liver biopsy.

30 s with forward 5′-GAGTGGTCCCCAGAAGACAG-3′ and reverse 5′-CACAGAGGCTGTGAAGGTCA-3′ primers. PCR products were analyzed using an ABI PRISM 3100 automated sequencer (Applied Biosystems, Foster City, CA) and the Big Dye Terminator reaction kit (Applera, Foster City, CA), according to the manufacturer's instructions. All primers were chosen using Primer3 software (http://primer3.sourceforge.net/).

DNAs were tested also for the rs12979860 polymorphism of the IL-28B genotype (Roche Diagnostics, Branchburg, NJ, USA).

Statistical Analysis

Continuous variables were summarized as mean and standard deviation, and categorical variables as absolute and relative frequencies. Differences in the mean values were evaluated by an unpaired Student t-test, and the chi-squared test was applied to categorical variables. Not normally distributed variables (AST, ALT, HCV viral load) were log-transformed before the analysis, and the mean values are shown in Tables 1 and 2. A p value <0.05 was considered to be statistically significant. All independent variablesat univariate analysis with a biological plausibility to the aim of the study were included in the multivariate analysis using a general linear model. The statistical analysis was performed using Statgraphics Centurion XV.II (Adalta, Arezzo, Italy; Statpoint Technologies Inc., Virginia, USA).

Results

The differences in the initial characteristics between the 53 subjects with PNALT and the 200 with abnormal ALT are shown in Table 1. Subjects in the PNALT group, compared with those in the abnormal ALT group, were older [mean± standard deviation (SD) 58.5±12 vs. 50.7±12.4 years, p = 0.001], more frequently female (66% vs. 42%, p = 0.003), with lower body mass index (BMI) (24.5±3.1 vs. 26.6±4.6, p = 0.003), and more frequently

Table 2. Demographic, biochemical and histological characteristics in HCV patients according to CB2 63 genotype variants.

	CB2 QQ	CB2 QR	CB2 RR
No. of patients	40	129	84
Males, no. (%)	19 (47.5)	68 (52.7)	47 (56)
Age, years (M ± SD)	55.4±12.2	51.6±12.1	51.9±13.6
BMI (M ± SD)	24.97±5.77	26.17±4.01	26.30+4.03
AST × n.v. (M ± SD)	1.61±1.54	1.56±1.22	1.58+1.37
ALT × n.v. (M ± SD)	1.76±1.85	1.71±2.12	1.95±1.34
Total cholesterol, mg/dl (M ± SD)	163±31	178+43	178±36
Triglycerides, mg/dl (M ± SD)	106±50	104+62	107±49
Iron, ug/dl (M ± SD)	138±51	108±43	111±58
Ferritin, ng/ml, (M ± SD)	160±72	154±126	129±123
Transferrin, (M ± SD)	313±53	289+36	278±58
gGT IU/ml, (M ± SD)	62±66	51±48	49±32
Glucose mg/dl, (M ± SD)	90±11	97±25	96±21
HCV RNA, IU×10³,(M ± SD)	2,394±2,470	2,109±3,872	3,620±8,239
HCV genotype, no. (%):			
1	27 (69.2)	83 (66.4)	50 (63.3)
2	7 (17.9)	27 (21.6)	22 (27.8)
3	3 (7.7)	14 (11.2)	5 (6.3)
4	2 (5.1)	1 (0.8)	2 (2.5)
Missing	1	4	5
Patients with LB, no. (%)	21 (52.5)	107 (82.9)	58 (69.04)
HAI score (M ± SD)	7.81±4.08[a]	5.60±3.33[b]	5.55±3.47[c]
Fibrosis score (M ± SD)	2.67±1.77	2.24±1.39	2.28±1.35
Steatosis score (M ± SD)	1.19±1.25	1.17±1.19	1.22±1.23
Patients with PNALT, no. (%)	18 (45)[d]	19 (14.7)[e]	16 (19.04)[f]
IL28-B, no. (%):			
CC	11 (27.5)	41 (31.8)	21 (25)
CT	24 (60)	77 (56.7)	47 (56)
TT	5 (12.5)	11 (8.5)	16 (19.04)

M: mean; SD: standard deviation; BMI: body mass index; AST: aspartate-aminotransferase; x n.v.: times normal value; ALT: alanine aminotransferase; gGT: g-glutamyltransferase; LB: liver biopsy.
Differences significant to the statistical analysis: a vs. b: p = 0.008; a vs. c: p = 0.017; d vs. e: p = 0.0001; d vs. f: p = 0.005.

with HCV genotype 2 (43.1% vs. 17.7%, p = 0.0002) and the CB2-63 QQ variant (34% vs. 11%, p = 0.0001). To confirm our CB2-63 data, we considered as two separate cohorts the two series of subjects with HCV chronic infection included at the two enrolling Liver Units and compared the results obtained. Similar prevalences of CB2-63 QQ variant were observed in these two cohorts, both in PNALT subjects (1st cohort 31% of 35 subjects; 2nd cohort 38% of 18 subjects) and chronic hepatitis patients (1st cohort 10.7% of 130 patients; 2nd cohort 11.4% of 70 patients).

Also the IL28-B CC genotype was more frequently observed in the PNALT than in the abnormal ALT group (37.7% vs. 26.5%), a small difference not significant to the statistical analysis (p = 0.1). Considering only patients with liver biopsy, the 15 in the PNALT group showed a lower histological activity index (HAI) (3.47±2.47 vs. 6.04±3.5, p = 0.0001), lower fibrosis (1.27±0.59 vs. 2.39±1.44, p = 0.0001) and lower steatosis scores (0.33±0.62 vs. 1.21±1.26, p = 0.0001) than the 171 patients in the abnormal ALT group (Table 1). The 118 patients with a BMI over 25 had a higher steatosis score than the 68 with a lower BMI (1.5±1.4 vs. 0.8±1.05).

Considering all 253 patients with chronic HCV infection in the present study, the prevalence of PNALT subjects was significantly higher in the CB2-63 QQ than in the QR and RR subgroups (45% vs. 14.7%, p<0.0001, and 19.04%, p<0.005, respectively), whereas no difference in demographic, biochemical, or virological data was observed between patients in the different CB2-63 subgroups (Table 2). No association of the HCV load with the PNALT status or a CB2-63 variant was found in the present study (Tables 1 and 2), which is in agreement with previous investigations never displaying HCV load associated with clinical, biochemical and histological findings [27–29]. In addition, no significant difference in the ALT serum values was observed between subgroups established on the basis of the CB2 variants, most probably due to the fact that of the 253 subjects investigated, 200 were chronic hepatitis patients with increased ALT values and only 53 were PNALT subjects with normal ALT, too small a number to influence substantially the mean ALT levels in the three CB2 subgroups. Also in the 600 normal controls, no significant difference in the ALT values was observed in the three CB2-63 variants.

Table 3. Logistic regression between CB2-63 variants and PNALT.

Analysis of Variance for PNALT					
Source	**Sum of Squares**	**df**	**Mean Square**	**F-Ratio**	***p*-Value**
Model	10.59271648	7	1.51324521	10.18	**0.0000**
Residual	22.60103352	152	0.14869101		
Total (Corr.)	33.19375	159			
Single factor contribution					
Source	**Sum of Squares**	**df**	**Mean Square**	**F-Ratio**	***p*-Value**
CB2-63 QQ vs non-QQ	2.451458816	2	1.225729408	8.24	**0.0004**
Age	1.125386271	1	1.125386271	7.57	**0.0067**
Sex	0.066793766	1	0.066793766	0.45	0.5037
BMI	3.335028877	1	3.335028877	22.43	**0.0000**
HCV genotype 2 vs non-2	2.708676302	1	2.708676302	18.22	**0.0000**

Of the 186 patients who underwent liver biopsy (171 in the abnormal ALT group and 15 in the PNALT group), the 21 with CB2-63 QQ showed a higher (mean±SD: 7.81±4.1) HAI than the 107 with CB2-63 QR (5.6±3.3, p = 0.008) and the 58 with CB2-63 RR (5.5±3.5, p = 0.017), whereas no statistically significant differences were observed in the degree of liver fibrosis and steatosis. This analysis was not performed separately for the abnormal ALT group and the PNALT group because the latter included only 15 patients with liver biopsy, of whom only 2 with the QQ and 3 with the QR variant.

The prevalence of subjects with PNALT was higher (45%) in the 40 with CB2-63 QQ than in the 129 with CB2-63 QR (14.7%, p<0.0001) and in the 84 with CB2-63 RR (19%, p = 0.005).

To confirm the association between the CB2-63 variants and the status of PNALT, a multivariate logistic regression analysis was performed (Table 3). The analysis included the CB2-63 QQ variant versus non-QQ, HCV genotype 2 versus non-2 and other potential confounding factors like age, sex and BMI. After all the confounding effects of the other risk factors were removed, the CB2-63 QQ variant, HCV genotype 2, older age and lower BMI were the only independent predictors of PNALT (p<0.00001).

Discussion

This study analyzed the role of a functional polymorphism of the cannabinoid receptor type 2 in a cohort of 253 patients with HCV chronic infection and found the CB2-63 QQ variant independently associated with the PNALT status. Besides the CB2-63 QQ variant, the multivariate analysis identified another three factors independently associated with the PNALT status: HCV genotype 2, an older age and a lower BMI. HCV genotype 2 and a lower BMI have been suggested as independent predictors of PNALT in previous studies [10,30,31], and confirmed in the present investigation. Instead, this is the first time the CB2-63 QQ variant and an older age have been cited as independent predictors of the PNALT status.

The association between the CB2-63 QQ variant and the status of HCV carrier with PNALT may be the result of a prolonged strong inhibition of the T cells with QQ variants, with a consequently less vigorous immune response against infected hepatic cells. Support for this hypothesis comes from an *in-vitro* study on the CB2-mediated inhibition of T-cell proliferation, normal with T cells deriving from CB2-63 QQ subjects and reduced two-fold with T cells from subjects with the RR homozygous variant [7]. In fact, aggressive autoimmune pathologies such as celiac disease and childhood immune thrombocytopenic purpura have been found to be associated with the CB2-63 RR variant [32,33].

It has been recently suggested that HCV-related proteins induce prolonged activation of liver Kupffer cells, leading to the accumulation of inflammatory cytokines that contributes to liver damage [34]. These cells, however, may also express a range of polarized phenotypes, including the M1proinflammatory phenotype and the M2 alternative phenotype involved in the resolution of inflammation and wound healing. It has beendemonstrated that CB2 stimulation inhibits pro-inflammatoryM1 polarization and favors the transition to the anti-inflammatory M2phenotype [35–37]. This transition might be more frequently expressed in CB2-63 QQ than in RR Kupffer cells due to the above-mentioned reduced inhibition of T-cell proliferation in subjects with CB2-63 RR. This transition may favor the progression from CHC to the PNALT status and explain, at least in part, the association observed between the QQ homozygous variant and the PNALT status.

The mean age of the PNALT subjects in the present study was 8 years older than that in the abnormal ALT group, suggesting that a substantial percentage of them may have reached the PNALT status through a variety of immunological conditions, from an active cellular immune response at the time of acute hepatitis C and in the initial stage of HCV carriage to a subsequent inhibition/failure of the cellular immune response favoring the progressionto the clinical and histological profile characteristic of PNALT. Such inhibition/failure of the immune response has been demonstrated to include type 1 helper T-cell (Th1) hyporesponsiveness, cytotoxic T lymphocyte (CTL) exhaustion, excessive function of regulatory T cells (Treg), and failure of lymphoid cells via direct binding and/or infection in B cells, T cells, natural killer cells and dendritic cells [38–43]. Since in CHC the liver damage is mainly induced by Th1- and/or CTL-related responses [44–46], we might presume that these responses are strongly suppressed in PNALT. In fact, immunosuppressive Treg are frequently present in HCV carriers, and the inhibitory activity has been demonstrated to be stronger in PNALT subjects than in patients with chronic active hepatitis [47]. Younger patients with

CHC investigated in a previous study [21] and in the present study showed that the QQ homozygous variant is associated with a high HAI, a finding further supporting our hypothesis that the PNALT status may represent the terminal phase of an HCV chronic infection, when the active cellular immune response to infected hepatocytes present in CHC has burned itself out.

Also in other models of liver disease, the CB2-63 QQ variant was associated with low ALT serum values. In 438 Italian obese children with ultrasound-proven liver steatosis, the ALT serum values were lower in the 27 with the CB2-63 QQ variant (24.4±8 6IU/ml) than in the 222 with the QR variant (32.3±16 4IU/ml) and in the 189 with the RR variant (37.2±21 4IU/ml) [48]. Considering that the above-mentioned CB2-mediated inhibition of T-cell proliferation was normal in CB2-63 QQ subjects and reduced in RR subjects [6,7], it has been hypothesized that the hepatic inflammation associated with liver steatosis is inhibited in CB2-63 QQ subjects [48], a hypothesis in good agreement with experimental observations showing the hepatoprotective properties of CB2 agonists in the mouse model of carbontetrachloride (CCl_4)-induced liver injury. In fact, CCl_4 induced acute hepatitis with higher serum ALT and AST levels and a more severe course in CB2 knock-out than in wild-type (WT) mice. In addition, ALT and AST levels were lower in CCl_4-treated WT mice receiving the CB2 agonist JWH-133 [49].

Moreover, the stimulation of CB2 favors the transition of the Th1/Th2 balance to an anti-inflammatory Th2 profile by increasing the IL-10 levels [50–52]. In a study evaluating IL-10 administration in 30 patients with HCV-related liver disease, Nelson et al showed that IL-10 caused a decrease in the number of HCV-specific CD4+ and CD8+ IFN-gamma secreting T cells and alterations in PBMC cytokine production towards a Th2 dominant profile, as well as an improvement in the ALT serum levels [53].

PNALT subjects compared to patients in the abnormal ALT group showed a significantly lower BMI associated with a lower degree of liver steatosis, in good agreement with the recent demonstration that the enzyme that metabolizes the endocannabinoid 2-AG increases with the increase in the BMI, whereas the levels of the enzyme for the 2-AG synthesis do not change. Therefore, the endogenous levels of cannabinoids are higher in leaner subjects, and possibly exert a stronger CB2-mediated inhibition of the immune response [54].

Some limitations of the present study should also be underlined. Although interesting, the data on the role of the CB2-63 polymorphism on the ALT levels need confirmation in a multicenter prospective study on a larger cohort of patients. Further *in-vitro* studies are also needed to extend our knowledge on the CB2-63 QQ-related mechanisms inducing a suppression of liver cell necrosis. For a global understanding of the impact of the CB2-63 QQ variant on HCV chronic infection, some data are needed on patients with acute hepatitis C, liver cirrhosis with or without HCC and on orthotopic liver-transplanted patients. All 253 patients investigated were Italians born in southern Italy, but the present data need confirmation in more extensive studies including other ethnic populations. Although liver biopsy was obtained in a high prevalence (75%) of cases, a misclassification might have occurred in some of the non-biopsied cases. The present study, however, has clinical importance since it is the first study presenting significant data on the CB2-63 QQ variant as a newly identified genetic factor associated with different aspects of the clinical presentation of chronic HCV infection. In addition, the possible therapeutic implications of this new genetic factor cannot be excluded.

The data presented in this study encourage us to start a prospective multicenter studyand experimental studies on the role of the CB2-63 QQ variant in the different stages of HCV infection.

Author Contributions

Conceived and designed the experiments: N. Coppola RZ EMDG FR. Performed the experiments: GB AB CM. Analyzed the data: LEA SM ES. Contributed reagents/materials/analysis tools: CS MS AM N. Capoluongo. Wrote the paper: N. Coppola RZ EMDG FR.

References

1. Pacher P, Batkai S, Kunos G (2006) The endocannabinoid system as an emerging target of pharmacotherapy. Pharmacol Rev 58: 389–462.
2. Tam J, Liu J, Mukhopadhyay B, Cinar R, Godlewski G, et al. (2011) Endocannabinoids in liver disease. Hepatology 53: 346–55.
3. Cabral GA, Griffin-Thomas (2008) Cannabinoids as therapeutic agents for ablating neuroinflammatory disease. Endocr Metab Immune Disord Drug Targets 8: 159–72.
4. Louvet A, Teixeira-Clerc F, Chobert MN, Deveaux V, Pavoine C, et al. (2011) Cannabinoid CB2 receptors protect against alcoholic liver disease by regulating Kupffer cell polarization in mice. Hepatology 54: 1217–26.
5. Basu PP, Aloysius MM, Shah NJ, Brown RS (2014) Review article: the endocannabinoid system in liver disease, a potential therapeutic target. Aliment Pharmacol Ther 39: 790–801.
6. Carrasquer A, Nebane NM, Williams WM, Song ZH (2010) Functional consequences of non synonymous single nucleotide polymorphisms in the CB2 cannabinoid receptor. Pharmacogenet Genomics 20: 157–166.
7. Sipe JC, Arbour N, Gerber A, Beutler E (2005) Reduced endocannabinoid immune modulation by a common cannabinoid 2 (CB2) receptor gene polymorphism: possible risk for autoimmune disorders. J Leukoc Biol 78: 231–8.
8. Wong JB, McQuillan GM, McHutchison JG, Poynard T (2000) Estimating future hepatitis C morbidity, mortality, and costs in the United States. Am J Public Health 90: 1562–1569.
9. Gentile I, Coppola N, Pasquale G, Liuzzi R, D'Armiento M, et al. (2013) A simple noninvasive score based on routine parameters can predict liver cirrhosis in patients with chronic hepatitis C. Hepat Mon 8; 13: e8352.
10. Prati D, Gasbarrini A, Mazzotta F, for AISF, SIMAST and SIMIT (2010) Practice guidelines for the treatment of hepatitis C: recommendations from an AISF/SIMIT/SIMAST Expert Opinion Meeting. Dig Liver Dis 42: 81–91.
11. Puoti C, Castellacci R, Montagnese F, Zaltron S, Stornaiuolo G, et al. (2002)Histological and virological features and follow-up of hepatitis C virus carriers with normal aminotransferase levels: the Italian prospective study of the asymptomatic C carriers (ISACC). J Hepatol 37: 117–23.
12. Pasquale G, Sagnelli E, Coppola N, Scarano F, Scolastico C, et al. (2003) Is the liver biopsy necessary for hepatitis C virus carriers with persistently normal aminotransferase levels? Eur J Gastroenterol Hepatol 15: 831–833.
13. Persico M, Persico E, Suozzo R, Conte S, De Seta M, et al. (2000) Natural history of hepatitis C virus carriers with persistently normal aminotransferase levels. Gastroenterology 118: 760–4.
14. Sagnelli E, Pisaturo M, Stanzione M, Messina V, Alessio L, et al. (2013) Presentation, outcomes, and response to therapy among patients with acute exacerbation of chronic hepatitis C. Clin Gastroenterol Hepatol 11: 1174–1180. e11.
15. Sagnelli E, Coppola N, Pisaturo M, Masiello A, Tonziello G, et al. (2009) HBV Superinfection in HCV Chronic Carriers: A Disease That Is Frequently Severe but Associated with the Eradication of HCV. Hepatology 49: 1090–7.
16. Benhamou Y, Di Martino V, Bochet M, Colombet G, Thibault V, et al. (2001) Factors affecting liver fibrosis in human immunodeficiency virus and hepatitis C virus-coinfected patients: impact of protease inhibitor therapy. Hepatology 34: 283–287.
17. Adinolfi LE, Gambardella M, Andreana A, Tripodi MF, Utili R, et al. (2001) Steatosis accelerates the progression of liver damage of chronic hepatitis C patients and correlates with specific HCV genotype and visceral obesity. Hepatology 33: 1358–64.
18. Ishida JH, Jin C, Bacchetti P, Tan V, Peters M, et al. (2008) Influence of cannabis use on severity of hepatitis C disease. Clin Gastroenterol Hepatol 6: 69–75.
19. Thomas DL, Thio CL, Martin MP, Qi Y, Ge D, et al. (2009) Genetic variation in IL28B and spontaneous clearance of hepatitis C virus. Nature 461: 798–801.
20. Ge D, Fellay J, Thompson AJ, Simon JS, Shianna KV, et al. (2009) Genetic variation in IL28B predicts hepatitis C treatment-induced viral clearance. Nature 461: 399–401.
21. Coppola N, Zampino R, Bellini G, Macera M, Marrone A, et al. (2014) Cannabinoid receptor 2-63 QQ variant is associated with severe necroinflammation in chronic hepatitis C. Clin Gastroenetrol Hep 12: 334–340.

22. Coppola N, Marrone A, Pisaturo M, Starace M, Signoriello G, et al. (2014) Role of interleukin 28-B in the spontaneous and treatment-related clearance of HCV infection in patients with chronic HBV-HCV dual infection. Eur J Clin Microbiol Infect Dis 33: 559–67.
23. Zampino R, Coppola N, Cirillo G, Boemio A, Pisaturo M, et al. (2013) Abdominal fat interacts with PNPLA3 I148M, but not with the APOC3 variant in the pathogenesis of liver steatosis in chronic hepatitis C. J Viral Hep 20: 517–523.
24. Ishak K, Baptista A, Bianchi L, Callea F, De Groote J, et al. (1995) Histological grading and staging of chronic hepatitis. J Hepatol 22: 696–699.
25. Kleiner DE, Brunt EM, Van Natta M, Behling C, Contos MJ, et al. (2005) Design and validation of a histological scoring system for nonalcoholic fatty liver disease. Hepatology 41: 1313–21.
26. Sagnelli E, Coppola N, Marrocco C, Onofrio M, Sagnelli C, et al. (2006) Hepatitis C virus superinfection in hepatitis B virus chronic carriers: A reciprocal viral interaction and a variable clinical course J Clin Virol 35: 317–20.
27. Romeo R, Colombo M, Rumi M, Soffredini R, Del Ninno E, et al. (1996) Lack of association between type of hepatitis C virus, serum load and severity of liver disease. J Viral Hepat 3: 183–90.
28. McGuinness PH, Bishop GA, Painter DM, Chan R, McCaughan GW (1996) Intrahepatic hepatitis C RNA levels do not correlate with degree of liver injury in patients with chronic hepatitis C. Hepatology 23: 676–87.
29. García F, Roldàn C, Hernàndez-Quero J, Bernal MC, Martínez MA, et al. (1996) Relationship between viral genotype and viral load in patients with chronic hepatitis C. Eur J Clin Microbiol Infect Dis 15: 884–7.
30. Shindo M, Arai K, Sokawa Y, Okuno T (1995) The virological and histological states of anti-hepatitis C virus-positive subjects with normal liver biochemical values. Hepatology 22: 418–25.
31. Uto H, Mawatari S, Kumagai K, Ido A, Tsubouchi H (2012) Clinical Features of Hepatitis C Virus Carriers With Persistently Normal Alanine Aminotransferase Levels. Hepat Mon 12: 77–84.
32. Rossi F, Mancusi S, Bellini G, Roberti D, Punzo F, et al. (2011) CNR2 functional variant (Q63R) influences childhood immune thrombocytopenic purpura. Haematologica 96: 1883–5.
33. Rossi F, Bellini G, Tolone C, Luongo L, Mancusi S, et al. (2012) The cannabinoid receptor type 2 Q63R variant increases the risk of celiac disease: implication for a novel molecular biomarker and future therapeutic intervention. Pharmacol Res 66: 88–94.
34. Shrivastava S, Mukherjee A, Ray R, Ray RB (2013) Hepatitis C Virus Induces Interleukin-1β (IL-1β)/IL-18 in Circulatory and Resident Liver Macrophages. J Virol 87: 12284–90.
35. Dixon LJ, Barnes M, Tang H, Pritchard MT, Nagy LE (2013) Kupffer cells in the liver. Compr Physiol 3: 785–97.
36. Wan J, Benkdane M, Teixeira-Clerc F, Bonnafous S, Louvet A, et al. (2014) M2 Kupffer cells promote M1 Kupffer cell apoptosis: A protective mechanism against alcoholic and non-alcoholic fatty liver disease. Hepatology 59(1): 130–42.
37. Luongo L, Guida F, Boccella S, Bellini G, Gatta L, et al. (2013) Palmitoylethanolamide reduces formalin-induced neuropathic-like behaviour through spinal glial/microglial phenotypical changes in mice. CNS NeurolDisord Drug Targets 12: 45–54.
38. Jinushi M, Takehara T, Kanto T, Tatsumi T, Groh V, et al. (2003) Critical role of MHC class I-related chain A and B expression on IFN-alpha-stimulated dendritic cells in NK cell activation: impairment in chronic hepatitis C virus infection. J Immunol 170: 1249–56.
39. Accapezzato D, Francavilla V, Paroli M, Casciaro M, Chircu LV, et al. (2004) Hepatic expansion of a virus-specific regulatory CD8(+) T cell population in chronic hepatitis C virus infection. J Clin Invest 113: 963–72.
40. Blackburn SD, Wherry EJ (2007) IL-10, T cell exhaustion and viral persistence. Trends Microbiol 15: 143–6.
41. Kondo Y, Sung VM, Machida K, Liu M, Lai M (2007) Hepatitis C virus infects T cells and affects interferon-gamma signaling in T cell lines. Virology 361: 161–73.
42. Machida K, Kondo Y, Huang JY, Chen YC, Cheng KT, et al. (2008) Hepatitis C virus (HCV)-induced immunoglobulin hypermutation reduces the affinity and neutralizing activities of antibodies against HCV envelope protein. J Virol 82: 6711–20.
43. Blackburn SD, Crawford A, Shin H, Polley A, Freeman GJ, et al. (2010) Tissue-specific differences in PD-1 and PD-L1 expression during chronic viral infection: implications for CD8 T-cell exhaustion. J Virol 84: 2078–89.
44. Nelson DR, Marousis CG, Davis GL, Rice CM, Wong J, et al. (1997) The role of hepatitis C virus-specific cytotoxic T lymphocytes in chronic hepatitis C. J Immunol 158: 1473–81.
45. Nelson DR, Marousis CG, Ohno T, Davis GL, Lau JY (1998) Intrahepatic hepatitis C virus-specific cytotoxic T lymphocyte activity and response to interferon alfa therapy in chronic hepatitis C. Hepatology 28: 225–30.
46. Schirren CA, Jung MC, Gerlach JT, Worzfeld T, Baretton G, et al. (2000) Liver-derived hepatitis C virus (HCV)-specific CD4(+) T cells recognize multiple HCV epitopes and produce interferon gamma. Hepatology 32: 597–603.
47. Itose I, Kanto T, Kakita N, Takebe S, Inoue M, et al. (2009) Enhanced ability of regulatory T cells in chronic hepatitis C patients with persistently normal alanine aminotransferase levels than those with active hepatitis. J Viral Hepat 16: 844–52.
48. Rossi F, Bellini G, Nobili B, Maione S, Perrone L, et al. (2011) Association of the cannabinoid receptor 2 (CB2) Gln63Arg polymorphism with indices of liver damage in obese children: an alternative way to highlight the CB2 hepatoprotective properties. Hepatology 54: 1102–1103.
49. Teixeira-Clerc F, Belot MP, Manin S, Deveaux V, Cadoudal T, et al. (2010) Beneficial paracrine effects of cannabinoid receptor 2 on liver injury and regeneration. Hepatology 52: 1046–1059.
50. Correa F, Hernangómez M, Mestre L, Loría F, Spagnolo A, et al. (2010) Anandamide enhances IL-10 production in activated microglia by targeting CB(2) receptors: roles of ERK1/2, JNK, and NF-kappa B. Glia 58: 135–47.
51. Singh UP, Singh NP, Singh B, Price RL, Nagarkatti M, et al. (2012) Cannabinoid receptor-2 (CB2) agonist ameliorates colitis in IL-10(−/−) mice by attenuating the activation of T cells and promoting their apoptosis. Toxicol Appl Pharmacol 258: 256–67.
52. Kozela E, Juknat A, Kaushansky N, Rimmerman N, Ben-Nun A, et al. (2013) Cannabinoids decrease the th17 inflammatory autoimmune phenotype. J Neuroimmune Pharmacol 8: 1265–76.
53. Nelson DR, Tu Z, Soldevila-Pico C, Abdelmalek M, Zhu H, et al. (2003) Long-term interleukin 10 therapy in chronic hepatitis C patients has a proviral and anti-inflammatory effect. Hepatology 38: 859–68.
54. Cable JC, Tan GD, Alexander SP, O'Sullivan SE (2011) The activity of the endocannabinoid metabolising enzyme fatty acid amide hydrolase in subcutaneous adipocytes correlates with BMI in metabolically healthy humans. Lipids Health Dis 10: 129.

Acute Hepatitis C in HIV-1 Infected Japanese Cohort: Single Center Retrospective Cohort Study

Masahiro Ishikane[1,5,6], Koji Watanabe[1,7], Kunihisa Tsukada[1], Yuichi Nozaki[2], Mikio Yanase[2], Toru Igari[3], Naohiko Masaki[2,4], Yoshimi Kikuchi[1], Shinichi Oka[1,7], Hiroyuki Gatanaga[1,7]*

1 AIDS Clinical Center, National Center for Global Health and Medicine, Tokyo, Japan, **2** Department of Gastroenterology, National Center for Global Health and Medicine, Tokyo, Japan, **3** Pathology Division of Clinical Laboratory, National Center for Global Health and Medicine, Tokyo, Japan, **4** Research Center for Hepatitis and Immunology, National Center for Global Health and Medicine, Tokyo, Japan, **5** Field Epidemiology Training Program Japan, Infectious Disease Surveillance Center, National Institute of Infectious Diseases, Tokyo, Japan, **6** Global Infectious Diseases of Infection and Epidemiology, Medical Sciences Doctoral Program, Graduate School of Medicine, Tohoku University, Miyagi, Japan, **7** Center for AIDS Research, Kumamoto University, Kumamoto, Japan

Abstract

Objectives: HCV co-infection is a poor prognostic factor in HIV-1-infected patients. Although the number of newly reported patients who show seroconversion is increasing, the clinical features are still unclear, especially in Asian countries.

Design: A single-center retrospective cohort study of patients diagnosed between 2001–2012.

Methods: Acute hepatitis C (AHC) was diagnosed upon detection of high serum ALT (>100 IU) followed by anti-HCV seroconversion. Clinical characteristics, HIV-1-related immunological status and IL-28B genotypes (rs12979860, rs8099917) were collected. We compared these variables between patients with and without spontaneous clearance of HCV and between responders and non-responders to treatment with pegylated interferon (PEG-IFN) plus ribavirin.

Results: Thirty-five patients were diagnosed with AHC during the study period. The majority (96.9%) were MSM. Three were lost to follow-up. Seventy-five percent of patients with AHC (24/32) were asymptomatic and found incidentally to have high serum ALT. Compared to those who did not show spontaneous clearance, patients with spontaneous HCV viral clearance showed more symptoms and more severe abnormalities related to acute hepatitis. Spontaneous clearance was seen in 4 out of 28 patients with CC+TT genotype, but not in 6 patients with IL-28B CT+TG genotype. PEG-IFN plus ribavirin treatment was initiated in 12 out of 28 cases without spontaneous clearance. The sustained virological response rate was high (81.8%, 9/11), even in cases with CT+TG genotype infected with HCV genotype 1b (SVR 2/2).

Conclusions: Careful attention to AHC is needed in HIV-1-infected MSM. Early diagnosis and PEG-IFN plus ribavirin treatment should be considered for AHC cases.

Editor: Golo Ahlenstiel, University of Sydney, Australia

Funding: This work was supported in part by Grants-in Aid for AIDS research from the Ministry of Health, Labor, and Welfare (H23-AIDS-001) and the Global COE Program (Global Education and Research Center Aiming at the Control of AIDS), MEXT, Japan. The funders had no role in study design, data collection and analysis, decision to publish, or preparation of the manuscript.

Competing Interests: The authors have declared that no competing interests exist.

* E-mail: higatana@acc.ncgm.go.jp

Introduction

The estimated worldwide prevalence of hepatitis C virus (HCV) infection is 2–3% [1]. HCV co-infection increases morbidity rate in HIV infected individuals, and previous meta-analysis reported mortality among patients co-infected with HCV was 1.35 times higher than that among patients with HIV-infection alone even in the highly active antiretroviral therapy (HAART) era [2]. In HIV-1/HCV co-infected patients, progression to liver cirrhosis and hepatocellular carcinoma (HCC) is faster than that in patients without HIV-1 infection [3]. Furthermore, the response to treatment with pegylated interferon (PEG-IFN) plus ribavirin (RBV) in HIV-positive patients with chronic HCV infection is poor (sustained virological response: SVR 19–40%), compared with patients infected with HCV alone (SVR 54–61%) [4–9].

The risk of HCV acquisition via heterosexual intercourse is estimated to be very low [10]. Recently, however, a high incidence of HCV seroconversion has been reported in HIV-1 infected men who have sex with men (MSM) [11–13]. These results suggest that new HCV infection can be a potential future problem in the clinical management of HIV-1 infected patients. On the other hand, a favorable response to treatment with PEG-IFN plus RBV for acute hepatitis C (AHC) relative to that for chronic one has been reported in HCV-infected (SVR 85–98%) [14,15] and HIV/HCV co-infected patients (SVR 60–80%) [16,17]. In this regard, the recent guidelines recommend PEG-IFN plus RBV treatment for AHC in HIV-1 co-infected patients [18–20]. However, data of AHC among HIV-1 infected patients is still limited, especially from Asian countries.

The response to treatment with PEG-IFN plus RBV is closely associated with the interleukin-28B (IL-28B) genotype, which encodes interferon-λ3 (IFN-λ3), in chronic HCV hepatitis, even in HIV-1 co-infected cases [21–23]. Furthermore, HCV mono-infected individuals with favorable IL-28B genotype (CC at rs12979860, TT at rs8099917) seem to achieve spontaneous clearance of HCV compared to those with non-favorable genotypes [21,22,24,25]. To our knowledge, there are no studies on the effect of IL-28B genotype on the natural course and response to treatment of AHC in HIV-1 infected individuals in Asian population [24,26,27].

In the last 12 years, 35 patients with HIV-1 infection were diagnosed with AHC in our hospital. In the present retrospective study, we report the results of analysis of data of 32 of these cases, and discuss the factors associated with spontaneous HCV clearance and response to treatment with PEG-IFN plus RBV (Fig. 1).

Methods

Study Design

This single-center retrospective cohort study was conducted in accordance with the ethical principles of the Declaration of Helsinki and of Good Clinical Practice. The ethics committee of National Center for Global Health and Medicine approved the study. All patients provided written informed consent.

Study Participants

The medical records of HIV-1 infected patients in our institution, the largest HIV clinic in Japan, admitted and treated between January 2001 and December 2012, were retrospectively reviewed. AHC was defined according to the following criteria; elevation of alanine transferase (ALT) >100 IU/L accompanied by seroconversion of anti-HCV antibody, and exclusion of other causes (e.g., acute hepatitis B and drug-induced hepatitis). Patients who were lost to follow-up within 1 year from the diagnosis of AHC were excluded from the analysis since they could not be assessed for clinical presentation including spontaneous clearance. Spontaneous clearance was defined as a decrease in HCV RNA to undetectable level without treatment within one year from the diagnosis and remaining as such thereafter. For patients receiving PEG-IFN plus RBV treatment, we assessed the SVR rate. SVR was defined as continued undetectable HCV RNA at 24 weeks

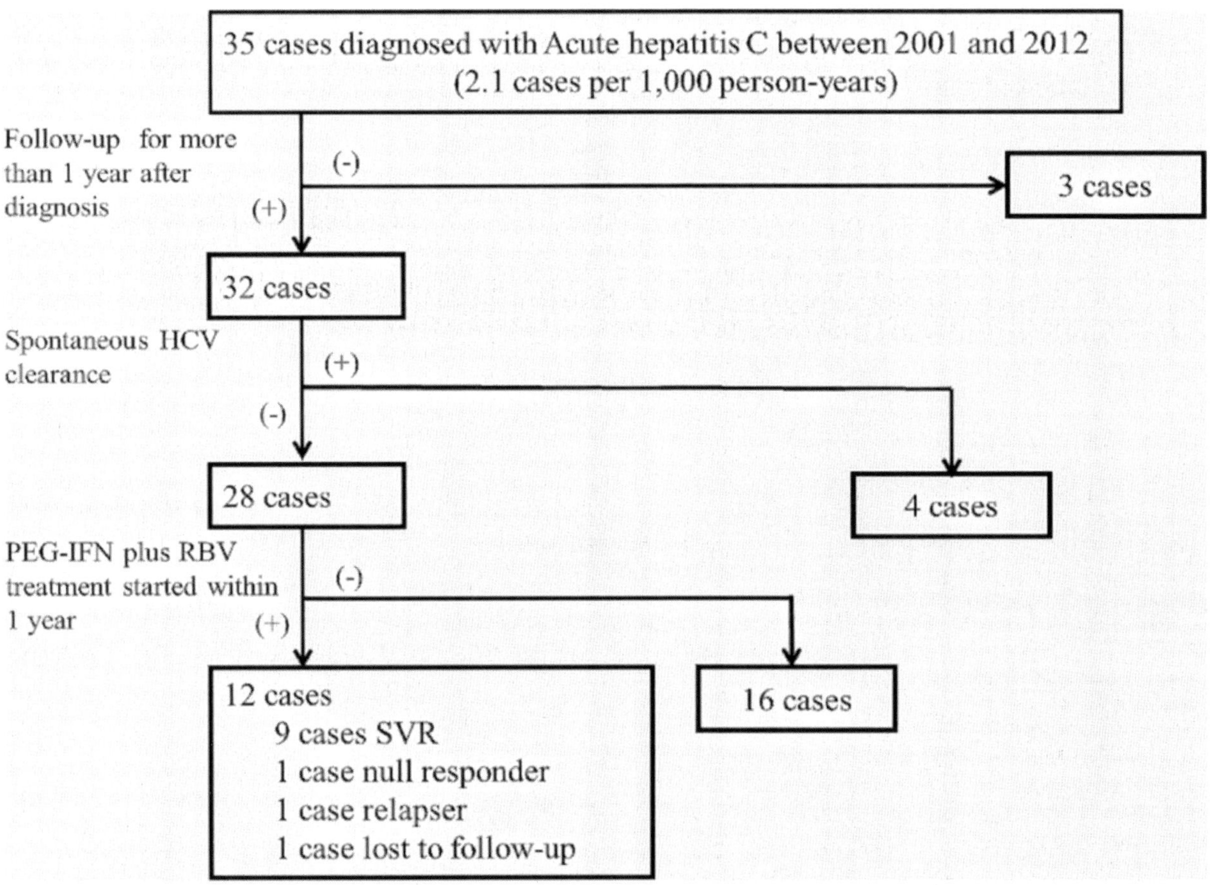

Figure 1. Patient enrollment process. Acute hepatitis C (AHC) was defined as elevation of alanine transaminase (ALT) >100 IU/L accompanied by seroconversion of anti-hepatitis C virus (HCV) antibody. Three patients could not be followed up for 1 year after diagnosis and were excluded from further analysis. HCV cleared spontaneously in 4 cases. PEG-IFN plus RBV treatment was initiated within 1 year of diagnosis of AHC in 12 out of 28 patients who did not show spontaneous clearance. One patient with missing treatment data following transfer to another clinic about two weeks after initiation of IFN plus RBV, was excluded from analysis related to the effect of PEG-IFN plus RBV. PEG-IFN: pegylated interferon, RBV: ribavirin.

Table 1. Characteristics of AHC patients (n = 32).

	All patients (n = 32)	Spontaneous clearance (n = 4)	Non-spontaneous clearance (n = 28)	P-value
Age (years)	40 [30–58]	44 [37–56]	40 [30–58]	0.361
Male sex	32 (100)	4 (100)	28 (100)	-
Men who have sex with men	31(96.9)	4 (100)	27 (96.4)	1.000
IL-28B genotypes (rs12979860+rs8099917)				
CC+TT genotype	26 (81.2)	4 (100)	22 (78.6)	0.416
CT+TG genotype	6 (18.8)	none	6 (21.4)	-
TT+GG genotype	none	none	none	-
Injecting drug users	4 (12.5)	none	4 (14.3)	1.000
Received ART at diagnosis	29 (90.6)	4 (100)	25 (89.3)	1.000
CD4 count at diagnosis (cells/μL)	420 [167–824]	317 [184–616]	424 [167–824]	0.424
HIV-RNA at diagnosis (copies/mL)	UD [UD−9.4×10^4]	50 [UD-50]	42.5 [UD-9.4×10^4]	0.737

Data are number (%) of patients or median [range].
ART, antiretroviral therapy; UD, undetectable.

after completion of therapy. Baseline characteristics, status of HIV-1 infection, history of injecting drug usage (IDU), symptoms related to AHC (fatigue and jaundice), laboratory data abnormalities from AHC (ALT, T-bil), treatment of HCV infection and histological findings of liver biopsy, where available, and were collected from the medical records. We compared these variables between patients with and without spontaneous clearance of HCV and between responders and non-responders to treatment with PEG-IFN plus RBV.

HCV Analysis

For each patient, titers of anti-HCV antibody were measured by a third-generation Latex aggregation assay (Ortho HCV Ab LPIA test III, Ortho Clinical Diagnostics, NJ) at first visit to our hospital and at diagnosis of AHC. Serum HCV RNA at each time point was extracted automatically (Cobas Ampliprep, Roche InVitro Diagnostics, Switzerland). Thereafter, cDNA was prepared and its titer was measured by quantitative polymerase chain reaction (Cobas TaqMan 48, Roche In Vitro Diagnostics). Direct sequencing was performed using DNA probe assay by ABI PRISM 3100 (Applied Biosystems, Foster City, CA). Finally, the

Table 2. Clinical presentation of AHC patients (n = 32).

	All patients (n = 32)	Spontaneous clearance (n = 4)	Non-spontaneous clearance (n = 28)	P-value
No symptoms	24 (75)	1 (25)	23 (82.1)	-
Symptoms	8 (25)	3 (75)	5 (17.9)	0.039
Fatigue	8 (25)	3 (75)	5 (17.9)	-
Jaundice	2 (6.25)	1 (25)	1(3.6)	-
Peak Alanine transaminase level (IU/L)	661 [117–2194]	707 [1237–2126]	614 [117–2194]	0.072
Peak total bilirubin level (mg/dL)	1.9 [0.7–17.0]	9.8 [4.2–17.0]	1.6 [0.7–6.8]	0.002
HCV genotype				
1a	1/27 (3.7)	None	1/2 (4.3)	-
1b	19/27 (70.4)	3/4 (75)	16/23 (69.6)	-
2a	4/27 (14.8)	1/4 (25)	3/23 (13)	-
2b	3/27 (11.1)	None	3/23 (13)	-
Not available	5	None	5	
HCV-RNA at diagnosis (Log IU/mL)	6.6 [1.9–7.8][¶]	6.6 [4.9–6.8][†]	6.6 [1.9–7.8][‡]	0.594
Latency to HCV clearance (wks)*	-	11 [7–31]	-	-

Data are number (%) of patients or median [range] values.
*Time between AHC diagnosis and HCV clearance (weeks).
¶Data of 6 patients not available for analysis.
†Data of 5 patients not available for analysis.
‡Data of 1 patient not available for analysis.

Table 3. Comparison of patients of the SVR and non-SVR groups.

	All patients (n = 11)	SVR (n = 9)	Non-SVR (n = 2)
Age (years)	38 [30–58]	38 [30–48]	52 [47–58]
Male sex	11 (100)	9 (100)	2 (100)
Men who have sex with men	11 (100)	9 (100)	2 (100)
IL-28B genotype			
CC+TT genotype	9 (81.8)	7 (77.8)	2 (100)
CT+TG genotype	2 (18.2)	2 (22.2)	None
Injecting drug users	1 (9.1)	None	1 (50)
Received ART before treatment	10 (90.9)	8 (88.9)	2 (100)
CD4 count before treatment (cells/μL)	382 [230–655]	440 [272–655]	238 [254–278]
HIV-RNA before treatment (copies/mL)	UD [UD-3.3×10⁴]	UD [UD-3.3×10⁴]	UD [305–610]
HCV genotype			
1b	10 (90.9)	8 (88.9)	2 (100)
2a	1 (9.1)	1 (11.1)	None
HCV-RNA before treatment (Log IU/mL)	6.3 [3.3–7.8]	6.3 [5–7.8]	5.7 [3.6–8.0]
Latency to AHC diagnosis (months)*	3.2 [0.9–6.9]	3.2 [0.9–6.9]	4.4 [3.7–5.1]
Duration of PEG-IFN+RBV therapy (wks)	43 [11–72]	43 [11–72]	36 [11–60]
Latency to HCV clearance (wks)¶	-	8 [3–16]	-
RVR	3 (27.2)	3 (33.3)	None
EVR	7 (63.6)	6 (66.7)	1 (50)
Histopathology positive for liver fibrosis			
F0	3/6	3	0
F1	2/6	1	1
F2	1/6	0	1
F3	0	0	0

Data are number (%) of patients or median [range] values.
*Time between AHC diagnosis and initiation of therapy (months).
¶Time between initiation of therapy and HCV clearance (weeks).
ART, antiretroviral therapy; UD, undetectable; PEG-IFN+RBV, pegylated interferon plus ribavirin; SVR, sustained viral response; EVR, early viral response; RVR, rapid viral response.

genotype was determined from the amino acid sequences of 5 – untranslated region [28].

Genotyping of IL-28b Alleles

Genomic DNA was isolated from peripheral blood mononuclear cells, using QIAamp DNA Mini Kit (Qiagen, Hilden, Germany). SNPs, rs12979860, and rs 8099917 were genotyped, using the TaqMan Drug Metabolism Assays by ABI PRISM 7900 HT sequence detection system (Applied Biosystems) according to the instructions provided by the manufacturer. The researchers responsible for genotyping were blinded to clinical data of the patients.

Statistical Analysis

The patients' characteristics and results of differences in viral clearance and virological response were compared using chi-square test (for qualitative variables) or Mann-Whitney U-test (for quantitative variables). Statistical significance was defined at two-sided p value of <0.05. All statistical analyses were performed with The Statistical Package for Social Sciences Version 21 (SPSS Inc, Chicago, IL).

Results

Patient Enrollment

A total of 35 patients were diagnosed with AHC during the study period. The incidence of AHC was 2.1 cases per 1,000 person-years. Three patients who were lost to follow-up within 1 year after diagnosis of AHC were excluded from the analysis. No deaths or fulminant hepatitis were recorded during the study period. Spontaneous HCV clearance was achieved by 4 patients, including 2 patients in whom HCV clearance was achieved within 3 months of diagnosis of AHC. The median time between diagnosis of AHC and HCV clearance was 11 weeks (range, 7–31 weeks). Among the 28 patients who did not show spontaneous HCV clearance, treatment with PEG-IFN plus RBV was initiated within 6 months of diagnosis in 9 patients and between 6 and 12 months of diagnosis of AHC in 3 patients (6.1, 6.4 and 6.9 months, respectively), whereas treatment was not initiated in the remaining 16 patients due to cost (n = 7) or other comorbidity (depression, history of epilepsy) (**Fig. 1**).

Patients' Characteristics and Clinical Presentations of AHC

The characteristics and clinical presentation of AHC patients are listed in **Tables 1** and **2**, respectively. All patients were

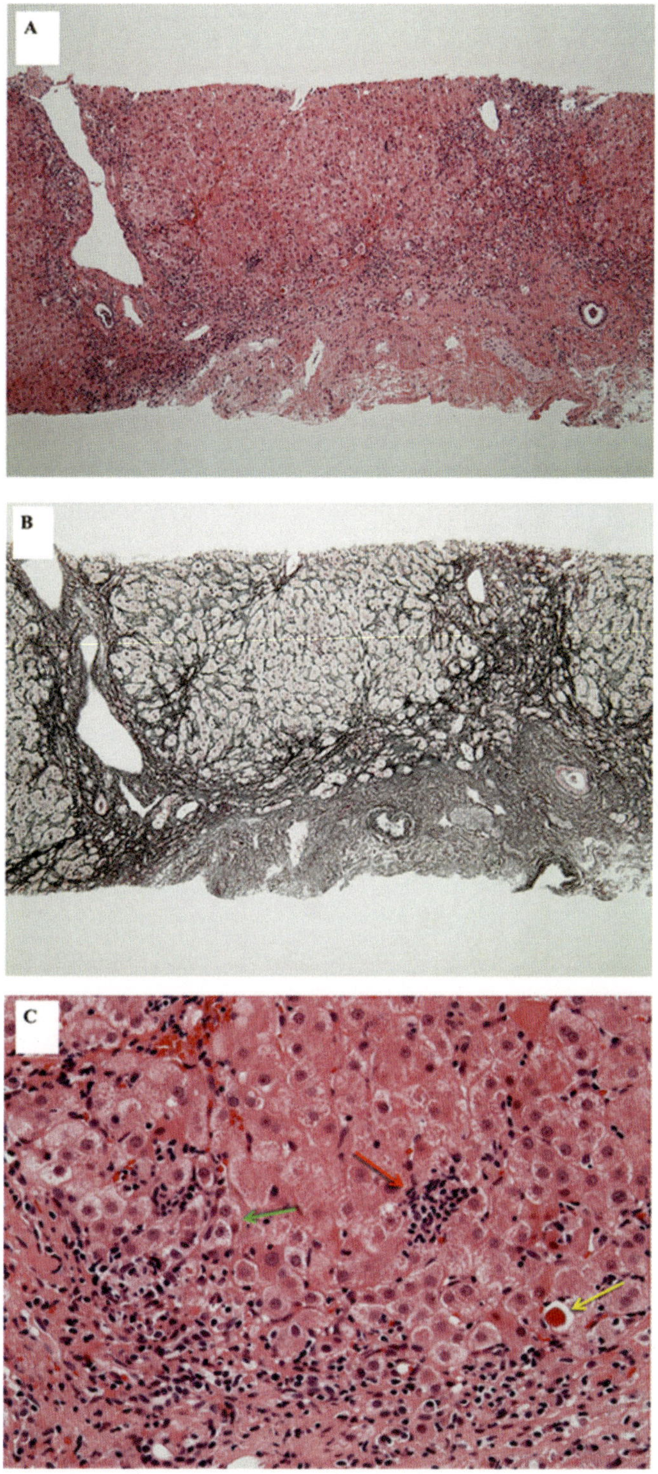

Figure 2. Histological findings in needle liver biopsy specimen from the patient who showed null-response (Table 3). The pre-treatment biopsy specimen obtained at 13 weeks after AHC diagnosis showed stage 2 fibrosis (F2) according to the classification of chronic hepatitis C (New Inuyama Classification). (A and B) Formation of bridging fibrosis by fibrous and cellular expansion in the portal tract. (C) Magnified view showing centrilobular piece-meal necrosis (green arrow), acid folic body (yellow arrow) and spotty necrosis (red arrow). (A) Hematoxylin-eosin stain, x100, (B) Silver impregnation stain, x100, (C) Hematoxylin-eosin stain, x400. PEG-IFN: pegylated interferon, RBV: ribavirin, AHC: acute C hepatitis.

Japanese men, including 31 (96.9%) MSM. Twenty nine patients (90.6%) received antiretroviral therapy (ART) and HIV-RNA was well suppressed in these patients. Four patients (12.5%) had a history of IDU, whereas none had a history of occupational exposure to HCV or blood transfusion. Although there was no significant difference between patients with and without spontaneous HCV clearance, the IL-28B CC+TT genotype was rs12979860 and rs8099917 in all 4 patients who showed spontaneous clearance and none of the patients with IL-28B CT+TG genotype showed spontaneous clearance (**Table 1**).

The majority of patients with AHC (24/32, 75%) were asymptomatic at the onset of AHC. High ALT was identified incidentally at routine visit for HIV-1 infection, with subsequent tests confirming the diagnosis of AHC. Compared to patients who did not show spontaneous clearance, patients with spontaneous clearance showed more severe clinical presentation of hepatitis (symptomatic, with higher serum total bilirubin and ALT value at diagnosis). The most frequent HCV genotype was 1b (70.4%). At diagnosis, HCV RNA was higher than 5.0 LC/mL in 24 out of 26 patients (**Table 2**).

Response to Treatment with PEG-IFN Plus RBV

Treatment with PEG-IFN plus RBV was initiated in 12 patients within 1 year of diagnosis of AHC (median interval from AHC diagnosis, 3.2 months). We assessed the response to treatment in only 11 patients; the other patient was lost to follow-up within two weeks of treatment initiation (**Fig. 1**, **Table 3**). SVR was achieved in 9 of 11 patients (81.8%) despite the high incidence of HCV genotype 1b and high viral load.

Two patients did not achieve SVR. Both patients were infected by genotype 1b with high viral load, and treatment was initiated within 6 months of diagnosis. One achieved viral clearance within 12 weeks (early virological response: EVR) but showed viral rebound at 15 weeks after completion of the treatment (relapser), whereas viral clearance was not achieved during treatment in the other patient (null-responder). Both patients were relatively older and their CD4 counts were lower, compared to those with SVR, although statistical analysis was not performed due to the small number of cases. In patients with SVR, the median time between initiation of therapy and clearance of HCV was 8 weeks (range, 3–16 weeks). Surprisingly, both patients with IL-28B CT+TG alleles achieved SVR despite genotype 1b and high viral load, although we could not compare the SVR rate among different genotypes since only one patient was infected with genotype 2a in this study.

Histological Findings of AHC in HIV-1 Co-infected Patients

HBs antigen was negative and ALT was within the normal range in the year preceding AHC in all 6 patients, whereas HBs Ab and/or HBc Ab was positive in 5 patients. No pre-existing factors of liver fibrosis other than HIV infection were evident before AHC. Liver biopsy was performed in 6 patients before treatment with PEG-IFN plus RBV. The median interval between diagnosis of AHC and biopsy was 4.3 months (range, 3.3–6.1 months). Fibrotic changes were confirmed in 3 cases by hematoxylin-eosin staining and silver impregnation staining (**Fig. 2**, **Table 3**). These lesions were paler-staining by Victoria Blue stain, indicating that the fibrotic areas did not reflect chronic changes.

Discussion

In the present study, we identified 35 cases of AHC during the study period and nearly all such patients (34/35) were MSM, and the most frequent HCV genotype was 1b (19/27). These findings are consistent with previous reports from other countries [11–13]. In this regard, a high incidence of HCV seroconversion in HIV-1 infected MSM was reported recently by two separate groups [11–13]. The same studies also reported that genotype 1b was the major genotype among their patients [11–13], and that HCV infection was frequently not detected during the acute phase and diagnosed only at the chronic stage mainly due to the lack of symptoms.

Similar to the previous reports on AHC, 75% of our cases were asymptomatic, and only 6.3% of the study population showed mild elevation of serum ALT (100 IU/L < ALT <150 IU/L). In this regard, ALT elevation during acute HCV infection is often relatively transient, and therefore could be easily missed during routine clinical care. The need of regular screening for anti-HCV antibody in HIV-1 infected MSM is controversial, and the recommendations are different in guidelines from different developed countries [29,30]. Our results emphasize the importance of regular ALT monitoring and HCV re-screening at the time of mild ALT elevation during follow-up, especially in high-risk populations such as sexually active MSM.

There are few reports on the relationship between IL-28B CC+TT genotype and spontaneous clearance of HCV [21,31]. In the present study, spontaneous HCV clearance was seen in 4 out of 26 patients with IL-28B CC+TT genotype, whereas no spontaneous HCV clearance was seen in all 6 patients with IL-28B CT+TG genotype. Although this difference could not be confirmed to be statistically significant due to the small number of patients (4 patients), this is, to our knowledge, the first report on the relation between IL-28B and spontaneous HCV clearance during AHC in HIV-1 co-infected patients in Asian population. Our study also showed that the severity of clinical symptoms was an important factor related to spontaneous HCV clearance. Further investigation is needed for a better understanding of the pathogenesis of AHC, especially factors involved in spontaneous clearance.

The use of PEG-IFN plus RBV treatment for AHC within 6 months of diagnosis is now recommended for HIV-1 co-infected cases [17–19] although data on the response of HIV-1 infected individuals with AHC to the PEG-IFN plus RBV remain limited. One study reported spontaneous clearance of HCV between 6 and 12 months of diagnosis [32]. In this regard, it is sometimes difficult in the clinical setting to start PEG-IFN plus RBV treatment within 6 months of diagnosis because some patients have comorbidities and complications other than HIV and HCV. In our analysis, 9 of 11 patients (81.8%), including 2 patients whose treatment was initiated between 6 and 12 months of diagnosis, achieved SVR despite high rate of genotype 1b infection (SVR 90.0% among those with genotype 1b virus). Furthermore, HCV genotype 1b-infected patients carrying the IL-28B CT+TG genotype (n = 2), which is a predictor of poor response to the treatment of chronic HCV infection, achieved SVR. These results emphasize the advantage of the PEG-IFN plus RBV treatment for AHC.

Little is known about the progression of AHC to liver fibrosis in patients with HIV/HCV co-infection [33], although rapid progression of liver fibrosis during the chronic phase is well recognized [3]. Fierer et al. [34] reported that the development of fibrosis occurs even in the acute phase of HCV infection in HIV-Infected men. In the present study with limited cross-sectional analysis of liver biopsies after AHC, fibrosis was detected in 3 out of 6 cases, which is consistent with the above report of Fierer et al. [34]. Moreover, SVR was not achieved in 2 out of 3 patients who showed liver fibrosis, whereas the other 3 patients without fibrosis achieved SVR (**Table 3**). These results emphasize the clinical importance of early diagnosis and early treatment for AHC in HIV-1 infected individuals.

In conclusion, the potential of AHC should always be considered in HIV-1 infected MSM, even in asymptomatic case, who present with mild ALT elevation. Favorable response can be expected if anti-HCV treatment is initiated during the early phase. Further investigation is needed to determine the predictor(s) of spontaneous HCV clearance, appropriate timing of treatment initiation, and duration of treatment.

Acknowledgments

We thank all the clinical staff at the AIDS Clinical Center, National Center for Global Health and Medicine, for the dedicated clinical practice and patient care.

Author Contributions

Conceived and designed the experiments: MI KW TK YK SO HG. Performed the experiments: MI KW TK YN MY TI NM. Analyzed the data: MI KW TK HG. Contributed reagents/materials/analysis tools: MI KW TK YN MY TI NM YK SO HG. Contributed to the writing of the manuscript: MI KW KT HG.

References

1. Alter MJ (2007) Epidemiology of hepatitis C virus infection. World J Gastroenterol 13: 2436–41.
2. Chen TY, Ding EL, Seage Iii GR, Kim AY (2009) Meta-analysis: increased mortality associated with hepatitis C in HIV-infected persons is unrelated to HIV disease progression. Clin Infect Dis 49: 1605–15.
3. Benhamou Y, Bochet M, Di Martino V, Charlotte F, Azria F, et al. (1999) Liver fibrosis progression in human immunodeficiency virus and hepatitis C virus coinfected patients. The Multivirc Group. Hepatology 30: 1054–8.
4. Sauleda S, Juarez A, Esteban JI, Altisent C, Ruiz I, et al. (2001) Interferon and ribavirin combination therapy for chronic hepatitis C in human immunodeficiency virus-infected patients with congenital coagulation disorders. Hepatology 34: 1035–40.
5. Landau A, Batisse D, Piketty C, Duonq Van Huyen JP, Bloch F, et al. (2001) Long-term efficacy of combination therapy with interferon-alpha 2b and ribavirin for severe chronic hepatitis C in HIV-infected patients. AIDS 15: 2149–55.
6. Nasti G, Di Gennaro G, Tavio M, Cadorin L, Tedeschi RM, et al. (2001) Chronic hepatitis C in HIV infection: feasibility and sustained efficacy of therapy with interferon alfa-2b and tribavirin. AIDS 15: 1783–7.
7. Fried MW, Shiffman ML, Reddy KR, Smith C, Marinos G, et al. (2002) Peginterferon alfa-2a plus ribavirin for chronic hepatitis C virus infection. N Engl J Med 347: 975–82.
8. Manns MP, McHutchison JG, Gordon SC, Rustgi VK, Shiffman M, et al. (2001) Peginterferon alfa-2b plus ribavirin compared with interferon alfa-2b plus ribavirin for initial treatment of chronic hepatitis C: a randomised trial. Lancet 358: 958–65.
9. Hadziyannis SJ, Cheinquet H, Morgan T, Diago M, Jensen DM, et al. (2002) Peginterferon alfa-2a (40 kD) (PEGASYS) in combination with ribavirin (RBV): efficacy and safety results from a phase III, randomized, double-blind, multicentre study examining effect of duration of treatment and RBV dose [Abstract]. J Hepatol 36: 3A.
10. Terrault NA, Dodge JL, Murphy EL, Tavis JE, Kiss A, et al. (2013) Sexual transmission of hepatitis C virus among monogamous heterosexual couples: the HCV partners study. Hepatology 57: 881–9.
11. van de Laar TJ, van der Bij AK, Prins M, Bruisten SM, Brinkman K, et al. (2007) Increase in HCV incidence among men who have sex with men in Amsterdam most likely caused by sexual transmission. J Infect Dis 196: 230–8.
12. van de Laar TJ, Matthews GV, Prins M, Danta M (2010) Acute hepatitis C in HIV-infected men who have sex with men: an emerging sexually transmitted infection. AIDS 24: 1799–812.
13. Lambers FA, Prins M, Thomas X, Molenkamp R, Kwa D, et al. (2011) Alarming incidence of hepatitis C virus re-infection after treatment of sexually acquired acute hepatitis C virus infection in HIV-infected MSM. AIDS 25: F21–7.
14. Kamal SM, Ismail A, Graham CS, He Q, Rasenack JW, et al. (2004) Pegylated interferon alpha therapy in acute hepatitis C: relation to hepatitis C virus-specific T cell response kinetics. Hepatology 39: 1721–31.

15. Deterding K, Grüner N, Buggisch P, Wieqand J, Galle PR, et al. (2013) Delayed versus immediate treatment for patients with acute hepatitis C: a randomised controlled non-inferiority trial. Lancet Infect Dis 13: 497–506.
16. Grebely J, Hellard M, Applegate T, Petoumenos K, Yeung B, et al. (2012) Virological responses during treatment for recent hepatitis C virus: potential benefit for ribavirin use in HCV/HIV co-infection. AIDS 26: 1653–61.
17. Boesecke C, Vogel M (2011) HIV and hepatitis C co-infection: acute HCV therapy. Current Opinion in HIV & AIDS 6: 459–464.
18. Lambers FA, Brinkman K, Schinkel J, Spijkerman IJ, Molenkamp R, et al. (2011) Treatment of acute hepatitis C virus infection in HIV-infected MSM: the effect of treatment duration. AIDS 25: 1333–6.
19. Piroth L, Larsen C, Binquet C, Alric L, Auperin I, et al. (2010) Treatment of acute hepatitis C in human immunodeficiency virus-infected patients: the HEPAIG study. Hepatology 52: 1915–1921.
20. Dore GJ, Hellard M, Matthews GV, Grebely J, Haber PS, et al. (2010) Effective treatment of injecting drug users with recently acquired hepatitis C virus infection. Gastroenterology 138: 123–35.
21. Grebely J, Petoumenos K, Hellard M, Matthews GV, Suppiah V, et al. (2010) Potential role for interleukin-28B genotype in treatment decision-making in recent hepatitis C virus infection. Hepatology 52: 1216–24.
22. van den Berg CH, Grady BP, Schinkel J, van de Laar T, Molenkamp R, et al. (2011) Female sex and IL28B, a synergism for spontaneous viral clearance in hepatitis C virus (HCV) seroconverters from a community-based cohort. PLoS One 6: e27555.
23. Rivero-Juarez A, Lopez-Cortes LF, Camacho A, Caruz A, Torres-Cornejo A, et al. (2013) The IL28B effect on hepatitis C virus kinetics among HIV patients after the first weeks of pegylated-interferon/ribavirin treatment varies according to hepatitis C virus-1 subtype. AIDS 27: 1941–7.
24. Grebely J, Page K, Sacks-Davis R, van der Loseff MS, Rice TM, et al. (2014) The effects of female sex, viral genotype, and IL28B genotype on spontaneous clearance of acute hepatitis C virus infection. Hepatology 59: 109–20.
25. Jiménez-Sousa MA, Fernández-Rodríguez A, Guzmán-Fulgencio M, García-Álvarez M, Resino S, et al. (2013) Meta-analysis: implications of interleukin-28B polymorphisms in spontaneous and treatment-related clearance for patients with hepatitis C. BMC Med 11: 1741-7015-11-6.
26. Boesecke C, Rockstroh JK (2011) Treatment of acute hepatitis C infection in HIV-infected patients. Curr Opin HIV AIDS 6: 278–84.
27. Nattermann J, Vogel M, Nischalke HD, Danta M, Mauss S (2011) Genetic variation in IL28B and treatment-induced clearance of hepatitis C virus in HIV-positive patients with acute and chronic hepatitis C. J Infect Dis 203: 595–601.
28. Germer JJ, Rys PN, Thorvilson JN (1999) Determination of hepatitis C virus genotype by direct sequence analysis of products generated with the Amplicor HCV test. J Clin Microbiol 37: 2625–30.
29. European AIDS Treatment Network (NEAT) Acute Hepatitis C Infection Consensus Panel (2011) Acute hepatitis C in HIV-infected individuals: HIV-infected individuals: recommendations from the European AIDS Treatment Network (NEAT) consensus conference. AIDS 25: 399–409.
30. Centers for Disease Control and Prevention (CDC); National Institutes of Health; HIV Medicine Association of the Infectious Diseases Society of America. Guidelines for prevention and treatment of opportunistic infections in HIV-infected adults and adolescents: recommendations from CDC, the National Institutes of Health, and the HIV Medicine Association of the Infectious Diseases Society of America. Available: http://aidsinfo.nih.gov/guidelines Accessed May 5, 2014.
31. Thomson EC, Fleming VM, Main J, Klenerman P, Weber J, et al. (2011) Predicting spontaneous clearance of acute hepatitis C virus in a large cohort of HIV-1-infected men. Gut 60: 837–45.
32. Ragonnet R, Boesecke C, Guiguet M, Lacombe K, Guedj J, et al. (2014) HCV Viral load kinetics during acute hepatitis C in HIV-infected patients: A model-based analysis [abstract 677]. In: Program and abstracts of the Conference on Retroviruses and Opportunistic Infections (Boston). San Francisco: International Antiviral Society-USA.
33. Boesecke C, Ingiliz P, Mandorfer M, Schwarze-Zander C, Berger A, et al. (2014) Is there long-term evidence of advanced liver fibrosis after acute hepatitis C in HIV coinfection? [abstract 644]. In: Program and abstracts of the Conference on Retroviruses and Opportunistic Infections (Boston). San Francisco: International Antiviral Society-USA.
34. Fierer DS, Uriel AJ, Carriero DC, Klepper A, Dieterich DT, et al. (2008) Liver fibrosis during an outbreak of acute hepatitis C virus infection in HIV-infected men: A prospective cohort study. J Infects Dis 198: 683–6.

The Effectiveness of Noninvasive Biomarkers to Predict Hepatitis B-Related Significant Fibrosis and Cirrhosis: A Systematic Review and Meta-Analysis of Diagnostic Test Accuracy

Xue-Ying Xu[1], Hong Kong[2], Rui-Xiang Song[3], Yu-Han Zhai[1], Xiao-Fei Wu[1], Wen-Si Ai[1], Hong-Bo Liu[1]*

1 School of Public Health, China Medical University, Shenyang, PR China, **2** Department of Clinical Laboratory, Shengjing Hospital of China Medical University, Shenyang, PR China, **3** Department of Urinary Surgery, Changhai Hospital, Shanghai, PR China

Abstract

Noninvasive biomarkers have been developed to predict hepatitis B virus (HBV)-related fibrosis owing to the significant limitations of liver biopsy. Those biomarkers were initially derived from evaluation of hepatitis C virus (HCV)-related fibrosis, and their accuracy among HBV-infected patients was under constant debate. A systematic review was conducted on records in PubMed, EMBASE and the Cochrane Library electronic databases, up until April 1st, 2013, in order to systematically assess the effectiveness and accuracy of these biomarkers for predicting HBV-related fibrosis. The questionnaire for quality assessment of diagnostic accuracy studies (QUADAS) was used. Out of 115 articles evaluated for eligibility, 79 studies satisfied the pre-determined inclusion criteria for meta-analysis. Eventually, our final data set for the meta-analysis contained 30 studies. The areas under the SROC curve for APRI, FIB-4, and FibroTest of significant fibrosis were 0.77, 0.75, and 0.84, respectively. For cirrhosis, the areas under the SROC curve for APRI, FIB-4 and FibroTest were 0.75, 0.87, and 0.90, respectively. The heterogeneity of FIB-4 and FibroTest were not statistically significant. The heterogeneity of APRI for detecting significant fibrosis was affected by median age ($P = 0.0211$), and for cirrhosis was affected by etiology ($P = 0.0159$). Based on the analysis we claim that FibroTest has excellent diagnostic accuracy for identification of HBV-related significant fibrosis and cirrhosis. FIB-4 has modest benefits and may be suitable for wider scope implementation.

Editor: Anand S. Mehta, Drexel University College of Medicine, United States of America

Funding: This research was supported by a National Natural Science Foundation Grant in China (No. 71073176) awarded to H.B.L. The funders had no role in study design, data collection and analysis, decision to publish, or preparation of the manuscript.

Competing Interests: The authors have declared that no competing interests exist.

* Email: hbliu@mail.cmu.edu.cn

Introduction

Chronic infection with hepatitis B virus (HBV) is an important global health problem. Approximately 350 million people are chronically infected with hepatitis B virus worldwide, especially in developing countries, 25% of whom will die from long term sequelae, such as cirrhosis, liver failure and hepatocellular carcinoma, resulting in 600,000 to one million deaths annually [1]. Patients who are suffering from significant hepatic inflammation and fibrosis are at high risk of those complications [2]. Assessment of liver significant fibrosis is critical to establishing effective clinical practice. It could be of great help for a doctor to determine patients' suitability and the optimal time for antiviral therapy to achieve the best curative effects as well as to prevent excessive medication [3]. In addition, early prediction of cirrhosis is beneficial to reducing complications in patients with chronic viral hepatitis [4].

Liver biopsy, an invasive technique, is the gold standard for the assessment of fibrosis. It has several disadvantages, such as patients' reluctance, pain, hemoperitoneum, and pneumothorax, etc. [5]. In addition, its accuracy in assessing fibrosis is questionable because of sampling errors and intra- and inter-observer variations [6]. Therefore, many people are beginning to realize the importance of prediction of liver fibrosis by noninvasive biomarkers.

Aspartate aminotransferase-to-platelet ratio index (APRI), the fibrosis index based on the 4 factors (FIB-4) and FibroTest are examples of noninvise biomarkers predicting liver fibrosis based on routinely available clinical parameters [7]. They were initially used in Western populations with hepatitis C virus (HCV) or HCV/human immunodeficiency virus (HIV) co-infection [8] and had good performance. The area under the receiver operating characteristic (AUROC) curve of FibroTest for detecting significant fibrosis peaked out at 0.85 [9], and the AUROC curve of APRI and FIB-4 reached 0.80 [10] and 0.81 [11] respectively. For detecting cirrhosis, FibroTest also has the best result, and its AUROC curve topped out at 0.90 [12]. The AUROC curve of APRI and FIB-4 are 0.83 [13] and 0.89 [14], respectively. These three markers can be considered as "good", even "better" markers, according to the criteria of Deeks JJ [15]. Consequently, the researchers were regularly conducting those markers to predict significant fibrosis and cirrhosis among HBV-infected patients. APRI was first used to predict significant fibrosis or cirrhosis in patients with HBeAg-negative chronic hepatitis B by Chrysanthos et al. [16]. They found APRI was strongly correlated to the fibrosis. Later FIB-4 and FibroTest were successively used to predict HBV-related fibrosis.

However, due to the fact that those markers were initially derived from evaluation of HCV-related fibrosis, their accuracy for HBV patients was under constant debate among the researchers. Some scholars indicated that all of those noninvasive markers were able to predict significant fibrosis or cirrhosis among HBV patients, and could potentially be used to decrease the number of liver biopsies [7]. Others maintained that those markers were not directly applicable to evaluation of HBV-related fibrosis because of the small AUROC curve [17]. Therefore, we decided to conduct this meta-analysis to assess the pooled performance of these biomarkers for prediction of significant fibrosis and cirrhosis among HBV-infected patients. It could provide the basis for future research and clinical application.

Methods

Literature Search

The review followed the Preferred Reporting Items for Systematic Reviews and Meta-Analyses (PRISMA) guidelines [18] (see Checklist S1 for PRISMA checklist). A protocol (see Text S1) was developed and systematic methods were used to identify relevant studies, assess study eligibility for inclusion, and evaluate study quality. Online database search was completed on PubMed, EMBASE and the Cochrane Library (01/2003-04/2013) for terms including the following: aspartate aminotransferase-to-platelet ratio index, APRI, fibrosis index based on the 4 factors, FIB-4, FibroTest, hepatitis B virus, HBV, Chronic hepatitis B, CHB, fibrosis and cirrhosis (see Text S2 for full search strategies). Additional studies were identified via a manual search for the referenced studies and review articles. EndNote X5 software was used to manage the references.

Selection Criteria

Studies were included if they met the following inclusion criteria: (a) The study evaluated the performance of the APRI and/or FIB-4 and/or FibroTest for the prediction of fibrosis and/or cirrhosis in HBV infected patients. Studies on patients with other etiologies of liver disease were also included if data for HBV-infected patients could be independently extracted. In addition, special populations of HBV patients (*e.g.*, HBV/HIV coinfection, HBV/HCV, and HBV/ hepatitis D virus [HDV]) were also included. (b) Liver biopsy was used to diagnose liver fibrosis as a golden standard. (c) Data could be extracted to construct at least one 2×2 table of test performance, based on some cutoff points of the APRI, FIB-4, and FibroTest for a fibrosis stage. (d) They assessed the diagnostic accuracy for fibrosis stage $F\geq2$ or $F\geq4$ according to METAVIR or a comparable staging system. (e) The study included at least 40 patients. Studies of smaller sample sizes were excluded due to concerns on their applicability.

Data Extraction and Quality Assessment

Two reviewers (XYX and RXS) screened the downloaded titles and abstracts against the inclusion criteria. Two reviewers (XYX and HK) independently evaluated study eligibility, graded the

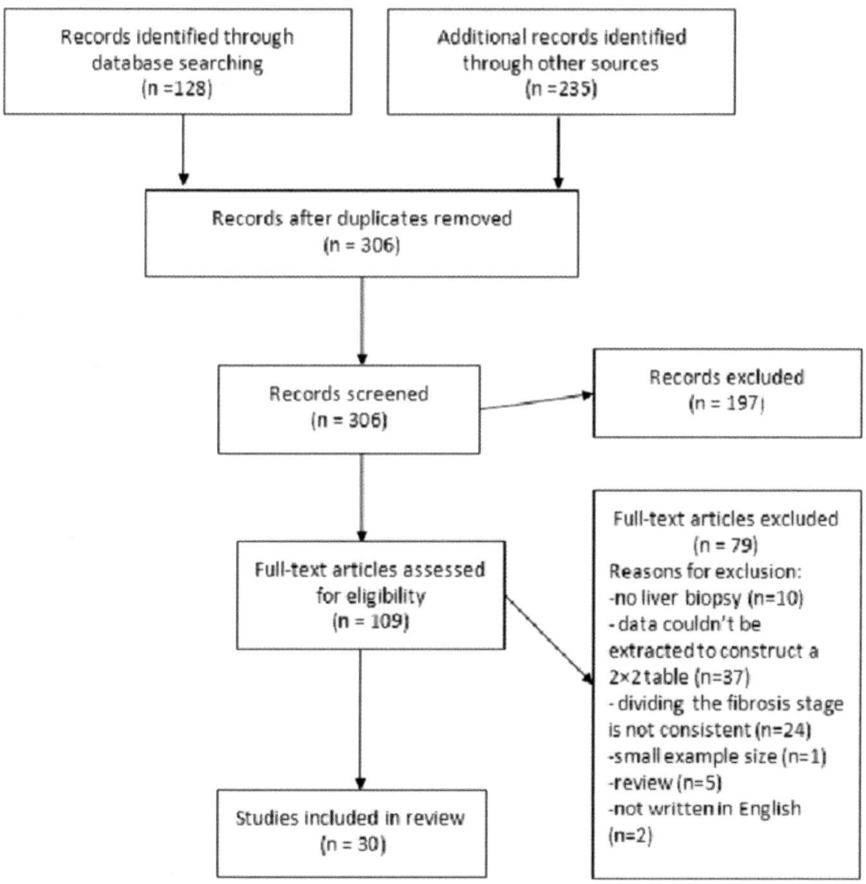

Figure 1. Flow diagram of article selection.

Table 1. Characteristics of the 31 Studies Included in the Meta-analysis.

Test	Author, Year, Regin	Study/Center Description	N	Interval Between Biopsy&Predictive index	Mean Age (%male)	Etiology	Liver biopsy System	length of liver specimen	Prevalence F2-4/F4	QUADAS Score
APRI	Zhou, 2010, China	Retrospective, 4 centers	146	Same time	35(84%)	HBV	Scheuer	>15 mm	58%,10%	13
APRI	Lin, 2008, TaiWan	Retrospective, one center	48	Unclear	56(83%)	HBV	METAVIR	Unclear	NA,38%	12
APRI	Shin, 2008, Korea	Retrospective, one center	264	Unclear	28(87%)	HBV	METAVIR	22 mm	53%,3%	13
APRI	Kim, 2007, Korea	Retrospective, 2 centers	346	Same time	34(90%)	HBV	Batts Ludwing	Unclear	75%,23%	13
APRI	Chrysanthos, 2005, Greece	Retrospective, one center	205	Same time	51(75%)	HBV(eAg-)	Ishak	≥15 mm	60%,27%	12
APRI	Liu, 2007, China	Retrospective, 2 centers	444	<1 week	30(71%)	HBV	Scheuer	>10 mm	29%,6%	14
APRI	Guzelbulut, 2011, Turkey	Retrospective, one center	250	Unclear	39(58%)	HBV	Ishak	Unclear	26%,16%	11
APRI	Lesmana, 2011, Indonesia	Retrospective, one center	117	Unclear	41(54%)	HBV	METAVIR	≥15 mm	62%,3%	13
FIB-4	Kim, 2009, Korea	Retrospective, one center	668	<2 days	39(66%)	HBV	Batts Ludwing	≥15 mm	79%,34%	12
FIB-4	Zhang, 2010, China	Retrospective, one center	212	Unclear	31(88%)	HBV	Scheuer	20 mm	76%,21%	11
FibroTest	Myers, 2003, France	Retrospective, one center	209	<6 months	39(70%)	HBV+HDV	METAVIR	Unclear	29%,9%	14
FibroTest	Miailhes, 2011, France	Prospective, 2 centers	59	Unclear	43(84%)	HBV+HIV	METAVIR	58%≥15 mm	61%,20%	14
FibroTest	Bottero, 2009, France	Cohort, multicenter	108	<6 months	42(90%)	HBV+HIV/HDV	METAVIR	17.0±7.3 mm	56%,15%	10
FibroTest	Kim, 2012, Korea	Retrospective, one center	194	Same time	47(61%)	HBV	Batts Ludwing	≥20 mm	85%,39%	14
FibroTest	Stibbe, 2011, The Netherlands	Retrospective, one center	48	<6 months	37(73%)	HBV	METAVIR	≥20 mm	46%,10%	12
FibroTest	Park, 2013, Korea	Retrospective, 3 centers	330	Same time	44(61%)	HBV	Batts Ludwing	≥20 mm	80%,24%	13
FibroTest	Gui, 2008, China	Retrospective, one center	100	Same time	35(78%)	HBV	Ishak	≥15 mm	39%,12%	14
FibroTest	Kim, 2012, Korea	Retrospective, one center	170	Same time	45(60%)	HBV	Batts Ludwing	≥20 mm	71%,28%	12
APRI/FIB-4	Seto, 2011, China	Prospective, one center	237	Same time	32(67%)	HBV	Ishak	15–20 mm	32%,2%	13
APRI/FIB-4	Liu, 2012, China	Retrospective, 2 centers	114	Same time	38(80%)	HBV	China hospital	15–20 mm	51%,11%	14
APRI/FIB-4	Zhu, 2011, China	Retrospective, one center	175	<7 days	37(78%)	HBV	METAVIR	>15 mm	45%,17%	14
APRI/FIB-4	Wu, 2010, China	Retrospective, one center	78	Unclear	33(85%)	HBV	METAVIR	18.2±3.4 mm	41%,12%	13
APRI/FIB-4	Wang, 2012, China	Retrospective, one center	231	Same time	34(68%)	HBV	Scheuer	≥15 mm	29%,7%	14
APRI/FIB-4	Ucar, 2013, Turkey	Retrospective, one center	73	Same time	45(64%)	HBV	METAVIR	Unclear	56%,11%	14
APRI/FIB-4	Gumusay, 2011, Turkek	Prospective, one center	58	Unclear	41(57%)	HBV	Ishak	≥20 mm	17%,NA	13
APRI/FIB-4	Basar, 2013, Turkey	Retrospective, one center	76	Same time	45(45%)	HBV	METAVIR	≥10 mm	67%,17%	14
APRI/FIB-4	Wang, 2012, China	Retrospective, multicenter	349	Same time	37(92%)	HBV(eAg-)	Scheuer	≥10 mm	60%,7%	13
APRI/FIB-4	Liu, 2011, china	Retrospective, one center	623	<1 week	32(55%)	HBV	METAVIR	≥10 mm	35%,6%	14
APRI/FT	Sebastiani, 2011, Italy	Retrospective, multicenter	253	Same time	44(73%)	HBV+HDV	METAVIR	Unclear	58%,8%	13
APRI/FT	Sebastiani, 2007, Italy	Retrospective, one center	110	Same time	43(73%)	HBV	METAVIR	≥15 mm	68%,20%	12
APRI/FIB-4/ FibroTest	Bonnard, 2010, France	Prospective, one center	59	Same time	35(69%)	HBV	METAVIR	21±6 mm	70%,24%	14

APRI, aspartate aminotransferase-to-platelet ratio index; FIB-4, fibrosis index based on the 4 factors; HBV, hepatitis B virus; HCV, hepatitis C virus; HDV, hepatitis D virus; QUADAS, The quality assessment of diagnostic accuracy studies.

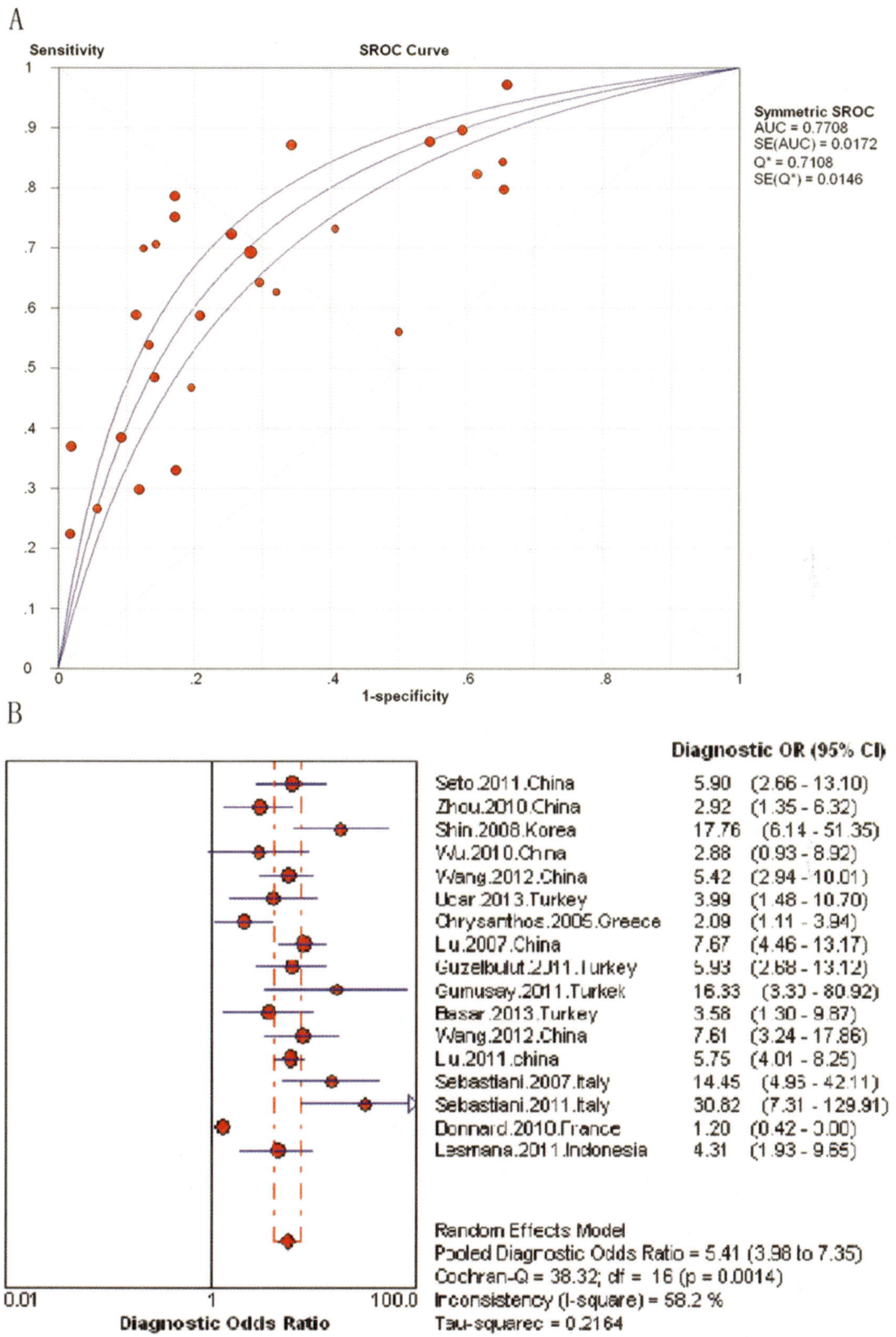

Figure 2. Meta-analysis of Hepatitis B-Related significant fibrosis. (A) SROC curve of the APRI; (B) Diagnostic odds ratio of the APRI.

Table 2. Diagnostic Accuracy of APRI for the Prediction of Significant Fibrosis in Various Studies.

Author,Year	Cutoff	Sensitivity	Specificity	PPV	NPV	AUROC(95%CI)
Sebastiani, 2011	1.5	36%	98%	96%	53%	0.64(0.58–0.70)
Seto, 2011	0.5	89%	41%	42%	89%	0.71(0.63–0.80)
	1.5	29%	88%	55%	72%	
Bonnard, 2010	1	56%	50%	72%	33%	0.61(0.46–0.76)
Zhou, 2010	0.5	82%	38%	54%	71%	0.72
	1.5	48%	86%	75%	66%	
Shin, 2008	0.5	97%	34%	63%	91%	0.86(0.82–0.91)
	1	87%	66%	75%	82%	
	1.4	78%	83%	84%	77%	
	1.5	75%	83%	83%	74%	
	2	58%	89%	86%	65%	
Wu, 2010	0.5	84%	35%	47%	76%	0.71(0.59–0.83)
	1.5	46%	80%	63%	68%	
Wang, 2012	0.5	58%	79%	54%	82%	0.77(0.71–0.84)
Ucar, 2013	0.54	73%	59%	70%	63%	0.66
Chrysanthos, 2005	0.5	79%	35%	65%	53%	NA
	1.5	33%	83%	75%	45%	
Liu, 2007	0.4	72%	75%	54%	87%	0.77
Guzelbulut, 2011	0.5	87%	45%	36%	91%	0.78(0.72–0.84)
	1.5	38%	91%	60%	81%	
Lesmana, 2011	0.24	64%	70%	78%	54%	0.69(0.60–0.79)
Gumusay, 2011	0.7	70%	87%	54%	93%	0.82
Basar, 2013	0.43	62%	68%	80%	47%	0.67(0.55–0.79)
Wang, 2012	0.5	53%	86%	86%	56%	0.78
	1.5	22%	98%	95%	46%	
Liu, 2011	0.3	69%	71%	56%	82%	0.76(0.73–0.8)
Sebastiani, 2007	0.5	70%	85%	91%	58%	0.72(0.58–0.86)
	1.5	26%	94%	91%	38%	

APRI, aspartate aminotransferase-to-platelet ratio index; AUROC, area under the receiver operating characteristic; PPV, positive predictive value; NPV, negative predictive value; 95%CI, 95% confidence interval.

study quality, and extracted data from the study. Any disagreements between the reviewers were resolved with detailed discussions between them together with a third reviewer (HBL). The parameters in our literature search included author, year of publication, region, method, patient gender, age, number of patients, underlying chronic liver disease etiology, histological scoring system, average length of liver specimen, time interval between biopsy and laboratory tests, prevalence of the fibrosis stage, as well as cutoff values to identify the fibrosis stage [13].

The quality of included studies was independently appraised by two reviewers (XYX and YHZ) using the quality assessment of diagnostic accuracy studies (QUADAS) questionnaire [19] (see Text S3). It could estimate the internal and external validity of diagnostic accuracy studies used in systematic reviews.

Statistical Analysis and Data Synthesis

We extracted and tabulated the data in a series of 2×2 tables, which included sensitivity, specificity, positive predictive value (PPV) and negative predictive value (NPV) at each threshold value. The primary outcome was the identification of significant fibrosis, defined by METAVIR [20], Batts and Ludwig [21], and Scheuer [22] for stages F2 through F4, and Ishak [23] for stages F3 through F6. This gauge was chosen because significant fibrosis is often considered a threshold for the initiation of antiviral therapy [24]. We also assessed cirrhosis (METAVIR, Batts and Ludwig, and Scheuer F4, and Ishak F5-6). In order to provide clinically meaningful results, the metrics of diagnostic test accuracy were examined.

The SROC curve, generated using linear regression, represents the relationship between the true positive rate and false positive rate across these studies, albeit they may have used different test thresholds [25]. In this analysis, the area under SROC curve was examined according to Moses et al. [26], and each study was weighted with its sample size and with adjustment for the number of thresholds within each study [27].

The diagnostic odds ratio (DOR) describes the odds of a positive test in true disease cases compared with cases of no disease [15]. The summary DOR was calculated using a DerSimonian and Laird random-effects model on a logarithmic scale with a corresponding test of heterogeneity [28]. Because such analyses require a single measure of accuracy for each study and many studies reported multiple test thresholds, we calculate the average DOR among all thresholds for a given study [29]. We also calculated summary sensitivities and specificities using the

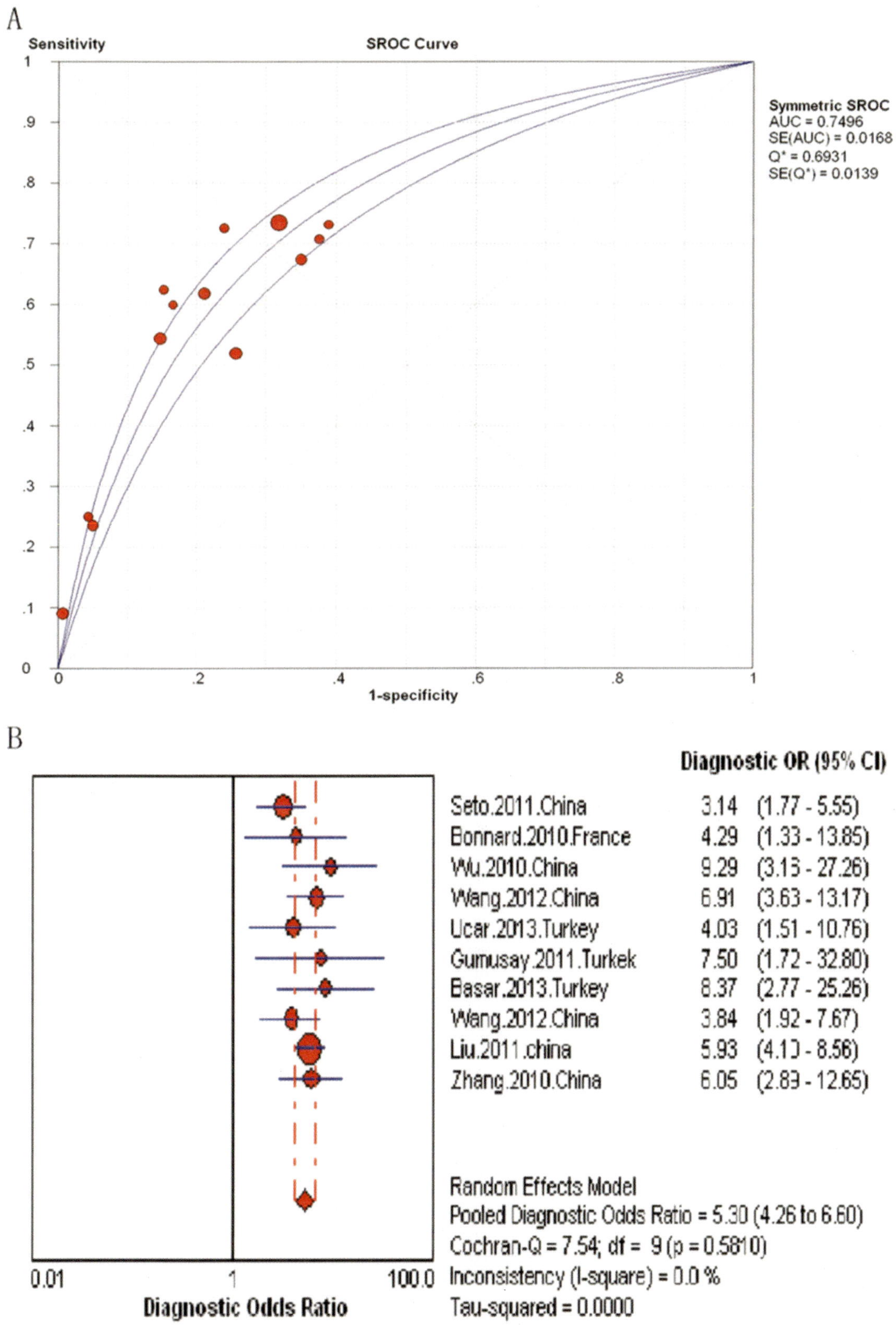

Figure 3. Meta-analysis of Hepatitis B-Related significant fibrosis. (A) SROC curve of the FIB-4; (B) Diagnostic odds ratio of the FIB-4.

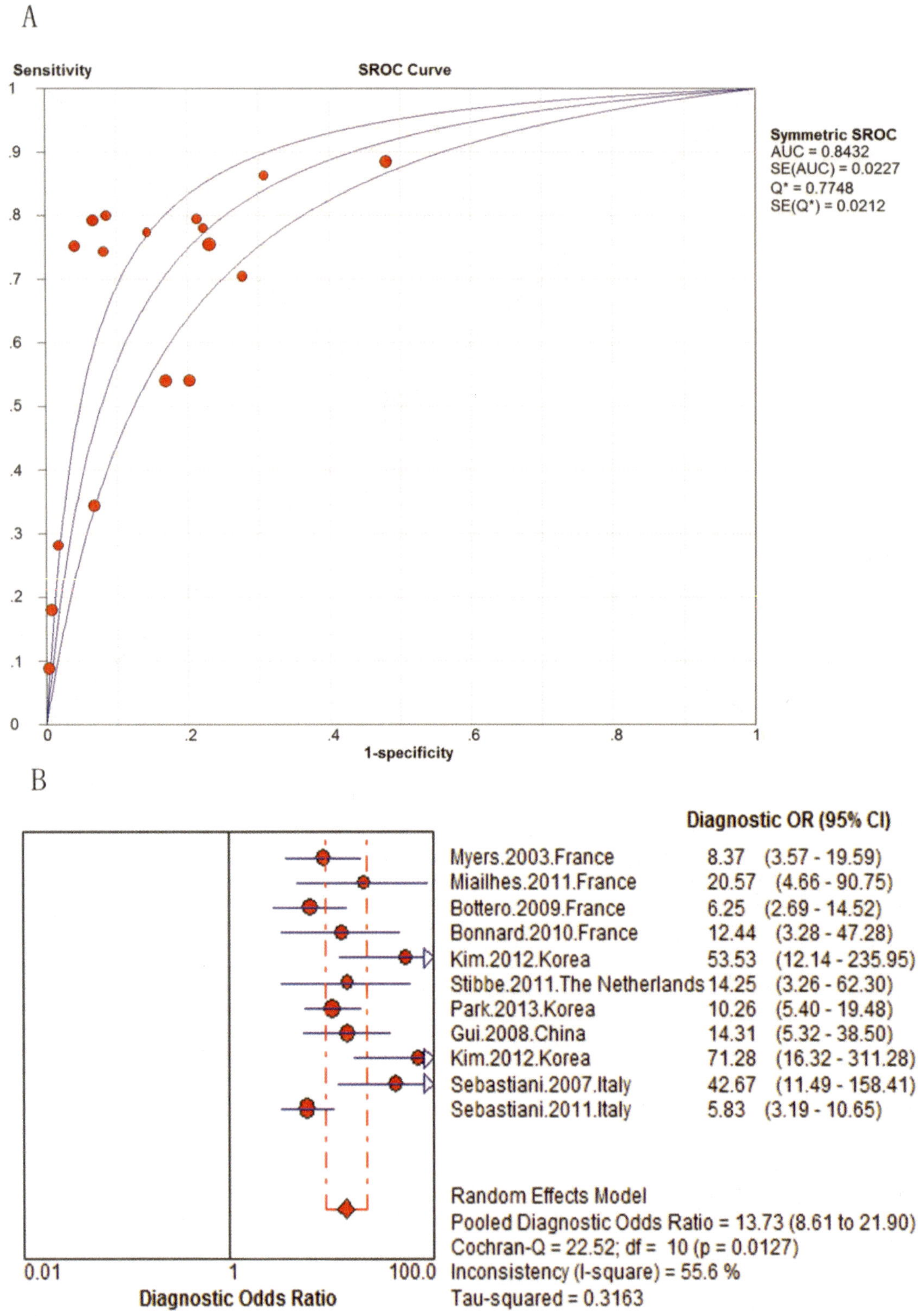

Figure 4. Meta-analysis of Hepatitis B-Related significant fibrosis. (A) SROC curve of the FibroTest; (B) Diagnostic odds ratio of the FibroTest.

bivariate meta-analytic approach [30]. Pairs of sensitivity and specificity for diagnostic thresholds are jointly analyzed, with any correlation that might exist between those two measures taken into account using a random-effects approach.

The heterogeneity (or the lack of homogeneity) of the results between studies was assessed statistically using the Cochran-Q and the quantity I2. I2 value describes the percentage of total variation across studies that is attributable to heterogeneity rather than

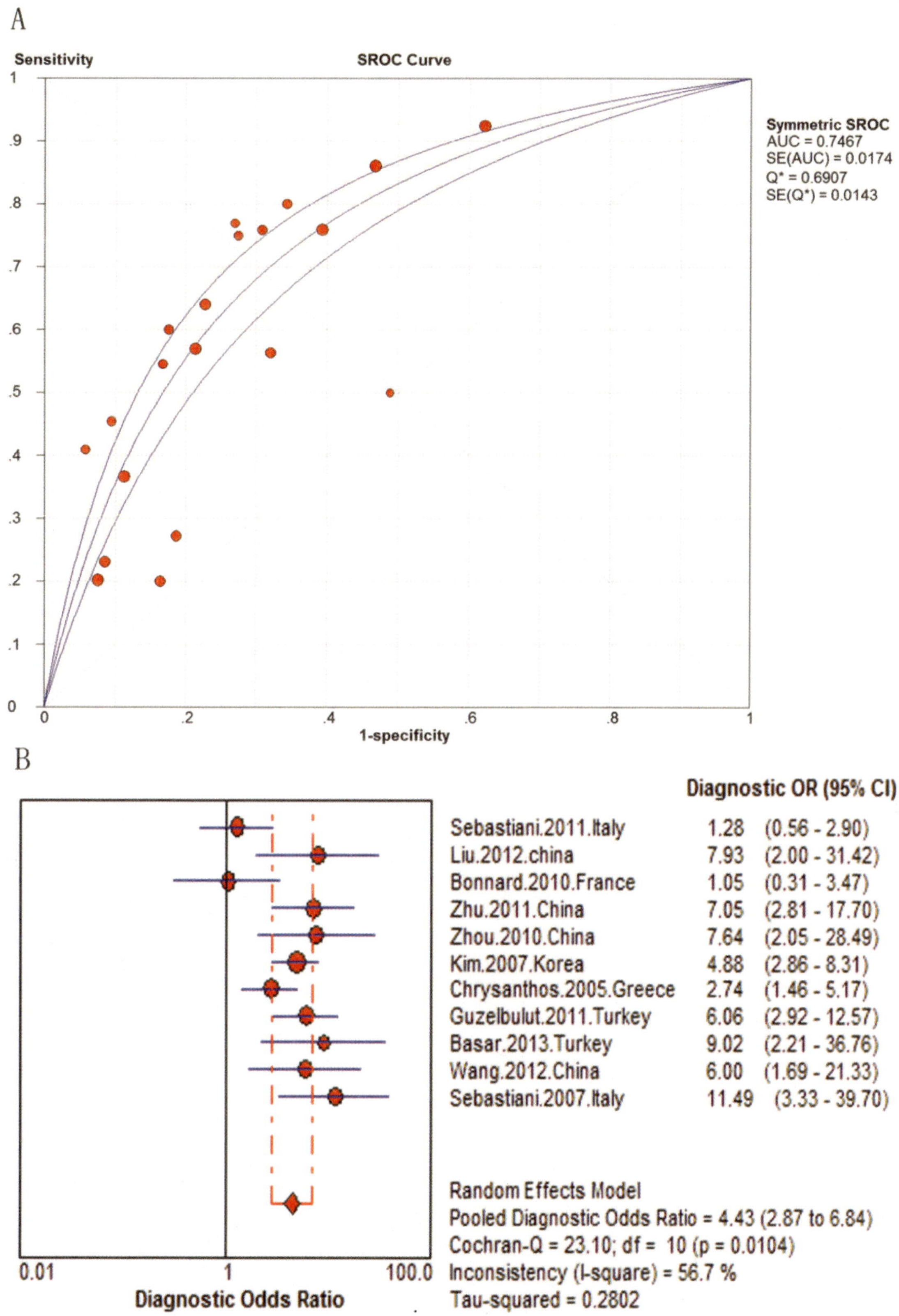

Figure 5. Meta-analysis of Hepatitis B-Related cirrhosis. (A) SROC curve of the APRI; (B) Diagnostic odds ratio of the APRI.

chance [31]. A meta-regression was conducted to further explore the covariates that may induce heterogeneity, according to the following predefined characteristics: (a) study design (retrospective or prospective); (b) etiology (HBV, HBV[HBeAg negative], or co-infection with other virus); (c) length of liver specimen (≥10 mm, ≥15 mm, ≥20 mm, or not); (d) liver biopsy scoring system

Table 3. Summary Sensitivities and Specificities of the APRI at Different Diagnostic Thresholds for the Prediction of Cirrhosis.

Test Threshold	Number of Studies	SROC	Summary Sensitivity(95%CI)	Summary Specificity(95%CI)
<1.0	5(1,228)	0.76	84% (79%–88%)	54% (51%–58%)
1	6(1,471)	0.76	62% (55%–68%)	75% (72%–77%)
2	6(1,409)	0.79	29% (23%–35%)	89% (87%–91%)

APRI, aspartate aminotransferase-to-platelet ratio index; 95%CI, 95% confidence interval.

(METAVIR, Ishak, Scheuer, Batts and Ludwig, and the Chinese Hospital System); (e) QUADAS score; (f) sample size; (g) median age (≤30, 31–40,41–50, or >50); (h) percentage of males; (i) location of study (Europe or Asia); (j) prevalence of significant fibrosis/cirrhosis.

The potential publication bias was assessed using the Deeks funnel plots (the logarithm of the DOR plotted against

$$1/\sqrt{\text{ESS}}$$

) [32].

$$1/\sqrt{\text{ESS}}$$

is proportional to the square root of (1/n1+1/n2), where n1 is the number diseased and n2 not diseased. Data analyses were performed using the Meta-Disc software (v. 1.4).

Results

Search Results

The study selection process is presented with a flow chart in Figure 1. 306 studies were retrieved with the described search strategies, of which 196 were excluded following title and abstract screening. The full texts of 110 potentially eligible reports were obtained for further assessment. Of those, 30 papers were included in the review following full-text screening (Table 1); 20 studies were related to the APRI [3,16,17,33-49], 13 studies related to the FIB-4 [3,7,17,39–46,48,50], and 11 studies related to the FibroTest [47–49,51–58].

Characteristics of the Included Studies

In the twenty APRI studies, a total of 4,208 patients (median age 36 yr, 72% male) were included. The overall prevalence of significant fibrosis and cirrhosis were 47% (ranged 17%–70%) and 11% (7%–27%), respectively. The liver biopsy scoring system used to classify the histology varied. 10 studies used a METAVIR score, 4 studies used an Ishak score, 4 studies used a Scheuer score, 1 study used a Batts and Ludwig score, and 1 study used the Chinese Hospital System. Nineteen of these studies (N = 3,955) included HBV-infected patients without comorbid conditions [3,16,17,33–48]. The one remaining study included special populations of patients such as HBV/HDV-coinfected patients (N = 253) [59]. According to the QUADAS scale, eight studies met all 14 requirements of this scale, nine studies met 13, two studies met 12, and one study met 11.

A total of 2,953 patients (median age 36 yr, 70% male) were included in the thirteen studies on FIB-4. The overall prevalence of significant fibrosis and cirrhosis were 53% (ranged 17%–76%) and 15% (11%–34%), respectively. All those studies (N = 2,953) included HBV-infected patients without comorbid conditions. The liver biopsy scoring system used to classify the histology varied. Six studies used a METAVIR score, three studies used a Scheuer score, two studies used an Ishak score, one study used a Batts and Ludwig score, and one study used the Chinese Hospital System. Seven studies met all 14 requirements of the QUADAS scale, 4 studies met 13, 1 study met 12, and one study met 11.

There were 1,640 patients (median age 42 yr, 69% male) used to assess the performance of FibroTest in eleven studies. The overall prevalence of significant fibrosis and cirrhosis were 63% (ranged 39%–85%) and 20% (8%–39%), respectively. Seven of these studies (N = 1,011) included HBV-infected patients without comorbid conditions [47,48,54–58]. The four remaining studies included special populations with HBV/HDV-coinfected patients (N = 462) [49,51], HBV/HIV-coinfected patients (N = 59) [52], and HBV/HDV/HIV-coinfected patients (N = 108) [53]. According to the Quality Assessment of Diagnostic Accuracy Studies scale, we can see that 5 studies met all 14 requirements of this scale, 2 study met 13, 3 studies met 12, and 1 study met 10.

Diagnostic Accuracy for the Prediction of Significant Fibrosis

In the seventeen studies assessing the APRI (N = 3,573), the AUROC curve ranged from 0.61 to 0.86. When combined, the area under the SROC curve was 0.77 08 (SE = 0.0172) (Figure 2A). The Pooled DOR was 5.41 (95% confidence interval [CI] 3.98–7.35) (Figure 2B). The Cochran-Q *and* I^2 value of all measures were 38.32 and 58.2%, indicating significant heterogeneity across the included studies (P = 0.001) (Figure 2B). The pooled sensitivities and specificities could not be assessed. Instead, the sensitivities and specificities of the APRI at various diagnostic thresholds in the seventeen studies are listed in Table 2. We used the meta-regression analysis to explore the heterogeneity of the APRI accuracy for detecting significant fibrosis, which was mainly affected by median age (P = 0.0211, see Text S4 for meta-regression). There was no significant correlation between other covariates and the DOR.

In the ten studies assessing the FIB-4 for the prediction of significant Fibrosis (N = 1,996), the AUROC curve ranged from 0.69 to 0.77. When combined, the area under the SROC curve was 0.75 (SE = 0.0168) (Figure 3A). The summary DOR was 5.3 (95% CI 4.3–6.6), and the score of Cochran-Q is 7.54 (P = 0.581) (Figure 3B). The result from the analysis of the heterogeneity was statistically insignificant. The summary sensitivities and specificities of the FIB-4 were 65.8% (95% CI 62.4%–69.1%) and 73.6% (95% CI 70.8%–76.3%), respectively (Figure S1–S2).

The AUROC curve ranged from 0.69 to 0.90 in the 11 studies assessing the FibroTest (N = 1.640). When combined, the area under the SROC curve was 0.84 (SE = 0.0227) (Figure 4A). The summary DOR was 13.73 (95% CI 8.61–21.90), and the score of Cochran-Q is 22.52, indicating significant heterogeneity across the included studies (P = 0.0127) (Figure 4B). We didn't find the cause of the heterogeneity of FibroTest accuracy according to the

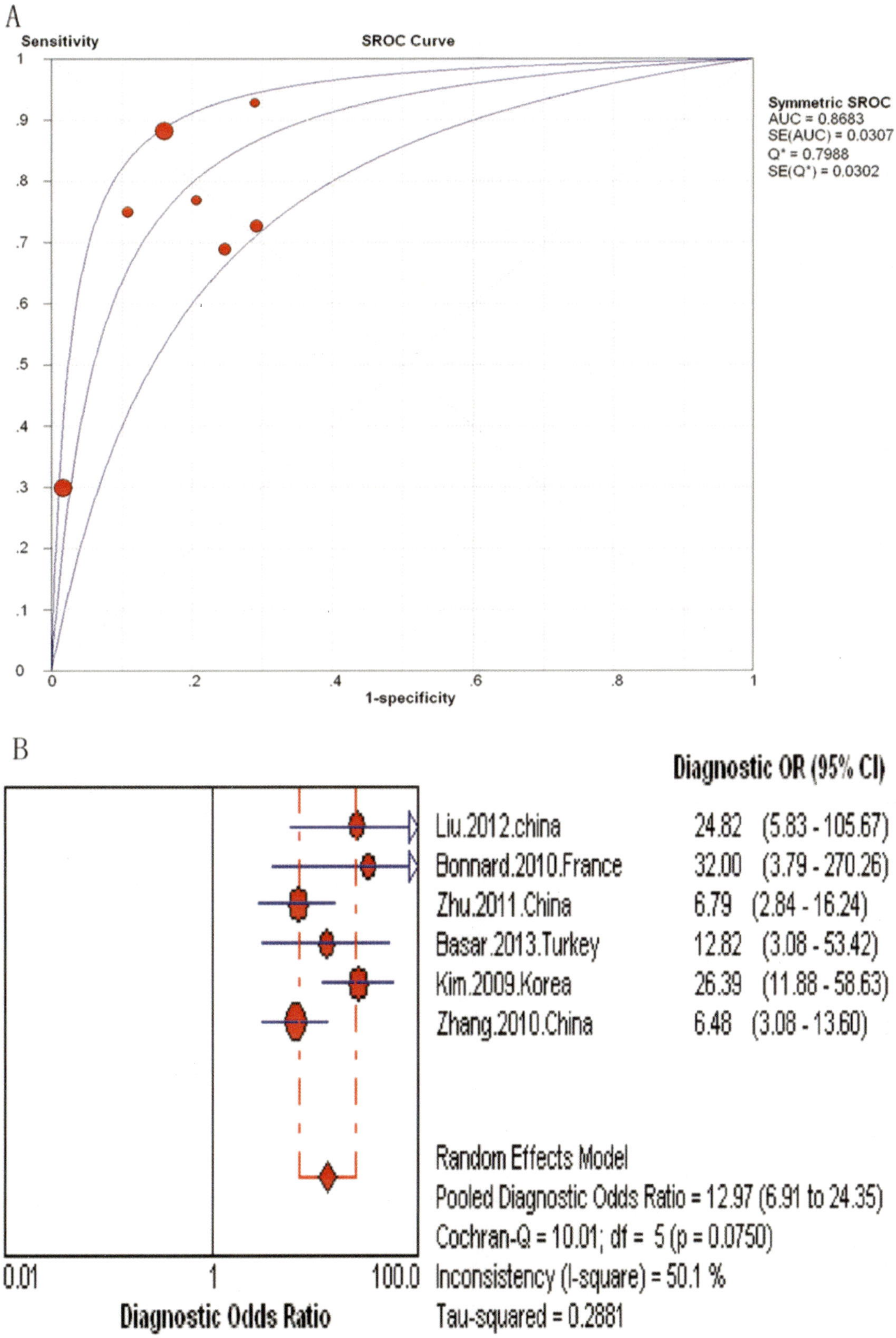

Figure 6. Meta-analysis of Hepatitis B-Related cirrhosis. (A) SROC curve of the FIB-4; (B) Diagnostic odds ratio of the FIB-4.

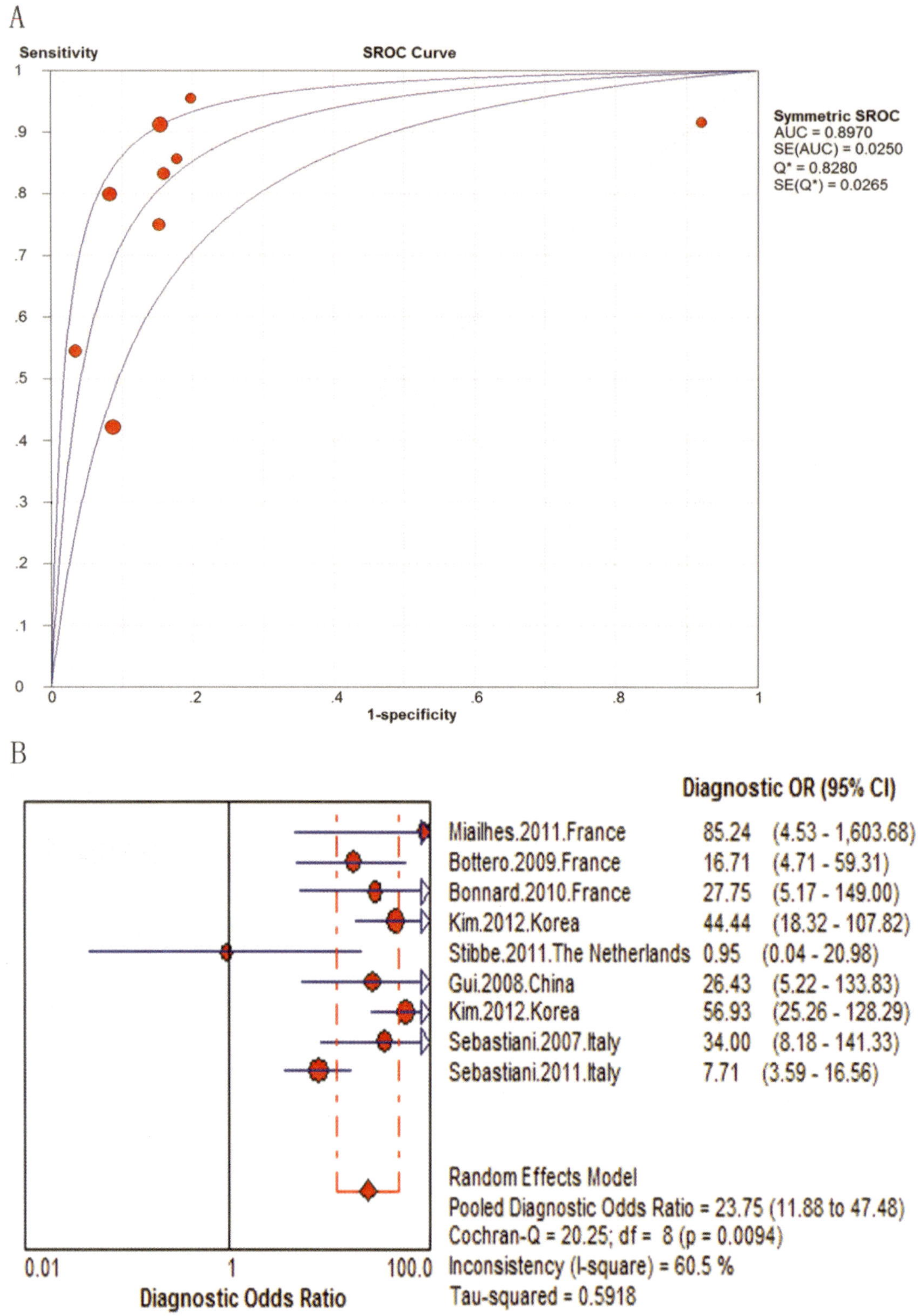

Figure 7. Meta-analysis of Hepatitis B-Related cirrhosis. (A) SROC curve of the FibroTest; (B) Diagnostic odds ratio of the FibroTest.

predefined characteristics. But center description might affect heterogeneity beyond the predefined design (See Text S5).

Diagnostic Accuracy for the Prediction of Cirrhosis

There were 11 studies on assessing the APRI for the predication of cirrhosis (N = 2,083). The AUROC curve of these studies ranged from 0.50 to 0.83. When combined, the area under the

Table 4. Diagnostic Accuracy of FibroTest for the Prediction of Significant Fibrosis and Cirrhosis in Various Studies.

Author,Year	Cutoff	Sensitivity	Specificity	PPV	NPV	AUROC(95%CI)
Significant Fibrosis						
Sebastiani, 2011	0.48	54%	83%	81%	57%	0.69(0.63–0.75)
Myers, 2003	0.2	89%	52%	43%	92%	0.78(0.74–0.82)
	0.4	54%	80%	52%	81%	
	0.6	34%	93%	68%	78%	
	0.8	18%	99%	92%	75%	
	1	8%	100%	100%	73%	
Miailhes, 2011	0.38	77%	85%	89%	72%	0.86(0.75–0.96)
Bottero, 2009	0.48	70%	72%	77%	65%	0.77(0.68–0.86)
Bonnard, 2010	0.37	78%	78%	89%	61%	0.79(0.66–0.91)
Kim, 2012	0.32	79%	93%	98%	45%	0.90(0.84–0.97)
Stibbe, 2011	0.31	86%	69%	70%	86%	NA
Park, 2013	0.32	75%	77%	93%	43%	NA
Gui, 2008	0.31	79%	79%	70%	86%	0.84(0.75–0.93)
	0.4	74%	92%	85%	85%	0.84(0.75–0.93)
	0.72	28%	98%	92%	68%	0.84(0.75–0.93)
Kim, 2012	0.31	75%	96%	98%	61%	0.9(0.85–0.94)
Sebastiani, 2007	F2	80%	91%	95%	68%	0.85(0.75–0.95)
Cirrhosis						
Sebastiani, 2011	0.75	42%	91%	51%	88%	0.68(0.63–0.73)
Miailhes, 2011	0.58	100%	81%	56%	100%	0.92(0.85–0.99)
Bottero, 2009	0.73	75%	85%	46%	95%	0.87(0.79–0.94)
Bonnard, 2010	0.5	86%	82%	60%	95%	0.85(0.74–0.96)
Kim, 2012	0.68	80%	92%	87%	87%	0.87(0.82–0.92)
Stibbe, 2011	0.75	100%	7%	11%	100%	NA
Gui, 2008	0.55	83%	84%	42%	97%	0.86(0.71–1.00)
Kim, 2012	0.67	91%	85%	85%	91%	0.88(0.83–0.94)
Sebastiani, 2007	F4	55%	97%	80%	89%	0.76(0.67–0.85)

SROC curve was 0.75 (SE = 0.0174) (Figure 5A). The summary DOR was 4.4 (95% CI 2.9–6.8). The heterogeneity occurred in the meta-analysis for the twelve studies assessing the APRI for the predication of cirrhosis, which was statistically significant ($Q = 23.10$, $P = 0.01$; $I^2 = 56.7\%$, Figure 5B). However, when we further conducted the meta-analysis at the different thresholds of <1.0, 1.0, and 2.0, we found that the heterogeneity wasn't statistically significant (Figure S3). The summary sensitivity and specificity of the APRI at different diagnostic thresholds are listed in Table 3.

According to the meta-regression analysis, the heterogeneity of APRI accuracy for detecting cirrhosis was mainly affected by etiology ($P = 0.0159$) (See Text S6), whereas the other covariates were not significant. After excluding the only one study which included HBV/HDV-coinfected patients, the pooled DOR was 5.03 (95% CI 3.45–7.35) and heterogeneity was no longer significant ($Q = 14.05$, $P = 0.1204$; $I^2 = 36.0\%$).(Figure S4) According to the meta-analysis, the pooled sensitivity and specificity were 60.9% (95% CI 55.0–66.6%) and 74.8% (72.4–77.1%), respectively (Figures S5–S6).

The AUROC curve in the six studies assessing the FIB-4 (N = 1,304) ranged from 0.74 to 0.93. When combined, the area under the SROC curve was 0.87 (SE = 0.0307) (Figure 6A). The summary DOR was 12.97 (95% CI 6.91–24.35) and the score of Cochran-Q is 10.01 ($P = 0.07$) (Figure 6B). The analysis showed that the heterogeneity was statistically insignificant. The summary sensitivities and specificities of the FIB-4 were 44.7% (95% CI 39.4%–50.2%) and 86.6% (95% CI 84.3%–88.7%), respectively (Figures S7–S8).

In the nine studies assessing the FibroTest (N = 1101), the AUROC curve ranged from 0.68 to 0.92. When combined, the area under the SROC curve was 0.90 (SE = 0.0250) (Figure 7A). The summary DOR was 23.75 (95% CI 11.88–47.48) and the score of Cochran-Q is 20.25 ($P = 0.0094$) (Figure 7B). The heterogeneity was statistically significant. The pooled sensitivities and specificities could not be assessed. Instead, the sensitivities and specificities of the FibroTest at various diagnostic thresholds in the nine studies are listed in Table 4.

According to the meta-regression analysis, the heterogeneity of FibroTest accuracy for detecting cirrhosis was mainly affected by sample size ($P = 0.0385$) and median age ($P = 0.0436$) (Text S7), whereas the other covariates were not significant.

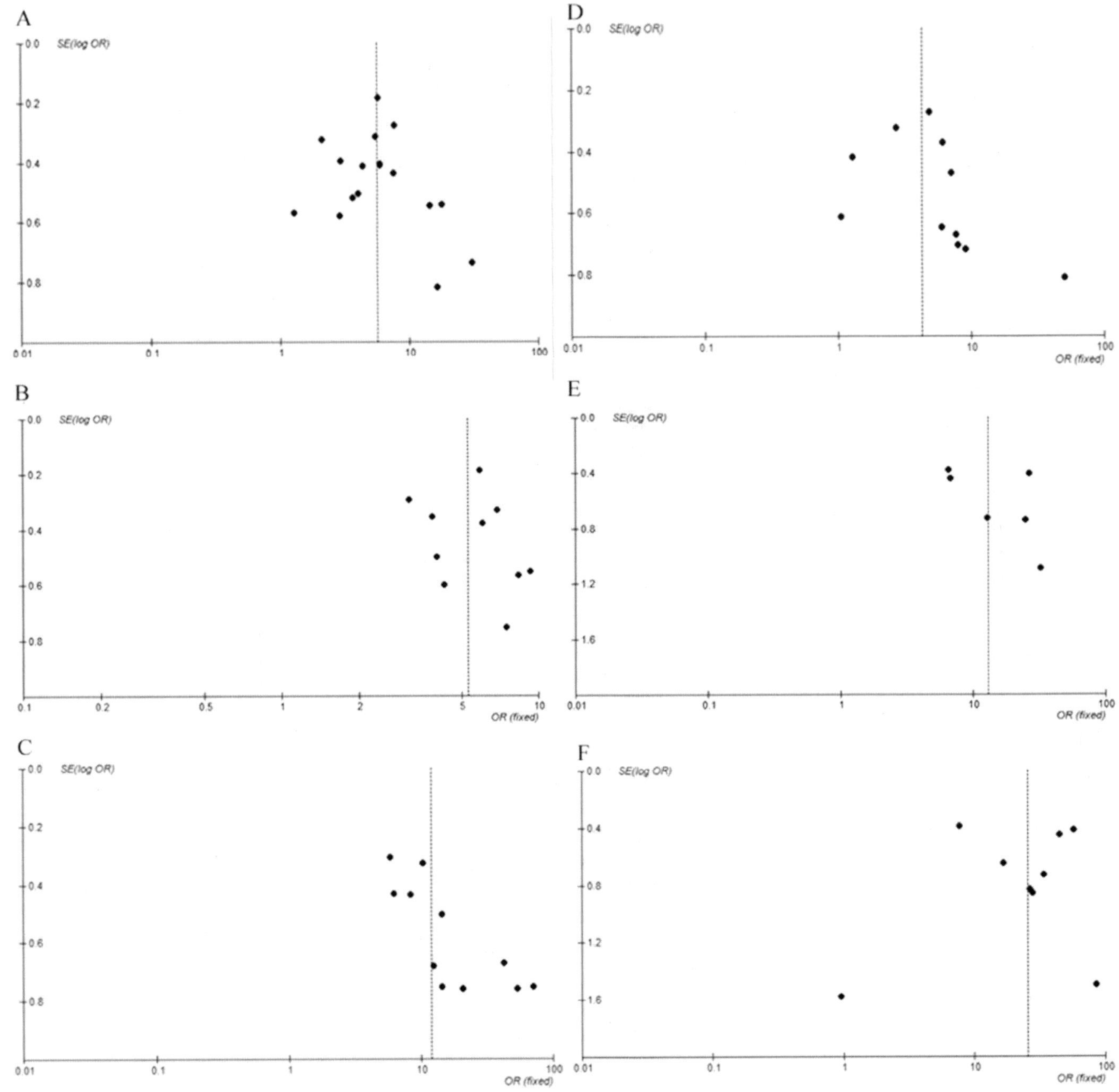

Figure 8. Funnel plot of publication bias. (A) APRI to predict significant fibrosis; (B) FIB-4 to predict significant fibrosis; (C) FibroTest to predict significant fibrosis; (D) APRI to predict cirrhosis; (E)FIB-4 to predict cirrhosis; (F) FibroTest to predict cirrhosis.

Publication Bias

Funnel plots of these three markers for assessing possible publication bias are illustrated in Figure 8. Mild asymmetry was noted in the funnel plots of the FIB-4 and FibroTest.

Discussion

Liver fibrosis progression is commonly found in HBV-infected patients. Cirrhosis develops in approximately one third of those cases, usually after an extensive period of time during which liver biochemical indices are found to be predominantly or even persistently abnormal [1]. Patients with significant fibrosis or cirrhosis should be considered for antiviral therapy, which can potentially reverse cirrhosis and reduce complications [60]. Considering the limitations and risks of biopsy, the researchers make persistent efforts in exploring some noninvasive markers in order to more accurately identify patients with significant fibrosis or cirrhosis. APRI, FIB-4 and FibroTest are such noninvasive markers gaining increasing acceptance in clinical practice. Those markers may reduce the need for liver biopsy and may help to monitor the efficacy of treatment [47].

In our systematic review, the diagnostic accuracy of the APRI, FIB-4 and FibroTest for HBV-related significant fibrosis and cirrhosis has been comprehensively evaluated and summarized on a large scale, and we confirmed the results of many individual studies. Our meta-analysis also included the description of multiple measures of test performance using confirmed meta-analytic techniques and formal assessment for publication bias and heterogeneity, as well as exploratory analysis. All results should be valid and reasonably reliable.

FibroTest had the best result in not only significant fibrosis but also cirrhosis. The area under the SROC curve of FibroTest is bigger and even reaches the standard of "better" on cirrhosis [15], and the summary sensitivity and specificity have reached 84% and 82%, respectively. A meta-analysis about HCV-infected patients showed that the area under the SROC curve of significant fibrosis and cirrhosis are 0.81 and 0.90 [12]. Evidently, the performance of FibroTest in evaluating HBV-related fibrosis is no worse than HCV-related. Therefore, FibroTest could be considered as a better marker in assessing fibrosis and cirrhosis of HBV-infected patients. The FibroTest, however, is calculated with alpha2 macroglobulin, alpha2 globulin (or haptoglobin), gamma globulin, apolipoprotein A1, GGT and total bilirubin [61]. Alpha2 macroglobulin and alpha2 globulin (or haptoglobin) are not routine clinical measurements, and those two indicators are not tested for patients in most hospitals. Furthermore they cost more than conventional indicators. Those factors may bring restrictions to the wider application of the FibroTest in clinical practice.

The calculation method of FIB-4 is simpler than that of FibroTest. The area under the SROC curve of FIB-4 predicting HBV-related significant fibrosis and cirrhosis are 0.75 and 0.87, respectively. FIB-4 also has a better performance of predicting fibrosis [7]. Its test items are easy to obtain in clinical practice, although its predictive results are not as good as FibroTest [11,14]. APRI shows lower diagnostic accuracy than FibroTest and Fib-4 to identify HBV-related significant fibrosis and cirrhosis. It has been introduced to assess HBV-related fibrosis the earliest because of its simple and easy practice. Presently, APRI is widely utilized in identifying the degree of fibrosis and cirrhosis of patients with hepatitis C and hepatitis B, particularly in regions with limited healthcare resources. Some scholars argue that the calculation method of APRI did not consider the factor of spleen size [35]. If patients were grouped by spleen size, the performance of APRI in predicting HBV-related fibrosis would be improved. Our meta-analysis revealed that the area under the SROC curve of APRI was small and the accuracy of the evaluation of HBV-related fibrosis was poor. Our results showed similar performance of APRI for staging of significant fibrosis and cirrhosis [62].

Meta-regression method was convenient and reliable to screen the factors of heterogeneity. The strength of our study is that meta-regression analysis has been used to explore several factors that may be responsible for heterogeneity. Liver biopsy scoring systems and percentage of males emerged from many relevant factors to provide heterogeneity to summary test result on APRI to predict significant fibrosis [62]. On the other hand, etiology of cirrhosis was found to be significantly associated with the heterogeneity on APRI to predict cirrhosis. But the heterogeneity of the meta-analysis of the FIB-4 and FibroTest to predict significant fibrosis and cirrhosis was not statistically significant. FIB-4 and FibroTest to predict fibrosis had better consistency, and summary test results were reasonably reliable.

However, there are several limitations in our systematic review. Firstly, we only focused our analysis on those patients with HBV-related fibrosis, without distinguishing between HBeAg negative and positive cases, or considering the virus replication rate due to the limited number of publications. Secondly, we included studies published in English and Chinese languages only, so the language bias may influence the results to some extent. Lastly, Fibroscan, a widely noninvasive tool, was not considered in this meta-analysis, because our focus was to compare the serum markers calculated by biochemical examination.

In summary, the FibroTest has excellent diagnostic accuracy for the identification of HBV-related significant fibrosis and cirrhosis. But FibroTest is seldom applied in clinical practice as a result of expensive cost. FIB-4, a relatively moderate marker, has better summary diagnostic accuracy and could be measured and calculated relatively easily. Furthermore, APRI shows some limited value in identifying hepatitis B-related significant fibrosis and cirrhosis. All of them have their own advantages and disadvantages. Future studies of novel fibrosis markers are needed to demonstrate improved accuracy and cost-effectiveness compared with those simple, economical, and widely available indeces.

Supporting Information

Figure S1 Sensitivity of FIB-4 detecting significant fibrosis.

Figure S2 Specificity of FIB-4 detecting significant fibrosis.

Figure S3 DOR of APRI cirrhosis (subgroup).

Figure S4 DOR of APRI cirrhosis excluded patients with HBV and HDV coinfected.

Figure S5 Sensitivity of APRI cirrhosis excluded patients with HBV and HDV coinfected.

Figure S6 Specificity of APRI cirrhosis excluded patients with HBV and HDV coinfected.

Figure S7 Sensitivity of Fib-4 detecting cirrhosis.

Figure S8 Specificity of Fib-4 detecting cirrhosis.

Checklist S1 PRISMA checklist of items.

Text S1 Systematic review protocol.

Text S2 Search strategies.

Text S3 Quadas checklist.

Text S4 Meta-regression of APRI detecting significant fibrosis.

Text S5 Meta-regression of FibroTest detecting significant fibrosis.

Text S6 Meta-regression of APRI detecting cirrhosis.

Text S7 Meta-regression of FibroTest detecting cirrhosis.

Author Contributions

Conceived and designed the experiments: HBL XYX. Analyzed the data: XYX WSA XFW HBL. Wrote the paper: HBL XYX HK RXS YHZ XFW WSA. Data collection: XYX HK RXS YHZ. First draft of the manuscript: XYX HBL.

References

1. Custer B, Sullivan SD, Hazlet TK, Iloeje U, Veenstra DL, et al. (2004) Global epidemiology of hepatitis B virus. J Clin Gastroenterol 38: S158–168.
2. Yu MW, Hsu FC, Sheen IS, Chu CM, Lin DY, et al. (1997) Prospective study of hepatocellular carcinoma and liver cirrhosis in asymptomatic chronic hepatitis B virus carriers. Am J Epidemiol 145: 1039–1047.
3. Gumusay O, Ozenirler S, Atak A, Sonmez C, Ozkan S, et al. (2013) Diagnostic potential of serum direct markers and non-invasive fibrosis models in patients with chronic hepatitis B. Hepatol Res 43: 228–237.
4. Liaw YF, Sung JJ, Chow WC, Farrell G, Lee CZ, et al. (2004) Lamivudine for patients with chronic hepatitis B and advanced liver disease. N Engl J Med 351: 1521–1531.
5. Bravo AA, Sheth SG, Chopra S (2001) Liver biopsy. N Engl J Med 344: 495–500.
6. Colloredo G, Guido M, Sonzogni A, Leandro G (2003) Impact of liver biopsy size on histological evaluation of chronic viral hepatitis: the smaller the sample, the milder the disease. J Hepatol 39: 239–244.
7. Kim BK, Kim do Y, Park JY, Ahn SH, Chon CY, et al. (2010) Validation of FIB-4 and comparison with other simple noninvasive indices for predicting liver fibrosis and cirrhosis in hepatitis B virus-infected patients. Liver Int 30: 546–553.
8. Sterling RK, Wegelin JA, Smith PG, Stravitz RT, Luketic VA, et al. (2010) Similar progression of fibrosis between HIV/HCV-infected and HCV-infected patients: Analysis of paired liver biopsy samples. Clin Gastroenterol Hepatol 8: 1070–1076.
9. Poynard T, Morra R, Halfon P, Castera L, Ratziu V, et al. (2007) Meta-analyses of FibroTest diagnostic value in chronic liver disease. BMC Gastroenterol 7: 40.
10. Corradi F, Piscaglia F, Flori S, D'Errico-Grigioni A, Vasuri F, et al. (2009) Assessment of liver fibrosis in transplant recipients with recurrent HCV infection: usefulness of transient elastography. Dig Liver Dis 41: 217–225.
11. Amorim TG, Staub GJ, Lazzarotto C, Silva AP, Manes J, et al. (2012) Validation and comparison of simple noninvasive models for the prediction of liver fibrosis in chronic hepatitis C. Ann Hepatol 11: 855–861.
12. Shaheen AA, Wan AF, Myers RP (2007) FibroTest and FibroScan for the prediction of hepatitis C-related fibrosis: a systematic review of diagnostic test accuracy. Am J Gastroenterol 102: 2589–2600.
13. Lin ZH, Xin YN, Dong QJ, Wang Q, Jiang XJ, et al. (2011) Performance of the aspartate aminotransferase-to-platelet ratio index for the staging of hepatitis C-related fibrosis: an updated meta-analysis. Hepatology 53: 726–736.
14. Martinez SM, Fernandez-Varo G, Gonzalez P, Sampson E, Bruguera M, et al. (2011) Assessment of liver fibrosis before and after antiviral therapy by different serum marker panels in patients with chronic hepatitis C. Aliment Pharmacol Ther 33: 138–148.
15. Deeks JJ (2001) Systematic reviews in health care: Systematic reviews of evaluations of diagnostic and screening tests. BMJ 323: 157–162.
16. Chrysanthos NV, Papatheodoridis GV, Savvas S, Kafiri G, Petraki K, et al. (2006) Aspartate aminotransferase to platelet ratio index for fibrosis evaluation in chronic viral hepatitis. Eur J Gastroenterol Hepatol 18: 389–396.
17. Wang H, Xue L, Yan R, Zhou Y, Wang MS, et al. (2013) Comparison of FIB-4 and APRI in Chinese HBV-infected patients with persistently normal ALT and mildly elevated ALT. J Viral Hepat 20: e3–10.
18. Moher D, Liberati A, Tetzlaff J, Altman DG (2009) Preferred reporting items for systematic reviews and meta-analyses: the PRISMA statement. PLoS Med 6: e1000097.
19. Whiting P, Rutjes AW, Reitsma JB, Bossuyt PM, Kleijnen J (2003) The development of QUADAS: a tool for the quality assessment of studies of diagnostic accuracy included in systematic reviews. BMC Med Res Methodol 3: 25.
20. Group TFMCS (1994) Intraobserver and interobserver variations in liver biopsy interpretation in patients with chronic hepatitis C. The French METAVIR Cooperative Study Group. Hepatology 20: 15–20.
21. Batts KP, Ludwig J (1995) Chronic hepatitis. An update on terminology and reporting. Am J Surg Pathol 19: 1409–1417.
22. Scheuer PJ (1991) Classification of chronic viral hepatitis: a need for reassessment. J Hepatol 13: 372–374.
23. Ishak K, Baptista A, Bianchi L, Callea F, De Groote J, et al. (1995) Histological grading and staging of chronic hepatitis. J Hepatol 22: 696–699.
24. Strader DB, Wright T, Thomas DL, Seeff LB (2004) Diagnosis, management, and treatment of hepatitis C. Hepatology 39: 1147–1171.
25. Walter SD (2002) Properties of the summary receiver operating characteristic (SROC) curve for diagnostic test data. Stat Med 21: 1237–1256.
26. Moses LE, Shapiro D, Littenberg B (1993) Combining independent studies of a diagnostic test into a summary ROC curve: data-analytic approaches and some additional considerations. Stat Med 12: 1293–1316.
27. Dukic V, Gatsonis C (2003) Meta-analysis of diagnostic test accuracy assessment studies with varying number of thresholds. Biometrics 59: 936–946.
28. DerSimonian R, Laird N (1986) Meta-analysis in clinical trials. Control Clin Trials 7: 177–188.
29. Doust JA, Glasziou PP, Pietrzak E, Dobson AJ (2004) A systematic review of the diagnostic accuracy of natriuretic peptides for heart failure. Arch Intern Med 164: 1978–1984.
30. Reitsma JB, Glas AS, Rutjes AW, Scholten RJ, Bossuyt PM, et al. (2005) Bivariate analysis of sensitivity and specificity produces informative summary measures in diagnostic reviews. J Clin Epidemiol 58: 982–990.
31. Higgins JP, Thompson SG, Deeks JJ, Altman DG (2003) Measuring inconsistency in meta-analyses. BMJ 327: 557–560.
32. Deeks JJ, Macaskill P, Irwig L (2005) The performance of tests of publication bias and other sample size effects in systematic reviews of diagnostic test accuracy was assessed. J Clin Epidemiol 58: 882–893.
33. Zhou K, Gao CF, Zhao YP, Liu HL, Zheng RD, et al. (2010) Simpler score of routine laboratory tests predicts liver fibrosis in patients with chronic hepatitis B. J Gastroenterol Hepatol 25: 1569–1577.
34. Shin WG, Park SH, Jang MK, Hahn TH, Kim JB, et al. (2008) Aspartate aminotransferase to platelet ratio index (APRI) can predict liver fibrosis in chronic hepatitis B. Dig Liver Dis 40: 267–274.
35. Kim BK, Kim SA, Park YN, Cheong JY, Kim HS, et al. (2007) Noninvasive models to predict liver cirrhosis in patients with chronic hepatitis B. Liver Int 27: 969–976.
36. Hongbo L, Xiaohui L, Hong K, Wei W, Yong Z (2007) Assessing routine and serum markers of liver fibrosis in CHB patients using parallel and serial interpretation. Clin Biochem 40: 562–566.
37. Guzelbulut F, Sezikli M, Akkan-Cetinkaya Z, Yasar B, Ozkara S, et al. (2012) AST-platelet ratio index in the prediction of significant fibrosis and cirrhosis in patients with chronic hepatitis B. Turk J Gastroenterol 23: 353–358.
38. Lesmana CR, Salim S, Hasan I, Sulaiman AS, Gani RA, et al. (2011) Diagnostic accuracy of transient elastography (FibroScan) versus the aspartate transaminase to platelet ratio index in assessing liver fibrosis in chronic hepatitis B: the role in primary care setting. J Clin Pathol 64: 916–920.
39. Seto WK, Lee CF, Lai CL, Ip PP, Fong DY, et al. (2011) A new model using routinely available clinical parameters to predict significant liver fibrosis in chronic hepatitis B. PLoS One 6: e23077.
40. Liu XD, Wu JL, Liang J, Zhang T, Sheng QS (2012) Globulin-platelet model predicts minimal fibrosis and cirrhosis in chronic hepatitis B virus infected patients. World J Gastroenterol 18: 2784–2792.
41. Zhu X, Wang LC, Chen EQ, Chen XB, Chen LY, et al. (2011) Prospective evaluation of FibroScan for the diagnosis of hepatic fibrosis compared with liver biopsy/AST platelet ratio index and FIB-4 in patients with chronic HBV infection. Dig Dis Sci 56: 2742–2749.
42. Wu SD, Wang JY, Li L (2010) Staging of liver fibrosis in chronic hepatitis B patients with a composite predictive model: a comparative study. World J Gastroenterol 16: 501–507.
43. Wang Y, Xu MY, Zheng RD, Xian JC, Xu HT, et al. (2013) Prediction of significant fibrosis and cirrhosis in hepatitis B e-antigen negative patients with chronic hepatitis B using routine parameters. Hepatol Res 43: 441–451.
44. Ucar F, Sezer S, Ginis Z, Ozturk G, Albayrak A, et al. (2013) APRI, the FIB-4 score, and Forn's index have noninvasive diagnostic value for liver fibrosis in patients with chronic hepatitis B. Eur J Gastroenterol Hepatol.
45. Basar O, Yimaz B, Ekiz F, Ginis Z, Altinbas A, et al. (2013) Non-invasive tests in prediction of liver fibrosis in chronic hepatitis B and comparison with post-antiviral treatment results. Clin Res Hepatol Gastroenterol 37: 152–158.
46. Liu HB, Zhou JP, Zhang Y, Lv XH, Wang W (2011) Prediction on liver fibrosis using different APRI thresholds when patient age is a categorical marker in patients with chronic hepatitis B. Clin Chim Acta 412: 33–37.
47. Sebastiani G, Vario A, Guido M, Alberti A (2007) Sequential algorithms combining non-invasive markers and biopsy for the assessment of liver fibrosis in chronic hepatitis B. World J Gastroenterol 13: 525–531.
48. Bonnard P, Sombie R, Lescure FX, Bougouma A, Guiard-Schmid JB, et al. (2010) Comparison of elastography, serum marker scores, and histology for the assessment of liver fibrosis in hepatitis B virus (HBV)-infected patients in Burkina Faso. Am J Trop Med Hyg 82: 454–458.
49. Sebastiani G, Castera L, Halfon P, Pol S, Mangia A, et al. (2011) The impact of liver disease aetiology and the stages of hepatic fibrosis on the performance of non-invasive fibrosis biomarkers: an international study of 2411 cases. Alimentary Pharmacology & Therapeutics 34: 1202–1216.
50. Zhang YF, Shi H, Chen LB, Xu QH (2010) [Value of FIB-4 for the diagnosis of liver fibrosis in chronic hepatitis B]. Zhonghua Shi Yan He Lin Chuang Bing Du Xue Za Zhi 24: 215–217.
51. Myers RP, Tainturier MH, Ratziu V, Piton A, Thibault V, et al. (2003) Prediction of liver histological lesions with biochemical markers in patients with chronic hepatitis B. J Hepatol 39: 222–230.
52. Miailhes P, Pradat P, Chevallier M, Lacombe K, Bailly F, et al. (2011) Proficiency of transient elastography compared to liver biopsy for the assessment of fibrosis in HIV/HBV-coinfected patients. J Viral Hepat 18: 61–69.

53. Bottero J, Lacombe K, Guechot J, Serfaty L, Miailhes P, et al. (2009) Performance of 11 biomarkers for liver fibrosis assessment in HIV/HBV co-infected patients. J Hepatol 50: 1074–1083.
54. Kim BK, Kim SU, Kim HS, Park JY, Ahn SH, et al. (2012) Prospective validation of FibroTest in comparison with liver stiffness for predicting liver fibrosis in Asian subjects with chronic hepatitis B. PLoS One 7: e35825.
55. Stibbe KJ, Verveer C, Francke J, Hansen BE, Zondervan PE, et al. (2011) Comparison of non-invasive assessment to diagnose liver fibrosis in chronic hepatitis B and C patients. Scand J Gastroenterol 46: 962–972.
56. Park MS, Kim BK, Cheong JY, Kim DJ, Park JY, et al. (2013) Discordance between liver biopsy and FibroTest in assessing liver fibrosis in chronic hepatitis B. PLoS One 8: e55759.
57. Gui HL, Xie Q, Wang H (2008) [FibroTest-ActiTest for predicting liver fibrosis and inflammatory activity in Chinese patients with chronic hepatitis B]. Zhonghua Gan Zang Bing Za Zhi 16: 897–901.
58. Kim BK, Kim HS, Park JY, Kim do Y, Ahn SH, et al. (2012) Prospective validation of ELF test in comparison with Fibroscan and FibroTest to predict liver fibrosis in Asian subjects with chronic hepatitis B. PLoS One 7: e41964.
59. Sebastiani G, Castera L, Halfon P, Pol S, Mangia A, et al. (2011) The impact of liver disease aetiology and the stages of hepatic fibrosis on the performance of non-invasive fibrosis biomarkers: an international study of 2411 cases. Aliment Pharmacol Ther 34: 1202–1216.
60. Lavanchy D (2004) Hepatitis B virus epidemiology, disease burden, treatment, and current and emerging prevention and control measures. J Viral Hepat 11: 97–107.
61. Imbert-Bismut F, Ratziu V, Pieroni L, Charlotte F, Benhamou Y, et al. (2001) Biochemical markers of liver fibrosis in patients with hepatitis C virus infection: a prospective study. Lancet 357: 1069–1075.
62. Jin W, Lin Z, Xin Y, Jiang X, Dong Q, et al. (2012) Diagnostic accuracy of the aspartate aminotransferase-to-platelet ratio index for the prediction of hepatitis B-related fibrosis: a leading meta-analysis. BMC Gastroenterol 12: 14.

29

Inhibition of C3 Convertase Activity by Hepatitis C Virus as an Additional Lesion in the Regulation of Complement Components

Hangeun Kim[1], Keith Meyer[1], Adrian M. Di Bisceglie[1,2], Ranjit Ray[1,2]*

1 Department of Internal Medicine, Saint Louis University, St. Louis, Missouri, United States of America, **2** Department of Molecular Microbiology & Immunology, Saint Louis University, St. Louis, Missouri, United States of America

Abstract

We have previously reported that *in vitro* HCV infection of cells of hepatocyte origin attenuates complement system at multiple steps, and attenuation also occurs in chronically HCV infected liver, irrespective of the disease stage. However, none of these regulations alone completely impaired complement pathways. Modulation of the upstream proteins involved in proteolytic processing of the complement cascade prior to convertase formation is critical in promoting the function of the complement system in response to infection. Here, we examined the regulation of C2 complement expression in hepatoma cells infected *in vitro* with cell culture grown virus, and validated our observations using randomly selected chronically HCV infected patient liver biopsy specimens. C2 mRNA expression was significantly inhibited, and classical C3 convertase (C4b2a) decreased. In separate experiments for C3 convertase function, C3b deposition onto bacterial membrane was reduced using HCV infected patient sera as compared to uninfected control, suggesting impaired C3 convertase. Further, iC3b level, a proteolytically inactive form of C3b, was lower in HCV infected patient sera, reflecting impairment of both C3 convertase and Factor I activity. The expression level of Factor I was significantly reduced in HCV infected liver biopsy specimens, while Factor H level remained unchanged or enhanced. Together, these results suggested that inhibition of C3 convertase activity is an additional cumulative effect for attenuation of complement system adopted by HCV for weakening innate immune response.

Editor: Neerja Kaushik-Basu, Rutgers, The State University of New Jersey, United States of America

Funding: This work was supported by research grants DK080812 from NIDDK, U54-AI057160 from the NAID to the Midwest Regional Center of Excellence (MRCE) for Biodefense and Emerging Infectious Diseases Research, and the Internal Blue Ribbon Fund of Saint Louis University. The funders had no role in study design, data collection and analysis, decision to publish, or preparation of the manuscript.

Competing Interests: The authors have declared that no competing interests exist.

* Email: rayr@slu.edu

Introduction

A significant number of people infected with HCV develop chronic infection [1,2]. Hepatocytes are the primary host for HCV replication and serve as a main source for complement synthesis. We previously examined the relationship between HCV infection and complement regulation, and have shown that HCV infection attenuates complement system by modulating multiple components, such as C3, C4, and C9 [3–5]. The complement system plays a central role in the innate immune system, as a first line of defense against pathogen infection. The complement system quickly detects antibody bound microbes for elimination. All three complement activation pathways (classical, lectin, and alternative), merge for the cleavage of C3 in to C3a and C3b by C3 convertase. Cleavage of C3 by C3 convertases results in the formation of C3b and the anaphylatoxin C3a. Further processing of C3b results in the formation of iC3b and C3f, and finally C3c and C3dg [6]. In this process, Factor I is a key serine protease that inactivates all complement pathways by degrading activated complement factors C4b and C3b. Factor I degrades C4b and C3b only in the presence of specific cofactors, such as Factor H, C4b binding protein (C4BP), membrane-cofactor protein (MCP), and complement receptor 1 (CR1) [7]. Deficiencies in complement predispose patients to infection via ineffective opsonization, and defects in membrane attack complex (MAC) mediated lysis activity [8,9]. Therefore, insights into the mechanisms of complement regulation are crucial for understanding disease pathology and therapies.

Complement component 2 (C2) is a 110 kDa serum glycoprotein that functions as part of the classical pathway of the complement system. The key function of C2 is the formation of the classical C3 convertase (C4b2a) together with C4b [8]. C2 deficiency (C2D) is the most common of the complement component deficiency. Hereditary C2D is an important susceptibility factor for invasive infections caused by encapsulated bacteria, such as pneumococci and haemophilus influenza type b [10–16]. C2D may also be a risk factor for development of atherosclerosis. However, many persons with C2D are apparently healthy. Complement component 3 (C3) plays an essential role in the complement pathways, including mediating convertase activity, opsonization, anaphylotoxin production, B cell activation, immunoglobulin production, immune-complex clearance. C2 is one of the C3 convertase components. C3 deficiency, either genetically determined or caused by deficiencies in the regulatory proteins factor H or factor I, include increased susceptibility to infection and rheumatic disorders [16,17]. In this study, we examined the effect of HCV upon C2 at the transcriptional level in HCV infected patient liver biopsies and in infected patient sera on the formation and activation of C3 convertase.

Materials and Methods

Reagents

Mouse monoclonal antibody to human C3 (Abcam, MA), goat anti-mouse secondary antibody (Sigma, MO), purified human complement component C3 protein (Quidel, CA) were purchased.

Patient materials

Paired serum samples and liver biopsy specimens from 12 chronically HCV infected patients [3,4] and 12 non-HCV liver disease patients were randomly selected for use in this study. Sera and liver samples were collected from subjects with their written consent, and the protocol was approved by the Saint Louis University Internal Review Board. The liver biopsy specimens were read by an experienced pathologist, and the severity of hepatitis was graded and staged according to a system described by Scheuer [18]. Liver biopsy tissue specimens were embedded in optimum cutting temperature (OCT) formulation and preserved at −70°C. Sera were prepared after storing on ice within a short time (2–3 h) to retain complement activity, aliquoted, and stored at −70°C. Each aliquot was thawed and tested once for complement related activity. Commercially available control liver RNAs were procured (Clonetics, CA; Clonetech, CA; and Lonza, NJ).

Cell culture grown HCV and infection of cells

Immortalized human hepatocytes (IHH) or human hepatoma cells were used to grow HCV genotype 1a, as previously described [19–20]. Cell culture grown HCV released in culture supernatant was filtered through a 0.45 μm cellulose acetate membrane (Nalgene, NY), aliquoted, and stored at −70°C for single use. RNA (IU/ml) was quantified by real-time PCR (Prism7500 real-time thermocycler; ABI) with the use of HCV analyte-specific reagents (ASR, Abbott) in the Pathology Clinical Laboratory at Saint Louis University. Infectious virus titer from cell culture supernatant was also measured by fluorescence-focus forming unit (FFU) using a NS5A specific monoclonal antibody. For virus infection, hepatocytes were incubated with 0.5 moi of cell culture grown HCV. After virus adsorption for ~8 h, cells were washed, incubated with fresh medium for 4 days, and used in subsequent experiment.

ELISA

HCV infected patient sera were used for C3 convertase (USCNK, TX) and iC3b (Quidel, CA) analyses by a commercially available enzyme-linked immunosorbent assay (ELISA) kit following manufacturer's protocol.

C3 cleavage assay

50 μg/ml of C3 purified protein was incubated with an indicated dose of human sera at 37°C for 30 min. Samples were separated under reducing conditions by SDS-PAGE. Proteins were transferred onto nitrocellulose membrane and treated with anti-human C3 antibody at 4°C overnight, followed by a mouse secondary antibody. The experiment was carried out three times, and a representative figure is shown. Densitometry was analyzed using Image J software.

C3b deposition assay

C3b deposition on gram-negative bacterial cell surface was performed similarly as described [21]. Briefly, *E. coli* DH5α (~1×10^7) was incubated with HCV infected patient serum or normal human serum (NHS) (10% sera in a final volume of 50 μl) at 37°C for 30 min. Purified C3 protein (20 μg/ml) was added in the bacteria and serum mixture. After washing with PBS, opsonized log-phase bacteria were plated onto 96-well EIA plates

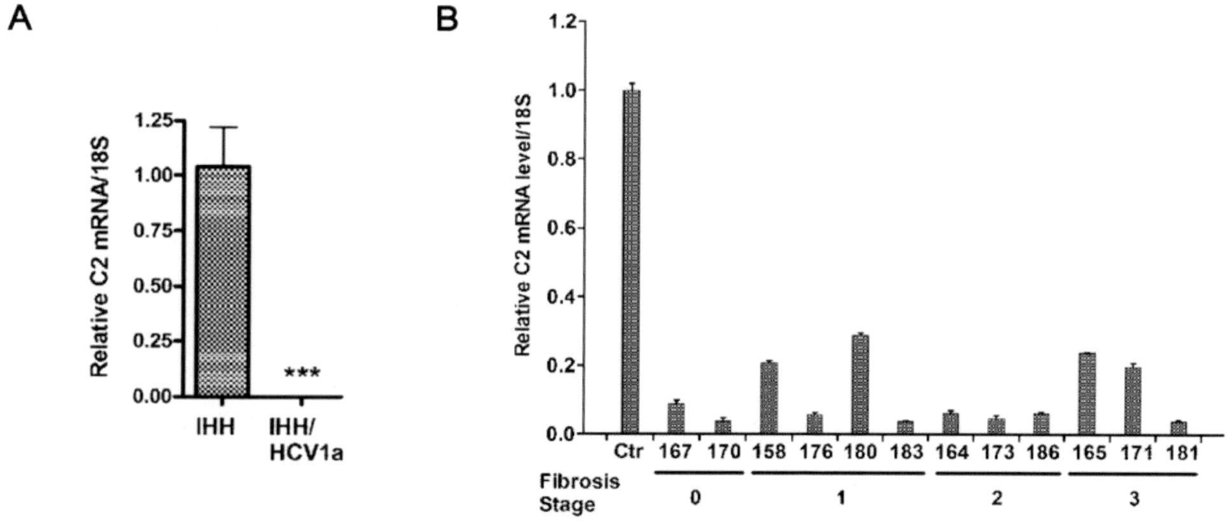

Figure 1. HCV infection inhibits mRNA expression of C2 complement component. (A) Real-time PCR analysis for C2 mRNA expression from HCV infected IHH and mock infected control cells. Results were normalized to endogenous 18S RNA. Asterisks denote: *$p<0.05$; **$p<0.01$; ***$p<0.001$ when compared to controls. (B) Real-time PCR analysis displaying HCV genotype 1a infection represses C2 expression in chronically infected liver biopsy specimens from patients (n = 12). Liver biopsy samples are each marked by 3-digit numbers at the bottom. Results are compared with non-HCV infected 3 control liver tissues arbitrarily set at 1. The error bars in individual samples are shown as variations form triplicate assays. All samples used in this study were significantly inhibited ($p<0.01$) as compared to negative controls.

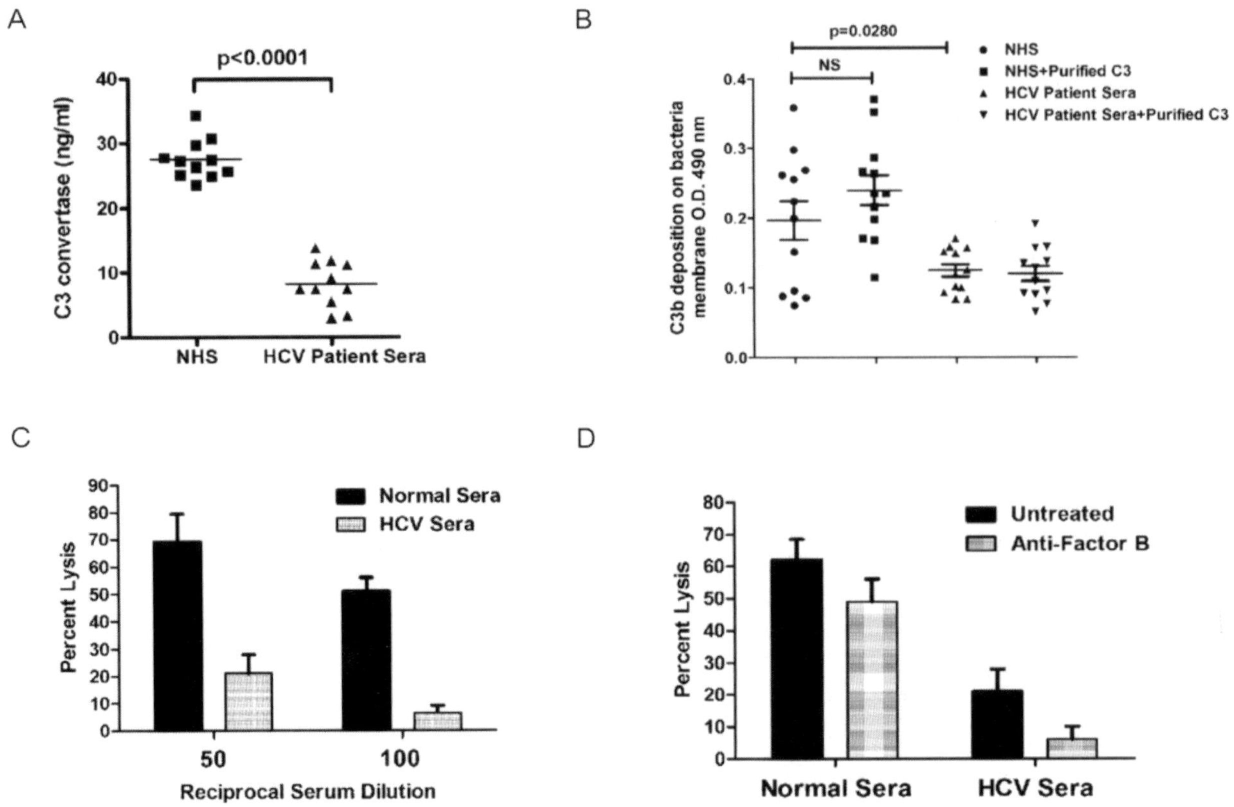

Figure 2. C3 convertase level reduces in HCV infected patient sera. (A) Comparison of serum C3 convertase level in randomly chosen HCV infected patient sera (n = 12) and normal human sera (NHS) from healthy donors (n = 12) using a commercially available ELISA kit. (B) HCV infected patient sera (n = 12) and NHS (n = 12) were subjected to analysis for comparison of C3b deposition on *E. coli* surface in the presence or absence of purified C3 protein. Asterisks denote: *p<0.05; **p<0.01; ***p<0.001 when compared to control. (C) Complement mediated lysis was inhibited in HCV infected patient sera. Normal sera (n = 6) and HCV infected patient sera (n = 6) were incubated with sheep RBC after treatment with EDTA. Sera from each test group were studied, with lysis of erythrocytes completed using EDTA treated guinea pig serum. (D) Sheep RBCs were incubated with sera in the presence or absence of anti-factor B antibody to separate out alternate pathway mediated lysis from classical antibody mediated lysis, and lysis was carried out as described above.

at ~5×10^6 per well and adhered by dry desiccation. Nonspecific binding sites were blocked with 0.5% BSA in PBS and incubated for 30 min at 37°C. After washing, the plates were sequentially incubated at room temperature with C3 antibody for 60 min, HRP-conjugated secondary antibody for 30 min, and finally substrate solution for visualizing HRP activity. The reaction was stopped with H_2SO_4 and color intensity measured at OD_{490}.

Convertase functional assay

Amboceptor sensitized sheep erythrocytes (EA) were purchased (Complement Technologies, Tyler, TX). Erythrocytes (5×10^8) were washed with dextrose gelatin veronal buffer (DGVB) buffer (2.5 mM veronal buffer, pH 7.3, 72 mM NaCl, 140 mM glucose, 0.1% gelatin, 1 mM $MgCl_2$, and 0.15 mM $CaCl_2$), EA suspensions were adjusted and lysed with 90 µl of water to have an absorbance value of ~1.5 at 405 nm.

For assessment of convertase function [22], 10 µl of EA were placed in a 96-well V-shape microplate (Nunc) and 40 µl of DGVB buffer containing a 2.0% HCV patient or healthy control serum was added to assemble convertases. The plate was kept in an incubator shaker at 30°C with 300 rpm shaking for 5 minutes for convertase formation. To initiate complement mediated lysis from existing convertase complexes, 50 µl of 40 mM EDTA-GVB buffer (40 mM EDTA, 5 mM veronal buffer, 0.1% gelatin, 145 mM NaCl) containing 1:40 guinea pig serum as a source of complement was added and the plate was incubated for another 30 minutes at 37°C on a 300 rpm shaker. Alternatively, lysis was developed with guinea pig complement deficient in C4 in 40 mM EDTA-GVB buffer. Cells were pelleted and 50 µl of the supernatant containing hemoglobin released from lysed EA were measured at 405 nm in a microplate reader.

Blocking of Factor B activity in a classical C5 convertase assay

To assess the contribution of the alternative convertases as an amplification loop of the classical pathway, we blocked Factor B activity during and after convertase formation. EA were mixed with 40 µl DGVB containing serum at a final concentration of 2% and 60 µg/ml of function blocking mouse anti-human FB antibody (Quidel, SanDiego) or control antibody. C5 convertase was allowed to assemble as previously described [22]. To initiate complement-mediated lysis, the same dilution of anti-Factor B antibody in 50 µl of DGVB was added and incubated in the presence of a 1:40 dilution of guinea pig complement. Cells were pelleted and supernatant containing hemoglobin released was measured at 405 nm.

Real-time PCR

C2, Factor I, or Factor H mRNA quantitation was performed by real-time PCR using specific primers and probes using a 7500

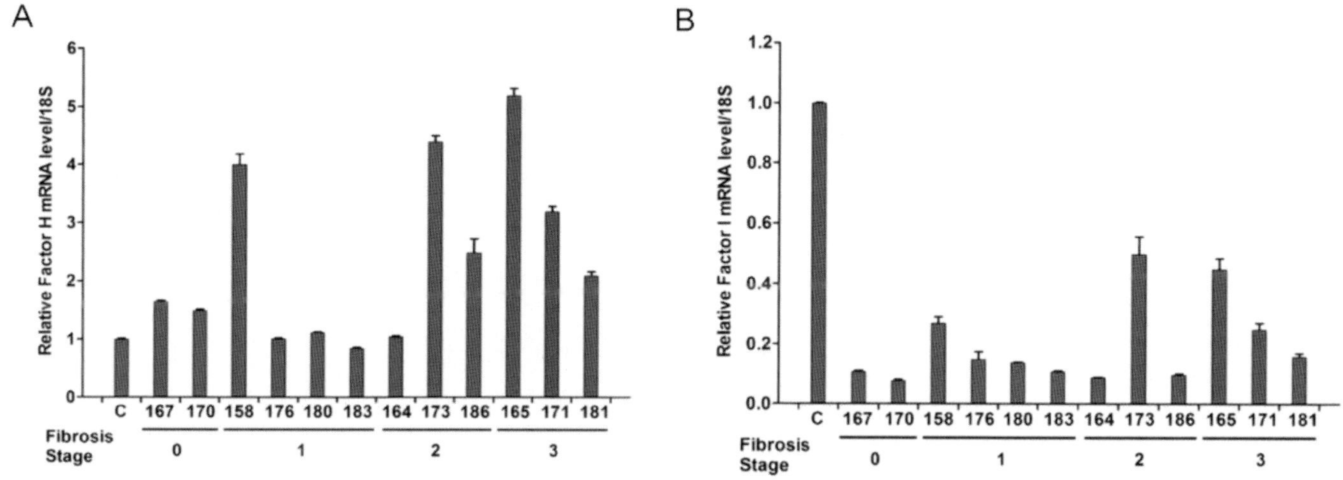

Figure 3. Factor H and Factor I expression are impaired in HCV infected patient sera. Real-time PCR analysis from HCV genotype 1a infected liver biopsy specimens from patients (n = 12) exhibiting Factor H (A) and Factor I (B) expression status are shown. Results were compared with non-HCV infected control liver RNAs (n = 3) arbitrarily set at 1. The error bars in individual samples are shown as variations form triplicate assays. Increase of Factor H was significant ($p<0.05$ in #186, 171, and 181; $p<0.01$ in #158, 173, and 165) as compared to control liver. Factor I inhibition was significant ($p<0.05$) in all tested samples.

Fast Real Time PCR system (Applied Biosystems, CA). RNA was isolated from experimental samples using TRIzol (Invitrogen, CA), and cDNA was synthesized using random hexamers and a SuperScript III first-strand synthesis kit (Invitrogen).

Statistical analysis

Results were expressed as the mean ± standard deviation (SD), and statistical analyses were performed using a two-tailed unpaired Student *t* test or one-way analysis of variance (ANOVA) in GraphPad Prism, version 5 (GraphPad, La Jolla, CA). A p values <0.05 was considered statistically significant.

Results

HCV infection inhibits C2 mRNA expression

We analyzed C2 mRNA expression in cells infected with cell culture-grown HCV. A significant reduction of C2 mRNA expression was observed in HCV genotype 1a infected IHH, as compared to mock-infected controls (Fig. 1, panel A). The results clearly indicated that HCV infection regulates C2 complement component at the transcriptional level at different magnitude based on HCV genotype.

In order to investigate the effect of HCV infection on C2 expression in chronically infected patients, C2 mRNA status was measured from liver biopsy samples. For this, RNA was extracted from randomly selected 12 liver biopsy patients infected with HCV genotype 1a [4,5]. Three unrelated human liver RNAs were included in this study for comparison. C2 mRNA expression was measured by real-time PCR. All HCV-infected liver biopsy specimens exhibited a significant reduction in C2 mRNA expression (>70%) as compared to control human liver RNAs (Fig. 1, panel B). Our results exhibited C2 repression in 12 liver biopsy specimens from chronically HCV infected patients. The C2 expression status was independent of their fibrotic stage, grade, presence, or absence of rheumatoid factor.

HCV infected patient sera exhibit reduced C3 convertase formation

The C3 convertase status of classical pathway in normal human sera (NHS) and HCV infected patient sera was examined by ELISA. A significant inhibition of C3 convertase complex in HCV infected patient sera as compared to NHS was observed (Fig. 2, panel A). We have previously shown that C4 serum level was lower in HCV infected patients as compared to normal human sera [3]. Together, our data suggests that the reduction of complement components C2 (Fig. 1) and C4 [3], may have a direct role on C3 convertase activity of classical pathway.

We examined the C3 convertase assembly of alternative pathway by analyzing C3b deposition on bacterial surface. After cleavage of C3, C3b is deposited on pathogen surface as an initial step in the formation of C3 convertase of alternative pathway or as part of the subsequent C5 convertase [23–24]. We performed a C3b deposition assay using *E. coli* DH5α. The level of C3b deposition on bacteria membrane was higher in NHS as compared to HCV infected patient sera (Fig. 2, panel B), indicating a low level of C3 convertase function in HCV infected patients. The limited C3 convertase formation from both pathways and impairment of C3b generation may additionally affect C5 convertase formation in HCV infected patients. When purified C3 protein was added to the reaction, NHS had a significantly increased C3b deposition, indicating the further potential for convertase activity. However, an increase in C3b deposition was not observed in the reaction using HCV infected patient sera with the addition of purified C3 protein (Fig. 2, panel B). This result suggests that HCV infected patient sera has limited factors related to C3 processing, and convertase function is limited due to the cumulative reduction of complement components at the initial stage of convertase formation, limiting downstream protease function. C3b deposition is a critical step for the complement cascade, especially in the formation of C5 convertase, which leads to membrane attack complex (MAC) formation. Thus, impairment of C3b deposition in HCV infected patient sera can affect MAC formation and pathogen killing activity.

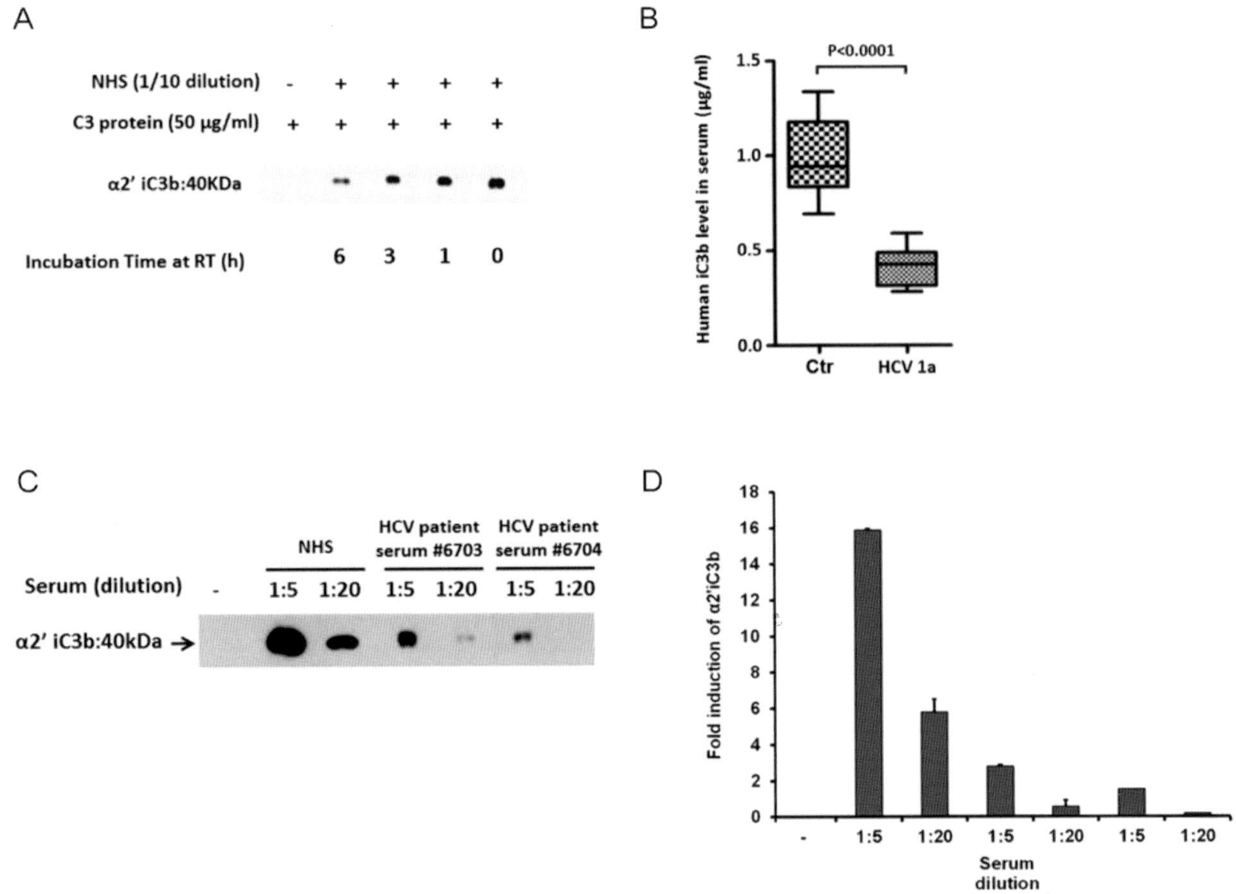

Figure 4. iC3b level decreases in HCV infected patient sera. (A) Undiluted NHS were incubated at room temperature for 1, 3, and 6 h. Purified C3 protein (50 μg/ml) was added to preincubated serum at 1:10 dilution at 37°C for 30 min. The α2'iC3b protein band was detected in samples by Western blot analysis. (B) Comparison of serum iC3b level in NHS (n = 12) and HCV infected patient sera (n = 12) using a commercially available ELISA kit. (C) NHS and HCV infected patient sera incubated with purified C3 protein (50 μg/ml) at 1:5 and 1:20 dilution. The protein band representing α2'iC3b was detected by Western blot and a representative figure is shown. (D) Densitometry analysis for α2'iC3b protein band intensity was done by ImageJ software after repeated experiments with NHS (n = 6) and HCV infected sera (n = 6).

Further examination revealed that a panel of chronically HCV infected patient sera display significantly reduced ability to lyse antibody sensitized sheep RBC as compared to NHS as control (Fig. 2, panel C). Initial convertase formation occurred using patient and control sera, with cell lysis from added guineapig complement treated with EDTA. This protocol allows for the analysis of upstream complement dysfunction, removing the effect prior noted with the modulation of complement C9 expression [5]. Lysis of amboreceptor sensitized sheep erythrocytes was significantly reduced when HCV patient sera were used to form initial convertase function. A neutralizing antibody to Factor B was utilized to inhibit RBC lysis derived from activity of the alternate pathway (2% serum concentration), and revealed that the majority of complement activity in these antibody sensitized erythrocytes occurred through the classical (antibody mediated) pathway (Fig. 2, panel D) in NHS. A similar reduction of alternate pathway mediated lysis was also apparent in HCV infected patient sera with the use of Factor B antibody. In the final analysis, the data indicate that the classical pathway mediated lysis analyzed in this system was compromised by a nearly 10 fold reduction in activity of HCV patient sera as compared to NHS. These results indicate that the expression and proteolytic processing of the early components of the complement convertase are significantly inhibited in HCV infected patients, with the potential to impair normal immune functions.

Factor H and Factor I are modulated in HCV infected patient sera

Factor H regulates complement activation on self-cells and surfaces by possessing both cofactor activity for the Factor I mediated C3b cleavage, and decay accelerating activity against the alternative pathway C3-convertase, C3bBb [25]. Factor I is a key serine protease that inactivates all complement pathways by degrading activated complement factors C4b and C3b [7]. In this study, we examined whether HCV modulates Factor H and Factor I to influence C3 convertase. Real-time PCR analysis suggested enhanced Factor H mRNA in liver biopsy specimens of patients infected with HCV genotype 1a (Fig. 3, panel A). Six out of 12 samples displayed a significant increase in Factor H mRNA level and others had modest alterations as compared to unrelated control liver specimens, and these changes did not correlate with fibrosis stage. On the other hand, Factor I levels in liver biopsy specimens were significantly inhibited in all examined samples irrespective of liver fibrosis stage, as compared to control (Fig. 3, panel B).

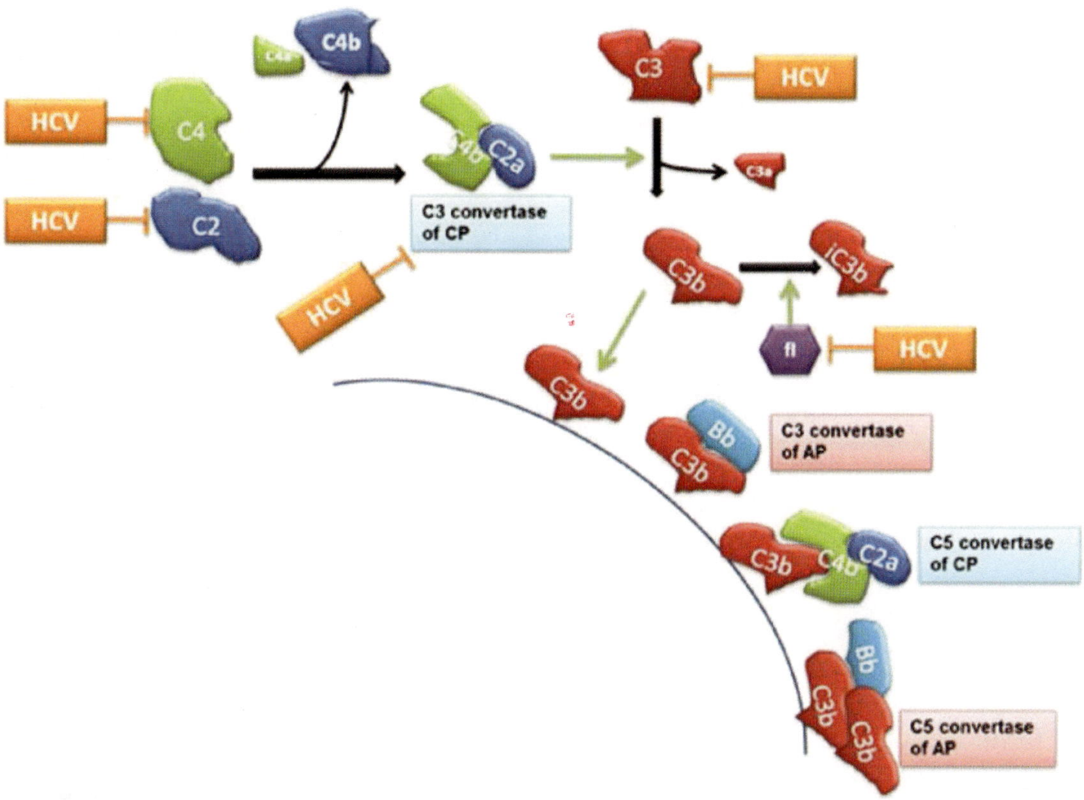

Figure 5. Schematic presentation of complement regulation by HCV. HCV infection inhibits C4 and C3 components expression [3,4] as well as C2 production (current study). Reduction of C4 and C2 synthesis by HCV affects C3 convertase formation in classical pathway, which results in the inhibition of C3 cleavage. Limited C3b generation affect C3b deposition onto pathogenic surface, and impairs another C3 convertase formation of alternative pathway and C5 convertase formation in both pathways. Together with the reduction of membrane attack complex formation [5], the impairment of C3 convertase activity may be a key event for HCV persistence. CP = classical pathway, AP = alternate pathway.

Decreased iC3b level in HCV infected patient sera

iC3b is generated by Factor I after formation of C3b. iC3b is a proteolytically inactive form of C3b that retains the ability to opsonize microbes, but cannot participate in convertase function. To examine the effect of time and temperature for C3 convertase, we incubated NHS at room temperature for various time and confirmed its C3 cleavage activity by observing iC3b generation. C3 convertase activity was not significantly altered by room temperature incubation up to 3 h (Fig. 4, panel A). Next, we evaluated iC3b levels in 12 chronically HCV genotype 1a infected patient sera by ELISA as an indicator of total complement activation, as C3b has a very short half-life. Six normal human sera were included as controls for comparison. The results indicated that iC3b levels were decreased at least 3 fold in HCV infected patient sera as compared to control (Fig. 4, panel B). This result suggests that C3 convertase activity was decreased in HCV infected patients. Serum iC3b level was much higher in NHS as compared to HCV infected patient sera incubated with a set concentration of purified C3 protein at the same dilution, such as 1:5 and 1:20 (Fig. 4, panel C). The iC3b level from 6 NHS and 6 HCV infected patient sera are represented as a fold induction after scanning of band intensity using ImageJ software (Fig. 4, panel D). These results indicated that Factor I activity is higher in NHS than in HCV infected patient sera. As we observed, Factor I quantity and/or activity is impaired in HCV infected patients, suggesting that the alternative pathway of complement leads to continuous generation of fluid-phase and cell-surface-deposited C3b by a self-amplification loop. However, C3b deposition on bacteria cell surface was limited (Fig. 2, panel B) and total C3 level was also lower in HCV infected patient sera as compared to NHS [4].

Discussion

The complement system plays a central role in the innate and adaptive immune response. The production of anaphylotoxins during complement convertase function results in complement induced T cell activation, with APC activation driving T cell differentiation, expansion and survival [25]. In the current study, we have shown impairment of C3 convertase in HCV infected patient sera. The effect of lower C3 convertase in the complement system leads to the impairment of downstream events including C5 convertase formation (Fig. 5). Previously, we have shown that HCV genotype 1a infected patients had a low level of C5b-9 in their sera, which resulted in impairment of MAC formation and bactericidal/virocidal activity [5]. Limited C3 convertase activity in HCV infected patients may affect C5 convertase generation and C5 cleavage. In the current study, we have shown C3b level was lower in HCV infected patient sera, suggesting that the formation of C5 convertase in classical pathway (C4b2a3b) is impaired. In addition, HCV inhibits C5 mRNA synthesis in hepatoma cells. These observations reinforce our previous results suggesting HCV impairs at multiple steps of the complement system to escape from complement mediated virocidal activity.

Factor I is a key serine protease that inactivates all complement pathways by degrading activated complement factors C4b and

C3b. Factor I does not cleave intact C4 or C3, and degrades C4b and C3b only in the presence of specific cofactors, such as Factor H, C4b binding protein (C4BP), membrane-cofactor protein (MCP), and complement receptor 1 (CR1) [7]. Interestingly, C4 has been shown to a cellular substrate of HCV NS3/4A protease and may also contribute to HCV persistence [26] The physiological importance of Factor I is shown by the fact that patients lacking Factor I have increased susceptibility to recurrent infection with encapsulated microorganisms, glomerulonephritis, and rheumatologic diseases [27,28]. In the absence of regulation by Factor I, the alternative pathway of complement leads to continuous generation of fluid-phase and cell-surface-deposited C3b by a self-amplification loop. Thus, lower level of iC3b from the current study suggests: (i) C3 cleavage occurs less in HCV infected patients because of limited C3 convertase activity, and (ii) increased iC3b level in NHS indicates the presence of activated factor I, while HCV infected patient sera has limited Factor I. Therefore, further knowledge on the mechanism of inhibition of Factor I expression by HCV may provide important information in understanding deregulation of complement activation. Factor H is a bifunctional and essential molecule for control of the alternative pathway of complement. Normal recognition of cell surface is required for effective protection. On the other hand, mutations and polymorphisms in Factor H gene may result in inadequate protection and disease. Abnormal recognition of host cell surfaces by Factor H has been associated with complement-mediated tissue damage and disease. In addition, unwanted recognition of pathogens and cancer cells by Factor H can be used as an immune evasion strategy [29]. At least 50% of HCV infected patients showed abnormal increase of Factor H and this suggest that HCV may use factor H to help escape immune surveillance, but more detailed studies are required.

Our current study suggests that HCV infection affects C3 convertase formation by modulating specific complement components and their activity. This results in an impairment of C3 processing and activation of complement dependent functions. In this manner, the effect HCV has on the innate immune system may carry over into further modulating host adaptive immune responses.

Acknowledgments

We thank Lin Cowick for preparation of the manuscript.

Author Contributions

Conceived and designed the experiments: HK RR. Performed the experiments: HK KM. Analyzed the data: HK AMD KM RR. Contributed reagents/materials/analysis tools: HK AMD KM RR. Contributed to the writing of the manuscript: HK KM RR.

References

1. Klenerman P, Gupta PK (2012) Hepatitis C virus: current concepts and future challenges. QJM 105: 29–32.
2. Petrovic D, Dempsey E, Doherty DG, Kelleher D, Long A (2012) Hepatitis C virus-T-cell responses and viral escape mutations. Eur J Immunol 42: 17–26.
3. Banerjee A, Mazumdar B, Meyer K, Di Bisceglie AM, Ray RB, et al. (2011) Transcriptional repression of C4 complement by hepatitis C virus proteins. J Virol 85: 4157–4166.
4. Mazumdar B, Kim H, Meyer K, Bose SK, Di Bisceglie AM, et al. (2012) Hepatitis C virus proteins inhibit C3 complement production. J Virol 86: 2221–2228.
5. Kim H, Meyer K, Di Bisceglie AM, Ray R (2013) Hepatitis C virus suppresses c9 complement synthesis and impairs membrane attack complex function. J Virol 87: 5858–5867.
6. Gros P, Milder FJ, Janssen BJ (2008) Complement driven by conformational changes. Nat Rev Immunol 8: 48–58.
7. Nilsson SC, Nita I, Månsson L, Groeneveld TW, Trouw LA, et al. (2010) Analysis of binding sites on complement factor I that are required for its activity. J Biol Chem 285: 6235–6245.
8. Qin X, Gao B (2006) The complement system in liver diseases. Cell Mol Immunol 3: 333–340.
9. Zipfel PF, Skerka C (2009) Complement regulators and inhibitory proteins. Nat Rev Immunol 9: 729–740. doi: 10.1038/nri2620.
10. Ricklin D, Hajishengallis G, Yang K, Lambris JD (2010) Complement: a key system for immune surveillance and homeostasis. Nat Immunol 11: 785–797. doi: 10.1038/ni.1923.
11. Day NK, L'Esperance R, Good RA, Michael AF, Hansen JA, et al. (1975) Hereditary C2 deficiency: Genetic studies and association with the HL-A system. J Exp Med 141: 1464–1469.
12. Figueroa JE, Densen P (1991) Infectious diseases associated with complement deficiencies. Clin Microbiol Rev 4: 359–395.
13. Pickering MC, Botto M, Taylor PR, Lachmann PJ, Walport MJ (2000) Systemic lupus erythematosus, complement deficiency, and apoptosis. Adv Immunol 76: 227–324.
14. Jönsson G, Truedsson L, Sturfelt G, Oxelius VA, Braconier JH, et al. (2005) Hereditary C2 deficiency in Sweden: frequent occurrence of invasive infection, atherosclerosis, and rheumatic disease. Medicine (Baltimore) 84: 23–34.
15. Tedesco F (2008) Inherited complement deficiencies and bacterial infections. Vaccine 26 (Suppl. 8): I3–I8.
16. Skattum L, van Deuren M, van der Poll T, Truedsson L (2011) Complement deficiency states and associated infections. Mol Immunol 48: 1643–1655.
17. Mayilyan KR (2012) Complement genetics, deficiencies, and disease associations. Protein Cell 3: 487–496.
18. Scheuer PJ (1991) Classification of chronic viral hepatitis: a need for reassessment. J. Hepatol. 13:372–4.
19. Ray RB, Meyer K, Ray R (2000) Hepatitis C virus core protein promotes immortalization of primary human hepatocytes. Virology, 271, 193–204.
20. Kanda T, Basu A, Steele R, Wakita T, Ryerse JS, et al. (2006) Generation of infectious hepatitis C virus in immortalized human hepatocytes. J Virol 80: 4633–4639.
21. Egan AM, Gordon DL (1996) Burkholderia pseudomallei activates complement and is ingested but not killed by polymorphonuclear leukocytes. Infect Immun 64: 4952–4959.
22. Okroj M, Holmquist E, King BC, Blom AM (2012) Functional Analyses of Complement Convertases Using C3 and C5-Depleted Sera. PLoS One 7: e47245.
23. Lambris JD, Ricklin D, Geisbrecht BV (2008) Complement evasion by human pathogens. Nat Rev Microbiol 6: 132–142.
24. Rodríguez de Córdoba S, Esparza-Gordillo J, Goicoechea de Jorge E, Lopez-Trascasa M, Sánchez-Corral P (2004) The human complement factor H: functional roles, genetic variations and disease associations. Mol Immunol 41: 355–367.
25. Kwan WH, van der Touw W, Heeger PS (2012) Complement regulation of T cell immunity. Immunol Res 54: 247–253.
26. Mawatari S, Uto H, Ido A, Nakashima K, Suzuki T, et al. (2013) Hepatitis C virus NS3/4A protease inhibits complement activation by cleaving complement component 4. PLoS One.8(12):e82094.
27. Amadei N, Baracho GV, Nudelman V, Bastos W, Florido MP, et al. (2001) Inherited complete factor I deficiency associated with systemic lupus erythematosus, higher susceptibility to infection and low levels of factor H. Scand J Immunol 53: 615–621.
28. Nilsson SC, Trouw LA, Renault N, Miteva MA, Genel F, et al. (2009) Genetic, molecular and functional analyses of complement factor I deficiency. Eur J Immunol 39: 310–323.
29. Ferreira VP, Pangburn MK, Cortés C (2010) Complement control protein factor H: the good, the bad, and the inadequate. Mol Immunol 47: 2187–2197.

Permissions

All chapters in this book were first published in PLOS ONE, by The Public Library of Science; hereby published with permission under the Creative Commons Attribution License or equivalent. Every chapter published in this book has been scrutinized by our experts. Their significance has been extensively debated. The topics covered herein carry significant findings which will fuel the growth of the discipline. They may even be implemented as practical applications or may be referred to as a beginning point for another development.

The contributors of this book come from diverse backgrounds, making this book a truly international effort. This book will bring forth new frontiers with its revolutionizing research information and detailed analysis of the nascent developments around the world.

We would like to thank all the contributing authors for lending their expertise to make the book truly unique. They have played a crucial role in the development of this book. Without their invaluable contributions this book wouldn't have been possible. They have made vital efforts to compile up to date information on the varied aspects of this subject to make this book a valuable addition to the collection of many professionals and students.

This book was conceptualized with the vision of imparting up-to-date information and advanced data in this field. To ensure the same, a matchless editorial board was set up. Every individual on the board went through rigorous rounds of assessment to prove their worth. After which they invested a large part of their time researching and compiling the most relevant data for our readers.

The editorial board has been involved in producing this book since its inception. They have spent rigorous hours researching and exploring the diverse topics which have resulted in the successful publishing of this book. They have passed on their knowledge of decades through this book. To expedite this challenging task, the publisher supported the team at every step. A small team of assistant editors was also appointed to further simplify the editing procedure and attain best results for the readers.

Apart from the editorial board, the designing team has also invested a significant amount of their time in understanding the subject and creating the most relevant covers. They scrutinized every image to scout for the most suitable representation of the subject and create an appropriate cover for the book.

The publishing team has been an ardent support to the editorial, designing and production team. Their endless efforts to recruit the best for this project, has resulted in the accomplishment of this book. They are a veteran in the field of academics and their pool of knowledge is as vast as their experience in printing. Their expertise and guidance has proved useful at every step. Their uncompromising quality standards have made this book an exceptional effort. Their encouragement from time to time has been an inspiration for everyone.

The publisher and the editorial board hope that this book will prove to be a valuable piece of knowledge for researchers, students, practitioners and scholars across the globe.

List of Contributors

Kyu Sik Jung, Young Eun Chon, Kyung Hyun Cheon, Sung Bae Kim, Sang Hoon Lee and Sung Soo Ahn
Department of Internal Medicine, Yonsei University College of Medicine, Seoul, Korea

Sang Hoon Ahn and Kwang-Hyub Han
Department of Internal Medicine, Yonsei University College of Medicine, Seoul, Korea
Institute of Gastroenterology, Yonsei University College of Medicine, Seoul, Korea
Liver Cirrhosis Clinical Research Center, Seoul, Korea
Brain Korea 21 Project of Medical Science, Seoul, Korea

Young Nyun Park
Department of Pathology, Yonsei University College of Medicine, Seoul, Korea

Beom Kyung Kim, Seung Up Kim, Jun Yong Park and Do Young Kim
Department of Internal Medicine, Yonsei University College of Medicine, Seoul, Korea
Institute of Gastroenterology, Yonsei University College of Medicine, Seoul, Korea
Liver Cirrhosis Clinical Research Center, Seoul, Korea

Baligh R. Yehia
Department of Medicine, University of Pennsylvania Perelman School of Medicine, Philadelphia, Pennsylvania, United States of America
Leonard Davis Institute of Health Economics, University of Pennsylvania, Philadelphia, Pennsylvania, United States of America
Center for Clinical Epidemiology and Biostatistics, Department of Biostatistics and Epidemiology, University of Pennsylvania Perelman School of Medicine, Philadelphia, Pennsylvania, United States of America

Asher J. Schranz
Department of Medicine, New York University School of Medicine, New York, United States of America

Craig A. Umscheid
Department of Medicine, University of Pennsylvania Perelman School of Medicine, Philadelphia, Pennsylvania, United States of America
Leonard Davis Institute of Health Economics, University of Pennsylvania, Philadelphia, Pennsylvania, United States of America
Center for Clinical Epidemiology and Biostatistics, Department of Biostatistics and Epidemiology, University of Pennsylvania Perelman School of Medicine, Philadelphia, Pennsylvania, United States of America
Center for Evidenced-Based Practice, University of Pennsylvania Health System, Philadelphia, Pennsylvania, United States of America

Vincent Lo Re III
Department of Medicine, University of Pennsylvania Perelman School of Medicine, Philadelphia, Pennsylvania, United States of America
Center for Clinical Epidemiology and Biostatistics, Department of Biostatistics and Epidemiology, University of Pennsylvania Perelman School of Medicine, Philadelphia, Pennsylvania, United States of America

Myrna L. Cozen, James C. Ryan, Hui Shen and Robert Lerrigo
Department of Medicine, Veterans Affairs Medical Center and University of California San Francisco, San Francisco, California, United States of America

Russell M. Yee
Department of Epidemiology, Mailman School of Public Health, Columbia University, New York, United States of America

Edward Sheen
Department of Medicine, Stanford University School of Medicine, Stanford, California, United States of America

Lucile Tran and Laure-Hélène Ouisse
INSERM U948, Nantes, France

Peggy Richard-Fiardo, Philippe R. Franken, Georges Vassaux and Jacques Darcourt
Faculté de Me´decine, Universite´ de Nice-Sophia-Antipolis, Nice, France
UMRE4320, CEA, Nice, France

Gaétan Cornilleau and Karim Benihoud
Université Paris-Sud, UMR 8203, Institut Gustave Roussy, Villejuif Cedex, France

Jan-Peter Sowa, Lars Peter Bechmann, Guido Gerken and Ali Canbay
Department of Gastroenterology and Hepatology, University Hospital, University Duisburg-Essen, Essen, Germany

Dominik Heider and Daniel Hoffmann
Department of Bioinformatics, Center for Medical Biotechnology, University Duisburg-Essen, Essen, Germany

Dongying Zhao, Lianshu Han and Zhengjuan He
XinHua Hospital, Shanghai Jiaotong University School of Medicine, Shanghai, China

Jun Zhang and Yongjun Zhang
XinHua Hospital, Shanghai Jiaotong University School of Medicine, Shanghai, China
MOE and Shanghai Key Laboratory of Children's Environmental Health, Shanghai, China

Valerio Nobili and Anna Alisi
Unit of Liver Research, Bambino Gesù Children's Hospital, Rome, Italy

Guido Carpino
Department of Movement, Human and Health Sciences, University of Rome "Foro Italico", Rome, Italy

Rita De Vito
Unit of Pathology, Bambino Gesù Children's Hospital, Rome, Italy

Antonio Franchitto
Department of Anatomical, Histological, Forensic Medicine and Orthopedics Sciences, Sapienza University of Rome, Rome, Italy
Eleonora Lorillard Spencer-Cenci Foundation, Rome, Italy

Gianfranco Alpini
Department of Medicine, Scott and White and Texas A&M Health Science Center College of Medicine, Temple, Texas, United States of America

Paolo Onori and Eugenio Gaudio
Department of Anatomical, Histological, Forensic Medicine and Orthopedics Sciences, Sapienza University of Rome, Rome, Italy

Weijie Li and Dongping Xu
Department of Microbiology, Peking University Health Science Center, Beijing, China
Institute of Infectious Diseases and Medical Center for Liver Failure, Beijing 302 Hospital, Beijing, China

Jingmin Zhao and Shuhong Liu
Department of Pathology, Beijing 302 Hospital, Beijing, China

Zhengsheng Zou, Yan Liu, Baosen Li, Ying Sun, Xiaodong Li, Shaoping Cai, Weimin Yao and Shaojie Xin
Institute of Infectious Diseases and Medical Center for Liver Failure, Beijing 302 Hospital, Beijing, China

Fengmin Lu
Department of Microbiology, Peking University Health Science Center, Beijing, China

Thomas Karlas
IFB Adiposity Diseases, Leipzig University Medical Center, Leipzig, Germany
Department of Medicine, Neurology and Dermatology, Division of Gastroenterology and Rheumatology, University Hospital Leipzig, Leipzig, Germany

David Petroff
IFB Adiposity Diseases, Leipzig University Medical Center, Leipzig, Germany
Clinical Trial Center, University of Leipzig, Leipzig, Germany

Nikita Garnov, Nicolas Linder and Alexander Schaudinn
IFB Adiposity Diseases, Leipzig University Medical Center, Leipzig, Germany
Department of Diagnostics and Interventional Radiology, University Hospital Leipzig, Leipzig, Germany

Stephan Böhm, Hannelore Tenckhoff, Manfred Wiese and Thomas Berg
Department of Medicine, Neurology and Dermatology, Division of Gastroenterology and Rheumatology, Section of Hepatology, University Hospital Leipzig, Leipzig, Germany

Christian Wittekind
Institute of Pathology, University Hospital Leipzig, Leipzig, Germany

Ingolf Schiefke
Clinic for Gastroenterology and Hepatology, Klinikum St. Georg, Leipzig, Germany

Harald Busse and Thomas Kahn
Department of Diagnostics and Interventional Radiology, University Hospital Leipzig, Leipzig, Germany

Joachim Mössner, Michael Tröltzsch and Volker Keim
Department of Medicine, Neurology and Dermatology, Division of Gastroenterology and Rheumatology, University Hospital Leipzig, Leipzig, Germany

Johannes Wiegand
IFB Adiposity Diseases, Leipzig University Medical Center, Leipzig, Germany
Department of Medicine, Neurology and Dermatology, Division of Gastroenterology and Rheumatology, University Hospital Leipzig, Leipzig, Germany
Department of Medicine, Neurology and Dermatology, Division of Gastroenterology and Rheumatology, Section of Hepatology, University Hospital Leipzig, Leipzig, Germany

Antonella Minutolo, Beatrice Conti and Carmela Viscomi
Laboratory of Molecular Virology and Oncology, Francesco Balsano Foundation, ex A. Cesalpino Foundation, Rome, Italy

Sandro Grelli
U.O.C. Clinical Microbiology, Tor Vergata Hospital, Rome, Italy

Giancarlo Labbadia
Department of Clinical and Medical Therapy, "Sapienza" University of Rome - Umberto I Hospital, Rome, Italy

Clara Balsano
Laboratory of Molecular Virology and Oncology, Francesco Balsano Foundation, ex A. Cesalpino Foundation, Rome, Italy
Institute of Biology and Molecular Pathology (IBPM) - CNR (National Research Council), Rome, Italy

Emilie Fugier, Hélène Marche, Zuzana Macek Jílková, Nicolas Van Campenhout and Evelyne Jouvin-Marche
INSERM, U823, Grenoble, France
Université Joseph Fourier, UMR-S823, Grenoble, France

Marie-Ange Thélu, Tania Dufeu-Duchesne, Vincent Leroy, Jean-Pierre Zarski and Patrice N. Marche
INSERM, U823, Grenoble, France
Université Joseph Fourier, UMR-S823, Grenoble, France
CHU-Grenoble, Clinique Universitaire d'Hépato-Gastroentérologie, Grenoble, France

Nathalie Sturm
INSERM, U823, Grenoble, France
Université Joseph Fourier, UMR-S823, Grenoble, France
CHU-Grenoble, Département d'Anatomie et de Cytologie Pathologiques, Grenoble, France

Jack X. Q. Pang, Steven J. Heitman, Gilaad G. Kaplan and Robert P. Myers
Liver Unit, Division of Gastroenterology and Hepatology, Department of Medicine, University of Calgary, Calgary, Alberta, Canada
Department of Community Health Sciences, University of Calgary, Calgary, Alberta, Canada

Scott Zimmer and Sophia Niu
Medical Services, Alberta Health Services, Calgary, Alberta, Canada

Pam Crotty, Jenna Tracey, Faruq Pradhan, Abdel Aziz M. Shaheen, Carla S. Coffin and Mark G. Swain
Liver Unit, Division of Gastroenterology and Hepatology, Department of Medicine, University of Calgary, Calgary, Alberta, Canada

Torsten Voigtländer, Michael P. Manns and Tim O. Lankisch
Department of Gastroenterology, Hepatology and Endocrinology, Hannover Medical School, Hannover, Germany
Integrated Research and Treatment Center - Transplantation (IFB-Tx), Hannover Medical School, Hannover, Germany

Sascha David and Kristina Thamm
Department of Nephrology and Hypertension, Hannover Medical School, Hannover, Germany

Jerome Schlué
Institute of Pathology, Hannover Medical School, Hannover, Germany

Jochen Metzger
Mosaiques diagnostics GmbH, Hannover, Germany

Lawrence M. Pfeffer, Chuan He Yang, Susan R. Pfeffer, Meiyun Fan, Joel Diament and Charles R. Handorf
Department of Pathology and Laboratory Medicine, and the Center for Cancer Research, University of Tennessee Health Science Center, Memphis, Tennessee, United States of America

Kui Li and Tony N. Marion
Department of Microbiology, Immunology and Biochemistry, University of Tennessee Health Science Center, Memphis, Tennessee, United States of America

Jaquelyn F. Fleckenstein
The Department of Medicine, Division of Gastroenterology, Washington University School of Medicine, St. Louis, Missouri, United States of America

Elizabeth Handorf
Biostatistics and Bioinformatics Facility, Fox Chase Cancer Center, Philadelphia, Pennsylvania, United States of America

Naim Alkhouri
Department of Pediatric Gastroenterology and Hepatology, Cleveland Clinic, Cleveland, Ohio, United States of America
Digestive Disease Institute, Cleveland Clinic, Cleveland, Ohio, United States of America

Sana Mansoor
Department of Pediatric Gastroenterology and Hepatology, Cleveland Clinic, Cleveland, Ohio, United States of America

Paola Giammaria, Daniela Liccardo and Valerio Nobili
The Liver Unit, Bambino Gesu Children's Hospital, Rome, Italy

Rocio Lopez
Department of Quantitative Health Sciences, Cleveland Clinic, Cleveland, Ohio, United States of America

Yuanyuan Li, Yu Chen and Ying Zhao
Department of Laboratory Medicine, The First Affiliated Hospital of the Medical College, Zhejiang University, Hangzhou, China

Wah-Kheong Chan and Sanjiv Mahadeva
Gastroenterology and Hepatology Unit, Gastrointestinal Endoscopy Unit, Department of Medicine, Faculty of Medicine, University of Malaya, Kuala Lumpur, Malaysia

Pavai Sthaneshwar
Division of Laboratory Medicine, Department of Pathology, Faculty of Medicine, University of Malaya, Kuala Lumpur, Malaysia

Nik Raihan Nik Mustapha
Department of Pathology, Hospital Alor Setar, Alor Setar, Kedah, Malaysia

Stella De Nicola and Alessio Aghemo
Department of Gastroenterology, Fondazione IRCCS Ca' Granda Ospedale Policlinico Milano, Milano, Italy

Paola Dongiovanni
Department of Internal Medicine, Fondazione IRCCS Ca' Granda Ospedale Policlinico Milano, Milano, Italy

Cristina Cheroni, Francesco Marabita, Lorena Donnici and Raffaele De Francesco
Virology Program, INGM - Istituto Nazionale di Genetica Molecolare "Romeo ed Enrica Invernizzi," Milano, Italy

Roberta D'Ambrosio and Massimo Colombo
Department of Gastroenterology, Fondazione IRCCS Ca' Granda Ospedale Policlinico Milano, Milano, Italy
Department of Pathophysiology and Transplantation, Università degli Studi di Milano, Milano, Italy

Michele Pedrazzini
Department of Pathophysiology and Transplantation, Università degli Studi di Milano, Milano, Italy

Marco Maggioni
Department of Pathology, Fondazione IRCCS Ca' Granda Ospedale Policlinico Milano, Milano, Italy

Silvia Fargion and Luca Valenti
Department of Internal Medicine, Fondazione IRCCS Ca' Granda Ospedale Policlinico Milano, Milano, Italy
Department of Pathophysiology and Transplantation, Università degli Studi di Milano, Milano, Italy

Partha K. Chandra, Feyza Gunduz, Sidhartha Hazari, Rajesh Panigrahi and Bret Poat and Tong Wu
Pathology and Laboratory Medicine, Tulane University Health Sciences Center, New Orleans, Louisiana, United States of America

Ramazan Kurt and Luis A. Balart
Department of Medicine, Gastroenterology and Hepatology, Tulane University Health Sciences Center, New Orleans, Louisiana, United States of America

David Bruce, Ari J. Cohen, Humberto E. Behorquez, Ian Carmody and George Loss
Transplant Surgery Section, Ochsner Medical Center, New Orleans, Louisiana, United States of America

Srikanta Dash
Pathology and Laboratory Medicine, Tulane University Health Sciences Center, New Orleans, Louisiana, United States of America
Department of Medicine, Gastroenterology and Hepatology, Tulane University Health Sciences Center, New Orleans, Louisiana, United States of America

Elżbieta Jabłonowska, Kamila Wójcik and Anna Piekarska
Department of Infectious Diseases and Hepatology, Medical University of Lodz, Łódź, Poland

Bożena Szymańska
Central Laboratory, Medical University of Lodz, Łódź, Poland

Aleksandra Omulecka
Department of Pathology, Biegański Provincial Specialistic Hospital, Łódź, Poland

Hanna Ćwiklińska
Laboratory of Neuroimmunology, Department of Neurology, Medical University of Łódź, Poland

Magdalena Ydreborg, Martin Lagging, Rune Wejstål, Gunnar Norkrans, Magnus Lindh and Johan Westin
Department of Infectious Diseases/Virology, Institute of Biomedicine, University of Gothenburg, Gothenburg, Sweden

Vera Lisovskaja
Department of Mathematical Sciences, Chalmers University of Technology and University of Gothenburg, Gothenburg, Sweden

Peer Brehm Christensen and Court Pedersen
Department of Infectious Diseases, Odense University Hospital, Odense, Denmark

Nina Langeland and Kristine Mørch
Department of Clinical Science, University of Bergen, Bergen, Norway

Mads Rauning Buhl
Department of Infectious Diseases, Aarhus University, Aarhus, Denmark

Martti Färkkilä
Institute of Clinical Medicine, Department of Gastroenterology, Helsinki University, Helsinki, Finland

Youichi Kawano
Department of Surgery, Nippon Medical School, Tokyo, Japan
Research Team for Geriatric Pathology, Tokyo Metropolitan Institute of Gerontology, Tokyo, Japan

Naoshi Ishikawa, Junko Aida, Naotaka Izumiyama-Shimomura, Ken-ichi Nakamura and Kaiyo Takubo
Research Team for Geriatric Pathology, Tokyo Metropolitan Institute of Gerontology, Tokyo, Japan

Yukihiro Sanada, Koichi Mizuta and Hideo Kawarasaki
Department of Transplant Surgery, Jichi Medical University, Tochigi, Japan

Steven S. S. Poon
Terry Fox Laboratory, British Columbia Cancer Research Centre, Vancouver, British Columbia, Canada

Koshi Matsumoto
Department of Clinical Pathology, Ebina General Hospital, Kanagawa, Japan

Eiji Uchida and Takashi Tajiri
Department of Surgery, Nippon Medical School, Tokyo, Japan

Qingsong Xie, Xiaohu Zhou, Pengfei Huang, Jianfeng Wei, Weilin Wang and Shusen Zheng
Division of Hepatobiliary and Pancreatic Surgery, Department of Surgery, First Affiliated Hospital, School of Medicine, Zhejiang University, Hangzhou, Zhejiang Province, China
Key Laboratory of Combined Multi- Organ Transplantation, Ministry of Public Health, Zhejiang Province, Hangzhou, China
Key laboratory of Organ Transplantation, Zhejiang Province, Hangzhou, China

Jun-Feng Li
The First Clinical Medical School, Lanzhou University, Lanzhou, China
Artificial Liver Center, Beijing YouAn Hospital, Capital Medical University, Beijing, China

Feng Qu and Jin-Lan Zhang
State Key Laboratory of Bioactive Substance and Function of Natural Medicines, Institute of Materia Medica, Chinese Academy of Medical Sciences and Peking Union Medical College, Beijing, China

Su-Jun Zheng, Hui-Li Wu, Mei Liu, Feng Ren, Yu Chen and Zhong-Ping Duan
Artificial Liver Center, Beijing YouAn Hospital, Capital Medical University, Beijing, China

Jin-Yu Ren
Evergreen Wellness Center, Kansas College of Chinese Medicine, Wichita, Kansas, United States of America

Hui Liu
Department of Pathology, Beijing YouAn Hospital, Capital Medical University, Beijing, China

Antonio Rivero-Juarez, Angela Camacho, Ana Gordon, Julian Torre-Cisneros and Antonio Rivero
Unidad de Enfermedades Infecciosas, Instituto Maimonides de Investigación Biomédica de Córdoba (IMIBIC), Hospital Universitario Reina Sofía de Córdoba, Córdoba, Spain

Luis F. López-Cortés, Almudena Torres-Cornejo, Rosa Ruiz-Valderas and Pompeyo Viciana
Unidad Clínica de Enfermedades Infecciosas, Microbiología y Medicina Preventiva, Instituto de Biomedicina de Sevilla (IBiS), Hospital Universitario Virgen del Rocío/CSIC/Universidad de Sevilla, Seville, Spain

Juan A. Pineda
Unidad de Enfermedades Infecciosas y Microbiología Clínica, Instituto de Biomedicina de Sevilla (IBiS), Hospital Universitario de Valme, Seville, Spain

Nicola Coppola, Nicolina Capoluongo, Carmine Minichini and Evangelista Sagnelli
Department of Mental Health and Public Medicine, Second University of Naples, Naples, Italy

Rosa Zampino, Aldo Marrone, Adriana Boemio and Luigi Elio Adinolfi
Internal Medicine and Hepatology, Second University of Naples, Naples, Italy

Caterina Sagnelli and Maria Stanzione
Department of Clinical and Experimental Medicine and Surgery, Second University of Naples, Naples, Italy

Giulia Bellini and Sabatino Maione
Department of Experimental Medicine, Second University of Naples, Naples, Italy

Emanuele Miraglia Del Giudice and Francesca Rossi
Department of Pediatrics, Second University of Naples, Naples, Italy

Masahiro Ishikane
AIDS Clinical Center, National Center for Global Health and Medicine, Tokyo, Japan
Field Epidemiology Training Program Japan, Infectious Disease Surveillance Center, National Institute of Infectious Diseases, Tokyo, Japan
Global Infectious Diseases of Infection and Epidemiology, Medical Sciences Doctoral Program, Graduate School of Medicine, Tohoku University, Miyagi, Japan

Kunihisa Tsukada and Yoshimi Kikuchi
AIDS Clinical Center, National Center for Global Health and Medicine, Tokyo, Japan

Yuichi Nozaki and Mikio Yanase
Department of Gastroenterology, National Center for Global Health and Medicine, Tokyo, Japan

Toru Igari
Pathology Division of Clinical Laboratory, National Center for Global Health and Medicine, Tokyo, Japan

Naohiko Masaki
Department of Gastroenterology, National Center for Global Health and Medicine, Tokyo, Japan
Research Center for Hepatitis and Immunology, National Center for Global Health and Medicine, Tokyo, Japan

Koji Watanabe, Shinichi Oka and Hiroyuki Gatanaga
AIDS Clinical Center, National Center for Global Health and Medicine, Tokyo, Japan
Center for AIDS Research, Kumamoto University, Kumamoto, Japan

Xue-Ying Xu, Yu-Han Zhai, Xiao-Fei Wu, Wen-Si Ai and Hong-Bo Liu
School of Public Health, China Medical University, Shenyang, PR China

Hong Kong
Department of Clinical Laboratory, Shengjing Hospital of China Medical University, Shenyang, PR China

Rui-Xiang Song
Department of Urinary Surgery, Changhai Hospital, Shanghai, PR China

Hangeun Kim and Keith Meyer
Department of Internal Medicine, Saint Louis University, St. Louis, Missouri, United States of America

Adrian M. Di Bisceglie and Ranjit Ray
Department of Internal Medicine, Saint Louis University, St. Louis, Missouri, United States of America
Department of Molecular Microbiology and Immunology, Saint Louis University, St. Louis, Missouri, United States of America

Index